Diagnosis and Emerging Treatments for Cystic Fibrosis

Diagnosis and Emerging Treatments for Cystic Fibrosis

Editor: Marvin Ward

AMERICAN
MEDICAL PUBLISHERS
www.americanmedicalpublishers.com

AMERICAN
MEDICAL PUBLISHERS
www.americanmedicalpublishers.com

Cataloging-in-Publication Data

Diagnosis and emerging treatments for cystic fibrosis / edited by Marvin Ward.
p. cm.
Includes bibliographical references and index.
ISBN 979-8-88740-054-9
1. Cystic fibrosis. 2. Cystic fibrosis--Diagnosis. 3. Cystic fibrosis--Treatment. 4. Fibrosis.
5. Lungs--Diseases. 6. Pancreas--Diseases. 7. Genetic disorders. I. Ward, Marvin.
RC858.C95 D53 2023
616.37--dc23

American Medical Publishers,
41 Flatbush Avenue,
1st Floor, New York,
NY 11217, USA

ISBN 979-8-88740-054-9 (Hardback)

Contents

Preface VII

Chapter 1 **Unraveling the Function of Lemur Tyrosine Kinase 2 Network** 1
Daniel F. Cruz, Carlos M. Farinha and Agnieszka Swiatecka-Urban

Chapter 2 **The Autophagy Inhibitor Spautin-1 Antagonizes Rescue of Mutant CFTR Through an Autophagy-Independent and USP13-Mediated Mechanism** 11
Emanuela Pesce, Elvira Sondo, Loretta Ferrera, Valeria Tomati, Emanuela Caci, Paolo Scudieri, Ilaria Musante, Mario Renda, Nesrine Baatallah, Nathalie Servel, Alexandre Hinzpeter, Diego di Bernardo, Nicoletta Pedemonte and Luis J. V. Galietta

Chapter 3 **Network Biology Identifies Novel Regulators of CFTR Trafficking and Membrane Stability** 27
Cláudia Almeida Loureiro, João D. Santos, Ana Margarida Matos, Peter Jordan, Paulo Matos, Carlos M. Farinha and Francisco R. Pinto

Chapter 4 **Human Primary Epithelial Cell Models: Promising Tools in the Era of Cystic Fibrosis Personalized Medicine** 40
Nikhil T. Awatade, Sharon L. Wong, Chris K. Hewson, Laura K. Fawcett, Anthony Kicic, Adam Jaffe and Shafagh A. Waters

Chapter 5 **Variable Responses to CFTR Correctors *in vitro:* Estimating the Design Effect in Precision Medicine** 51
Elizabeth Matthes, Julie Goepp, Carolina Martini, Jiajie Shan, Jie Liao, David Y. Thomas and John W. Hanrahan

Chapter 6 **Identification and Characterization of Novel CFTR Potentiators** 60
Maarten Gees, Sara Musch, Steven Van der Plas, Anne-Sophie Wesse, Ann Vandevelde, Katleen Verdonck, Oscar Mammoliti, Tzyh-Chang Hwang, Kathleen Sonck, Pieter Stouten, Andrew M. Swensen, Mia Jans, Jan Van der Schueren, Luc Nelles, Martin Andrews and Katja Conrath

Chapter 7 **Emerging microRNA Therapeutic Approaches for Cystic Fibrosis** 72
Pauline Bardin, Florence Sonneville, Harriet Corvol and Olivier Tabary

Chapter 8 **Role of the SLC26A9 Chloride Channel as Disease Modifier and Potential Therapeutic Target in Cystic Fibrosis** 83
Anita Balázs and Marcus A. Mall

Chapter 9 **Adapting Proteostasis and Autophagy for Controlling the Pathogenesis of Cystic Fibrosis Lung Disease** 92
Manish Bodas and Neeraj Vij

Chapter 10 **TMEM16A in Cystic Fibrosis: Activating or Inhibiting?**......105
Karl Kunzelmann, Jiraporn Ousingsawat, Inês Cabrita, Tereza Doušová, Andrea Bähr, Melanie Janda, Rainer Schreiber and Roberta Benedetto

Chapter 11 **Anion-Transport Mechanism of a Triazole-Bearing Derivative of Prodigiosine: A Candidate for Cystic Fibrosis Therapy**......123
Claudia Cossu, Michele Fiore, Debora Baroni, Valeria Capurro, Emanuela Caci, Maria Garcia-Valverde, Roberto Quesada and Oscar Moran

Chapter 12 ***In vitro* Methods for the Development and Analysis of Human Primary Airway Epithelia**......136
Ambra Gianotti, Livia Delpiano and Emanuela Caci

Chapter 13 **Peripheral Protein Quality Control as a Novel Drug Target for CFTR Stabilizer**......148
Ryosuke Fukuda and Tsukasa Okiyoneda

Chapter 14 **Challenges Facing Airway Epithelial Cell-Based Therapy for Cystic Fibrosis**......157
Andrew Berical, Rhianna E. Lee, Scott H. Randell and Finn Hawkins

Chapter 15 **Use of a Primary Epithelial Cell Screening Tool to Investigate Phage Therapy in Cystic Fibrosis**......169
Stephanie Trend, Barbara J. Chang, Mark O'Dea, Stephen M. Stick and Anthony Kicic

Chapter 16 **Trial Refresh: A Case for an Adaptive Platform Trial for Pulmonary Exacerbations of Cystic Fibrosis**......180
Andre Schultz, Julie A. Marsh, Benjamin R. Saville, Richard Norman, Peter G. Middleton, Hugh W. Greville, Matthew I. Bellgard, Scott M. Berry and Tom Snelling

Chapter 17 **Gene Therapy for Cystic Fibrosis Lung Disease: Overcoming the Barriers to Translation to the Clinic**......188
Martin Donnelley and David W. Parsons

Chapter 18 **Elucidating the Interaction of CF Airway Epithelial Cells and Rhinovirus: Using the Host-Pathogen Relationship to Identify Future Therapeutic Strategies**......196
Kak-Ming Ling, Luke W. Garratt, Timo Lassmann, Stephen M. Stick and Anthony Kicic

Chapter 19 **Animal Models in the Pathophysiology of Cystic Fibrosis**......209
Anna Semaniakou, Roger P. Croll and Valerie Chappe

Permissions

List of Contributors

Index

Preface

It is often said that books are a boon to mankind. They document every progress and pass on the knowledge from one generation to the other. They play a crucial role in our lives. Thus I was both excited and nervous while editing this book. I was pleased by the thought of being able to make a mark but I was also nervous to do it right because the future of students depends upon it. Hence, I took a few months to research further into the discipline, revise my knowledge and also explore some more aspects. Post this process, I begun with the editing of this book.

Cystic fibrosis (CF) is a genetic disorder, which influences the liver, lungs, pancreas, intestine and kidneys. The long-term effects of this disorder include trouble in respiration, and coughing up mucus because of regular lung infections. There can be other symptoms such as fatty stool, sinus infections, infertility in most males, poor growth and clubbing of the fingers and toes. CF is hereditary in an autosomal recessive manner. It occurs due to the presence of mutations in both the replicas of the gene for cystic fibrosis transmembrane conductance regulator (CFTR) protein. There is currently no treatment for cystic fibrosis. Antibiotics are used in the treatment of lung infections, which can be taken orally, inhaled or given intravenously. Antibiotic azithromycin is used in severe cases for long time duration. Inhaled hypertonic saline and salbutamol can also provide relief. If the lung functioning is constantly deteriorating, lung transplantation can be done. Emerging medicines for the treatment of this disorder, include powdered versions of tobramycin and colistin, nebulized aztreonam and mannitol for inhalation. This book unravels the recent studies on cystic fibrosis. It will help the readers in keeping pace with the diagnosis and emerging treatments of this medical condition.

I thank my publisher with all my heart for considering me worthy of this unparalleled opportunity and for showing unwavering faith in my skills. I would also like to thank the editorial team who worked closely with me at every step and contributed immensely towards the successful completion of this book. Last but not the least, I wish to thank my friends and colleagues for their support.

Editor

1

Unraveling the Function of Lemur Tyrosine Kinase 2 Network

Daniel F. Cruz[1,2]*, *Carlos M. Farinha*[1] *and Agnieszka Swiatecka-Urban*[2]

[1] *Biosystems and Integrative Sciences Institute, Faculty of Sciences, University of Lisboa, Campo Grande, Portugal,*
[2] *Department of Nephrology, Children's Hospital of Pittsburgh, Pittsburgh, PA, United States*

***Correspondence:**
Daniel F. Cruz
dfcruz@fc.ul.pt

Lemur Tyrosine Kinase 2 (LMTK2) is a recently clonec transmembrane protein, actually a serine/threonine kinase named after the Madagascar primate lemur due to the long intracellular C-terminal tail. LMTK2 is relatively little known, compared to other kinases but its role has been increasingly recognized. Published data show that LMTK2 regulates key cellular events, including endocytic trafficking, nerve growth factor signaling, apoptosis, and Cl^- transport. Abnormalities in the expression and function of LMTK2 are associated with human disease, such as neurodegeneration, cancer and infertility. We summarized the current state of knowledge on LMTK2 structure, regulation, interactome, intracellular localization, and tissue expression and point out future research directions to better understand the role of LMTK2.

Keywords: LMTK2, PP1, kinase, phosphorylation, signaling pathway

INTRODUCTION

Protein phosphorylation is an important post-translational modification regulating protein–protein interactions and signal transduction (Manning et al., 2002a; Ubersax and Ferrell, 2007; Ardito et al., 2017). Indeed, the activity of enzymes and receptors is controlled by specific kinases and phosphatases. Kinases are responsible for protein phosphorylation, a reversible process that consists of the addition of a phosphate group PO_4 from the adenosine 5′-triphosphate (ATP) or guanosine 5′-triphosphate (GTP) to a polar group of various amino acids. This addition modifies the protein from hydrophobic apolar to hydrophilic polar, allowing a conformational change during interaction with other molecules (Ubersax and Ferrell, 2007; Cheng et al., 2011; Ardito et al., 2017). Most protein phosphorylation events occur on hydroxyl groups at the side chain of serine (S), threonine (T), and tyrosine (Y) residues (Ubersax and Ferrell, 2007; Schwartz and Murray, 2011; Ardito et al., 2017). In turn, phosphatases remove the PO_4 group from phosphoproteins by hydrolyzing phosphoric acid monoesters (Barford, 1996; Zhang, 2002; Ardito et al., 2017).

The human kinome comprises 518 protein kinases and 20 lipid kinases encoded by genes that correspond to 1.7% of the human genome (Manning et al., 2002b; Heath et al., 2003; Duong-Ly and Peterson, 2013). Lemur Tyrosine Kinase 2 (LMTK2) is one of the most recently cloned serine/threonine (S/T) kinases. It is also known as cyclin-dependent kinase-5 (cdk5)/p35 regulated kinase (cprk), kinase/phosphatase/inhibitor-2 (KPI2), brain-enriched kinase (BREK), and apoptosis-associated tyrosine kinase (AATYK)-2. LMTK2 was found almost simultaneously by three different groups. In 2002, Wang and Brautigan aimed to understand the protein complex composed of Inhibitor 2 (Inh2) and Protein Phosphatase 1 (PP1), specifically if Inh2 binds to other partners besides PP1, and identified LMTK2 as one of the interacting proteins by yeast two-hybrid assay (Wang and Brautigan, 2002). In 2003, Kesavapany et al. (2003) found LMTK2 as a binding partner of the cdk5/p35 kinase. In 2004, Kawa et al. (2004) identified LMTK2 as a novel kinase expressed in the brain, using *in silico* search, confirmed by reverse-transcription polymerase chain reaction (RT-PCR) and Northern blot analysis. Here, we present a comprehensive review of published data on LMTK2, identify knowledge gaps, and point out research directions to better understand the role of LMTK2 in physiology and human disease.

STRUCTURE, SPECIFICITY, REGULATION, AND LOCALIZATION OF LMTK2

Lemur Tyrosine Kinase 2 is composed of 1503 amino acid residues forming a short soluble N-terminal domain, followed by two hydrophobic transmembrane helices (residues 11–29 and 46–63), and a kinase domain (residues 137–407) with the ATP binding site (residues 143–168) (Wang and Brautigan, 2002; Nixon et al., 2013) (**Figure 1**). N- and C-terminal domains as well as the kinase active site are located in the cytosol (Nixon et al., 2013).

Naming of LMTK2 resulted from the sequence homology of the kinase domain with tyrosine kinases. The bioinformatics analysis revealed 60% homology between the kinase domain of LMTK2 and AATYK (Wang and Brautigan, 2002). LMTK2 also shares a putative autophosphorylation site with Src-family kinases, the Y^{295} residue, while the D^{265}LALRN motif in LMTK2 is also present in non-Src tyrosine kinases (Kawa et al., 2004). Despite the initial naming, LMTK2 was found to be a serine/threonine kinase (Wang and Brautigan, 2002, 2006). First, phospho-amino acid analysis demonstrated that LMTK2 undergoes auto-phosphorylation on serine and threonine residues, while tyrosine phosphorylation was not observed (Wang and Brautigan, 2002). Second, immunoblotting with anti-phospho-threonine and anti-phospho-serine antibodies showed reactivity with LMTK2 (Wang and Brautigan, 2002). Last, phosphorylation of myelin basic protein (MBP) by LMTK2 was mostly located at serine residues, with a trace at threonine residues; once again, no tyrosine phosphorylation was found (Wang and Brautigan, 2002). Similar results were obtained using a peptide microarray, which demonstrated that LMTK2 interacts with phosphorylated serine and threonine sites in peptides from bovine MBP (Wang and Brautigan, 2006). In fact, the peptide microarray demonstrated that LMTK2 phosphorylates serine and threonine residues preceded or followed by proline (P) residues (Wang and Brautigan, 2006), suggesting similarity with proline-directed kinases. Although these kinases, such as cyclin-dependent kinase (cdk) or glycogen synthase kinase 3 beta (GSK3-β) phosphorylate only those serine/threonine residues that are followed by proline [(S/T)-P-x] (Pelech, 1995; Wang and Brautigan, 2006). LMTK2 also differs from the proline-directed kinases because it is not exclusively specific to proline sites; actually, many of the LMTK2 reactive sites have neighboring basic residues (Wang and Brautigan, 2006).

The C-terminal domain of LMTK2 contains a V^{1355}TF motif that binds the catalytic subunit of PP1 (PP1c) necessary for inhibition of PP1 activity (Wang and Brautigan, 2002). The C-terminal domain is also rich in proline residues conforming to seven PxxP-motifs, where x is a variable amino acid (Kawa et al., 2004). The PxxP domains may be involved in regulation of LMTK2 activity, intracellular localization, or substrate recognition, through interaction with SH3 domains of LMTK2-interacting proteins; however, specific SH3 domain containing partners of LMTK2 have not been identified yet.

Tissue Expression and Subcellular Localization

According to the Human Protein Atlas (HPA) database[1], LMTK2 is ubiquitously expressed in human tissues (The Human Protein Atlas, 2018a). Northern blot analysis demonstrated high levels of the LMTK2 mRNA in human skeletal muscle while low levels were observed in the brain and pancreas (Wang and Brautigan, 2002). LMTK2 protein was also experimentally detected in human bronchial epithelial (HBE) cells (Luz et al., 2014) and prostate epithelial cells (Shah and Bradbury, 2015b). LMTK2 transcripts were detected in mice, with the most prominent signal found in telenchepalon (Kawa et al., 2004). Indeed, mouse LMTK2 mRNA levels were much higher in the brain than in the skeletal muscle, in contrast to human LMTK2 (Wang and Brautigan, 2002). LMTK2 expression in the mouse brain was detected at all developmental stages, with increased expression during the early postnatal age (weeks 0–2). Similar to human, LMTK2 was found in mouse primary prostate epithelial cells (Shah and Bradbury, 2015b).

Concerning subcellular localization, LMTK2 is enriched on intracellular membranes, especially in organelles involved in the endocytic and recycling pathways (Nixon et al., 2013). Specifically, LMTK2 was found on transferrin-, Rab5-, EEA1-, and Rab11-positive vesicles (Kawa et al., 2004; Chibalina et al., 2007). Confocal imaging and subcellular fractionation studies detected LMTK2 in nuclear and non-nuclear compartments in prostate cancer cells (Shah and Bradbury, 2015b). In differentiated and undifferentiated PC12 cells, derived from pheochromocytoma of the rat adrenal medulla, LMTK2 was enriched at juxta-membranous regions while in differentiated PC12 cells it was also enhanced at the growth cone (Kawa et al., 2004). LMTK2 can also localize at the plasma membrane. It was detected at the apical and basolateral membrane domain in primary differentiated HBE cells derived from cystic fibrosis (CF) lungs and in immortalized CFBE41o- cells, a human CF bronchial epithelial cell line derived from a CF patient homozygous for the F508del-CFTR mutation (Luz et al., 2014). In HeLa cells, LMTK2 was present at the plasma membrane as well as throughout the cytoplasm and it was enriched in cellular extensions and the perinuclear region (Chibalina et al., 2007).

Regulation of *lmtk2* Gene Expression

The *lmtk2* gene promoter regulates expression of endogenous LMTK2 (Dey and Bradbury, 2017). The sequence GGTGAGTCAGTG upstream of the transcription initiation site of the *lmtk2* gene, conforms to the phorbol 12-myristate 13-acetate (TPA) response element (TRE) (Dey and Bradbury, 2017). Exposure of HEK293, HeLa, and CFBE41o- cells to low

[1] https://www.proteinatlas.org/

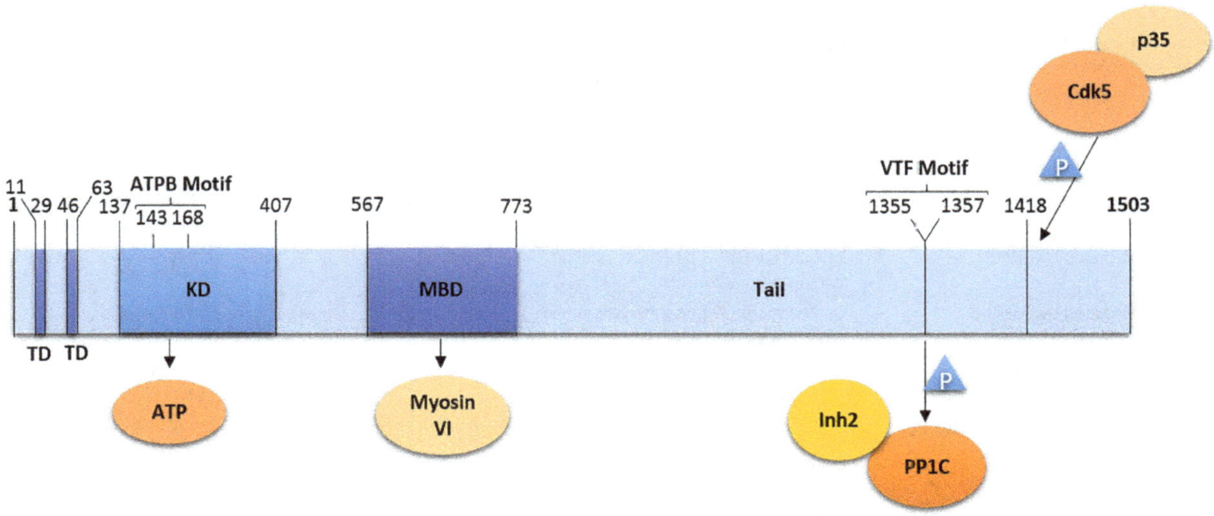

FIGURE 1 | Domain organization of LMTK2. LMTK2 contains two transmembrane domains (TD), followed by a kinase domain (KD) with an ATP binding (ATPB) motif, a Myosin VI binding domain (MBD), and a tail domain. The kinase domain residue K^{168} is critical for LMTK2 catalytic activity. LMTK2 interacts with PP1c via its VTF motif (residues 1355–1357). LMTK2 is phosphorylated in its residue S^{1418}, by the complex Cdk5/p35. Numbers indicate amino acid residues.

concentrations of TPA significantly increased LMTK2 mRNA and protein levels, that were not further increased with higher concentrations of TPA. In fact, exposure to high concentrations of TPA, in CFBE cells, decreased the LMTK2 protein expression below basal levels (Dey and Bradbury, 2017). Phorbol esters regulate gene expression by altering the protein kinase C (PKC) activity. Inhibition of PKC blunted the upregulation of LMTK2 expression by low concentrations of TPA while prolonged exposure of cells to high concentrations of phorbol esters downregulated PKC activity and inhibited LMTK2 expression (Castagna et al., 1982; Sanders and Stern, 1996; Dey and Bradbury, 2017). TPA induces binding of the transcriptional AP-1 complex c-Jun and c-Fos protein families to the TRE in *lmtk2* promoter and these proteins modulate TPA effects on LMTK2 in a PKC dependent manner (Angel and Karin, 1991; Dey and Bradbury, 2017).

Biosynthetic Processing of LMTK2

Synthesis of membrane proteins occurs on ribosomes associated with the rough ER followed by export in the coat protein complex II (COPII)-coated vesicles. To facilitate this process, LMTK2 contains three arginine residues R^8RR, located upstream of the first hydrophobic sequence, which functions as a signal peptide targeting LMTK2 to the endoplasmic reticulum (ER) and secretory pathway (Peterson et al., 2003; Kawa et al., 2004; Owji et al., 2018).

Endoplasmic reticulum export is also regulated by specific amino acid residues located in the protein cytoplasmic domain (Butler and Bradbury, 2015). One of the previously identified ER export motifs is characterized by two acidic residues separated by a variable amino acid [(D/E)×(D/E)] (Sevier et al., 2000; Butler and Bradbury, 2015). The di-acidic motif is localized within the cytosolic domain of the protein, facilitating interactions with COPII components (Butler and Bradbury, 2015).This motif, first found in the vesicular stomatitis virus glycoprotein (VSVG) (Sevier et al., 2000), was later demonstrated in the Cystic Fibrosis Transmembrane Conductance Regulator (CFTR) and subsequently in other mammalian proteins (Fu and Sztul, 2003; Wang et al., 2004). Sequence alignment of various mammalian orthologs of LMTK2 revealed presence of a canonical di-acidic motif in the distal portion of the C-terminal tail, with a proximal upstream tyrosine residue, as observed in VSVG sequence in all species (Sevier et al., 2000; Butler and Bradbury, 2015).

Mutations of the di-acidic ER export motif D^{1110}-S-E, with D^{1110} and E^{1112} substituted with alanines (A^{1110}SA), caused retention of LMTK2 in the ER; however, a small amount of mutant LMTK2 was exported, suggesting presence of another ER export signal (Butler and Bradbury, 2015). The A^{1110}SA mutation increased stability of LMTK2 protein compared to the wild type (WT) kinase (half-life ~3.5 h vs. ~2.5 h, respectively) (Butler and Bradbury, 2015). Increased half-life of the A^{1110}SA mutant suggests that its targeting to the ER-associated protein degradation (ERAD) pathway is reduced, compared to the WT LMTK2. The ER export motif is located downstream of the catalytic and membrane spanning domains, thus proper folding of the mutant LMTK2 may prevent targeting to ERAD, leading to ER accumulation and subsequent increase of the half-life (Butler and Bradbury, 2015).

THE LMTK2 INTERACTOME

Lemur Tyrosine Kinase 2 has been described to interact with different protein partners, as summarized in **Table 1**. Validation of such protein–protein interactions with endogenously expressed proteins or *in vivo* models confirms the relevance of the LMTK2 interactome in human health and disease.

TABLE 1 | LMTK2 interactome.

Interactors	Type of interaction	Function	Cell line	Reference
PP1	Phosphorylation of PP1c-T^{320}	Inhibition of PP1c	HeLa, COS7	Manser et al., 2012a,b; Wang and Brautigan, 2002
Inh2	Direct binding (dependent of PP1c)	Regulation of PP1c	HeLa, COS7	Wang and Brautigan, 2002
Cdk5/p35	Phosphorylation of LMTK2-S^{1418}	Activation of LMTK2	HeLa, CHO, rat cortical neurons, COS	Kesavapany et al., 2003; Manser et al., 2012b
GSK3-β	Mediated by PP1c	Inhibition of GSK3-β phosphorylation, leading to its activation	HeLa	Manser et al., 2012a
KLC2	Mediated by GSK3-β	Decreases KLC2 phosphorylation and promotes binding to Smad2	HeLa	Manser et al., 2012a
Myosin VI	Direct binding (no phosphorylation)	Regulation of endocytic trafficking pathway	HeLa	Chibalina et al., 2007; Inoue et al., 2008
CFTR	Phosphorylation of CFTR-S^{737}	Regulation of CFTR endocytosis	Calu-3, CFBE41o^{-}	Luz et al., 2014; Wang and Brautigan, 2006
NGF	Phosphorylation of LMTK2	Down-regulation of LMTK2 activity	PC12	Kawa et al., 2004
BCL2/BCL-xL	Indirect interaction (cell-type dependent)	Regulation of expression of anti- and pro-apoptotic proteins	HME, MCF10A, HCT116, DLD-1	Conti et al., 2017
BIM	Indirect interaction (cell-type dependent)	Regulation of expression of anti- and pro-apoptotic proteins	HME, MCF10A, HCT116, DLD-1	Conti et al., 2017
AR	Direct binding	Inhibition of AR transcriptional activity	LNCaP, Human prostate tissue, HEK293	Shah and Bradbury, 2015b

PP1, protein phosphatase 1; Inh2, inhibitor 2; Cdk5, cyclin-dependent kinase-5; GSK3-β, glycogen synthase kinase 3 beta; KLC2, kinesin-1 light chain 2; CFTR, cystic fibrosis transmembrane conductance regulator; NGF, nerve growth factor; BCL, B-cell lymphoma; BIM, Bcl-2-interacting mediator of cell death; AR, androgen receptor.

PP1, Cdk5/p35, and Cell Signaling

Protein Phosphatase 1 is an ubiquitous serine/threonine phosphatase regulating many distinct processes, including gene transcription, cell cycle progression, protein synthesis, carbohydrate metabolism, neuronal signaling, and muscle contraction (Kelker et al., 2009). The PP1 holoenzyme is composed of PP1c and diverse regulatory subunits that are cell type and subcellular compartment specific (Pelech, 1995). LMTK2 binds directly to PP1c via the C-terminal VTF motif, resulting in an inhibitory phosphorylation of the T^{320} residue in PP1c (Wang and Brautigan, 2002; Manser et al., 2012a,b). LMTK2 interacts with one of the regulatory subunits of PP1c, Inh2 (Wang and Brautigan, 2002; Bollen et al., 2010). The Inh2–LMTK2 interaction is dependent on PP1c, because both PP1 and Inh2 demonstrated default binding in cell extracts (Wang and Brautigan, 2002). In view of this finding, it was suggested that LMTK2 inhibits PP1c activity through phosphorylation of its residue PP1c-T^{320} or through the interaction with Inh2 (Wang and Brautigan, 2002). It was subsequently shown that the LMTK2 kinase activity is required to inactivate PP1c. Studies conducted in Chinese hamster ovary (CHO) cells, HeLa cells and in cultured rat cortical neurons demonstrated that phosphorylation of LMTK2 on the S^{1418} residue, in mouse sequence, activates the kinase (Manser et al., 2012b). In human sequence, this residue corresponds to S^{1450}, however, we will always mention as LMTK2-Ser^{1418} to remain consistent with the literature and to a better understanding. A bioinformatic analysis, using NetPhosK database, predicted that cdk5/p35 phosphorylates S^{1418} with the highest score. This prediction was corroborated with the observation that the LMTK2-S^{1418} precedes a proline and thus is phosphorylated by proline-directed kinases, such as the cdk5/p35 complex. Bioinformatics analysis also predicted that GSK3-β and p38 phosphorylate LMTK2-S^{1418}, although these predictions have not been experimentally validated (Manser et al., 2012b). *In vitro* studies confirmed that modulation of the cdk5/p35 activity alters LMTK2-S^{1418} phosphorylation. Studies in HeLa cells, where cdk5 is present in an inactive form due to absence of p35, demonstrated that transfection of p35 increased LMTK2-S^{1418} phosphorylation. However, LMTK2-S^{1418} was also phosphorylated at low levels in the absence of the cdk5/p35 complex, suggesting that other kinases may also phosphorylate LMTK2-S^{1418} in non-neuronal cells (Manser et al., 2012b). Although the LMTK2-S^{1418} is located only 91 amino acid (90 aminoacids in human sequence) residues apart from the PP1c-binding motif, mutation of this residue only affects the phosphorylation of PP1c-T^{320} and does not prevent the LMTK2–PP1c interaction (Manser et al., 2012b). Based on the data, a model has been proposed where cdk5/p35 activates LMTK2 by phosphorylating the S^{1418} residue that in turn stimulates LMTK2 binding and inhibition of PP1 by phosphorylation of the PP1c-T^{320} (Manser et al., 2012b).

Kinesin 1 and the TGF-β Signaling Pathway

Lemur Tyrosine Kinase 2 controls the kinesin-1 mediated transport along microtubule filaments, including the canonical TGF-β mediator, Smad2. Kinesin-1 is a heterotetramer composed of two motor subunits also known as kinesin-1 heavy chains (KHC) and two associated kinesin-1 light chains (KLC) (Rahman et al., 1998; DeBoer et al., 2008). GSK3-β phosphorylates one of the KLC, KLC2, leading to release of the protein cargo and inhibition of kinesin-1 mediated transport (Morfini et al., 2002).

The signaling pathway that controls GSK3-β phosphorylation of KLC2 involves cdk5/p35-mediated inhibitory phosphorylation of PP1c-T^{320}, which in turn induces inhibitory phosphorylation of GSK3-β-S^{9}. Several lines of evidence support the role of LMTK2 in this pathway. First, LMTK2 contains the PP1c-binding motif. Second, transfection of LMTK2 indirectly increased GSK3-β-S^{9} phosphorylation by mediating the inhibitory phosphorylation of PP1c-T^{320}. Third, transfection of LMTK2 decreased KLC2 phosphorylation and promoted binding of a known KLC2 cargo, Smad2, necessary for activation of the canonical TGF-β signaling pathway (Manser et al., 2012a).

Myosin VI and Endocytic Trafficking

Lemur Tyrosine Kinase 2 interacts with myosin VI, the minus-end directed actin-associated motor protein critical for trafficking in the endocytic and secretory pathway (Chibalina et al., 2007; Inoue et al., 2008). LMTK2 is the first transmembrane protein and kinase identified to directly bind to myosin VI. The myosin VI binding site in LMTK2 is located in a region downstream of the kinase domain (residues 567–773), first discovered by an yeast two-hybrid screen and later confirmed in cultured cells (Chibalina et al., 2007; Inoue et al., 2008). The LMTK2 role in endocytic trafficking does not involve phosphorylation of myosin VI (Tumbarello et al., 2013).

Lemur Tyrosine Kinase 2 binds to the WWY motif in the C-terminal tail of myosin VI and shares the binding site with the multifunctional adaptor protein Disabled-2 (Dab2) (Chibalina et al., 2007; Inoue et al., 2008). Myosin VI recruits Dab2 and LMTK2 to different vesicular compartments. Recruitment of myosin VI to the clathrin-coated structures requires Dab2 while LMTK2 recruitment is necessary for transport from early endosomes to the recycling compartment (Morris et al., 2002; Chibalina et al., 2007; Spudich et al., 2007). LMTK2 is present on endocytic and recycling vesicles, namely a subset of early endosomes, where it colocalizes with Rab5, early endosomal antigen 1 (EEA1) and Rab11, while myosin VI is restricted to Rab5-positive early endosomes (Hasson, 2003; Chibalina et al., 2007). Knockdown of LMTK2 resulted in enlargement, swelling, ring-like appearance, and altered function of vesicles involved in the endocytic trafficking pathways in HeLa cells (Chibalina et al., 2007). Moreover, LMTK2 binding to myosin VI was required for endocytic trafficking of the transferrin receptor (Inoue et al., 2008). Loss of LMTK2 in the appropriate vesicular regions, induced by the ER export motif mutation A^{1110}SA, affected membrane trafficking, characterized by reduced recycling of transferrin from the cells without affecting its endocytosis (Butler and Bradbury, 2015). The impact of A^{1110}SA on transferrin trafficking was similar to the results obtained after LMTK2 knockdown (Chibalina et al., 2007).

CFTR and Cl^- Transport

Lemur Tyrosine Kinase 2 interacts with CFTR and mediates its inhibitory phosphorylation and endocytosis, and inhibits the CFTR-mediated Cl^- transport. CFTR is a member of the ATP binding cassette (ABC) transporter family that functions as a cAMP-activated Cl^- ion channel (Riordan et al., 1989; Gregory et al., 1990). CFTR was identified as an interacting partner of LMTK2 through a microarray where the peptide containing the S^{737} residue, corresponding to a sequence in the regulatory domain of CFTR, showed the strongest reactivity with LMTK2 (Wang and Brautigan, 2006).

The interaction between CFTR and LMTK2 was predicted to occur at the plasma membrane (Wang and Brautigan, 2006). The prediction was later experimentally validated in human airway epithelial Calu-3 cells where the endogenous LMTK2 co-immunoprecipitated with endogenous CFTR specifically at the apical plasma membrane (Luz et al., 2014). Additionally, depletion of LMTK2 increased the steady-state plasma membrane abundance and activity of CFTR in the primary HBE cells. Increased CFTR expression at the plasma membrane, after LMTK2 knockdown resulted from decreased CFTR endocytosis, suggesting that endogenous LMTK2 decreases the CFTR-mediated Cl^- secretion, at least in part by decreasing density of the CFTR Cl^- channels at the cell surface. This is the first evidence that CFTR endocytosis can be regulated, explaining the mechanism of phospho-dependent inhibitory effect of CFTR-S^{737} on the CFTR mediated Cl^- secretion (Wilkinson et al., 1997). LMTK2 depletion increased the efficacy of the CFTR corrector VX-809 (Lumafactor), currently a component of Orkambi, a FDA approved drug for CF patients homozygous for the most common disease-causing mutation F508del (Luz et al., 2014). These data suggest that interfering with the LMTK2 mediated inhibitory phosphorylation of CFTR may increase efficacy of CF-directed therapy.

The Nerve Growth Factor (NGF) and Neuronal Differentiation

Lemur Tyrosine Kinase 2 interaction with NGF inhibits neuronal differentiation. The specific distribution and phosphorylation of LMTK2 in the brain tissue first suggested that it may regulate early postnatal brain function (Kawa et al., 2004). Endogenous LMTK2 is phosphorylated upon stimulation with NGF in PC12 cells, possibly by a PKC-dependent mechanism, although a direct interaction between LMTK2 and PKC has not been demonstrated (Kawa et al., 2004). The NGF-stimulated phosphorylation down-regulates LMTK2 activity, resulting in activation of extracellular-signal-regulated kinases (ERK), leading to neurite outgrowth (Kawa et al., 2004).

The B-Cell Lymphoma (BCL) Proteins and Apoptosis

It has been suggested that LMTK2 inhibits cytotoxicity by interacting with the apoptotic and survival pathways. A high-throughput siRNA-based screen recently identified LMTK2 as a novel anti-apoptotic sensor (Conti et al., 2017). LMTK2 knockdown reduced the expression of anti-apoptotic B-cell lymphoma-2 (BCL2) and B-cell lymphoma-extra-large (BCL-xL) proteins and increased the expression of pro-apoptotic BCL2-interacting mediator of cell death (BIM) protein. While LMTK2-dependent regulation of BIM was more evident in non-cancer cell lines, other members of the BCL2 family, such as BCL2 and BCL-xL, were regulated by LMTK2 mainly in fully transformed cancer cells. Furthermore, LMTK2 knockdown enhanced the cytotoxic effect of apoptosis inducing ligands, such as the tumor necrosis factor-related apoptosis-inducing ligand (TRAIL) and etoposide, among others (Conti et al., 2017).

The Androgen Receptor (AR) and Prostate Development

Lemur Tyrosine Kinase 2 interacts with AR and inhibits its transcriptional activity (Shah and Bradbury, 2015a,b). AR promotes cell growth and plays an important role in prostate development (Chang et al., 1988; Mangelsdorf et al., 1995). The LMTK2–AR interaction was demonstrated by co-immunoprecipitation and Proximity Ligation Assay (PLA) in LNCaP cells, an androgen-sensitive human prostate adenocarcinoma cell line. Localization of the complex was dependent on the androgen ligands: under androgen deprivation, it was predominantly extra-nuclear and in presence of androgens the complex translocated to the nucleus. The LMTK2–AR complex was also detected in human prostate tissue (Shah and Bradbury, 2015b). Inhibition of the AR transcriptional activity by LMTK2 was demonstrated by luciferase reporter assay in HEK293 cells (Shah and Bradbury, 2015b).

ROLE OF LMTK2 IN HUMAN DISEASE: POTENTIAL BIOMARKER AND THERAPEUTIC TARGET

The role of LMTK2 in cell signaling, endocytic trafficking, apoptosis, and Cl^- transport explains why its dysregulation is associated with neurodegeneration, cancer, and infertility. Below, we discuss the role of LMTK2 in human disease and its potential to become a biomarker and a therapeutic target.

Prostate Cancer

The role of LMTK2 in prostate cancer is well established (Eeles et al., 2008; Guy et al., 2009; Waters et al., 2009; Harries et al., 2010; Wang et al., 2013; Shui et al., 2014; Shah and Bradbury, 2015a,b; Hao et al., 2016; Jiang et al., 2016). The *lmtk2* gene was identified as one of seven *loci* associated with prostate cancer in a genome-wide association study (GWAS) using blood DNA from 1854 individuals with prostate cancer detected before 60 years of age or with a family history of the disease (Eeles et al., 2008; Guy et al., 2009). The LMTK2 expression had no significant ethnic heterogeneity, as demonstrated in multi-ethnic prostate cancer populations from California with African and Latino background, or from Hawaii from native, Japanese or European descent (Waters et al., 2009). Furthermore, the LMTK2 single nucleotide polymorphism (SNP), rs6465657 was inversely associated with the risk of non-fatal prostate cancer and the cancer-specific mortality (Shui et al., 2014).

The expression of *lmtk2* gene was studied in benign prostate hyperplasia (BPH) and prostate cancer cells by RT-PCR. The *lmtk2* gene expression was decreased by 68% in tissue with prostate adenocarcinoma, when compared to BPH (Harries et al., 2010). In addition, LMTK2 protein abundance was undetectable or low in prostate cancer tissues, compared to very high expression in non-malignant tissue (Shah and Bradbury, 2015b). Additionally, a direct association between LMTK2 and tumor forming capacity was assessed in LNCaP cells. LMTK2 knockdown demonstrated significantly higher colony-forming capacity and increased cell viability, suggesting that LMTK2 plays a role in the regulation of cell proliferation (Shah and Bradbury, 2015b). This idea is corroborated by the fact that LMTK2 regulates the expression of several proteins involved in apoptosis, as described above.

In view of the above data, LMTK2 has a potential to serve as a novel biomarker in prostate cancer that, in contrast to the prostate specific antigen (PSA), can distinguish between BPH and prostate cancer. Furthermore, targeted activation of LMTK2 in the prostate tissues by small molecules could decrease the AR-proliferative activity, preventing the prostate cancer cell growth.

Other Cancers

The role of LMTK2 in apoptosis suggests that its dysregulation may be involved in other forms of cancer as well. In fact, LMTK2 mRNA is expressed in all cancer tissues according to The Cancer Genome Atlas (TCGA) (The Human Protein Atlas, 2018b). The LMTK2 protein levels differ in a variety of cancer cells. Levels are high in colorectal and ovarian cancer while they are low in lymphoma, lung, testis and renal cancer (The Human Protein Atlas, 2018b). Thus, LMTK2 has a potential to serve as a prognostic biomarker (The Human Protein Atlas, 2018b). For example, in renal cancer, LMTK2 indicates favorable prognosis because higher expression correlated with higher survival probability. By contrast, higher LMTK2 levels were associated with reduced survival in ovarian cancer (The Human Protein Atlas, 2018b).

Whole-exome sequencing (WES) followed by the Protein Variation Effect Analyzer (PROVEAN) modeling in pulmonary sarcomatoid carcinoma (PSC) cells identified deleterious effects of mutations in the *lmtk2* gene in 2 of 10 patients (Liu et al., 2016). PSC is an aggressive and poorly differentiated, non-small-cell lung carcinoma responsible for 0.1–0.4% of all lung cancer cases (Brambilla et al., 2001; Liu et al., 2016; Karim et al., 2018). A mutation in the *lmtk2* gene was also found in patients with lung adenocarcinoma (Seo et al., 2012). Future studies are needed to experimentally validate the diagnostic and prognostic potential of LMTK2 in different forms of cancer.

Male Infertility and Contraception

Animal studies suggest a strong association between LMTK2 and male fertility (Kawa et al., 2006; Sakugawa et al., 2009). Studies conducted with LMTK2 knockout (KO) mice demonstrated that LMTK2 plays an essential role in spermatogenesis. Although the KO animals had normal phenotype at birth and experienced normal growth, they had azoospermia (Kawa et al., 2006). Normal number and morphology of testicular somatic cells and intact hormonal levels in the LMTK2 KO mice suggest that impaired spermatogenesis was directly caused by a defect in germ cells. Indeed, it was observed that the first step of spermatogenesis – the differentiation of spermatogonia to round spermatids – occurred normally in these animals; however, further differentiation of spermatids was largely suppressed (Kawa et al., 2006). Thus, it has been hypothesized that LMTK2 is necessary for the morphological progression of postmeiotic germ cells, a process that includes mitochondrial compaction and expulsion of the cytoplasm. This hypothesis was experimentally validated by examination of the wild-type mice, in which LMTK2 expression was higher between 2 and 3 weeks after birth, the time of the late phase spermatogenesis, possibly after the generation of round spermatids (Kawa et al., 2006). Additionally, the *lmtk2* gene was predicted as a target for heat-sensitive micro (mi)RNAs in pachytene spermatocytes (Yadav et al., 2018). However, a study that examined the association of LMTK2 and infertility in humans demonstrated that the nine SNPs in exon 11 of the *lmtk2* gene identified in 18 Japanese men with azoospermia were not causative (Sakugawa et al., 2009).

Lemur Tyrosine Kinase 2 is a known inhibitor of PP1 that regulates sperm motility (Chakrabarti et al., 2007; Fardilha et al., 2011). Hence, LMTK2 emerges as a potential target for both reproductive contraceptives, such as an inhibitor of sperm motility, and infertility treatment in men, by regulating the activity of PP1. However, more studies are needed to better understand how LMTK2 regulates spermatogenesis.

Cystic Fibrosis

Cystic fibrosis (CF) is the most common lethal autosomal recessive disease in Caucasians (Grody and Desnick, 2001). The most common disease-associated mutation in the *cftr* gene F508del, is caused by the in-frame deletion of three nucleotides encoding phenylalanine at position 508. This mutation, present in 90% of CF patients in at least one allele, leads to an intracellular processing defect and retention of CFTR in the ER. The corrector VX-809 (part of the FDA-approved drug Orkambi) partially rescues the processing defect of F508del-CFTR and allows maturation while passing through the Golgi complex and trafficking to the cell membrane in cultured cells (Van Goor et al., 2011, 2014; Clancy et al., 2012; Ren et al., 2013; Wainwright et al., 2015). F508del-CFTR forms a Cl^- channel regulated by cAMP but has dramatically different gating properties compared to the wild-type CFTR (Dalemans et al., 1991; Swiatecka-Urban et al., 2005). The FDA-approved drug Kalydeco^{TM} (Ivacaftor; VX-770) potentiated membrane-resident F508del-CFTR channel "open" probability (Accurso et al., 2014). Clinical trials show that the combined use of corrector VX-809 and potentiator VX-770 (Orkambi) improved the percent of predicted forced expiratory volume in 1 second (FEV1), decreased the rate of pulmonary exacerbations, and reduced the rate of events leading to hospitalization or use of intravenous antibiotics in patients with two F508del copies (Wainwright et al., 2015). Clinical trial evaluating a different corrector VX-661 (Tezacaftor) with VX-770 in patients with two F508del copies showed results similar to Orkambi [Donaldson et al., 2013; Two Phase 3 Studies of the Tezacaftor/Ivacaftor Combination Treatment Met Primary Endpoints with Statistically Significant Improvements in Lung Function (FEV1) in People with Cystic Fibrosis, 2017] – with this combination also securing FDA approval under the brand name Symdeko. Although this is seen as a very important step forward, improved treatment efficacy is still needed for these patients.

While at the cell membrane, the corrector-rescued F508del-CFTR has reduced membrane residence and current therapies do not improve this defect (Swiatecka-Urban et al., 2005). LMTK2 depletion facilitates the VX-809 mediated trafficking of F508del-CFTR to the apical plasma membrane and rescue of the CFTR-mediated Cl^- secretion across human bronchial epithelial cells (Luz et al., 2014). Since LMTK2 facilitates CFTR endocytosis, these effects could result from decreased CFTR endocytosis after LMTK2 depletion. Thus, targeting the LMTK2-mediated inhibitory phosphorylation of CFTR-S^{737} could serve as a novel approach to study the plasma membrane stability defect of F508del-CFTR. It could also help to design new pharmacological approaches to stabilize rescued F508del-CFTR and improve the efficacy of the corrector/potentiator strategy (Luz et al., 2014).

Neurodegeneration

Neurodegeneration represents an irreversible structural and functional damage of neurons that can lead to cell death. It is the hallmark of several central nervous system disorders, including Alzheimer's and Parkinson's diseases (Przedborski et al., 2003). Bencze et al. (2018) recently reviewed the role of LMTK2 in neurodegeneration. The authors proposed three LMTK2-dependent mechanisms of neurodegeneration: (i) disruption of axonal transport, mediated by aberrant LMTK2–kinesin-1 interaction; (ii) hyperphosphorylation of Tau protein by LMTK2, mediated by cdk5 and GSK3-β; and (iii) regulation of apoptosis by LMTK2 (Bencze et al., 2018). The authors proposed that modulation of LMTK2 expression could be considered as a promising novel therapeutic target for neurodegenerative states, such as Alzheimer disease (Bencze et al., 2018).

CONCLUSION

Although LMTK2 is still incompletely characterized, its role in key biological functions has been well established by strong scientific evidence. LMTK2 works as a multifunctional adaptor, being involved on very distinct signaling pathways and cell mechanisms, such as endocytosis, apoptosis, channel trafficking and cell differentiation. Improved characterization of LMTK2 holds the potential to enhance our knowledge about the molecular basis of human disease and discover novel diagnostic and prognostic biomarkers. Targeting the LMTK2 interactome could also advance treatment for cancer, neurodegeneration, infertility, and cystic fibrosis and create novel strategies for contraception.

AUTHOR CONTRIBUTIONS

DC was involved in the planning and writing of the review manuscript. CF and AS-U were involved in the planning, writing and review process.

FUNDING

This work was supported by the Portuguese FCT fellowship grant from BioSys (PD/BD/114384/2016) to DC, Portuguese FCT grant UID/MULTI/04046/2013 to CF, the NIH grants R01DK104847 and R56HL127202, and the CFF grant SWIATE18G0 to AS-U.

REFERENCES

Accurso, F. J., Van Goor, F., Zha, J., Stone, A. J., Dong, Q., Ordonez, C. L., et al. (2014). Sweat chloride as a biomarker of CFTR activity: proof of concept and ivacaftor clinical trial data. *J. Cyst. Fibros* 13, 139–147. doi: 10.1016/j.jcf.2013.09.007

Angel, P., and Karin, M. (1991). The role of Jun, Fos and the AP-1 complex in cell-proliferation and transformation. *Biochim. Biophys. Acta* 1072, 129–157. doi: 10.1016/0304-419X(91)90011-9

Ardito, F., Giuliani, M., Perrone, D., Troiano, G., Muzio, L., and Lo. (2017). The crucial role of protein phosphorylation in cell signaling and its use as targeted therapy (Review). *Int. J. Mol. Med.* 40, 271–280. doi: 10.3892/ijmm.2017.3036

Barford, D. (1996). Molecular mechanisms of theprotein serine/threonine phosphatases. *Trends Biochem. Sci.* 21, 407–412. doi: 10.1016/S0968-0004(96)10060-8

Bencze, J., Mórotz, G. M., Seo, W., Bencs, V., Kálmán, J., Miller, C. C. J., et al. (2018). Biological function of Lemur tyrosine kinase 2 (LMTK2): implications in neurodegeneration. *Mol. Brain* 11:20. doi: 10.1186/s13041-018-0363-x

Bollen, M., Peti, W., Ragusa, M. J., and Beullens, M. (2010). The extended PP1 toolkit: designed to create specificity. *Trends Biochem. Sci.* 35, 450–458. doi: 10.1016/j.tibs.2010.03.002

Brambilla, E., Travis, W. D., Colby, T. V., Corrin, B., and Shimosato, Y. (2001). The new world health organization classification of lung tumours. *Eur. Respir. J.* 18, 1059–1068. doi: 10.1183/09031936.01.00275301

Butler, E. C., and Bradbury, N. A. (2015). Signal dependent ER export of lemur tyrosine kinase 2. *BMC Cell Biol.* 16:26. doi: 10.1186/s12860-015-0072-6

Castagna, M., Takai, Y., Kaibuchi, K., Sano, K., Kikkawa, U., and Nishizuka, Y. (1982). Direct activation of calcium-activated, phospholipid-dependent protein kinase by tumor-promoting phorbol esters. *J. Biol. Chem.* 257, 7847–7851.

Chakrabarti, R., Cheng, L., Puri, P., Soler, D., and Vijayaraghavan, S. (2007). Protein phosphatase PP1 gamma 2 in sperm morphogenesis and epididymal initiation of sperm motility. *Asian J. Androl.* 9, 445–452. doi: 10.1111/j.1745-7262.2007.00307.x

Chang, C. S., Kokontis, J., and Liao, S. T. (1988). Molecular cloning of human and rat complementary DNA encoding androgen receptors. *Science* 240, 324–326. doi: 10.1126/science.3353726

Cheng, H.-C., Qi, R. Z., Paudel, H., and Zhu, H.-J. (2011). Regulation and function of protein kinases and phosphatases. *Enzyme Res.* 2011, 1–3. doi: 10.4061/2011/794089

Chibalina, M. V., Seaman, M. N. J., Miller, C. C., Kendrick-Jones, J., and Buss, F. (2007). Myosin VI and its interacting protein LMTK2 regulate tubule formation and transport to the endocytic recycling compartment. *J. Cell Sci.* 120, 4278–4288. doi: 10.1242/jcs.014217

Clancy, J. P., Rowe, S. M., Accurso, F. J., Aitken, M. L., Amin, R. S., Ashlock, M. A., et al. (2012). Results of a phase IIa study of VX-809, an investigational CFTR corrector compound, in subjects with cystic fibrosis homozygous for the F508del-CFTR mutation. *Thorax* 67, 12–18. doi: 10.1136/thoraxjnl-2011-200393

Conti, A., Majorini, M. T., Fontanella, E., Bardelli, A., Giacca, M., Delia, D., et al. (2017). Lemur tyrosine kinase 2 (LMTK2) is a determinant of cell sensitivity to apoptosis by regulating the levels of the BCL2 family members. *Cancer Lett.* 389, 59–69. doi: 10.1016/j.canlet.2016.12.025

Dalemans, W., Barbry, P., Champigny, G., Jallat, S., Dott, K., Dreyer, D., et al. (1991). Altered chloride ion channel kinetics associated with the delta F508 cystic fibrosis mutation. *Nature* 354, 526–528. doi: 10.1038/354526a0

DeBoer, S. R., You, Y., Szodorai, A., Kaminska, A., Pigino, G., Nwabuisi, E., et al. (2008). Conventional kinesin holoenzymes are composed of heavy and light chain homodimers. *Biochemistry* 47, 4535–4543. doi: 10.1021/bi702445j

Dey, I., and Bradbury, N. A. (2017). Activation of TPA-response element present in human Lemur Tyrosine Kinase 2 (lmtk2) gene increases its expression. *Biochem. Biophys. Rep.* 12, 140–150. doi: 10.1016/j.bbrep.2017.09.006

Donaldson, S., Pilewski, J., Griese, M., Dong, Q., and Lee, P.-S. (2013). WS7.3 VX-661, an investigational CFTR corrector, in combination with ivacaftor, a CFTR potentiator, in patients with CF and homozygous for the F508Del-CFTR mutation: interim analysis. *J. Cyst. Fibros.* 12:S14. doi: 10.1016/S1569-1993(13)60042-9

Duong-Ly, K. C., and Peterson, J. R. (2013). The human kinome and kinase inhibition. *Curr. Protoc. Pharmacol.* Chap. 2:Unit9.2. doi: 10.1002/0471141755.ph0209s60

Eeles, R. A., Kote-Jarai, Z., Giles, G. G., Olama, A. A., Al, Guy, M., et al. (2008). Multiple newly identified loci associated with prostate cancer susceptibility. *Nat. Genet.* 40, 316–321. doi: 10.1038/ng.90

Fardilha, M., Esteves, S. L. C., Korrodi-Gregório, L., Pelech, S., da Cruz, E., Silva, O. A. B., et al. (2011). Protein phosphatase 1 complexes modulate sperm motility and present novel targets for male infertility. *Mol. Hum. Reprod.* 17, 466–477. doi: 10.1093/molehr/gar004

Fu, L., and Sztul, E. (2003). Traffic-independent function of the Sar1p/COPII machinery in proteasomal sorting of the cystic fibrosis transmembrane conductance regulator. *J. Cell Biol.* 160, 157–163. doi: 10.1083/jcb.200210086

Gregory, R. J., Cheng, S. H., Rich, D. P., Marshall, J., Paul, S., Hehir, K., et al. (1990). Expression and characterization of the cystic fibrosis transmembrane conductance regulator. *Nature* 347, 382–386. doi: 10.1038/347382a0

Grody, W. W., and Desnick, R. J. (2001). Cystic fibrosis population carrier screening: here at last—Are we ready? *Genet. Med.* 3, 87–90. doi: 10.1097/00125817-200103000-00001

Guy, M., Kote-Jarai, Z., Giles, G. G., Al Olama, A. A., Jugurnauth, S. K., Mulholland, S., et al. (2009). Identification of new genetic risk factors for prostate cancer. *Asian J. Androl.* 11, 49–55. doi: 10.1038/aja.2008.18

Hao, Q., Wei, D., Zhang, Y., Chen, X., Yang, F., Yang, Z., et al. (2016). Systematic meta-analyses of gene-specific genetic association studies in prostate cancer. *Oncotarget* 7, 22271–22284. doi: 10.18632/oncotarget.7926

Harries, L. W., Perry, J. R. B., McCullagh, P., and Crundwell, M. (2010). Alterations in LMTK2, MSMB and HNF1B gene expression are associated with the development of prostate cancer. *BMC Cancer* 10:315. doi: 10.1186/1471-2407-10-315

Hasson, T. (2003). Myosin VI: two distinct roles in endocytosis. *J. Cell Sci.* 116, 3453–3461. doi: 10.1242/jcs.00669

Heath, C. M., Stahl, P. D., and Barbieri, M. A. (2003). Lipid kinases play crucial and multiple roles in membrane trafficking and signaling. *Histol. Histopathol.* 18, 989–998. doi: 10.14670/HH-18.989

Inoue, T., Kon, T., Ohkura, R., Yamakawa, H., Ohara, O., Yokota, J., et al. (2008). BREK/LMTK2 is a myosin VI-binding protein involved in endosomal membrane trafficking. *Genes Cells* 13, 483–495. doi: 10.1111/j.1365-2443.2008.01184.x

Jiang, X., Zhang, M., Bai, X.-Y., Li, S., and Wu, H. (2016). Association between 17q25.3-rs6465657 polymorphism and prostate cancer susceptibility: a meta-analysis based on 19 studies. *Onco. Targets. Ther.* 9, 4491–4503. doi: 10.2147/OTT.S104775

Karim, N. A., Schuster, J., Eldessouki, I., Gaber, O., Namad, T., Wang, J., et al. (2018). Pulmonary sarcomatoid carcinoma: University of Cincinnati experience. *Oncotarget* 9, 4102–4108. doi: 10.18632/oncotarget.23468

Kawa, S., Fujimoto, J., Tezuka, T., Nakazawa, T., and Yamamoto, T. (2004). Involvement of BREK, a serine/threonine kinase enriched in brain, in NGF signalling. *Genes Cells* 9, 219–32. doi: 10.1111/j.1356-9597.2004.00714.x

Kawa, S., Ito, C., Toyama, Y., Maekawa, M., Tezuka, T., Nakamura, T., et al. (2006). Azoospermia in mice with targeted disruption of the Brek/Lmtk2 (brain-enriched kinase/lemur tyrosine kinase 2) gene. *Proc. Natl. Acad. Sci. U.S.A.* 103, 19344–19349. doi: 10.1073/pnas.0603603103

Kelker, M. S., Page, R., and Peti, W. (2009). Crystal structures of protein phosphatase-1 bound to nodularin-R and tautomycin: a novel scaffold for structure-based drug design of serine/threonine phosphatase inhibitors. *J. Mol. Biol.* 385, 11–21. doi: 10.1016/j.jmb.2008.10.053

Kesavapany, S., Lau, K.-F., Ackerley, S., Banner, S. J., Shemilt, S. J. A., Cooper, J. D., et al. (2003). Identification of a novel, membrane-associated neuronal kinase, cyclin-dependent kinase 5/p35-regulated kinase. *J. Neurosci.* 23, 4975–4983. doi: 10.1523/JNEUROSCI.23-12-04975.2003

Liu, X., Jia, Y., Stoopler, M. B., Shen, Y., Cheng, H., Chen, J., et al. (2016). Next-generation sequencing of pulmonary sarcomatoid carcinoma reveals high frequency of actionable MET gene mutations. *J. Clin. Oncol.* 34, 794–802. doi: 10.1200/JCO.2015.62.0674

Luz, S., Cihil, K. M., Brautigan, D. L., Amaral, M. D., Farinha, C. M., and Swiatecka-Urban, A. (2014). LMTK2-mediated phosphorylation regulates CFTR endocytosis in human airway epithelial cells. *J. Biol. Chem.* 289, 15080–15093. doi: 10.1074/jbc.M114.563742

Mangelsdorf, D. J., Thummel, C., Beato, M., Herrlich, P., Schütz, G., Umesono, K., et al. (1995). The nuclear receptor superfamily: the second decade. *Cell* 83, 835–839. doi: 10.1016/0092-8674(95)90199-X

Manning, G., Plowman, G. D., Hunter, T., and Sudarsanam, S. (2002a). Evolution of protein kinase signaling from yeast to man. *Trends Biochem. Sci.* 27, 514–20. doi: 10.1016/S0968-0004(02)02179-5

Manning, G., Whyte, D. B., Martinez, R., Hunter, T., and Sudarsanam, S. (2002b). The protein kinase complement of the human genome. *Science* 298, 1912–1934. doi: 10.1126/science.1075762

Manser, C., Guillot, F., Vagnoni, A., Davies, J., Lau, K.-F., McLoughlin, D. M., et al. (2012a). Lemur tyrosine kinase-2 signalling regulates kinesin-1 light chain-2 phosphorylation and binding of Smad2 cargo. *Oncogene* 31, 2773–2782. doi: 10.1038/onc.2011.437

Manser, C., Vagnoni, A., Guillot, F., Davies, J., and Miller, C. C. J. (2012b). Cdk5/p35 phosphorylates lemur tyrosine kinase-2 to regulate protein phosphatase-1C phosphorylation and activity. *J. Neurochem.* 121, 343–348. doi: 10.1111/j.1471-4159.2012.07650.x

Morfini, G., Szebenyi, G., Elluru, R., Ratner, N., and Brady, S. T. (2002). Glycogen synthase kinase 3 phosphorylates kinesin light chains and negatively regulates kinesin-based motility. *EMBO J.* 21, 281–293. doi: 10.1093/emboj/21.3.281

Morris, S. M., Arden, S. D., Roberts, R. C., Kendrick-Jones, J., Cooper, J. A., Luzio, J. P., et al. (2002). Myosin VI binds to and localises with Dab2, potentially linking receptor-mediated endocytosis and the actin cytoskeleton. *Traffic* 3, 331–341. doi: 10.1034/j.1600-0854.2002.30503.x

Nixon, A., Jia, Y., White, C., and Bradbury, N. A. (2013). Determination of the membrane topology of lemur tyrosine kinase 2 (LMTK2) by fluorescence protease protection. *Am. J. Physiol. Cell Physiol.* 304, C164–C169. doi: 10.1152/ajpcell.00288.2012

Owji, H., Nezafat, N., Negahdaripour, M., Hajiebrahimi, A., and Ghasemi, Y. (2018). A comprehensive review of signal peptides: structure, roles, and applications. *Eur. J. Cell Biol.* 97, 422–441. doi: 10.1016/j.ejcb.2018.06.003

Pelech, S. L. (1995). Networking with proline-directed protein kinases implicated in tau phosphorylation. *Neurobiol. Aging* 16, 247–56; discussion 257–261. doi: 10.1016/0197-4580(94)00187-6

Peterson, J. H., Woolhead, C. A., and Bernstein, H. D. (2003). Basic amino acids in a distinct subset of signal peptides promote interaction with the signal recognition particle. *J. Biol. Chem.* 278, 46155–46162. doi: 10.1074/jbc.M309082200

Przedborski, S., Vila, M., and Jackson-Lewis, V. (2003). Neurodegeneration: what is it and where are we? *J. Clin. Invest.* 111, 3–10. doi: 10.1172/JCI17522

Rahman, A., Friedman, D. S., and Goldstein, L. S. (1998). Two kinesin light chain genes in mice. Identification and characterization of the encoded proteins. *J. Biol. Chem.* 273, 15395–15403. doi: 10.1074/jbc.273.25.15395

Ren, H. Y., Grove, D. E., De La Rosa, O., Houck, S. A., Sopha, P., Van Goor, F., et al. (2013). VX-809 corrects folding defects in cystic fibrosis transmembrane conductance regulator protein through action on membrane-spanning domain 1. *Mol. Biol. Cell* 24, 3016–3024. doi: 10.1091/mbc.E13-05-0240

Riordan, J. R., Kerem, B., Alon, N., Rozmahel, R., Grzelczak, Z., et al. (1989). Identification of the cystic fibrosis gene: cloning and characterization of complementary DNA. *Science* 8, 1066–1073. doi: 10.1126/science.2475911

Sakugawa, N., Miyamoto, T., Tsujimura, A., Koh, E., Miyagawa, Y., Sato, H., et al. (2009). LMTK2 and PARP-2 gene polymorphism and azoospermia secondary to meiotic arrest. *J. Assist. Reprod. Genet.* 26, 545–552. doi: 10.1007/s10815-009-9347-1

Sanders, J. L., and Stern, P. H. (1996). Expression and phorbol ester-induced down-regulation of protein kinase C isozymes in osteoblasts. *J. Bone Miner. Res.* 11, 1862–1872. doi: 10.1002/jbmr.5650111206

Schwartz, P. A., and Murray, B. W. (2011). Protein kinase biochemistry and drug discovery. *Bioorg. Chem.* 39, 192–210. doi: 10.1016/j.bioorg.2011.07.004

Seo, J.-S., Ju, Y. S., Lee, W.-C., Shin, J.-Y., Lee, J. K., Bleazard, T., et al. (2012). The transcriptional landscape and mutational profile of lung adenocarcinoma. *Genome Res.* 22, 2109–2119. doi: 10.1101/gr.145144.112

Sevier, C. S., Weisz, O. A., Davis, M., and Machamer, C. E. (2000). Efficient export of the vesicular stomatitis virus G protein from the endoplasmic reticulum requires a signal in the cytoplasmic tail that includes both tyrosine-based and di-acidic motifs. *Mol. Biol. Cell* 11, 13–22. doi: 10.1091/mbc.11.1.13

Shah, K., and Bradbury, N. A. (2015a). Kinase modulation of androgen receptor signaling: implications for prostate cancer. *Cancer Cell Microenviron.* 2:e123. doi: 10.14800/ccm.1023

Shah, K., and Bradbury, N. A. (2015b). Lemur tyrosine kinase 2, a novel target in prostate cancer therapy. *Oncotarget* 6, 14233–14246. doi: 10.18632/oncotarget.3899

Shui, I. M., Lindström, S., Kibel, A. S., Berndt, S. I., Campa, D., Gerke, T., et al. (2014). Prostate cancer (PCa) risk variants and risk of fatal PCa in the national cancer institute breast and prostate cancer cohort consortium. *Eur. Urol.* 65, 1069–1075. doi: 10.1016/j.eururo.2013.12.058

Spudich, G., Chibalina, M. V., Au, J. S.-Y., Arden, S. D., Buss, F., and Kendrick-Jones, J. (2007). Myosin VI targeting to clathrin-coated structures and dimerization is mediated by binding to Disabled-2 and PtdIns(4,5)P2. *Nat. Cell Biol.* 9, 176–183. doi: 10.1038/ncb1531

Swiatecka-Urban, A., Brown, A., Moreau-Marquis, S., Renuka, J., Coutermarsh, B., Barnaby, R., et al. (2005). The short apical membrane half-life of rescued {Delta}F508-cystic fibrosis transmembrane conductance regulator (CFTR) results from accelerated endocytosis of {Delta}F508-CFTR in polarized human airway epithelial cells. *J. Biol. Chem.* 280, 36762–36772. doi: 10.1074/jbc.M508944200

The Human Protein Atlas (2018a). *LMTK2*. Available at: https://www.proteinatlas.org/ENSG00000164715-LMTK2/tissue [accessed January 5, 2018].

The Human Protein Atlas (2018b). *LMTK2 in Pathology*. Available at: https://www.proteinatlas.org/ENSG00000164715-LMTK2/pathology [accessed January 5, 2018].

Tumbarello, D. A., Kendrick-Jones, J., and Buss, F. (2013). Myosin VI and its cargo adaptors – Linking endocytosis and autophagy. *J. Cell Sci.* 126, 2561–2570. doi: 10.1242/jcs.095554

Two Phase 3 Studies of the Tezacaftor/Ivacaftor Combination Treatment Met Primary Endpoints with Statistically Significant Improvements in Lung Function (FEV1) in People with Cystic Fibrosis (2017). *Vertex Press Release*. Available at: https://investors.vrtx.com/news-releases/news-release-details/two-phase-3-studies-tezacaftorivacaftor-combination-treatment.

Ubersax, J. A., and Ferrell, J. E. Jr. (2007). Mechanisms of specificity in protein phosphorylation. *Nat. Rev. Mol. Cell Biol.* 8, 530–541. doi: 10.1038/nrm2203

Van Goor, F., Hadida, S., Grootenhuis, P. D. J., Burton, B., Stack, J. H., Straley, K. S., et al. (2011). Correction of the F508del-CFTR protein processing defect in vitro by the investigational drug VX-809. *Proc. Natl. Acad. Sci. U.S.A.* 108, 18843–18848. doi: 10.1073/pnas.1105787108

Van Goor, F., Yu, H., Burton, B., and Hoffman, B. J. (2014). Effect of ivacaftor on CFTR forms with missense mutations associated with defects in protein processing or function. *J. Cyst. Fibros* 13, 29–36. doi: 10.1016/j.jcf.2013.06.008

Wainwright, C. E., Elborn, J. S., and Ramsey, B. W. (2015). Lumacaftor-ivacaftor in patients with cystic fibrosis homozygous for Phe508del CFTR. *N. Engl. J. Med.* 373, 1783–1784. doi: 10.1056/NEJMc1510466

Wang, H., and Brautigan, D. L. (2002). A novel transmembrane Ser/Thr kinase complexes with protein phosphatase-1 and inhibitor-2. *J. Biol. Chem.* 277, 49605–49612. doi: 10.1074/jbc.M209335200

Wang, H., and Brautigan, D. L. (2006). Peptide microarray analysis of substrate specificity of the transmembrane Ser/Thr kinase KPI-2 reveals reactivity with cystic fibrosis transmembrane conductance regulator and phosphorylase. *Mol. Cell. Proteomics* 5, 2124–2130. doi: 10.1074/mcp.M600188-MCP200

Wang, N., Wang, J., Shi, X., Zhang, Y., Liu, M., Wang, X., et al. (2013). [Association of TET2, LMTK2 and FAM84B gene expression with prostate cancer risk in Chinese patients]. *Zhonghua Zhong Liu Za Zhi* 35, 262–267.

Wang, X., Matteson, J., An, Y., Moyer, B., Yoo, J.-S., Bannykh, S., et al. (2004). COPII-dependent export of cystic fibrosis transmembrane conductance regulator from the ER uses a di-acidic exit code. *J. Cell Biol.* 167, 65–74. doi: 10.1083/jcb.200401035

Waters, K. M., Le Marchand, L., Kolonel, L. N., Monroe, K. R., Stram, D. O., Henderson, B. E., et al. (2009). Generalizability of associations from prostate cancer genome-wide association studies in multiple populations. *Cancer Epidemiol. Biomarkers Prev.* 18, 1285–1289. doi: 10.1158/1055-9965.EPI-08-1142

Wilkinson, D. J., Strong, T. V., Mansoura, M. K., Wood, D. L., Smith, S. S., Collins, F. S., et al. (1997). CFTR activation: additive effects of stimulatory and inhibitory phosphorylation sites in the R domain. *Am. J. Physiol.* 273, L127–L133. doi: 10.1152/ajplung.1997.273.1.L127

Yadav, S. K., Pandey, A., Kumar, L., Devi, A., Kushwaha, B., Vishvkarma, R., et al. (2018). The thermo-sensitive gene expression signatures of spermatogenesis. *Reprod. Biol. Endocrinol.* 16:56. doi: 10.1186/s12958-018-0372-8

Zhang, Z.-Y. (2002). Protein tyrosine phosphatases: structure and function, substrate specificity, and inhibitor development. *Annu. Rev. Pharmacol. Toxicol.* 42, 209–234. doi: 10.1146/annurev.pharmtox.42.083001.144616

2

The Autophagy Inhibitor Spautin-1 Antagonizes Rescue of Mutant CFTR Through an Autophagy-Independent and USP13-Mediated Mechanism

*Emanuela Pesce[1†], Elvira Sondo[1†], Loretta Ferrera[1], Valeria Tomati[1], Emanuela Caci[1], Paolo Scudieri[2], Ilaria Musante[2], Mario Renda[2], Nesrine Baatallah[3,4], Nathalie Servel[3,4], Alexandre Hinzpeter[3,4], Diego di Bernardo[2], Nicoletta Pedemonte[1] and Luis J. V. Galietta[2]**

[1] U.O.C. Genetica Medica, IRCCS Istituto Giannina Gaslini, Genoa, Italy, [2] Telethon Institute of Genetics and Medicine, Pozzuoli, Italy, [3] INSERM, U1151, Institut Necker Enfants Malades, Paris, France, [4] Université Paris Descartes, Paris, France

***Correspondence:**
Luis J. V. Galietta
l.galietta@tigem.it

† These authors have contributed equally to this work

The mutation F508del, responsible for a majority of cystic fibrosis cases, provokes the instability and misfolding of the CFTR chloride channel. Pharmacological recovery of F508del-CFTR may be obtained with small molecules called correctors. However, treatment with a single corrector *in vivo* and *in vitro* only leads to a partial rescue, a consequence of cell quality control systems that still detect F508del-CFTR as a defective protein causing its degradation. We tested the effect of spautin-1 on F508del-CFTR since it is an inhibitor of USP10 deubiquitinase and of autophagy, a target and a biological process that have been associated with cystic fibrosis and mutant CFTR. We found that short-term treatment of cells with spautin-1 downregulates the function and expression of F508del-CFTR despite the presence of corrector VX-809, a finding obtained in multiple cell models and assays. In contrast, spautin-1 was ineffective on wild type CFTR. Silencing and upregulation of USP13 (another target of spautin-1) but not of USP10, had opposite effects on F508del-CFTR expression/function. In contrast, modulation of autophagy with known activators or inhibitors did not affect F508del-CFTR. Our results identify spautin-1 as a novel chemical probe to investigate the molecular mechanisms that prevent full rescue of mutant CFTR.

Keywords: CFTR, chloride channel, cystic fibrosis, autophagy, ubiquitination, spautin-1

INTRODUCTION

CFTR, a plasma membrane chloride channel with a main role in epithelial cells, is mutated in cystic fibrosis (CF), one of the most frequent genetic diseases (Stoltz et al., 2015; Castellani and Assael, 2017). Loss of CFTR-dependent chloride transport affects multiple organs, including lungs, pancreas, liver, and sweat glands. Among the many types of mutations that affect the *CFTR* gene, the loss of phenylalanine 508 (F508del) is the most frequent. F508del impairs the folding and stability of CFTR protein (Lukacs and Verkman, 2012). Consequently, F508del-CFTR trafficking to the cell surface is severely altered. The mutant protein is retained in the endoplasmic reticulum and degraded by the ubiquitin-proteasome system (Lukacs and Verkman, 2012). A small fraction of the protein may reach the plasma membrane where, however, it is rapidly removed and eliminated by peripheral quality control mechanisms (Sharma et al., 2001; Okiyoneda et al., 2010; Fu et al., 2015).

Recently, pharmacological correctors of F508del defect have been developed (Galietta, 2013; Quon and Rowe, 2016). Such molecules favor F508del-CFTR trafficking with different mechanisms. One of the most advanced molecules is the corrector VX-809 (Van Goor et al., 2011). This small molecule partially rescues F508del-CFTR by possibly binding to the mutant protein itself (Ren et al., 2013; Hudson et al., 2017). VX-809 is presently used, in combination with the potentiator VX-770, to treat CF patients homozygous for the F508del mutation (Wainwright et al., 2015). However, the extent of clinical benefit obtained with the VX-809/VX-770 combination is relatively modest. The low efficacy of the combination is believed to be due to the partial activity of VX-809 as a corrector (Okiyoneda et al., 2013). A negative interaction between VX-809 and VX-770 can be also involved (Cholon et al., 2014; Veit et al., 2014). It has been shown that more marked levels of F508del-CFTR rescue can be obtained with combinations of correctors having complementary mechanisms of action (Farinha et al., 2013; Okiyoneda et al., 2013). Such other correctors may work by binding to a second site in the CFTR protein or by modulation of the cell machinery responsible for CFTR processing and degradation. Several proteins, including RNF5/RMA1, gp78, CHIP, CAL, Dab2, and cCBL, have been identified to affect CFTR processing but the list is probably far from being complete (Cheng et al., 2002; Younger et al., 2006; Morito et al., 2008; Okiyoneda et al., 2010; Ye et al., 2010; Fu et al., 2015; Tomati et al., 2015, 2018; Sondo et al., 2017). It has been shown that the ubiquitin specific peptidase 10 (USP10) is an important factor that controls CFTR degradation (Bomberger et al., 2009). Interestingly, a small molecule inhibitor of USP10, spautin-1, has been recently described. This compound also inhibits another ubiquitin peptidase, USP13 (Liu et al., 2011). By inhibiting USP10 and USP13, spautin-1 is also an inhibitor of autophagy, a process that has a possible important relationship with CFTR (Luciani et al., 2010). Therefore, we were interested in evaluating spautin-1 as a possible pharmacological tool to perturb CFTR processing. We found that spautin-1 antagonizes the rescue by VX-809 causing a rapid rundown of F508del-CFTR at the functional and molecular level. This effect may involve USP13 inhibition but is independent from autophagy block. USP13 appears as an important protein regulating the fate of mutant CFTR while spautin-1 may become an interesting probe for mechanistic studies and the search of new therapeutic agents.

RESULTS

CFBE41o- cells expressing F508del-CFTR and the halide-sensitive yellow fluorescent protein (HS-YFP) were treated for 24 h with 1 μM VX-809 or vehicle (DMSO) alone. F508del-CFTR function was then determined with the HS-YFP assay in microplate reader. The treatment with VX-809 caused a nearly three-fold increase in F508del-CFTR function, as indicated by the faster fluorescence quenching caused by iodide influx (**Figure 1A**). We tested spautin-1 at 10 μM, the concentration previously found to affect USP10 and USP13 activity (Liu et al., 2011). When spautin-1 was added in the last 3 h of incubation, the rescue induced by VX-809 was reduced by nearly 40% (**Figure 1A**). The decrease in CFTR function by spautin-1 was paralleled by an altered pattern of F508del-CFTR maturation as indicated by immunoblot experiments. In lysates from untreated cells, the mutant CFTR migrates as a core-glycosylated protein (band B) with an apparent size of 150 kDa (**Figure 1B** and **Supplementary Datasheet 2**). Treatment with the corrector VX-809 is known to improve F508del-CFTR maturation with appearance of a fully glycosylated version of the protein (band C) with mobility corresponding to 170 kDa. VX-809 also increases band B abundance. Importantly, treatment with spautin-1 for 3 h antagonized the rescue by VX-809 as evident from the downregulation of band C and of total CFTR (band C plus band B; **Figure 1B**). Interestingly, the ratio band C/band B was not altered since both bands were downregulated by spautin-1 to a similar extent.

Using the HS-YFP functional assay, we determined the time-dependence of spautin-1 effect. Treatments with spautin-1 (10 μM) as short as 5–15 min were enough to cause a significant inhibition (20–30%) of F508del-CFTR function (**Figure 1C**). Larger effects were observed with longer incubations.

To estimate spautin-1 potency, we tested multiple concentrations in the range 0.08–20 μM. We found that micromolar concentrations were needed to inhibit F508del-CFTR function, with 20 μM causing a nearly total reversal of VX-809 rescue (**Figure 2A**). A similar dose-dependence was found by examining F508del-CFTR protein maturation (**Figure 2B**). Importantly, at the same concentrations, spautin-1 caused no inhibition of wild type CFTR activity, irrespective of presence or absence of VX-809 (**Supplementary Figure 1A**). This result was consistent with unaltered pattern of CFTR protein maturation even with 20 μM of spautin-1 (**Supplementary Figure 1B**).

F508del-CFTR can be also rescued by cell incubation at low temperature. Cells were incubated for 21 h at 32°C, a condition that increases F508del-CFTR function as a result of enhanced expression on cell surface (Sondo et al., 2011). Then, cells were kept for three additional hours at 32°C or at 37°C, with and without spautin-1 (20 μM). As shown in **Figure 2C**, spautin-1 inhibited F508del-CFTR function also in cells rescued by hypothermia.

We also investigated F508del-CFTR protein expression by cell surface biotinylation. Intact cells were labeled with biotin and then lysed. Biotinylated proteins were isolated by pull-down and then revealed by immunoblot. Spautin-1 decreased F508del-CFTR but not Na^+/K^+-ATPase expression on cell surface (**Supplementary Figure 2**). It may be noted that both bands C and B are revealed by this method. The presence of core-glycosylated F508del-CFTR on cell surface, due to an unconventional route of trafficking, has already been shown in CFBE41o- cells (Gee et al., 2011; Tomati et al., 2015). In this respect, absence of calnexin and 14-3-3 proteins in the biotinylated fraction indicates that intracellular proteins were not labeled by our procedure.

We asked whether spautin-1 effects could be due to a block in protein synthesis. CFBE41o- cells were treated with VX-809 for 24 h and, in the last 3 or 6 h, with cycloheximide (CHX)

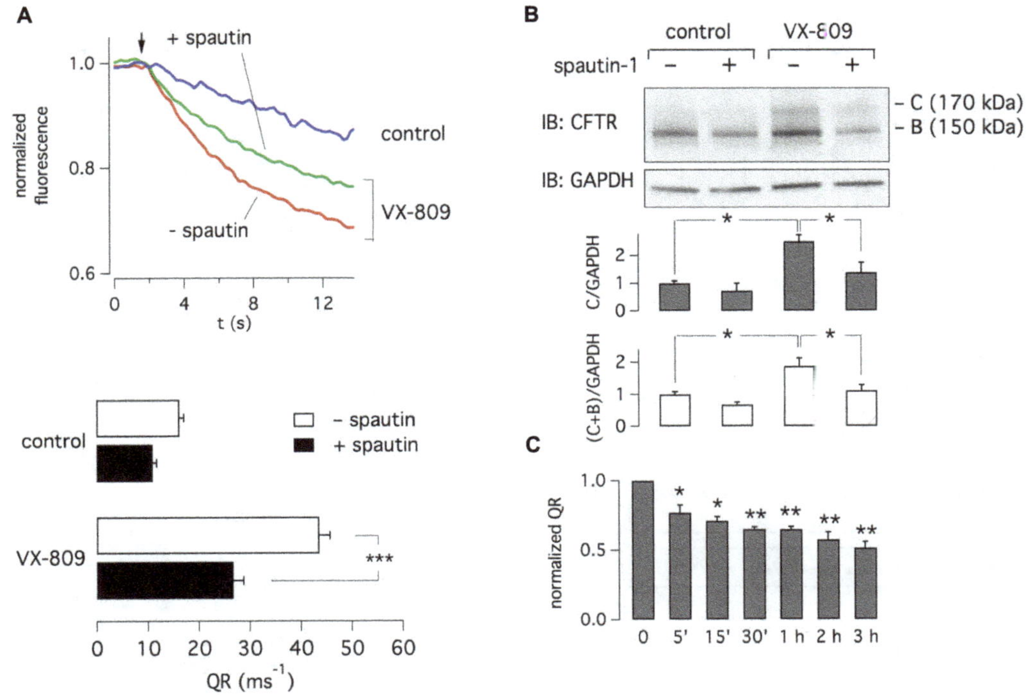

FIGURE 1 | Inhibition of F508del-CFTR function and expression by spautin-1. **(A)** Representative traces and bar graphs showing F508del-CFTR activity measured with the HS-YFP microplate reader assay. The arrow indicates the time of addition of extracellular I^-. CFBE41o- cells were treated for 24 h with vehicle (DMSO) or VX-809 (1 μM). In the last 3 h, cells also received spautin-1 (10 μM) or vehicle. Data in the graph are reported as quenching rate (QR) of HS-YFP fluorescence (n = 14–23 independent experiments; *** $p < 0.001$). **(B)** Immunoblot analysis of F508del-CFTR expression. The image shows that both band C and band B, particularly in VX-809 treated cells, are decreased by spautin-1 (10 μM, 3 h). The bar graphs show the densitometric analysis of band C or band C plus band B, normalized for GAPDH (n = 3 independent experiments; * $p < 0.05$). **(C)** Time-course of spautin-1 effect. Bars report the normalized QR of HS-YFP fluorescence in cells treated with VX-809 for 24 h and then with spautin-1 (10 μM) for the indicated time (n = 3 independent experiments; * $p < 0.05$; ** $p < 0.01$).

plus/minus spautin-1. In the presence of CHX and VX-809, we noted a strong reduction in both band C and band B levels (**Figure 3A**). However, the immature form was more markedly affected. It is interesting to note that the smear of F508del-CFTR signal, evident in cells treated with VX-809 alone, disappeared in CHX-treated cells. We interpret such results as an effect of rapid F508del-CFTR degradation (despite the presence of the corrector) that is not compensated by novel protein synthesis. Importantly, in the presence of CHX, spautin-1 was able to further decrease F508del-CFTR expression (**Figure 3A**).

We also investigated the effect of spautin-1 on F508del-CFTR ubiquitination (**Figure 3B**). After immunoprecipitation of F508del-CFTR, ubiquitin levels were assessed by immunoblot. Treatment with the proteasome inhibitor MG-132 increased the levels of ubiquitinated F508del-CFTR, also in cells corrected with VX-809. The lysosome inhibitor bafilomycin A1 was instead ineffective. Surprisingly, spautin-1 decreased the ubiquitin signal despite the presence of MG-132 or both inhibitors together (**Figure 3B**). This finding suggests that the F508del-CFTR disappearance elicited by spautin-1 may still occur independently of proteasome and lysosome.

The effect of spautin-1 was also checked on other cell types and with other assays. We studied FRT cells with expression of F508del-CFTR (**Figure 4A**). Such cells form tight epithelia when seeded on porous membranes (Snapwell supports). Therefore, the function of F508del-CFTR in the plasma membrane can be simply evaluated by measuring transepithelial electrical resistance (TEER), which is then converted, for convenience, to transepithelial electrical conductance, TEEC (Xue et al., 2014). Indeed, a rescue of F508del-CFTR results in higher number of chloride-conducting channels and therefore increased TEEC. It should be noted that this method measures both membranes, apical and basolateral, as two electrical resistances in series. Therefore, the detection of a drop or increase in resistance, reflecting activation or inhibition of CFTR respectively, does not distinguish whether this occurs on one or the other membrane. In this respect, it is known that CFTR traffics to both membranes in FRT cell (Sheppard et al., 1994). Therefore, TEEC changes are a reasonably good indicator of CFTR function in the plasma membrane (Xue et al., 2014).

For TEEC measurements, FRT cells were incubated for 24 h with and without VX-809 to rescue F508del-CFTR. In the last 3 h, cells were treated with or without spautin-1. At the time of the experiment, TEEC was measured under resting conditions, after maximal stimulation of F508del-CFTR with forskolin (20 μM) plus genistein (50 μM), and finally after block with PPQ-102 (30 μM), a CFTR inhibitor. **Supplementary Figure 3** precisely describes the procedure. F508del-CFTR function was reported as ΔTEEC, i.e., the difference between TEEC measured with forskolin plus genistein and TEEC measured after PPQ-102

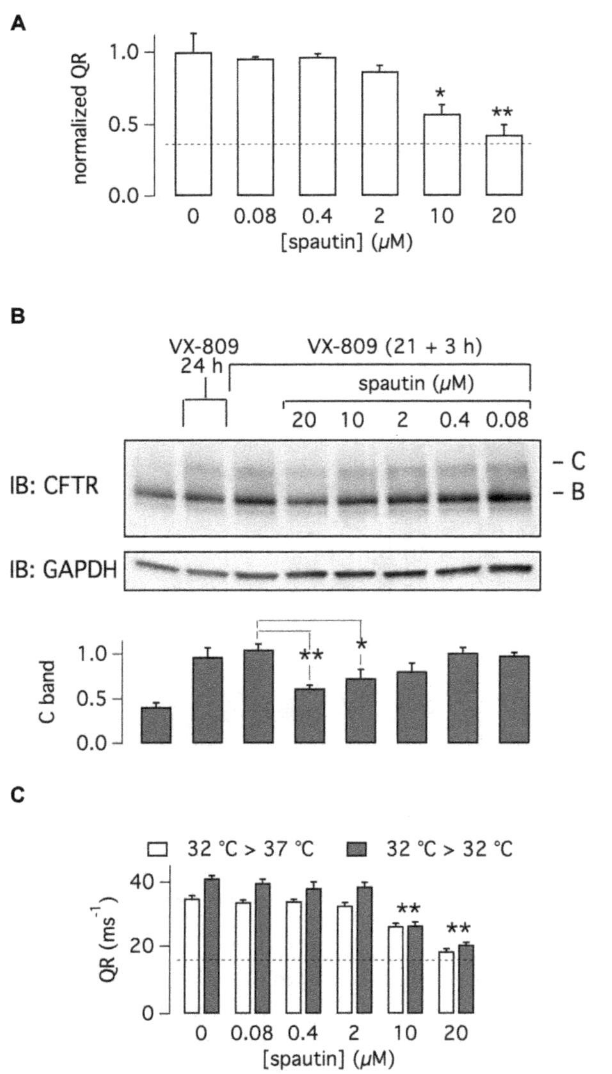

FIGURE 2 | Characterization of spautin-1 effect. **(A)** Dose-response of spautin-1. The graph reports the normalized QR of HS-YFP in CFBE41o- cells treated with VX-809 (1 μM) and then, in the last 3 h, with vehicle or spautin-1 at the indicated concentrations (n = 5 independent experiments; *$p < 0.05$; **$p < 0.01$). The dashed line indicates the level of F508del-CFTR activity in uncorrected cells (no VX-809). **(B)** Immunoblot analysis of F508del-CFTR expression (representative image and densitometric analysis of band C; n = 3 independent experiments). CFBE41o- cells were treated with the indicated conditions (*$p < 0.05$; **$p < 0.01$). **(C)** F508del-CFTR activity (QR) in CFBE41o- cells incubated at 32°C. In the last 3 h, cells were kept at 32°C or shifted to 37°C and treated with vehicle or the indicated concentrations of spautin-1 (n = 3 independent experiments; **$p < 0.01$ vs. vehicle).

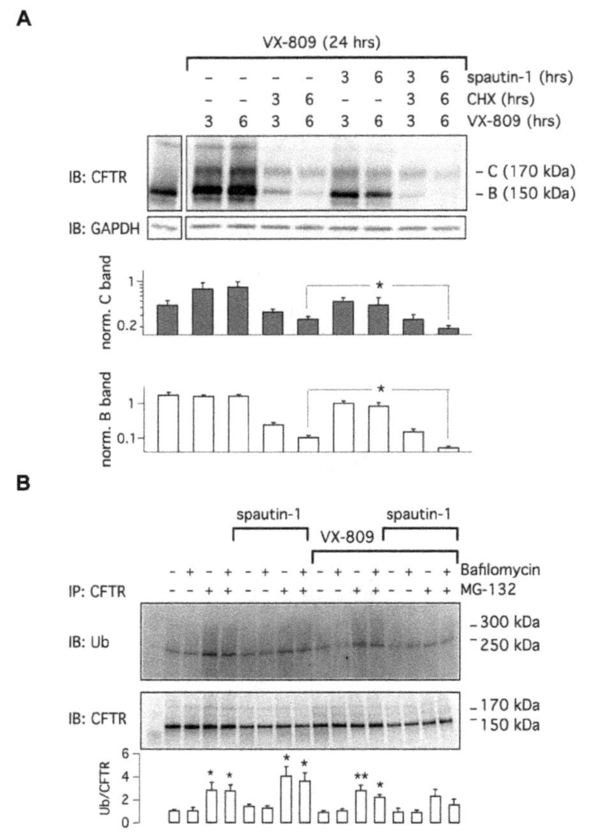

FIGURE 3 | Analysis of spautin-1 mechanism of action. **(A)** Spautin-1 in the presence of protein synthesis block. The image shows a representative western blot experiment done on lysates of CFBE41o- cells treated with VX-809 (1 μM) for 24 h and, in the last 3 or 6 h, with CHX (150 μg/ml), with spautin-1 (20 μM), or with both compounds together. To apply the different conditions, the entire medium was replaced at 3 or 6 h with fresh medium containing the required compounds, including VX-809. Therefore, the times indicate for VX-809 (3 and 6 h) simply indicate the time of medium replacement (the total time of VX-809 treatment was kept at 24 h). The pattern of lysates from cells treated with vehicle alone (no corrector) for 24 h is also shown (first separate lane on the left). Bar graphs show densitometry of bands C and B, normalized for GAPDH intensity, from three independent experiments. Spautin-1 caused a significant downregulation of F508del-CFTR signal in CHX-treated cells (*$p < 0.05$). **(B)** Evaluation of spautin-1 on ubiquitinated F508del-CFTR. The image shows immunodetection of CFTR and ubiquitin in cell lysates after immunoprecipitation using an anti-CFTR antibody. Where indicated, cells where treated with VX-809 (1 μM) for 24 h and, in the last 3 h, with MG-132 (10 μM), bafilomycin A1 (100 nM), and/or spautin-1 (20 μM). The image is representative of three similar experiments. The bar graph shows the ratio of ubiquitin to CFTR signals (n = 3 separate experiments; *$p < 0.05$; **$p < 0.01$ vs. corresponding condition without MG-132 and bafilomycin).

addition. Treatment with VX-809 increased ΔTEEC by more than three-fold, reflecting F508del-CFTR rescue (**Figure 4A**). Spautin-1 decreased the effect of VX-809 by nearly 75 and 95% at 10 and 20 μM, respectively (**Figure 4A**).

Effect on spautin-1 in FRT cells was also assessed using the patch-clamp technique in the whole-cell configuration (**Figure 4B**, top part). FRT cells expressing F508del-CFTR were treated with VX-809 (1 μM) for 24 h. During whole-cell patch-clamp recordings, F508del-CFTR was activated with forskolin (20 μM) plus genistein (50 μM). We monitored membrane currents for 15 min to check that they were stable. Then, we added spautin-1 (20 μM) by extracellular perfusion. We observed a progressive decline in F508del-CFTR function that reached a stable level (nearly 30% of original value) in 30–40 min (**Figure 4B**). This decline was not observed in experiments in which membrane currents were monitored for a comparable time

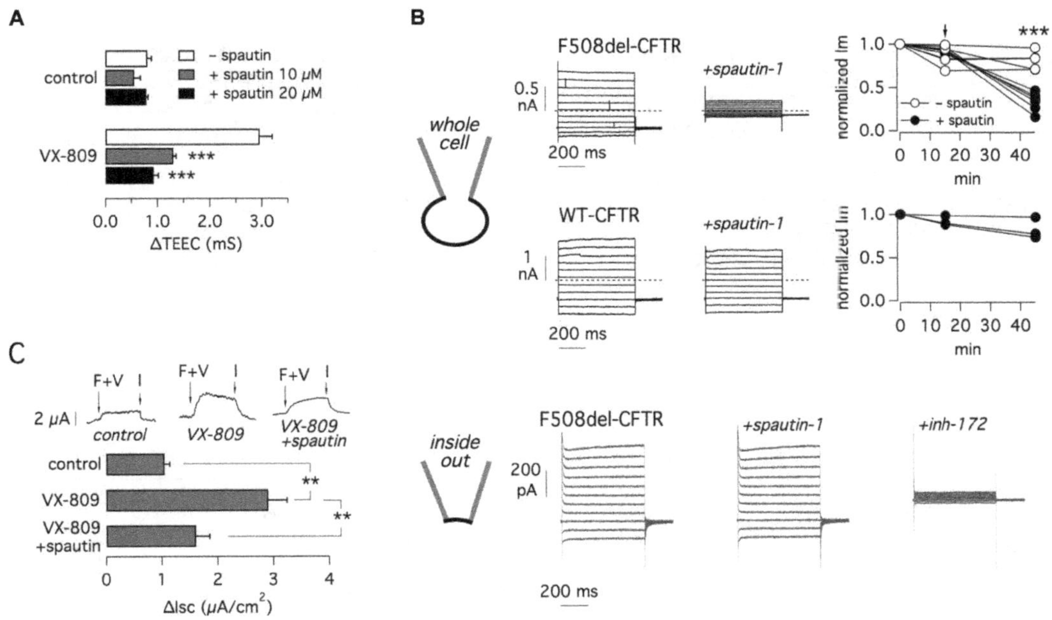

FIGURE 4 | Electrophysiological evaluation of F508del-CFTR inhibition by spautin-1. **(A)** TEEC measurement in FRT cells expressing F508del-CFTR. Cells were treated with or without VX-809 (1 μM) and, in the last 3 h, with spautin-1 (10 or 20 μM) or vehicle. The graph reports the ΔTEEC value, i.e., the difference between TEEC after maximal stimulation with forskolin plus genistein and TEEC after block with PPQ-102 (see text and **Supplementary Figure 3** for further details). Data are from four independent experiments (***$p < 0.001$). **(B)** Results from patch-clamp experiments. The top part shows data obtained in the whole-cell configuration on FRT cells expressing F508del or wild type CFTR (representative traces and graphs reporting the normalized current measured at +100 mV). Cells expressing mutant CFTR were previously treated for 24 h with VX-809 (1 μM). During experiments, cells were acutely stimulated with forskolin (20 μM) plus genistein (50 μM). After full stimulation of mutant or wild type CFTR, the currents were measured for 15 min to check that the activity was stable. Then spautin-1 (20 μM) was added to the extracellular solution and the currents were measured for further 30–40 min. Spautin-1 elicited a significant decrease in membrane currents in F508del-CFTR but not in wild type CFTR cells. The graphs show the currents measured at the three relevant time points. Arrow shows the time of spautin-1 addition. Spautin-1 caused a significant decrease in F508del-CFTR currents (***$p < 0.001$). The bottom part of panel B shows representative currents obtained in the inside-out configuration on FRT cells expressing F508del-CFTR. Currents were significantly inhibited by $CFTR_{inh}$-172 (10 μM) but not by spautin-1 (data are representative of three similar experiments). **(C)** Effect of spautin-1 (20 μM) on human bronchial epithelial cells from a F508del-CFTR patient. Representative traces show short-circuit recordings from epithelia treated with/without VX-809 (1 μM) for 24 h. Where indicated, spautin-1 was added in the last 3 h. During recordings, F508del-CFTR was activated with 20 μM forskolin plus 1 μM VX-770 (F+V) and then blocked with 10 μM $CFTR_{inh}$-172 (I). The graph reports the amplitude of the current drop elicited by the CFTR inhibitor ($n = 4$ separate experiments per condition; **$p < 0.01$).

in the absence of spautin-1 (**Figure 4B**). Addition of $CFTR_{inh}$-172 (10 μM), another specific inhibitor of CFTR channel, strongly blocked the residual current (not shown). We also tested spautin-1 on cells expressing wild type CFTR (**Figure 4B**). In agreement with HS-YFP data, spautin-1 was largely ineffective on the normal protein (**Figure 4B**).

To check the dependence of spautin-1 on an intact intracellular environment, we carried out patch-clamp experiments in the inside-out configuration (**Figure 4B**, bottom part). After excision of the membrane patch, F508del-CFTR channels were activated by phosphorylation. Subsequent addition of spautin-1 (20 μM), kept for the duration of the recording (up to 30 min) did not significantly inhibit the current. Membrane currents were 370 ± 79 and 403 ± 113 pA before and after spautin-1 ($n = 3$), respectively. After spautin-1, block by $CFTR_{inh}$-172 demonstrated that the recorded currents were in large part due to CFTR activity (**Figure 4B**, bottom).

Spautin-1 was also tested in primary bronchial epithelial cells from a F508del/F508del patient (**Figure 4C**). F508del-CFTR function was determined with short-circuit current recordings. The ENaC sodium channel was first blocked with amiloride (10 μM) and then F508del-CFTR was stimulated with CPT-cAMP (100 μM) and VX-770 (1 μM). Stimulation resulted in an increase in transepithelial current due to F508del-CFTR function which was subsequently blocked with $CFTR_{inh}$-172 (10 μM). The amplitude of the current blocked by $CFTR_{inh}$-172 indicates the amount of functional F508del-CFTR in the plasma membrane. This value increased from nearly 1 to 2.9 μA/cm^2 after treatment for 24 h with VX-809 (1 μM). Rescue by VX-809 was decreased by 70% in cells treated for 3 h with 10 μM spautin-1 (**Figure 4C**).

To elucidate the mechanism of action of spautin-1, we separately silenced USP10 and USP13, the possible targets of this small molecule. We transfected CFBE41o- cells with three different DsiRNAs against USP13 or control DsiRNA. Cells were then treated with VX-809. Two of the anti-USP13 molecules caused a significant decrease in anion transport (**Figure 5A**). In particular, USP13A DsiRNA decreased the corrector-dependent fraction of F508del-CFTR function by ~50%. Importantly, the functional effect on mutant CFTR correlated with the extent

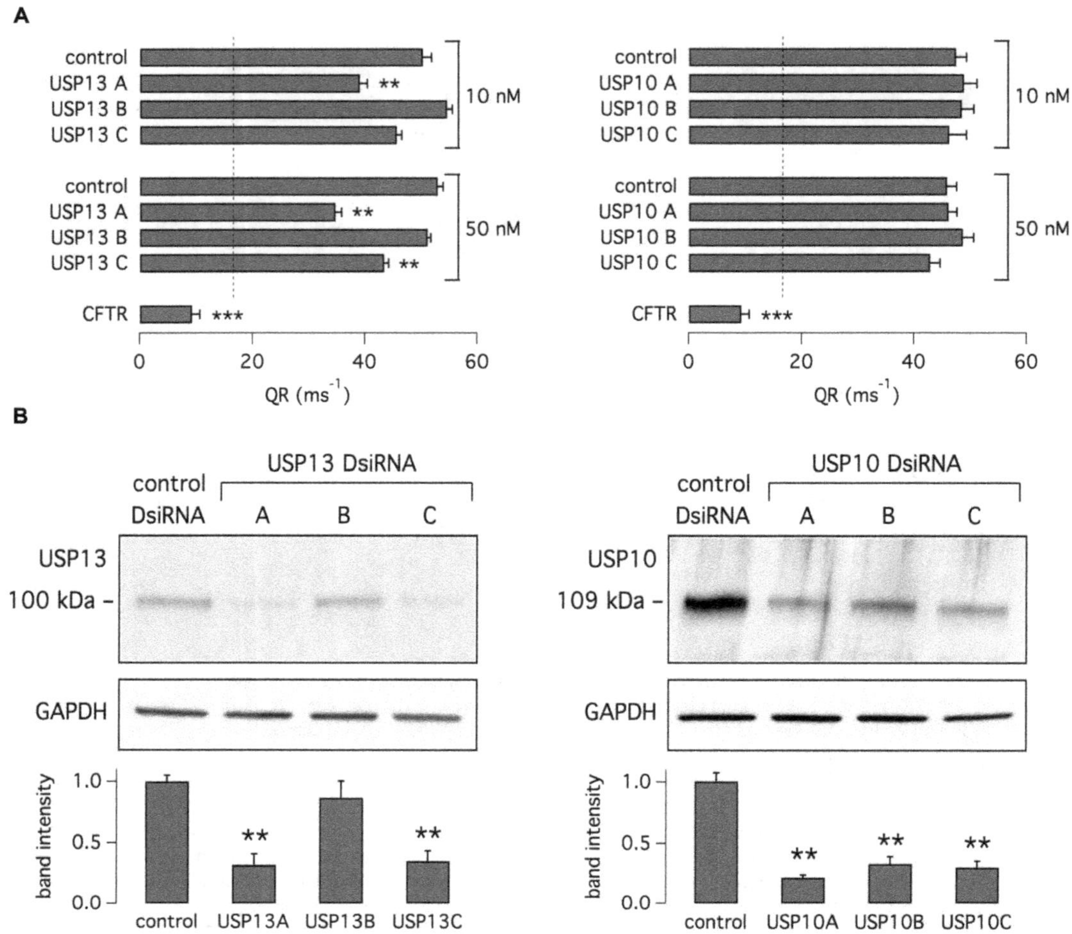

FIGURE 5 | Analysis of USP13 and USP10 relationship with F508del-CFTR expression and function. **(A)** Evaluation of F508del-CFTR activity in CFBE41o- cells treated with VX-809 (1 μM). Data were obtained with the HS-YFP assay after transfection of cells with DsiRNAs (10 or 50 nM) against USP13, USP10, or CFTR. Non-silencing DsiRNA was also used as control. Dashed line reports the value of activity in cells without VX-809 treatment. Silencing of USP13 but not of USP10 significantly decreased F508del-CFTR function. Silencing of CFTR also caused a marked decrease in activity (n = 4–7 independent experiments; $^{**}p < 0.01$; $^{***}p < 0.001$). **(B)** Immunoblot analysis of USP13 and USP10 expression in cells transfected with indicated DsiRNAs (50 nM). Bar graphs report densitometric analysis of USP13 and USP10 bands normalized for GAPDH (n = 3 separate experiments; $^{**}p < 0.01$ vs. control).

of USP13 protein knockdown as revealed by western blot experiments (**Figure 5B**). We also transfected CFBE41o- cells with DsiRNAs against USP10. Unexpectedly, given that USP10 has been shown to control CFTR processing (Bomberger et al., 2009), USP10 knockdown (confirmed by western blot) did not affect F508del-CFTR function (**Figures 5A,B**). As a control, cells were also treated with siRNAs against CFTR. Anion transport was reduced by more than 80% following CFTR knockdown (**Figure 5A**).

The possible role of USP13 and USP10 was also investigated by transfection in CFBE41o- cells. For this purpose, we used plasmids coding for USP13 and USP10 tagged with the mCherry red fluorescent protein. Therefore, the HS-YFP assay was carried out with a microscope and fluorescence quenching, reflecting F508del-CFTR activity, was analyzed in mCherry-positive cells. Cells were treated with VX-809 or vehicle alone. Importantly, overexpression of USP13 did not rescue F508del-CFTR by itself but significantly amplified the effect of VX-809 (**Figure 6A**). In contrast, overexpression of USP10 was ineffective (**Figure 6A**). Importantly, the effect of USP13 overexpression on F508del-CFTR function was nearly abolished by spautin-1 (**Figure 6B**).

The relationship between F508del-CFTR and USP13 was further investigated by analyzing their subcellular localization with immunofluorescence. Endogenous USP13 appeared to be expressed in nucleus and cytosol (**Figure 7A**), in agreement with previous studies (Zhang et al., 2013; Li et al., 2017). Interestingly, cytosolic USP13 showed significant co-localization with F508del-CFTR. In particular, in cells treated with VX-809, regions of the cell periphery showing F508del-CFTR expression also showed staining for USP13 (**Figure 7A**, arrows). We also noticed peripheral regions with USP13 and no F508del-CFTR (**Figure 7A**, arrowheads) but not the opposite situation, thus suggesting that mutant CFTR at the plasma membrane or close compartments is always accompanied by USP13. The dot plots in **Figure 7B** show that peripheral colocalization of USP13

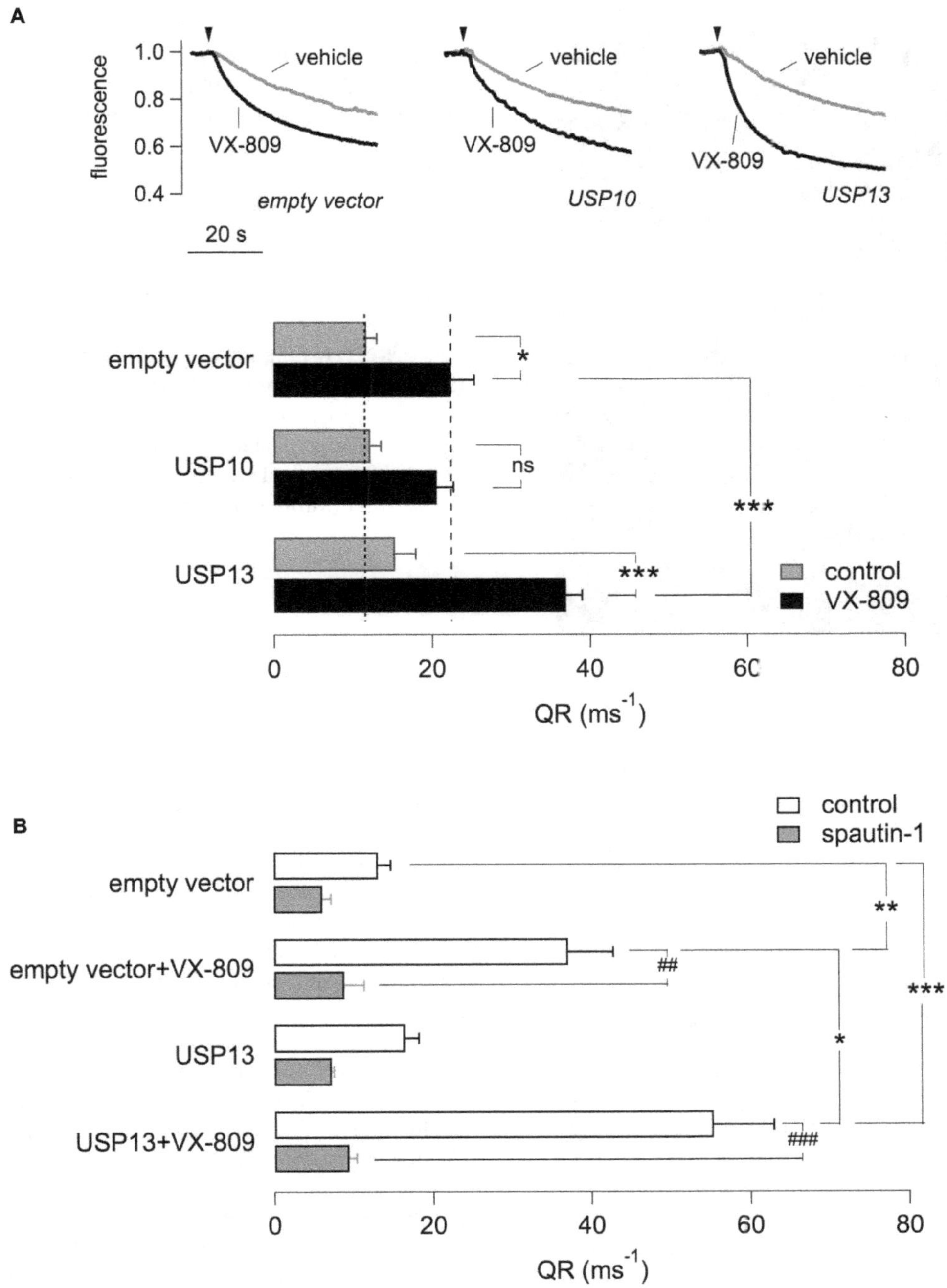

FIGURE 6 | Effect of USP13 or USP10 overexpression. **(A)** Functional analysis in CFBE41o- transiently transfected with plasmids expressing USP13/USP10 or with a control plasmid. Cells also stably expressed F508del-CFTR and the HS-YFP. After transfection, cells were treated with VX-809 (1 μM) or with vehicle. The figure shows representative traces (top) and summary of QR for the different conditions (n = 4 independent experiments; *$p < 0.05$; ***$p < 0.001$). **(B)** Effect of spautin-1 on cells transfected with USP13 and treated with/without VX-809. Data obtained with the HS-YFP assay. Spautin-1 markedly abolishes F508del-CFTR function in USP13-transfected cells (n = 4–7 independent experiments; *$p < 0.05$; ##/**$p < 0.01$; ###/***$p < 0.001$).

and F508del-CFTR is significantly increased following VX-809 treatment (**Figure 7B**).

It has been reported that spautin-1 is an autophagy inhibitor through the ubiquitin-dependent degradation of beclin-1, a subunit of the Vps34 PI3K complex (Liu et al., 2011). On the other hand, F508del-CFTR trafficking was connected to autophagy (Luciani et al., 2010). Therefore, to further investigate the mechanism of action of spautin-1 on F508del-CFTR, we also used SAR-405, another recently identified autophagy inhibitor (Ronan et al., 2014). While spautin-1 causes degradation of Vps34 complex, SAR-405 directly inhibits the catalytic activity of Vps34. Importantly, SAR-405, tested at concentrations between 10 nM

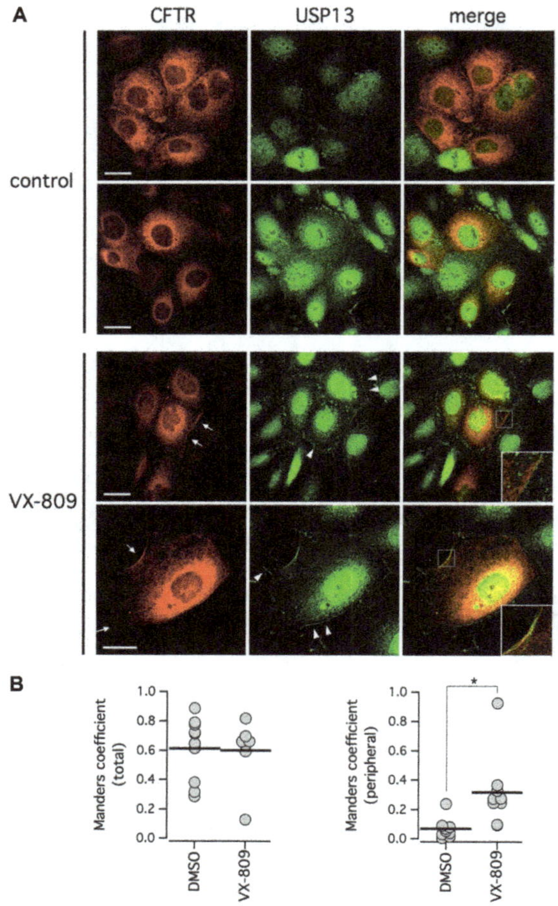

FIGURE 7 | Subcellular localization of F508del-CFTR and endogenous USP13. **(A)** Confocal microscope images taken from CFBE41o- cells stained with antibodies against CFTR and USP13. Cells were treated with VX-809 (1 μM) or vehicle. Arrows indicate examples of cells with peripheral co-localization of F508del-CFTR and USP13. Arrowheads show peripheral regions with USP13 alone. Insets depict magnified cell areas of cell periphery with colocalization of USP13 and F508del-CFTR. **(B)** Colocalization analysis of F508del-CFTR and USP13 in cells treated with vehicle alone (DMSO) or with VX-809. Analysis was done on total cell area (left) or on cell periphery (right; $^{*}p < 0.05$).

and 10 μM did not affect the function of F508del-CFTR rescued by VX-809 (**Figure 8A**). In agreement with functional data, the expression of F508del-CFTR protein was also not affected by SAR-405 in contrast to spautin-1 (**Figure 8B**). To further explore the link between autophagy and F508del-CFTR, we used torin-1 as an autophagy inducer (Thoreen et al., 2009). Torin-1, tested at multiple concentrations, did not alter F508del-CFTR rescue (**Figure 9A**) despite being effective in increasing the expression of LC3-II, a marker of autophagy (**Figure 9B**). In separate experiments, we confirmed that spautin-1 and SAR-405, as autophagy inhibitors, antagonize the effect of torin-1 on LC3-II (**Figure 9C**).

To check the effect of autophagy modulators, we also used an assay based on monodansylcadaverine (MDC). This fluorescent probe is a specific marker for autolysosomes (Biederbick et al., 1995). Indeed, MDC is accumulated inside autophagosomes. After autophagosomes fusion with lysosomes, MDC fluorescence increases due to the acidic environment (Biederbick et al., 1995; Munafó and Colombo, 2001). As shown by representative images (**Figure 10A**) and bar graphs (**Figure 10B**), torin-1 markedly increases the signal of MDC, in particular the total number and brightness of spots. This effect is significantly inhibited by spautin-1, SAR405, and wortmannin, another autophagy inhibitor acting on the Vps34 complex. Similarly to SAR405, and in contrast to spautin-1, wortmannin did not affect F508del-CFTR function (**Supplementary Figure 4A**). Also, the silencing of beclin 1, confirmed at the protein level, did not reduce F508del-CFTR function and expression in VX-809 treated cells (**Supplementary Figures 4B–D**).

In a further attempt to elucidate spautin-1 mechanism of action, we investigated the effect of dynasore, an endocytosis inhibitor. Treatment with this compound did not block the effect of spautin-1 (**Supplementary Figure 5**).

DISCUSSION

Our study reveals novel mechanisms that affect the therapeutic correction of mutant CFTR. There is a strong interest in the development of novel strategies to maximize the rescue of CFTR with the F508del mutation. This is particularly important for CF patients with a single copy of the mutation. Indeed, the drug available for clinical use, VX-809, is only modestly effective on F508del homozygotes (in combination with the potentiator VX-770) and ineffective on individuals with a single F508del allele (Rowe et al., 2017). As shown previously, F508del-CFTR, even in the presence of VX-809 or other correctors, is still intrinsically unstable and therefore recognized by quality control mechanisms and eliminated (He et al., 2013). Enhanced rescue could be obtained by combining VX-809 (or another similarly active compound) with another small molecule acting on a second site in the F508del-CFTR protein (Farinha et al., 2013; Okiyoneda et al., 2013). Alternatively, pharmacological modulation of another protein that is responsible for mutant CFTR elimination could improve the efficacy of correctors.

In the present study, we have investigated spautin-1 as a possible probe to perturb F508del-CFTR rescue. There were two reasons for testing this small molecule. First, spautin-1 is an inhibitor of USP10 (Liu et al., 2011), a deubiquitinating enzyme that is important for CFTR homeostasis (Bomberger et al., 2009). Second, spautin-1, by acting on USP10 and USP13, is also an inhibitor of autophagy (Liu et al., 2011), a cell process that has been proposed to be crucial for F508del-CFTR fate and CF pathogenesis (Luciani et al., 2010).

Short-term pre-incubation of cells with spautin-1 significantly decreased the activity of F508del-CFTR in cells treated with VX-809 or low temperature. An acute effect of spautin-1 was also observed during electrophysiological recordings of rescued F508del-CFTR activity. Importantly, we found no inhibitory effect of spautin-1 in cells expressing wild type CFTR. This finding indicates that spautin-1 is not acting as a direct blocker of CFTR or by interfering with the process of CFTR channel

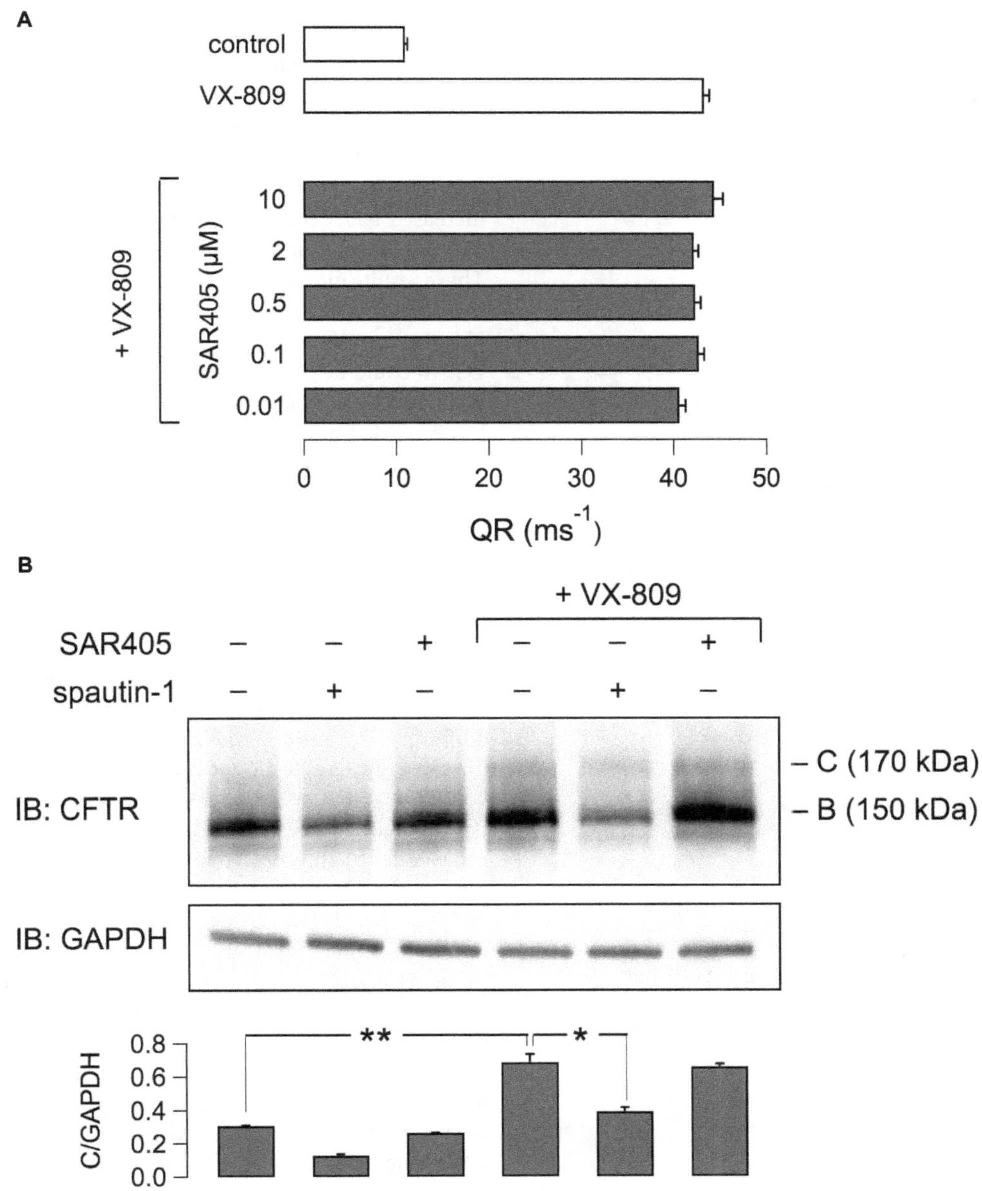

FIGURE 8 | Evaluation of SAR405 on F508del-CFTR expression and function. **(A)** F508del-CFTR activity determined as QR with the HS-YFP assay. CFBE41o- cells expressing F508del-CFTR were treated with VX-809 (1 µM) and various concentrations of SAR405 or vehicle. **(B)** Immunoblot analysis of F508del-CFTR expression in cells treated (3 h) with spautin-1 or SAR405 in the presence or absence of VX-809 (1 µM, 24 h). Bar graph shows normalized densitometric analysis of band C for the different conditions (*n* = 3 independent experiments; **p* < 0.05; ***p* < 0.01).

opening but with a mechanism that is linked with the intrinsic instability of F508del-CFTR. We also found that spautin-1 is effective in different cell types, including primary CF bronchial epithelial cells, and using different assays.

We investigated the effect of spautin-1 at the protein level. In agreement with functional data, spautin-1 altered the expression of F508del-CFTR but not of wild type CFTR. In particular, spautin-1 decreased the expression of both mature and immature forms of the mutant protein. This type of effect was also observed when the protein in the plasma membrane was detected by cell surface biotinylation. The presence of partially glycosylated F508del-CFTR (i.e., band B) in the plasma membrane is not surprising since it has been attributed to an unconventional route of protein trafficking that bypasses the Golgi (Gee et al., 2011; Tomati et al., 2015). Therefore, the decrease in F508del-CFTR function caused by spautin-1 could be explained with a decreased expression of both forms of F508del-CFTR in the plasma membrane, either by reduced trafficking to the cell surface and/or accelerated internalization. In this respect, it is particularly interesting to note the results from patch-clamp experiments. In the whole-cell configuration, spautin-1 caused a significant decrease in the activity of F508del-CFTR. This

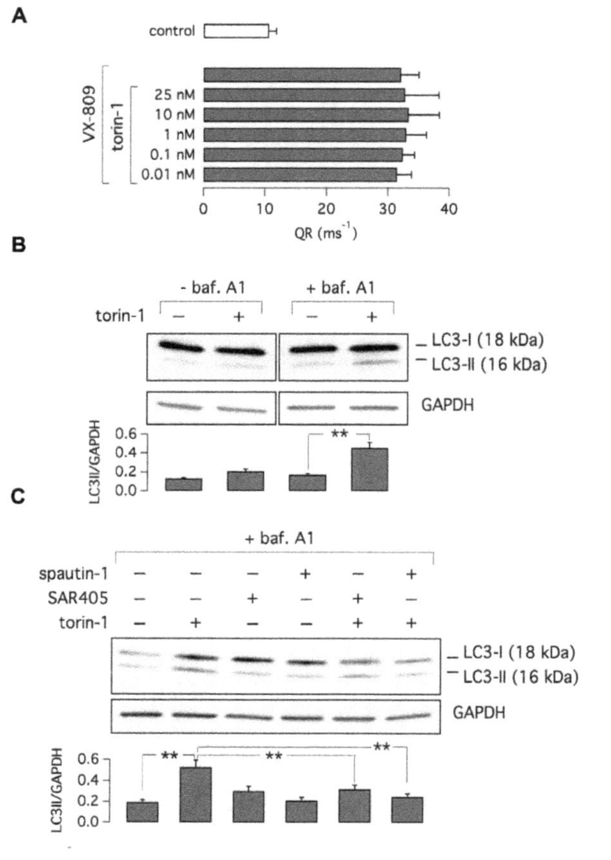

FIGURE 9 | Evaluation of torin-1 as an autophagy inducer. **(A)** Test of different torin-1 concentrations on F508del-CFTR function. Cells were treated with VX-809 (1 μM) or vehicle (n = 3 separate experiments). **(B)** Analysis of LC3-I and LC3-II expression in cells treated with/without torin-1, to induce autophagy, and bafilomycin A1, to block lysosome-dependent degradation. **(C)** Analysis of LC3-I and LC3-II expression in cells treated with torin-1 (or vehicle) in presence/absence of SAR405 or spautin-1. Bar graphs in **(B,C)** show normalized densitometry analysis of LC3-II (n = 3 separate experiments; ** $p < 0.01$).

effect was not detected in inside-out patch recordings from the same cell type. Such results indicate that inhibition by spautin-1 requires an intracellular machinery that is lost upon membrane patch excision. The fast effect induced by spautin-1, with a decrease in function starting a few minutes from compound addition, is intriguing. It is possible that this initial effect is due to rapid internalization of F508del-CFTR protein. However, we could not block the effect of spautin-1 with dynasore. Therefore, if internalization is involved, it should occur through a mechanism insensitive to dynasore. Another possibility is that the initial decrease in function is caused by F508del-CFTR channel inactivation by ubiquitination at the plasma membrane.

We investigated the involvement of USP10 and USP13 in the effect of spautin-1 on mutant CFTR. We silenced USP10 and USP13 expression by transfection with specific DsiRNAs of cells that were also treated with VX-809. Surprisingly, USP10 knockdown did not result in alteration of F508del-CFTR activity. This seems to be in contrast with previous studies in which function of USP10 was found to be important in CFTR trafficking at the cell periphery (Bomberger et al., 2009). However, those studies were done on cells expressing wild type CFTR. Therefore, it is possible that USP10 is much less involved in mutant CFTR processing. Instead, we found that silencing of USP13 inhibited F508del-CFTR function. In agreement with RNAi transfection experiments, overexpression of USP13, but not of USP10, increased F508del-CFTR function above the level achieved with VX-809 incubation and this effect was blocked by spautin-1. These results indicate that USP13 is an important deubiquitinase that controls the extent of F508del-CFTR expression in the plasma membrane. Consequently, inhibition of endogenous USP13 could be the mechanism through which spautin-1 affects F508del-CFTR function and processing. It should be emphasized, however, that most small molecules are rarely absolutely specific for a single target. Therefore, we cannot exclude that spautin-1 also acts on another deubiquitinase. This issue will require further studies.

By inhibiting a deubiquitinase, spautin-1 treatment should result in increased F508del-CFTR ubiquitination, an effect that should lead to enhanced degradation. However, combined inhibition with MG-132 and bafilomycin did not prevent spautin-1 effect. In particular, MG-132 alone was sufficient to markedly enhance ubiquitination of F508del-CFTR. However, addition of spautin-1 did not further enhance ubiquitination but actually had the opposite effect. This unexpected finding could suggest that F508del-CFTR, similarly to other proteins, is also eliminated through a proteasome- and lysosome-independent pathway (Donoso et al., 2005; Mbonye et al., 2008; Lee et al., 2014). Alternatively, it should be noted that pro-collagen was found to be degraded by the lysosome with a non-conventional mechanism insensitive to bafilomycin (Omari et al., 2018). This issue needs further investigation to clarify the molecular mechanisms involved in this type of protein degradation.

We also asked whether spautin-1 affects F508del-CFTR by inhibiting autophagy. In a recently published paper, which investigated the molecular mechanisms of unconventional CFTR trafficking, spautin-1 was found to decrease F508del-CFTR in the plasma membrane (Noh et al., 2018). This effect was interpreted as an evidence of the involvement of autophagy machinery in CFTR trafficking. According to this model, autophagosomes could be used, under particular conditions, to transport immature CFTR to the plasma membrane (Noh et al., 2018). In our study, we tested two other small molecules, torin-1 (Thoreen et al., 2009) and SAR405 (Ronan et al., 2014), which act respectively as an activator and an inhibitor of autophagy. Importantly, neither SAR405 and wortmannin, as autophagy inhibitors, nor torin-1, as autophagy activator, affected F508del-CFTR in a positive or negative way. In particular, SAR405 and wortmannin act at the same early stage of autophagic process as spautin-1 (Vps34 complex). Therefore, we conclude that the effect of spautin-1 on F508del-CFTR is independent of autophagic machinery. In general, our results also indicate that pharmacological modulation of autophagy does not affect *per se* the function/trafficking of F508del-CFTR nor its rescue by VX-809.

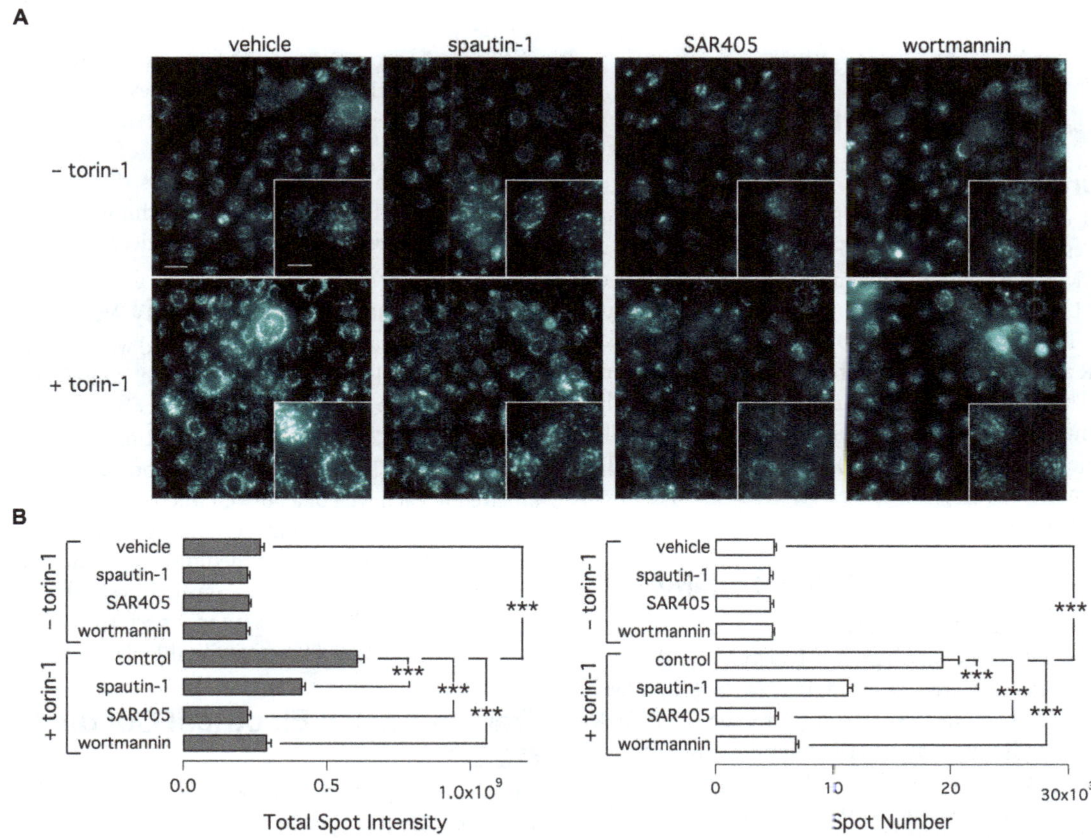

FIGURE 10 | Determination of autophagy with MDC. **(A)** Representative microscopy images of CFBE41o- cells exposed to indicated treatments (torin-1, spautin-1, SAR405). Cells were stained with MDC. **(B)** Data (total spot intensity, left, and spot numer, right) obtained from MDC-stained cells ($n = 3$ separate experiments; $^{***}p < 0.001$).

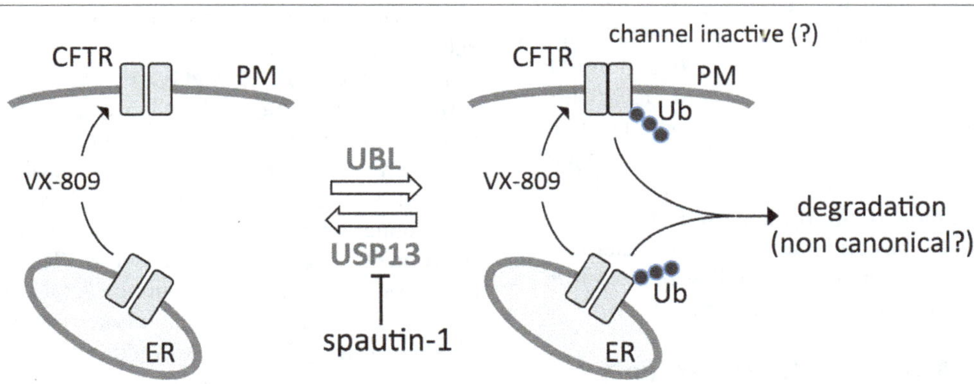

FIGURE 11 | Postulated model for spautin-1 mechanism of action. F508del-CFTR is ubiquitinated at the ER and plasma membrane by ubiquitin ligases. At the plasma membrane, ubiquitination may cause internalization and, possibly, as an initial effect, also channel inactivation. Mutant CFTR is partially protected from degradation by the activity of USP13. Inhibition of USP13 with spautin-1 blocks deubiquitination thus increasing the fraction of F508del-CFTR undergoing elimination.

Summarizing, our results reveal spautin-1 as an interesting probe that works as an "anti-corrector." In the presence of this compound, the effect of VX-809 and of another rescue maneuver, low temperature incubation, is significantly diminished. A possible explanation is that spautin-1 blocks a protective mechanism, possibly deubiquitination by USP13, which shields F508del-CFTR from degradation through a still unknown process (**Figure 11**). Therefore, spautin-1 can be used to reveal the underlying degradation mechanisms that limit F508del-CFTR rescue. In future studies, elucidation of spautin-1 mechanism of action may lead to the identification of novel therapeutic targets to improve rescue of F508del-CFTR and to the discovery of novel biological pathways involved in protein degradation.

MATERIALS AND METHODS

Cell Culture Conditions

The bronchial epithelial cell line CFBE41o- with and without stable co-expression of F508del-CFTR or wild type CFTR was cultured with MEM medium supplemented with 10% fetal calf serum, 2 mM L-glutamine, 100 U/ml penicillin, and 100 μg/ml streptomycin. The generation of CFBE41o- cells co-expressing F508del-CFTR and the HS-YFP was previously described (Sondo et al., 2011). The FRT cells expressing F508del-CFTR and HS-YFP (Pedemonte et al., 2010) were cultured in Coon's modified Ham's F-12 medium (Sigma-Aldrich) supplemented with 10% fetal calf serum, 2 mM L-glutamine, 100 U/ml penicillin, and 100 μg/ml streptomycin.

Fluorescence Assay for CFTR Activity (Microplate Reader Version)

CFBE41o- cells with co-expression of F508del-CFTR or wt-CFTR and the HS-YFP were treated for 24 h with DMSO or VX-809 1 μM. In some experiments, rescue of F508del-CFTR was obtained by incubation at low temperature for 24 h. Where needed, spautin-1 was added at different concentrations in the last 3 h of incubation. Shorter times of incubation with spautin-1 were also tested. After treatments, cells were washed with PBS (containing: 137 mM NaCl, 2.7 mM KCl, 8.1 mM Na_2HPO_4, 1.5 mM KH_2PO_4, 1 mM $CaCl_2$, 0.5 mM $MgCl_2$) and then stimulated for 30 min with forskolin (20 μM) and genistein (50 μM). Cells were then transferred to a microplate reader (FLUOstar Galaxy; BMG Labtech) for CFTR activity determination. The plate reader was equipped with high-quality excitation (HQ500/20X: 500 ± 10nm) and emission (HQ535/30M: 535 ± 15 nm) filters for YFP (Chroma Technology). Each assay consisted of a continuous 14 s fluorescence reading including 2 s before and 12 s after injection of an iodide-containing solution (PBS with Cl^- replaced by I^-; final I^- concentration 100 mM). Data were normalized to the initial background-subtracted fluorescence. To determine I^- influx rate, the last 11 s of data for each well were fitted with an exponential function to extrapolate initial slope (dF/dt).

Fluorescence Assay for CFTR Activity (Microscope Version)

CFBE41o- cells with stable co-expression of F508del-CFTR and HS-YFP, were transfected 6 h after plating with plasmids coding for USP13 or USP10 tagged with the mCherry red fluorescence protein (Origene). The day after, the cells were treated with DMSO or VX-809 (1 μM) for 24 h and, where needed, spautin-1 (20 μM) was added in the last 3 h of incubation. At the time of the assay, cells were stimulated with forskolin (20 μM) and genistein (50 μM) for 30 min and transferred to a fluorescence microscope (IX50 Olympus) equipped with a 20× objective and excitation/emission optical filters for YFP and mCherry. Images of HS-YFP fluorescence were taken with a digital camera (CoolSNAP; Photometrics) at four frames per second for a total of 40 s. At 5 s from beginning of acquisition, the high I^- solution was added in the well (same volumes and concentrations as indicated for the plate reader assay). A single image of mCherry-expressing cells was taken at the end of assay. For analysis of results, the MetaMorph software was used to determine the time-course of HS-YFP fluorescence quenching in mCherry-positive cells. For each well, 10 cells were considered for analysis.

Gene Silencing With DsiRNAs

CFBE41o- cells were reverse transfected with DsiRNAs (Origene) at the time of plating. For this purpose, complexes were formed by combining DsiRNAs at the desired concentration with 0.25 μl Lipofectamine 2000 in 50 μl of Optimem synthetic medium for each well. The DsiRNA-lipofection agent complexes were pipetted in each well of a 96-well microplate together with 100 μl of MEM without antibiotics containing 50,000 cells. After 24 h of cell incubation at 37°C, the medium was removed and replaced with fresh MEM plus serum and antibiotics. After additional 24 h, the functional YFP-based assay was performed to determine the extent of F508del-CFTR activity in the plasma membrane.

Transepithelial Electrical Conductance (TEEC)

FRT cells expressing F508del-CFTR were plated on HTS Transwell-24 well permeable supports (Code 3379, Corning Life Sciences) at a density of 200,000 cells/well. After 6 days, cells were incubated for 24 h with vehicle (DMSO) or VX-809 (1 μM) in both basolateral (800 μl) and apical (300 μl) culture medium. Where needed, spautin-1 was included in the last 3 h of treatment. After treatment, the culture medium was removed and replaced on both sides with a saline solution (100 μl apical, 800 μl basolateral) containing (in mM): 130 NaCl, 2.7 KCl, 1.5 KH_2PO_4, 1 $CaCl_2$, 0.5 $MgCl_2$, 10 glucose, 10 Na-Hepes (pH 7.4). The 24-well tray with cells was placed on a block heater (SBH 130D, Stuart) to keep the temperature at 37°C during the entire experiment. After 10 min, the basal TEER across each layer of FRT cells was measured with a STX100C electrode pair connected to an EVOM2 voltohmeter (World Precision Instruments). To stimulate F508del-CFTR, each well received (apical side) 50 μl of saline solution containing 60 μM forskolin and 150 μM genistein (final concentrations: 20 μM forskolin, 50 μM genistein). Forskolin was added to the basolateral medium to obtain the 20 μM concentration. After 10 min, TEER was measured again in each well. To block F508del-CFTR function, the inhibitor PPQ-102 was used at the final concentration of 30 μM. To achieve the desired concentration, 75 μl of the apical solution in each well was replaced with an equal volume of saline solution containing 20 μM forskolin, 50 μM genistein, and 60 μM PPQ-102. After further 10 min, the TEER was measured. All values of TEER were converted to TEEC using the formula TEEC = 1/TEER. The parameter to indicate activity of F508del-CFTR in each well, ΔTEEC was calculated from the difference in TEEC measured after maximal stimulation of F508del-CFTR with forskolin plus genistein and after block with PPQ-102 (see

Supplementary Figure 3). Two particular conditions used in these experiments need to be discussed in detail. These conditions were defined during the setting of this technique. First, we used genistein instead of VX-770 as a potentiator. Indeed, the very high potency and "stickiness" of VX-770 caused problems of contamination and carry over due to adhesion to electrodes. Second, we used PPQ-102, instead of $CFTR_{inh}$-172, to block CFTR, because the former compound is more water soluble. Therefore, it is more adequate for a procedure in which the CFTR inhibitor has to be prepared in a saline solution at three times the final concentration. For $CFTR_{inh}$-172, this would mean 30 μM, which appeared to cause problems of solubility.

Whole-Cell and Inside-Out Patch-Clamp Recordings

Experiments were done on FRT cells stably expressing F508del-CFTR or wild type CFTR. For whole-cell experiments, the extracellular (bath) solution had the following composition: 150 mM NaCl, 1 mM $CaCl_2$, 1 mM $MgCl_2$, 10 mM glucose, 10 mM mannitol, and 10 mM Na-Hepes (pH 7.4). The pipette (intracellular) solution instead contained 120 mM CsCl, 10 mM TEA-Cl, 0.5 mM EGTA, 1 mM $MgCl_2$, 40 mM mannitol, 1 mM ATP, and 10 mM Cs-Hepes (pH 7.2). Acute stimulation was done by perfusion with forskolin (20 μM) plus genistein (50 μM).

For inside-out experiments, the bath solution contained: 150 mM NMDG-Cl, 2 mM $MgCl_2$, 10 mM EGTA, 1 mM MgATP, 10 mM HEPES (pH 7.35). The bath solution also contained 5 μg/ml (125 nM) of protein kinase A catalytic subunit of (PKA, Promega). The pipette was instead filled with: 150 mM NMDG-Cl, 3 mM $CaCl_2$, 2 mM $MgCl_2$, 10 mM HEPES (pH 7.35). After excision of inside-out membrane patches, CFTR Cl^- channels were activated by the activity of the kinase.

During experiments, the membrane capacitance and series resistance were analogically compensated using the circuitry provided by the EPC7 patch-clamp amplifier. The usual protocol for stimulation consisted in 600 ms-long voltage steps from −100 to +100 mV in 20 mV increments starting from a holding potential of −60 mV. The waiting time between steps was 4 s. Membrane currents were filtered at 1 kHz and digitized at 5 kHz with an ITC-16 (InstruTech) AD/DA converter. Data were analyzed using the Igor software (Wavemetrics) supplemented by custom software kindly provided by Dr. Oscar Moran.

Short-Circuit Current Recordings on Human Bronchial Epithelial Cells

Human bronchial epithelial cells obtained from a CF patient (F508del/F508del genotype) were plated on Snapwell inserts (Code 3603, Corning Life Sciences) at a density of 500,000 cells per insert. Cells were cultured for 2 weeks in a differentiating medium whose compositions has been previously described (Scudieri et al., 2012). For the first week, the medium was kept on both apical and basolateral sides of inserts (liquid–liquid condition). For the second week, the apical medium was removed (air-liquid condition, ALC). At the end of second week, cells were treated for 24 h in the basolateral medium with vehicle (DMSO) or VX-809 (1 μM). Where needed, spautin-1 was added in the medium for the last 3 h. After treatment, Snapwell inserts carrying differentiated bronchial epithelia were mounted in a vertical chamber resembling an Ussing system with internal fluid circulation. Both apical and basolateral hemichambers were filled with 5 ml of a Krebs bicarbonate solution containing (in mM): 126 NaCl, 0.38 KH_2PO_4, 2.13 K_2HPO_4, 1 $MgSO_4$, 1 $CaCl_2$, 24 $NaHCO_3$, and 10 glucose. Both sides were continuously bubbled with a gas mixture containing 5% CO_2 − 95% air and the temperature of the solution was kept at 37°C. The transepithelial voltage was short-circuited with a voltage-clamp (DVC-1000, World Precision Instruments) connected to the apical and basolateral chambers via Ag/AgCl electrodes and agar bridges (1 M KCl in 1% agar). The offset between voltage electrodes and the fluid resistance were canceled before experiments. The short-circuit current was recorded with a PowerLab 4/25 (ADInstruments) analogical to digital converter connected to a Macintosh computer. During recordings, cells were sequentially treated with: amiloride (10 μM, apical side) to block Na^+ absorption through ENaC channel; CPT-cAMP (100 μM, apical and basolateral side) plus VX-770 (1 μM) to stimulate F508del-CFTR activity; $CFTR_{inh}$-172 (10 μM, apical side) to inhibit F508del-CFTR. The difference between the current measured with CPT-cAMP plus potentiator and the current remaining after $CFTR_{inh}$-172 activity was taken as the parameter reflecting F508del-CFTR expression in the apical membrane.

Labeling of Autophagic Vacuoles With Monodansylcadaverine (MDC)

CFBE41o- cells stably expressing F508del-CFTR and the HS-YFP were plated (50,000 cells/well) on high quality clear-bottom 96-well black microplates suitable for high-content imaging. After 24 h, cells were treated with test compounds or DMSO (as negative control). After 24 h, cells were washed and incubated with 50 μM MDC (Sigma-Aldrich) in PBS at 37°C for 10 min (Biederbick et al., 1995). After incubation, cells were washed three times with PBS and immediately analyzed. High-content imaging and data analysis were performed using an Opera Phenix (PerkinElmer) high-content screening system. Wells were imaged in confocal mode, using a 40X water-immersion objective with high numerical aperture. MDC signal was laser excited at 405 nm and the emission was collected between 435 and 550 nm.

Data analysis of MDC signal spots was performed using the Harmony software (version 4.5) of the Opera Phenix high-content system. Briefly, for each field of view, the analysis algorithm detected the signal spots, and quantified the total number of spots, single spot intensity, and total spot intensity.

Western Blot

Cells were grown to confluence on 60-mm diameter dishes and lysed in RIPA buffer containing a complete protease inhibitor (Roche). Cell lysates were centrifuged at 12000 rpm at 4°C for 10 min. Supernatant protein concentration was calculated using the BCA assay (Euroclone) following the manufacturer's instructions. Equal amounts of protein (30 μg) were separated onto gradient (4–15% or 4–20% depending on target protein molecular weight) Criterion TGX Precast gels (Bio-Rad Laboratories Inc.), transferred to nitrocellulose membrane with *Trans*-Blot Turbo system (Bio-Rad Laboratories Inc.) and analyzed by Western blotting. Primary antibodies and dilutions were: mouse monoclonal anti-CFTR (596, Cystic Fibrosis Foundation Therapeutics, University of North Carolina, Chapel Hill) 1:5000; mouse monoclonal anti Na^+/K^+-ATPase α1 (cl. C464.6; Millipore) 1:6000; mouse monoclonal anti-GAPDH (cl.6C5; Santa Cruz Biotechnology, Inc.) 1:10000; rabbit polyclonal anti-USP13 (Abcam) 1:1000; rabbit polyclonal anti-USP10 (Abcam) 1:1000; rabbit monoclonal anti-calnexin (Abcam) 1:5000; rabbit polyclonal anti-14-3-3 epsilon (Abcam) 1:1000; rabbit polyclonal anti-LC3B (Sigma, L7543) 1:1000; rabbit polyclonal anti-Beclin-1 (Cell Signaling Technology, 3738) 1:1000. As secondary antibodies, we used anti-rabbit HRP-conjugated antibody (Abcam) diluted 1:5000 and anti-mouse HRP-conjugated secondary antibody (Ab 97023, Abcam) diluted 1:10000. Results were subsequently visualized by chemiluminescence using the SuperSignal West Femto Substrate (Thermo Scientific) and the Molecular Imager ChemiDoc XRS System. Images were analyzed with ImageJ software (National Institutes of Health). Intensity of bands was analyzed as Region-Of-Interest (ROI). The background was subtracted sand intensity was normalized against the GAPDH loading control. Data are presented as mean ± SEM of independent experiments.

Detection of CFTR Ubiquitination

CFBE41o- cells stably expressing F508del-CFTR were grown to confluence on 60-mm diameter dishes, treated for 24 h with VX809 (1 μM) and in the last 3 h with MG132 (10 μM), bafilomicyn A1 (100nM) and/or spautin-1 (20 μM). Then, cells were rinsed twice with ice-cold Ca^{2+}/Mg^{2+}-free PBS and then lysed with IP Lysis Buffer (#87788 Thermo Sci.) containing EDTA-free complete protease inhibitor (Roche), N-ethylmaleimide (5 mM) and MG-132 (20 mM). Nuclei were pelleted by centrifugation at 12000 rpm at 4°C for 20 min. Supernatant protein concentration was calculated using the BCA assay (Euroclone) following the manufacturer's instructions. An aliquot of supernatant corresponding to 500 μg of protein was incubated for 1 h with 2 μg/sample of mouse monoclonal anti-CFTR R24-1 antibody (R&D), rocking at room temperature. Antibody-antigen mixture was precipitated with 25 μl/sample of Pierce Protein A/G Magnetic Beads (Thermo Sci.) for 1 h rocking at RT, following supplier instructions. Immunoprecipitated proteins were eluted from the resin under reducing conditions with 100 μl Laemli Sample Buffer 1X, at RT. Equal amount of IP products (20 μl) were subjected to SDS-PAGE for immunoblotting analysis. Detection of CFTR and ubiquitin was performed using mouse monoclonal anti-CFTR (596, Cystic Fibrosis Foundation Therapeutics, University of North Carolina, Chapel Hill) 1:5000 and anti mouse monoclonal anti-ubiquitin (ub-P4D1, Santa Cruz Biotechnology) 1:1000. As secondary antibody, we used anti mouse-HRP-conjugated secondary antibody (Ab 97023, Abcam).

Cell Surface Biotinylation

CFBE41o- cells were processed as previously described (Tomati et al., 2015). Briefly, cells were seeded on 100 mm dishes and treated with 1 μM VX-809 (or vehicle) for 24 h and with 20 μM spautin-1 (or vehicle) in the last 3 h. At the end of treatments, cells were washed twice with ice-cold PBS and incubated with biotin (0.35 mg/ml in PBS) for 25 min each time on a shaker at 4°C. After three washes in PBS, biotin was quenched with two washes of 50 mM NH_4Cl in PBS (15 min each) on a shaker at 4°C. Cells were then washed three times in PBS without Ca^{2+} and Mg^{2+} and then scraped into Lysis Buffer (50 mM Hepes pH 7, 150 mM NaCl, 1% Glycerol, 1% Triton X-100, 1.5 mM $MgCl_2$, 5 mM EGTA). Cell lysates were collected in an Eppendorf tube and rocked for 30 min at 4°C. Nuclei were then pelleted by centrifugation at 10,000 rpm at 4°C for 20 min. Supernatant protein concentration was calculated using the BCA assay (Euroclone) according to manufacturer's instructions. An aliquot of supernatant corresponding to 600 μg of proteins was precipitated by rotation at 4°C for 6 h using high capacity streptavidin agarose resin (Thermo Fischer Scientific Inc.), following the manufacturer's recommendation. The resin was then washed with the following solutions: once with Lysis Buffer, twice with Buffer 1 (150 mM NaCl, 20mM Tris-HCl, pH 8, 5 mM EDTA, 1% Triton X-100, 0.2% BSA), once with Buffer 3 (150 mM NaCl, 20 mM Tris-HCl, pH 8, 5 mM EDTA, 0.5% Triton X-100), and once with Buffer 4 (50 mM Tris–HCl, pH 8). Biotinylated proteins were eluted from the resin with reducing Sample Buffer 4X and 30 μl of each sample were separated on a 4–15% or 4–20% gradient Criterion TGX gel (Biorad) and analyzed by Western blotting.

Immunofluorescence Detection of CFTR and USP13

CFBE41o- cells seeded in a 12-well μ-chamber (81201, Ibidi) at a density of 25.000 cells per well and treated with VX-809 and spautin-1 as for functional assays, were rinsed with PBS and fixed by adding 100 μl per well of 10% neutral buffered formalin for 5 min at room temperature. After three washes with 300 μl of PBS, cells were permeabilized with PBS-Triton X-100 0.3% for 5 min, blocked with PBS-BSA 1% for 2 h, and then incubated overnight at 4°C with 100 μl of primary antibodies diluted in blocking solution. The following antibodies and dilutions were used: ab570 mouse IgG1 anti-CFTR (J. R. Riordan, University of North Carolina at Chapel Hill, and Cystic Fibrosis Foundation Therapeutics) at 1:250 and ab99421 rabbit anti-USP13 (Abcam) at 1:200. Following incubation with primary antibodies, cells were rinsed three times with PBS and incubated with 100 μl of a solution of secondary goat anti-rabbit Alexa Fluor-488 and goat anti-mouse Alexa Fluor-546 antibodies (Invitrogen) diluted in PBS-BSA 1% for 1 h in the dark. After three further washes in PBS, cells were covered with mounting medium and coverslip, and then analyzed using a laser-scanning confocal microscope SPE (Leica Microsystems). Image analysis was performed using Leica and ImageJ software. Fractional overlap between CFTR and USP13 was quantified via Manders' colocalization coefficient in total cell ROIs or in peripheral ROIs by using Coloc2 plugin.

Statistics

Data are shown as representative traces/images or as a mean values and SEM of independent experiments. Significance of differences was established with ANOVA (with Tukey or Dunnett *post hoc* tests, as appropriate) except for experiments shown in **Figures 4B**, **7B** in which Student's *t*-test was used. Analysis was done with InStat (GraphPad) software.

ETHICS STATEMENT

The protocols to isolate, culture, store, and study bronchial epithelial cells from patients undergoing lung transplant (described in Scudieri et al., 2012) were approved by the Regional Ethical Committee (Comitato Etico Regionale) under the supervision of the Italian Ministry of Health (registration number: ANTECER, 042-09/07/2018). Informed and written informed consent was obtained from all patients using a form that was also approved by the same Ethical Committee.

AUTHOR CONTRIBUTIONS

EP, ES, NP, AH, and LG conceived the study. EP, ES, LF, VT, EC, PS, IM, MR, NB, NS, DdB, and NP investigated and validated the data. EP, ES, NP, AH, and LG wrote the manuscript. NP and LG acquired the funding. NP, DB, AH, and LG provided the resources.

FUNDING

This study was supported by grants from Telethon Foundation (TMLGCBX16TT), from Fondazione Italiana per la Ricerca sulla Fibrosi Cistica (FFC#2/2017, grant adopted by FFC delegations from Bologna and Ferrara), from ERA-Net for Research Programmes on Rare Diseases (01GM1601), and from "Ricerca Corrente" from the Italian Ministry of Health (Linea 1).

ACKNOWLEDGMENTS

We thank Dr. John Riordan (University of North Carolina - Chapel Hill), and Cystic Fibrosis Foundation Therapeutics for kindly providing us with anti-CFTR antibodies.

REFERENCES

Biederbick, A., Kern, H. F., and Elsässer, H. P. (1995). Monodansylcadaverine (MDC) is a specific in vivo marker for autophagic vacuoles. *Eur. J. Cell Biol.* 66, 3–14.

Bomberger, J. M., Barnaby, R. L., and Stanton, B. A. (2009). The deubiquitinating enzyme USP10 regulates the post-endocytic sorting of cystic fibrosis transmembrane conductance regulator in airway epithelial cells. *J. Biol. Chem.* 284, 18778–18789. doi: 10.1074/jbc.M109.001685

Castellani, C., and Assael, B. M. (2017). Cystic fibrosis: a clinical view. *Cell. Mol. Life Sci.* 74, 129–140. doi: 10.1007/s00018-016-2393-9

Cheng, J., Moyer, B. D., Milewski, M., Loffing, J., Ikeda, M., Mickle, J. E., et al. (2002). A Golgi-associated PDZ domain protein modulates cystic fibrosis transmembrane regulator plasma membrane expression. *J. Biol. Chem.* 277, 3520–3529. doi: 10.1074/jbc.M110177200

Cholon, D. M., Quinney, N. L., Fulcher, M. L., Esther, C. R. Jr., Das, J., Dokholyan, N. V., et al. (2014). Potentiator ivacaftor abrogates pharmacological correction of ΔF508 CFTR in cystic fibrosis. *Sci. Transl. Med.* 6:246ra96. doi: 10.1126/scitranslmed.3008680

Donoso, G., Herzog, V., and Schmitz, A. (2005). Misfolded BiP is degraded by a proteasome-independent endoplasmic-reticulum-associated degradation pathway. *Biochem. J.* 387, 897–903. doi: 10.1042/BJ20041312

Farinha, C. M., King-Underwood, J., Sousa, M., Correia, A. R., Henriques, B. J., Roxo-Rosa, M., et al. (2013). Revertants, low temperature, and correctors reveal the mechanism of F508del-CFTR rescue by VX-809 and suggest multiple agents for full correction. *Chem. Biol.* 20, 943–955. doi: 10.1016/j.chembiol.2013.06.004

Fu, L., Rab, A., Tang, Lp., Bebok, Z., Rowe, S. M., Bartoszewski, R., et al. (2015). ΔF508 CFTR surface stability is regulated by DAB2 and CHIP-mediated ubiquitination in post-endocytic compartments. *PLoS One* 10:e0123131. doi: 10.1371/journal.pone.0123131

Galietta, L. J. (2013). Managing the underlying cause of cystic fibrosis: a future role for potentiators and correctors. *Paediatr. Drugs* 15, 393–402. doi: 10.1007/s40272-013-0035-3

Gee, H. Y., Noh, S. H., Tang, B. L., Kim, K. H., and Lee, M. G. (2011). Rescue of ΔF508-CFTR trafficking via a GRASP-dependent unconventional secretion pathway. *Cell* 146, 746–760. doi: 10.1016/j.cell.2011.07.021

He, L., Kota, P., Aleksandrov, A. A., Cui, L., Jensen, T., Dokholyan, N. V., et al. (2013). Correctors of ΔF508 CFTR restore global conformational maturation without thermally stabilizing the mutant protein. *FASEB J.* 27, 536–545. doi: 10.1096/fj.12-216119

Hudson, R. P., Dawson, J. E., Chong, P. A., Yang, Z., Millen, L., Thomas, P. J., et al. (2017). Direct binding of the corrector VX-809 to human CFTR NBD1: evidence of an allosteric coupling between the binding site and the NBD1:CL4 Interface. *Mol. Pharmacol.* 92, 124–135. doi: 10.1124/mol.117.108373

Lee, C. M., Lee, B. S., Arnold, S. L., Isoherranen, N., and Morgan, E. T. (2014). Nitric oxide and interleukin-1β stimulate the proteasome-independent degradation of the retinoic acid hydroxylase CYP2C22 in primary rat hepatocytes. *J. Pharmacol. Exp. Ther.* 348, 141–152. doi: 10.1124/jpet.113.209841

Li, Y., Luo, K., Yin, Y., Wu, C., Deng, M., Li, L., et al. (2017). USP13 regulates the RAP80-BRCA1 complex dependent DNA damage response. *Nat. Commun.* 8:15752. doi: 10.1038/ncomms15752

Liu, J., Xia, H., Kim, M., Xu, L., Li, Y., Zhang, L., et al. (2011). Beclin1 controls the levels of p53 by regulating the deubiquitination activity of USP10 and USP13. *Cell* 147, 223–234. doi: 10.1016/j.cell.2011.08.037

Luciani, A., Villella, V. R., Esposito, S., Brunetti-Pierri, N., Medina, D., Settembre, C., et al. (2010). Defective CFTR induces aggresome formation and lung inflammation in cystic fibrosis through ROS-mediated autophagy inhibition. *Nat. Cell Biol.* 12, 863–875. doi: 10.1038/ncb2090

Lukacs, G. L., and Verkman, A. S. (2012). CFTR: folding, misfolding and correcting the ΔF508 conformational defect. *Trends Mol. Med.* 18, 81–91. doi: 10.1016/j.molmed.2011.10.003

Mbonye, U. R., Yuan, C., Harris, C. E., Sidhu, R. S., Song, I., Arakawa, T., et al. (2008). Two distinct pathways for cyclooxygenase-2 protein degradation. *J. Biol. Chem.* 283, 8611–8623. doi: 10.1074/jbc.M710137200

Morito, D., Hirao, K., Oda, Y., Hosokawa, N., Tokunaga, F., Cyr, D. M., et al. (2008). Gp78 cooperates with RMA1 in endoplasmic reticulum-associated degradation of CFTRDeltaF508. *Mol. Biol. Cell* 19, 1328–1336. doi: 10.1091/mbc.E07-06-0601

Munafó, D. B., and Colombo, M. I. (2001). A novel assay to study autophagy: regulation of autophagosome vacuole size by amino acid deprivation. *J. Cell Sci.* 114, 3619–3629.

Noh, S. H., Gee, H. Y., Kim, Y., Piao, H., Kim, J., Kang, C. M., et al. (2018). Specific autophagy and ESCRT components participate in the unconventional secretion of CFTR. *Autophagy* 14, 1761–1778. doi: 10.1080/15548627.2018.1489479

Okiyoneda, T., Barrière, H., Bagdány, M., Rabeh, W. M., Du, K., Höhfeld, J., et al. (2010). Peripheral protein quality control removes unfolded CFTR from the plasma membrane. *Science* 329, 805–810. doi: 10.1126/science.1191542

Okiyoneda, T., Veit, G., Dekkers, J. F., Bagdany, M., Soya, N., Xu, H., et al. (2013). Mechanism-based corrector combination restores ΔF508-CFTR folding and function. *Nat. Chem. Biol.* 9, 444–454. doi: 10.1038/nchembio.1253

Omari, S., Makareeva, E., Roberts-Pilgrim, A., Mirigian, L., Jarnik, M., Ott, C., et al. (2018). Noncanonical autophagy at ER exit sites regulates procollagen turnover. *Proc. Natl. Acad. Sci. U.S.A.* 115, E10099–E10108. doi: 10.1073/pnas.1814552115

Pedemonte, N., Tomati, V., Sondo, E., and Galietta, L. J. (2010). Influence of cell background on pharmacological rescue of mutant CFTR. *Am. J. Physiol.* 298, C866–C874. doi: 10.1152/ajpcell.00404.2009

Quon, B. S., and Rowe, S. M. (2016). New and emerging targeted therapies for cystic fibrosis. *BMJ* 352:i859. doi: 10.1136/bmj.i859

Ren, H. Y., Grove, D. E., De La Rosa, O., Houck, S. A., Sopha, P., Van Goor, F., et al. (2013). VX-809 corrects folding defects in cystic fibrosis transmembrane conductance regulator protein through action on membrane-spanning domain 1. *Mol. Biol. Cell* 24, 3016–3024. doi: 10.1091/mbc.E13-05-0240

Ronan, B., Flamand, O., Vescovi, L., Dureuil, C., Durand, L., Fassy, F., et al. (2014). A highly potent and selective Vps34 inhibitor alters vesicle trafficking and autophagy. *Nat. Chem. Biol.* 10, 1013–1019. doi: 10.1038/nchembio.1681

Rowe, S. M., McColley, S. A., Rietschel, E., Li, X., Bell, S. C., Konstan, M. W., et al. (2017). Lumacaftor/ivacaftor treatment of patients with cystic fibrosis heterozygous for F508del-CFTR. *Ann. Am. Thorac. Soc.* 14, 213–219. doi: 10.1513/AnnalsATS.201609-689OC

Scudieri, P., Caci, E., Bruno, S., Ferrera, L., Schiavon, M., Sondo, E., et al. (2012). Association of TMEM16A chloride channel overexpression with airway goblet cell metaplasia. *J. Physiol.* 590, 6141–6155. doi: 10.1113/jphysiol.2012.240838

Sharma, M., Benharouga, M., Hu, W., and Lukacs, G. L. (2001). Conformational and temperature-sensitive stability defects of the delta F508 cystic fibrosis transmembrane conductance regulator in post-endoplasmic reticulum compartments. *J. Biol. Chem.* 276, 8942–8950. doi: 10.1074/jbc.M009172200

Sheppard, D. N., Carson, M. R., Ostedgaard, L. S., Denning, G. M., and Welsh, M. J. (1994). Expression of cystic fibrosis transmembrane conductance regulator in a model epithelium. *Am. J. Physiol.* 266, L405–L413. doi: 10.1152/ajplung.1994.266.4.L405

Sondo, E., Pesce, E., Tomati, V., Marini, M., and Pedemonte, N. (2017). RNF5, DAB2 and friends: novel drug targets for cystic fibrosis. *Curr. Pharm. Des.* 23, 176–186. doi: 10.2174/1381612822666161006161033

Sondo, E., Tomati, V., Caci, E., Esposito, A. I., Pfeffer, U., Pedemonte, N., et al. (2011). Rescue of the mutant CFTR chloride channel by pharmacological correctors and low temperature analyzed by gene expression profiling. *Am. J. Physiol.* 301, C872–C885. doi: 10.1152/ajpcell.00507.2010

Stoltz, D. A., Meyerholz, D. K., and Welsh, M. J. (2015). Origins of cystic fibrosis lung disease. *N. Engl. J. Med.* 372, 351–362. doi: 10.1056/NEJMra1300109

Thoreen, C. C., Kang, S. A., Chang, J. W., Liu, Q., Zhang, J., Gao, Y., et al. (2009). An ATP-competitive mammalian target of rapamycin inhibitor reveals rapamycin-resistant functions of mTORC1. *J. Biol. Chem.* 284, 8023–8032. doi: 10.1074/jbc.M900301200

Tomati, V., Pesce, E., Caci, E., Sondo, E., Scudieri, P., Marini, M., et al. (2018). High-throughput screening identifies FAU protein as a regulator of mutant cystic fibrosis transmembrane conductance regulator channel. *J. Biol. Chem.* 293, 1203–1217. doi: 10.1074/jbc.M117.816595

Tomati, V., Sondo, E., Armirotti, A., Caci, E., Pesce, E., Marini, M., et al. (2015). Genetic inhibition of the ubiquitin ligase Rnf5 attenuates phenotypes associated to F508del cystic fibrosis mutation. *Sci. Rep.* 5:12138. doi: 10.1038/srep12138

Van Goor, F., Hadida, S., Grootenhuis, P. D., Burton, B., Stack, J. H., Straley, K. S., et al. (2011). Correction of the F508del-CFTR protein processing defect in vitro by the investigational drug VX-809. *Proc. Natl. Acad. Sci. U.S.A.* 108, 18843–18848. doi: 10.1073/pnas.1105787108

Veit, G., Avramescu, R. G., Perdomo, D., Phuan, P. W., Bagdany, M., Apaja, P. M., et al. (2014). Some gating potentiators, including VX-770, diminish ΔF508-CFTR functional expression. *Sci. Transl. Med.* 6:246ra97. doi: 10.1126/scitranslmed.3008889

Wainwright, C. E., Elborn, J. S., Ramsey, B. W., Marigowda, G., Huang, X., Cipolli, M., et al. (2015). Lumacaftor-ivacaftor in patients with cystic fibrosis homozygous for Phe508del CFTR. *N. Engl. J. Med.* 373, 220–231. doi: 10.1056/NEJMoa1409547

Xue, X., Mutyam, V., Tang, L., Biswas, S., Du, M., Jackson, L. A., et al. (2014). Synthetic aminoglycosides efficiently suppress cystic fibrosis transmembrane conductance regulator nonsense mutations and are enhanced by ivacaftor. *Am. J. Respir. Cell Mol. Biol.* 50, 805–816. doi: 10.1165/rcmb.2013-0282OC

Ye, S., Cihil, K., Stolz, D. B., Pilewski, J. M., Stanton, B. A., and Swiatecka-Urban, A. (2010). c-Cbl facilitates endocytosis and lysosomal degradation of cystic fibrosis transmembrane conductance regulator in human airway epithelial cells. *J. Biol. Chem.* 285, 27008–27018. doi: 10.1074/jbc.M110.139881

Younger, J. M., Chen, L., Ren, H. Y., Rosser, M. F., Turnbull, E. L., Fan, C. Y., et al. (2006). Sequential quality-control checkpoints triage misfolded cystic fibrosis transmembrane conductance regulator. *Cell* 126, 571–582. doi: 10.1016/j.cell.2006.06.041

Zhang, J., Zhang, P., Wei, Y., Piao, H. L., Wang, W., Maddika, S., et al. (2013). Deubiquitylation and stabilization of PTEN by USP13. *Nat. Cell Biol.* 15, 1486–1494. doi: 10.1038/ncb2874

3

Network Biology Identifies Novel Regulators of CFTR Trafficking and Membrane Stability

Cláudia Almeida Loureiro[1,2†], João D. Santos[1,3†], Ana Margarida Matos[1,2†], Peter Jordan[1,2†], Paulo Matos[1,2†], Carlos M. Farinha[1,3†] and Francisco R. Pinto[1,3]*

[1] BioISI—Biosystems & Integrative Sciences Institute, Faculty of Sciences, University of Lisbon, Lisbon, Portugal, [2] Department of Human Genetics, National Health Institute "Dr. Ricardo Jorge," Lisbon, Portugal, [3] Department of Chemistry and Biochemistry, Faculty of Sciences, University of Lisbon, Lisbon, Portugal

***Correspondence:**
Francisco Pinto
frpinto@fc.ul.pt

†These authors have contributed equally to this work.

In cystic fibrosis, the most common disease-causing mutation is F508del, which causes not only intracellular retention and degradation of CFTR, but also defective channel gating and decreased membrane stability of the small amount that reaches the plasma membrane (PM). Thus, pharmacological correction of mutant CFTR requires targeting of multiple cellular defects in order to achieve clinical benefit. Although small-molecule compounds have been identified and commercialized that can correct its folding or gating, an efficient retention of F508del CFTR at the PM has not yet been explored pharmacologically despite being recognized as a crucial factor for improving functional rescue of chloride transport. In ongoing efforts to determine the CFTR interactome at the PM, we used three complementary approaches: targeting proteins binding to tyrosine-phosphorylated CFTR, protein complexes involved in cAMP-mediated CFTR stabilization at the PM, and proteins selectively interacting at the PM with rescued F508del-CFTR but not wt-CFTR. Using co-immunoprecipitation or peptide–pull down strategies, we identified around 400 candidate proteins through sequencing of complex protein mixtures using the nano-LC Triple TOF MS technique. Key candidate proteins were validated for their robust interaction with CFTR-containing protein complexes and for their ability to modulate the amount of CFTR expressed at the cell surface of bronchial epithelial cells. Here, we describe how we explored the abovementioned experimental datasets to build a protein interaction network with the aim of identifying novel pharmacological targets to rescue CFTR function in cystic fibrosis (CF) patients. We identified and validated novel candidate proteins that were essential components of the network but not detected in previous proteomic analyses.

Keywords: CFTR, interactome, membrane traffic, network biology, plasma membrane

INTRODUCTION

CFTR is a polytopic integral membrane protein that belongs to the ATP-binding cassette (ABC) transporter superfamily functioning as cAMP- and phosphorylation-regulated chloride and bicarbonate at the apical membrane of epithelial cells. Mutations in the *CFTR* gene cause cystic fibrosis, the most common autosomal recessive disorder among Caucasians (Riordan, 2008). The most prevalent CF-causing mutation is F508del, which is present in about 90% of CF patients and generates a mutant protein recognized by endoplasmic reticulum (ER) quality control (ERQC) mechanisms (Farinha and Amaral, 2005; Farinha et al., 2013; Farinha and Canato, 2017) and targeted for proteasomal degradation (Jensen et al., 1995).

Although most F508del-CFTR protein is only detected as a non-native (misfolded) core-glycosylated ER-specific intermediate, a small amount reaches the plasma membrane (PM) and is partially functional as a channel (Dalemans et al., 1991; Swiatecka-Urban et al., 2005). Thus, one important focus of basic research in CF involves attempts to rescue F508del-CFTR to the PM, by identifying either the key molecular factors involved in its ER retention or small molecules that promote its folding and release from the ERQC. Recent advances in the field allowed the identification of small molecules with potential to treat the basic defect in CF—either correctors, promoting the relocation of F508del-CFTR from the ER to the PM or potentiators, promoting channel activity (for variants already located at the PM). Among these, the potentiator VX-770 alone or its combinations with the correctors VX-809 or VX-661 made their way to the clinical practice, securing approval from the EMA and the FDA. However, results of these modulators in patients bearing F508del suggest that a physiologically relevant restoration of function will require additional small molecules with distinct corrective properties (Farinha and Matos, 2016). This may be due to the fact that F508del-CFTR, despite its partial pharmacological rescue of intracellular retention and impaired channel regulation, still presents decreased stability at the PM (Sharma et al., 2004; Swiatecka-Urban et al., 2005). Whereas the retention and the gating defects have been extensively studied, and both small-molecule correctors and potentiators are available, CFTR membrane stability is a less understood aspect, albeit crucial to restore F508del-CFTR to levels that correspond to clinical benefit.

CFTR traffic and activity at the PM is the result of numerous interactions that function as molecular switches (Amaral, 2005; Farinha et al., 2013) modulating channel activity and controlling the number of channel present at the membrane, through regulation of the secretory and membrane recycling pathways. This complex network of proteins is the last step in the control of the overall biogenesis/function of the protein and includes other transporters, channels, and trafficking machinery components (Rab GTPases, SNAREs, PDZ-domain-containing proteins) as well as different types of molecular switches (such as kinases, phosphatases, and small GTPases) (Guggino and Stanton, 2006; Farinha et al., 2013; Farinha and Canato, 2017).

Several mechanisms have been described to regulate CFTR anchoring and trafficking at the PM, which include CFTR phosphorylation by different kinases, interaction with cAMP sensors, or response to small GTPase signaling.

Phosphorylation in the regulatory region of CFTR is known for long to be required for its activity and it involves protein kinases A (PKA) and C (PKC) (Schultz et al., 1999). Together with PDZ-domain containing proteins, phosphorylation is responsible for the formation of multiprotein signaling complexes that provide spatial and temporal specificity to CFTR function (Guggino and Stanton, 2006). Besides this well-documented role on function, phosphorylation by spleen tyrosine kinase (Syk) in NBD1 (Luz et al., 2011; Mendes et al., 2011) or by lemur tyrosine kinase 2 LMTK2 in the R region (Luz et al., 2014) was shown to control the levels of CFTR at the PM.

cAMP levels in the cell lead to PKA activation and hence promote CFTR function, as described above. cAMP also activates members of guanine nucleotide-exchange factors, called EPACs (exchange proteins directly activated by cAMP), whose activation does not lead to PKA activation (Bos, 2006). Activation of EPAC1, the most abundant EPAC family member expressed in the lung, promotes its interaction with CFTR, leading to its stabilization at the PM through interaction with the PDZ-containing anchor protein NHERF-1 (Lobo et al., 2016).

Overexpression of NHERF1 promotes apical expression of the F508del-CFTR mutant channel (Guerra et al., 2005). This effect relies on the activation of endogenous RAC1 signaling and may also contribute to the increase of F508del-CFTR PM levels (Moniz et al., 2013; Loureiro et al., 2015).

Here, we used network biology to identify relevant protein nodes that may connect the interactomes obtained by analyzing different mechanisms regulating CFTR stability, namely, through phosphorylation by SYK or activation of EPAC1 or RAC1. We focused the network analysis on proteins never described to interact with or regulate CFTR and show that this approach is a valid strategy for finding novel regulators of CFTR function and traffic. Network biology thus proves to be a tool capable of contributing insights into the etiology of other human diseases linked to chloride transport or membrane protein traffic.

MATERIALS AND METHODS

Protein Interaction Networks

Human physical protein–protein interaction data were extracted from HuRI (Human Reference Protein Interactome Mapping Project) (interactome.baderlab.org) (Rual et al., 2005; Venkatesan et al., 2009; Yu et al., 2011; Rolland et al., 2014; Yang et al., 2016) and APID (Agile Protein Interaction DataAnalyzer) (apid.dep.usal.es) (Alonso-Lopez et al., 2016) databases (accessed in June 2018). APID gathers literature-reported protein interactions, while HuRI results from unbiased large-scale screens for binary interactions. We constructed undirected and unweighted networks using Igraph R-package (Csardi and Nepusz, 2006). Loop and multiple edges were eliminated and only the main component of the network was selected. The network was further filtered to contain only proteins that are not exclusively located in nucleus, mitochondria, or peroxisomes. Gene ontology cellular component annotations obtained from UNIPROT were used to define protein subcellular location. This filter was necessary since the relevant interactions affecting CFTR stability at the PM should not occur within these three cellular compartments. The resulting operational network contained 17,218 proteins and 252,472 interactions.

Network Analysis

Candidate proteins were selected through a neighbor enrichment test and a bridge score. The neighbor enrichment test evaluates if the set of direct neighbors of a candidate protein is enriched in members of an input protein set using a hypergeometric test. The bridging score quantifies for every node in a network its relevance in connecting two other nodes (provided as inputs) through short paths of length 2, 3, or 4. It counts the fraction of paths of length 2, 3, or 4 linking the two input nodes that contain a candidate node. These fractions for each length are used in a weighted sum where paths of length 2 have weight 1, paths of length 3 have weight 0.5, and paths of length 4 have weight 0.25. Both methods are implemented as R functions (*specific_neighbors* and *bridge_score*, respectively) publicly available in the NetSetStat repository (github.com/GamaPintoLab/NetSetStat). Proteins selected through both methods were analyzed for biological process enrichment using the DAVID tool (Huang Da et al., 2009a; Huang Da et al., 2009b) with the *Homo sapiens* genome as background and testing terms from the FAT subset of the Biological Process branch of Gene Ontology. Enriched GO terms were considered significant with a False Discovery Rate lower than 0.05 and were excluded if their background frequency was greater than 10% or lower than 5%.

Preparation of siRNA-Coated 96-Well Plates

Two siRNAs against each of the following targets (CUL3, GABARAP, GABARAPL1, GABARAPL2, ILK, IQGAP1, LRRK2, NF2, NOS2, SMURF1, and UBASH3B) were acquired as a cherry-pick siGenome library (Dharmacon, Cambridge, UK); 96-well plates were coated with customized siRNAs for solid-phase reverse transfection. For that, a transfection mixture of 300 µl was prepared containing 161.5 µl of the Lipofectamine 2000 (Invitrogen #11668019) and 138.5 µl of 0.4 M sucrose in OptiMEM solution. Then, 1.25 µl of siRNA 20 µM was added per well into 96-conic well plates (siRNA plate); 1.75 µl of transfection mix was added per well to siRNA plate, followed by mixing and centrifugation for 1 min at 50×*g*. After 30 min incubation at room temperature, 1.75 µl of 0.2% (w/v) gelatin solution was added to the siRNA plate and centrifuged at 50×*g*. Then, the total of 4.25 µl of the mix in siRNA plate (siRNA plus transfection mix plus gelatin) was diluted 1:50 in a 96-conic well plate using double-distilled water. Finally, 50 µl from the diluted mix was lyophilized and stored in an anhydrous atmosphere before cell seeding.

Reverse Transfection With siRNA

CFBE cells expressing an inducible doxycycline promotor for mCherry-Flag-CFTR (kind gift of Prof. Margarida Amaral, Lisbon) were grown to confluence and split. Then, after 24 h, cells were seeded in a siRNA-coated 96-well plate (100 µl of cell suspension/well, 7×10^{7} cells/well) using a Multidrop™ Combi Reagent Dispenser (Thermo Scientific #5840300). After 24 h of reverse transfection, CFTR expression was induced for 24 h for wt-CFTR and 48 h for F508del-CFTR, using 1 µg/ml doxycycline (Sigma #9891) in antibiotic-free medium.

CFTR Trafficking Assay

The CFTR trafficking assay was performed as previously documented (Almaca et al., 2011; Botelho et al., 2015). This assay uses a double-tagged version of CFTR with mCherry at the N-terminus and FLAG at the fourth extracellular loop. Usage of the mCherry tag allows for quantification of the total amount of CFTR protein expressed by each individual cell. The Flag tag allows one to quantify CFTR that is exclusively localized at the cell surface by usage of an antibody applied extracellularly without cell permeabilization. Hence, 72 h after seeding and siRNA knockdown, cells were washed once with cold $PBS^{+/+}$ (1× PBS supplemented with 0.9 mM $CaCl_2$, 0.5 mM $MgCl_2$, pH 7.2) using Tecan Hydrospeed™ and immunostained for the extracellular Flag-tag (in non-permeabilized cells) for 1 h at 4°C with 1:500 anti-Flag® M2 monoclonal antibody (Sigma-Aldrich #F1804). Then, cells were washed three times in ice with cold $PBS^{+/+}$ and incubated 20 min with 3% (w/v) paraformaldehyde (PFA) at 4°C. Cells were then washed three times in ice with cold $PBS^{+/+}$ and incubated with anti-mouse Cy5 conjugated secondary antibody (Invitrogen, #A10524). Cells were washed three times in ice with cold $PBS^{+/+}$ and incubated for 1 h with 1:5000 Hoechst 33342 solution (Sigma #B2261) for nucleus staining. Finally, cells were washed in ice with cold $PBS^{+/+}$ and immersed in $PBS^{+/+}$. All solutions were prepared in $PBS^{+/+}$ and primary and secondary antibodies were diluted in $PBS^{+/+}$ supplemented with 1% (v/v) BSA.

Image Acquisition

Cell imaging was performed at room temperature with an inverted wide-field fluorescence microscope Leica DMI6000 equipped with a 12-bit 1,344 × 1,024 pixel resolution DFC360FX camera (Leica) and a 10× objective. Exposure times at maximum light brightness for Hoechst, mCherry, and Cy5 were 50, 1,300, and 8,000 ms, respectively. The Hoechst channel was used for contrast-based autofocus. The experiment was conducted in triplicate and five images per well were collected.

Image Analysis

Automatic image analysis was performed using open-source software tools [cell image analysis software CellProfiler[1] (Carpenter et al., 2006) and R[2]] and a pipeline to measure CFTR traffic efficiency developed previously (Botelho et al., 2015). Using this pipeline, the background subtraction was first applied to each image to correct the image illumination and background fluorescence. Then, a quality control was also applied for each image to exclude cells that do not significantly express CFTR, present abnormal morphology, or contain a significant number of saturated pixels. Finally, CFTR traffic was measured in each cell using the fluorescence quantification according to the following formula:

$$\text{CFTR Traffic Efficiency} = \frac{\text{PM CFTR}}{\text{Total CFTR}} = \frac{\text{Cy5 Integrated Fluorescence}}{\text{mCherry Integrated Fluorescence}} \quad \text{(Formula 1)}$$

CFTR traffic efficiency was calculated using the median CFTR traffic efficiency for all cells in the image. Using this pipeline, we

[1] CellProfiler, http://cellprofiler.org/ (last accessed October 19, 2017).
[2] R program, https://www.r-project.org/ (last accessed March 09, 2018).

also remove out-of-focus images, images with high background fluorescence, and images with a lower number of cells (less than 20 cells). Then, the average of CFTR traffic efficiency for all images in wells transfected with siRNAs, which passed the quality control (traffic efficiency test), was compared with the one measured under control conditions—siRNA EGFP (Traffic $\text{Efficiency}_{\text{control}}$) according to the following formula:

$$\text{Deviation Score} = \frac{\text{Traffic Efficiency}_{\text{test}} - \text{Traffic Efficiency}_{\text{control}}}{2 \times \text{SEM}_{\text{control}}} \quad \text{(Formula 2)}$$

The standard error of the mean for the Traffic Efficiency is given by the $\text{SEM}_{\text{control}}$ recorded for siRNA EGFP. Deviation scores (DSs) that are positive or negative correspond to traffic enhancers or inhibitors, respectively. The DS equation normalizes the Traffic Efficiency measures to the mean and variation of the negative controls included in the same 96-well plate. This normalization facilitates the comparison between independent replicates, as all values are relative to the mean and standard error of the mean (SEM) of the negative controls in the respective plate. A DS of 1 is the double of the negative control SEM, which means that the latter has a normalized value of 0.5.

Analysis of siRNA Knock-Down Efficiency

CFBE cells constitutively expressing F508del-CFTR were seeded in 96-well dishes and transfected with the panel of siRNAs described above (Dharmacon, Cambridge, UK), using Lipofectamine 2000 (Invitrogen). All cells were incubated for 48 h at 37°C with 5% CO_2 and then RNA was extracted with the NucleoSpin RNA kit (Macherey Nagel, Düren, Germany). For cDNA synthesis, 0.5 µg of total RNA was then reverse transcribed using random primers (Invitrogen/Life Technologies) and Ready-to-Go You-Prime beads (GE Healthcare, Buckinghamshire, UK). Real-time PCR quantification (qPCR) was performed as previously described (Matos et al., 2008). Primers used in qPCR for each of the targeted transcripts are described in **Table 1**. Each cDNA sample was diluted fivefold to guarantee accurate pipetting and 5 µl was added to each real-time reaction together with 250 nM primers and SYBR Green Master Mix (Applied Biosystems/Life Technologies). Data were analyzed with the ABI Prism 7000 SDS 1.1 RQ Software (ΔΔCT method, Applied Biosystems/Life Technologies).

CFTR Functional Assay by Halide-Sensitive YFP (HS-YFP)

CFBE cells constitutively expressing wt- or F508del-CFTR together with HS-YFP-F46L/H148Q/I152L (Galietta et al., 2001) were seeded in eight-well chamber slides. F508del-CFTR cells were seeded in duplicate slides. Cells were then transfected with either siLUC (Eurofins MWG Operon), siGABARAP_1, siSMURF1_2, or siENOS_2 (Dharmacon) using Lipofectamine 2000 (Invitrogen). All cells were incubated for 48 h and VX-809 (3 µM; Gentaur) was added to one of the F508del-CFTR cell sets. Cells were carefully washed twice with isomolar PBS (WPBS: 137 mM NaCl, 2.7 mM KCl, 0.7 mM $CaCl_2$, 1.1 mM $MgCl_2$, 1.5 mM KH_2PO_4, 8.1 mM Na_2HPO_4, pH 7.4), and wt-CFTR cells were incubated for 15 min in WPBS containing 1 µM indomethacin to reduce endogenous cAMP levels. Cells were then transferred to a Leica TCS-SPE confocal microscope for time-lapse analysis. Each well was assayed individually for iodide influx by recording fluorescence continuously (500 ms per point), first for 10 s (baseline) and then for 60 s after the rapid (≤1 s) addition of isomolar PBS, containing either 5 µM Forskolin (Fsk) (wt-CFTR cells) or 5 µM Fsk plus 20 µM Gen (F508del-CFTR cells), in which 137 mM Cl^- was replaced by I^- (IPBS; final NaI concentration of 100 mM/plate well). Cells were kept at 37°C up until being assayed at room temperature. After background subtraction, HS-YFP fluorescence recordings (F) were normalized to the initial average value measured before addition of I^- (F_0). Quantification of fluorescence decay was performed on at least 24 individual cells per well, using ImageJ (NIH) as previously described (Matos et al., 2018). The average fluorescence decay was fitted to an exponential decay function to derive the maximal slope $[d(F/F_0)/dt, \text{at } t = 0]$ that is proportional to the initial influx of I^- into the cells. (Loureiro et al., 2015).

Protein Thermal Destabilization Assay (Thermal Shift Assay, TS)

After Dox-induced CFTR expression (1 µg/ml; Sigma-Aldrich), mCherry-Flag-F508del-CFTR CFBE cells were transfected with either siLUC (Eurofins MWG Operon) or siGABARAP_1 (Dharmacon), using Lipofectamine 2000. Cells were then incubated for 24 h with VX-809 (3 µM; Gentaur) at 37°C and then moved for another 24 h to 30°C, to increase the thermal stability of rescued F508del-CFTR

TABLE 1 | Primers used for qPCR quantification of siRNA efficiency.

Gene name	Transcript_id	Forward primer sequence	Reverse primer sequence
CUL3	NM_003590.4	ACAGCTATGGTGATGATTAGAGAC	TACGACTTCTCCTTTCCGCT
GABARAP	NM_007278.1	GGCTCCCAAAGCTCGGATAG	GCAGCTTCACAGACCGTAGA
GABARAPL1	NM_001363598	TGCCTGATCTGGACAAGAGG	AACGCATCTAGAACAAGGGCT
GABARAPL2	NM_007285.6	TGTTCAAGGAGGACCACTCG	CCACAAACAGGAAGATCGCC
ILK	NM_004517.3	GCTTGGGGTTCATCCTCCTT	TTACATTGATCCGTGCCCCC
IQGAP1	NM_003870.3	GCACTGGCTAAGACGGAAGT	CGGATAGCACGTCTCTGCAT
LRRK2	XM_005268629.4	GGCCCTCCTCACTGAGACTA	TGCATCAGCATGGAGAGCAT
NF2	NM_181832.2	AGAGGAGCTGGTTCAGGAGA	GCCAAAAATCCCCGCTTGTG
NOS2	NM_000625.4	CCTCGCTCTGGAAAGACCAG	GGGACAGGACGTAGTTCAGC
SMURF1	NM_181349.2	CGTGGGGAAGAAGGTTTGGA	AAGCCCCCGTTGATGTAGTG
UBASH3B	NM_032873.4	TGGACGTGCTCCTCTCCAT	GGGGAAGATGTTGTGTGCCT

at the PM and allow its accumulation at the cell surface. For the thermal shift assay, cells were again transferred to 37°C for 4 h to induce F508del-CFTR thermal destabilization and PM removal, as described previously (Okiyoneda et al., 2010). Cells were then placed on ice, washed three times with ice-cold WPBS, and left 5 min in cold WPBS to fully arrest CFTR trafficking. Afterwards, they were incubated on ice with anti-Flag M2 Ab (F3165, Sigma-Aldrich) in WPBS for 1 h at 4°C, without permeabilization. Cells were washed three times with ice-cold WPBS and incubated with anti-mouse Alexa Fluor 488 secondary Ab (Thermo Fisher Scientific) for 1 h at 4°C. Cells were then fixed with 4% formaldehyde for 15 min, thoroughly washed in PBS containing DAPI (4′,6-diamidino-2-phenylindole, Sigma-Aldrich), mounted on microscope slides with Vectashield (Vector Laboratories), and analyzed by confocal microscopy.

Confocal Microscopy Imaging

Slides of mCherry-Flag-F508del-CFTR CFBE cells immunolabeled with anti-Flag followed by Alexa Fluor 488 were analyzed by confocal microscopy. Images were acquired on a Leica TCS-SPE confocal microscope, where mCherry fluorescence is proportional to the total amount of CFTR, Alexa Fluor 488 fluorescence is proportional to the amount of CFTR present at the cell surface, and nuclei were stained with DAPI. A 0.2-µm Z-stack of 1-Airy confocal images was acquired to select the best *XY* plane to analyze the CFTR protein at the cell surface. ImageJ software (NIH) was then used to delimitate each single cell as individual ROIs (regions of interest, to allow measurement of mCherry and Alexa488 fluorescence signal intensities). Quantification of fluorescence was performed on at least 24 individual cells per field, as previously described (Matos et al., 2018), and expressed as mean ± SEM fold variation over control cells.

Statistical Analysis

Multiple treatment data analysis—Statistical significance of the observed variations between different treatments was assessed using two-tailed Kruskal–Wallis tests, followed by paired comparisons using the Mann–Whitney *U* test, considering a 0.05 significance level for both tests. All observations were confirmed in at least three independent experiments, each with two replicates for each individual condition tested.

Statistical analysis of CFTR trafficking assay—Each siRNA was used to measure traffic efficiency of wild-type CFTR, F508del-CFTR, and F508del-CFTR rescued with VX-809. For each siRNA and CFTR type, three independent replicate DSs were obtained. The DS mean was considered a measure of the siRNA capacity to influence the traffic efficiency of a particular CFTR type ($<DS_i>$, i corresponding to CFTR type), and the sum of the three DS mean absolute values ($\Sigma|<DS_i>|$) was considered a global measure of the siRNA effect. To evaluate statistical significance of these effects, a random permutation test was performed, where the data matrix containing all the individual DS (all replicates for all CFTR types and all siRNAs, including siRNAs without knockdown effect, functioning as additional controls) was randomly shuffled 10,000 times. Full matrix permutation is possible because all DS values are normalized by EGFP control traffic efficiency mean and SEM values. For each random matrix, each siRNA random $\Sigma|<DS_i>|$ was computed, generating distributions according to the null hypothesis that siRNAs have no effect. Null hypotheses were rejected when the fraction of random values greater than or equal to the observed $\Sigma|<DS_i>|$ was lower than 0.05.

RESULTS

Network Connectivity between CFTR Interactors Potentially Modulating Stability at the PM

Studies from our team have identified five sets of CFTR interactors through three parallel approaches (under consideration elsewhere): a) proteins selectively interacting at the PM with either wt-CFTR (set 1: wt) or rescued F508del-CFTR (set 2: rescued), b) protein complexes involved in cAMP-mediated CFTR stabilization (set 3: EPAC), and c) adaptor proteins binding to tyrosine-phosphorylated (set 4: pep-py) or un-phosphorylated (set 5: pep-wt) CFTR peptide (unpublished data). All these complementary approaches were designed to identify potential modulators of CFTR PM stability through different pathways. We hypothesized that proteins simultaneously interacting with these different pathways may also have a significant influence on CFTR stability at the PM.

First, we mapped these sets of interactors on a human protein physical interaction network and explored how strongly they were connected through this network (**Table 2**). To evaluate the statistical significance of network connectivity, we had to consider that these interactor sets were selected by their presence in immunoprecipitated CFTR complexes. Therefore, we generated 500 random sets of interactors (for each of the five observed sets), with the same number of proteins at each observed network distance from CFTR. For each connectivity property (number of overlapping proteins between sets, number of direct interactions between set members, and number of common direct neighbors between sets), we recorded the average value across the 500 randomizations and a *p* value, which corresponds to the fraction of random set pairs showing a value higher than that observed with the experimental sets. The five sets have a low number of proteins in common, although 8 out of 10 pairs have a significantly higher overlap than expected by chance. The strong connectivity between these CFTR interactor sets is much more evident by looking at the numbers of direct physical interactions and common neighbors that are much higher than randomly expected and reach statistical significance for all set pairs. This strong connectivity supports our attempt to find new proteins simultaneously interacting with multiple CFTR PM stability-related pathways.

Specific Common Neighbors of CFTR Interactor Sets

We have identified 4411 proteins that have direct physical interactions with proteins in at least two CFTR interactor sets (2,420, 1,161, and 443 with direct neighbors in at least 3, 4, and 5 sets, respectively). However, to increase the likelihood that perturbations in one of these proteins will have an effect in these

TABLE 2 | Overlap, direct interactions, and common neighbors between CFTR interactor sets.

CFTR interactor sets		Overlap		Direct interactions		Common neighbors	
		Observed (expected)	*p*	Observed (expected)	*p*	Observed (expected)	*p*
wt	rescued	7 (1.2)	<0.002	183 (48.1)	<0.002	2,092 (1,244)	<0.002
	EPAC	3 (0.4)	0.004	54 (16.9)	<0.002	1,138 (692)	0.006
	pep-py	2 (0.3)	0.024	82 (15.3)	<0.002	1,535 (661)	<0.002
	pep-wt	0 (0.2)	0.547	28 (5.6)	<0.002	888 (310)	0.002
Rescued	EPAC	8 (1.1)	<0.002	164 (44.8)	<0.002	1,818 (1,191)	0.006
	pep-py	6 (0.9)	0.002	359 (41.8)	<0.002	2,300 (1,153)	<0.002
	pep-wt	3 (0.3)	0.002	113 (15.3)	<0.002	1,364 (515)	<0.002
EPAC	pep-py	1 (0.2)	0.117	57 (14.0)	<0.002	1,140 (636)	0.002
	pep-wt	2 (0.1)	0.002	23 (5.2)	<0.002	758 (301)	0.008
pep-py	pep-wt	4 (0.1)	<0.002	94 (5.0)	<0.002	1,473 (294)	<0.002

specific neighbor pathways and, consequently, on CFTR PM stability, we should require that these proteins are enriched in direct interactions with these CFTR interactor sets. With that aim, we performed a hypergeometric test to determine if these proteins are enriched in interactions with each of the five sets. As we performed this test to all proteins with neighbors in each of the five interactor sets, choosing a trivial *p* value cutoff may be associated with many false positives. To avoid this multiple testing problem, we selected for each set of CFTR interactors the 5% proteins with the lowest hypergeometric *p* values as specific neighbors of that set, and additionally required the selected proteins to have at least three interactions with two or more CFTR interactor sets. This strategy resulted in the selection of 478 proteins. We ranked these proteins by summing the ranks of their neighbor enrichment *p* values for all sets, discarding sets where the protein was not in the top 5% of significantly enriched proteins (protein list and associated statistics are available in **Supplementary Table 1** and the selection process is depicted in **Figure 1**).

Important Mediators of CFTR Interaction With EPAC, NHERF1, EZRIN, and SYK

The CFTR interactor sets were experimentally detected under conditions that modulate CFTR PM stability through the influence of factors such as EPAC, NHERF1, EZRIN, and SYK, previously known to be involved in the stabilization process (Mendes et al., 2011; Loureiro et al., 2015; Lobo et al., 2016). To uncover novel proteins that most likely influence CFTR PM stability, we aimed to quantify the contribution of a given protein to interfere (either positively or negatively) with the formation of complexes including CFTR and one of the referred stability factors.

For this purpose, we developed a bridge score that measures the fraction of short length paths (with two to four interactions) connecting two proteins of interest (CFTR and the stability factor) that are mediated by a candidate protein. Mediation of shorter paths is given a higher weight/score. The perturbation of proteins with high bridge scores will disrupt a higher fraction of short network paths linking the two proteins of interest. If the interactions in these paths stabilize or facilitate the assembly of the complex containing the two proteins of interest, the bridging protein may have a positive effect on the functional interaction between the two proteins. Reversely, if the interactions in the short paths compete with the formation of the complex, the bridging protein may negatively affect the functional interaction between the two proteins.

To compute the bridge score, we assembled a connected subnetwork containing CFTR, the four stability factors, and the common neighbors identified in the previous section (process described in **Figure 1**). The resulting subnetwork contained 482 proteins and 16,481 interactions. We considered a protein to be an important mediator between CFTR and one stability factor if its bridge score was in the top 25% of all scores with the corresponding stability factor. This procedure allowed the identification of 194 strong mediator proteins (**Supplementary Table 1**). Gene ontology analysis (**Supplementary Table 2**) showed that the two biological processes most significantly enriched within these 194 proteins were "protein localization to organelle" (GO:0033365, 54 proteins) and "regulation of protein modification process" (GO:0031399, 71 proteins), which supports their hypothetical role in the modulation of CFTR PM stability.

Hit Selection

To assess the impact of protein networks in CFTR trafficking, we selected hits for validation from the list of 478 proteins significantly enriched in neighbors from at least two CFTR interactor sets.

From the list of specific common neighbors of CFTR interactors, we started by excluding any proteins detected in the three initial experimentally derived interactor sets. Then, we focused on the top 25% of the list (proteins with higher neighbor enrichment rank sum as defined above). Then, we used data from Human Protein Atlas and excluded proteins with low expression in the "bronchus" (keeping thus only those with medium, high, or n/a protein expression). As we were interested in assessing CFTR PM stability, we then excluded proteins with annotation as ribosomal proteins/ elongation or transcription factors/HNRNP/RNA processing/ nuclear proteins. The next step was to exclude proteins already detected as CFTR interactors in previous studies (Wang et al., 2006; Pankow et al., 2015). This refined our list from 478 to 44 proteins. Finally, we used literature mining and refined this list to 25%, selecting 11 possible hits for validating the proteins listed in **Table 3**.

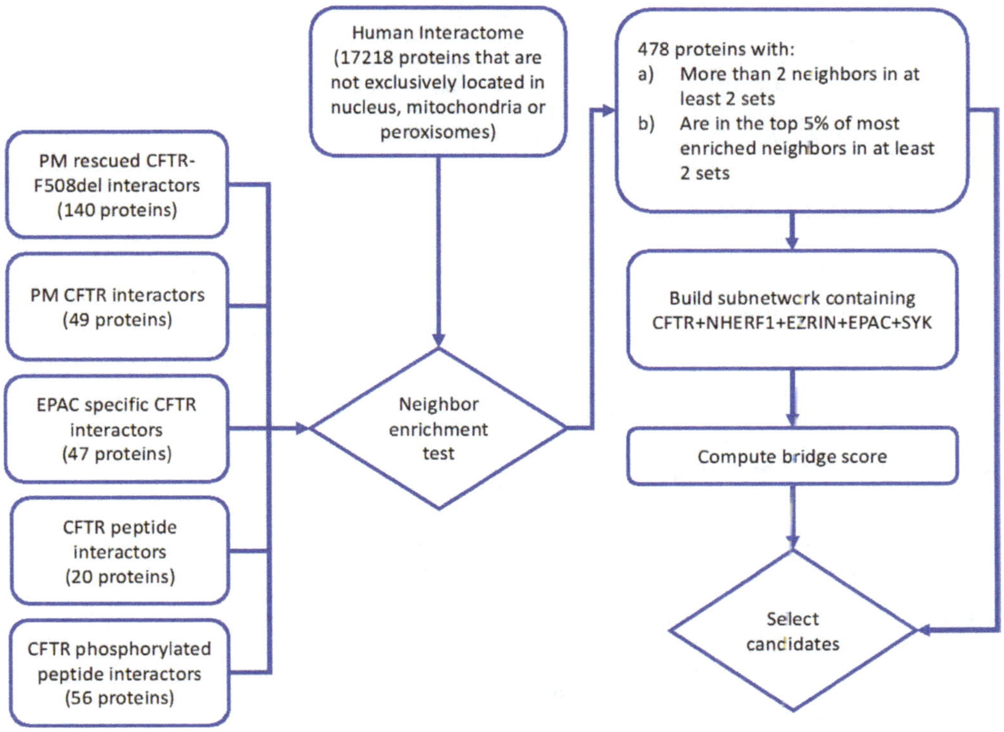

FIGURE 1 | Diagram of the network analysis procedures. CFTR interactor sets were mapped on a human protein physical interaction network, filtered for protein subcellular location to guarantee plausible interactions with CFTR. Proteins in the network were submitted to a neighbor enrichment test to select specific common neighbors of the CFTR interactor sets. A subnetwork containing the selected specific neighbors, CFTR, and related stability factors (EPAC, NHERF1, EZRIN, and SYK) was assembled and a bridge score was computed to identify strong network mediators of CFTR interaction with the referred stability factors. The ranking of neighbor specificity and bridge score were used to select candidates for experimental validation of CFTR PM stability modulation.

Assessment of CFTR Trafficking Under Knockdown of Selected Hits

We ordered two different siRNAs for each of the putative hit proteins from Dharmacon's siGenome library (see Materials and methods). We then used qPCR to assess the knockdown efficiency of the targeted transcript by each siRNA in CFBE cells (**Figure S1**). We verified that most siRNA pairs exhibited considerable differences in their ability to knock down the abundance of the mRNAs coding for the targeted proteins. Notwithstanding, we observed that the siRNAs GABARAP_1, GABARAPL2_1, IQGAP1_1, LRRK2_2, NF2_2, NOS2_2, and SMURF1_2 were able to significantly ($p < 0.05$) downregulate the hit mRNAs that they targeted (**Figure S1**), and these were chosen for further analysis on CFTR trafficking (wt-, F508del-, and F508del-CFTR rescued with VX-809). We used CFBE cell lines stably expressing a double-tagged (mCherry and FLAG) version of CFTR under the control of a doxycycline-inducible promoter so that CFTR expression could be induced 24 h after transfection with siRNA and immunofluorescence be performed at 24 h post-induction. CFTR at the PM is monitored by the Flag (Cy5) signal and total CFTR by mCherry fluorescence. CFTR trafficking is given by the ratio of PM CFTR to total CFTR (Botelho et al., 2015).

For this assay, cells were also transfected with two previously validated siRNAs targeting CFTR and COPBI (Botelho et al. 2015), as controls of the transfection efficiency and trafficking inhibition, respectively.

Results showed that the different proteins affected differently the three CFTR conditions tested (**Figure 2**). **Table 4** summarizes the top seven siRNAs that, when transfected into the three cell lines, promoted the largest increases in CFTR trafficking efficiency.

Altogether, we observed that siRNAs GABARAP_1, NOS2_2, and SMURF1_2 elicited consistent increments in the trafficking and overall PM levels of VX-809-rescued F508del-, wt-, and untreated F508del-CFTR, respectively (**Figure 2**), prompting us to analyze their impact on overall CFTR function in CFBE cells.

Knockdown of GABARAP and NOS2 Modulates wt- and VX-809 Rescued F508del-CFTR Function in Opposite Ways

To test the effect of knocking down the expression of the three selected candidates on CFTR function, we used a widely used and previously validated functional assay, based on the ability of iodide to quench the fluorescence of the halide-sensitive YFP-F46L/H148Q/I152L mutant (HS-YFP) (Loureiro et al., 2015; Matos et al., 2018). As shown in **Figure 3**, knockdown of either SMURF1, NOS2, or GABARAP had no apparent

TABLE 3 | Hits selected for validation.

UniProt identifier	Gene	Protein	Specific neighbor of	Strong mediator of CFTR with
Q9H0R8	GABARAPL1	Gamma-aminobutyric acid receptor-associated protein-like 1 (Early estrogen-regulated protein) (GABA(A) receptor-associated protein-like 1) (Glandular epithelial cell protein 1) (GEC-1)	All sets	EZRIN, NHERF1, SYK
O95166	GABARAP	Gamma-aminobutyric acid receptor-associated protein (GABA(A) receptor-associated protein) (MM46)	All sets	NHERF1
P60520	GABARAPL2	Gamma-aminobutyric acid receptor-associated protein-like 2 (Early estrogen-regulated protein) (GABA(A) receptor-associated protein-like 2) (Glandular epithelial cell protein 2)	All sets	EPAC, EZRIN, NHERF1, SYK
P35228	NOS2	Nitric oxide synthase, inducible (EC 1.14.13.39) (Hepatocyte NOS) (HEP-NOS) (Inducible NO synthase) (Inducible NOS) (iNOS) (NOS type II) (Peptidyl-cysteine *S*-nitrosylase NOS2)	All sets	NHERF1
Q5S007	LRRK2	Leucine-rich repeat serine/threonine-protein kinase 2 (EC 2.7.11.1) (Dardarin)	All sets	EPAC, EZRIN, NHERF1, SYK
P35240	NF2	Merlin (Moesin-ezrin-radixin-like protein) (Neurofibromin-2) (Schwannomerlin) (Schwannomin)	All sets	EZRIN, NHERF1
Q13418	ILK	Integrin-linked protein kinase (EC 2.7.11.1) (59 kDa serine/threonine-protein kinase) (ILK-1) (ILK-2) (p59ILK)	All sets except pep-wt	
Q9HCE7	SMURF1	E3 ubiquitin-protein ligase SMURF1 (hSMURF1) (EC 2.3.2.26) (HECT-type E3 ubiquitin transferase SMURF1) (SMAD ubiquitination regulatory factor 1) (SMAD-specific E3 ubiquitin-protein ligase 1)	All sets except wt	NHERF1, SYK
Q8TF42	UBASH3B	Ubiquitin-associated and SH3 domain-containing protein B (EC 3.1.3.48) (Cbl-interacting protein p70) (Suppressor of T-cell receptor signaling 1) (STS-1) (T-cell ubiquitin ligand 2) (TULA-2) (Tyrosine-protein phosphatase STS1/TULA2)	All sets except wt	SYK
Q13618	CUL3	Cullin-3 (CUL-3)	All sets	EZRIN, NHERF1, SYK
P46940	IQGAP1	Ras GTPase-activating-like protein IQGAP1 (p195)	All sets except pep-py	EZRIN, NHERF1, SYK

effect on HS-YFP fluorescence in untreated F508del-CFTR cells, compared to control cells (siLUC). In contrast, following VX-809 treatment of cells to allow some F508del-CFTR protein to reach the PM, the downregulation of GABARAP produced a moderate but clear effect on HS-YFP quenching (**Figure 3A**), corresponding to a significant ($p < 0.05$) 1.4-fold increase in the initial iodide influx rate, as calculated from the exponential decay fit of quantified fluorescence values (**Figure 3A**). Interestingly, whereas the downregulation of either SMURF1 or NOS2 appeared to have no significant effect on rescued F508del-CFTR, the knockdown of NOS2 produced an apparent 40% decrease in influx rate, when compared to control (siLUC) cells (**Figure 3B**). Notably, similar and statistically significant opposite effects were observed upon the downregulation of GABARAP and NOS2 in wt-CFTR cells (**Figure 3A** and **C**). Moreover, despite showing no observable consequence in the trafficking assay, the increment produced by GABARAP knockdown in these cells was clearly pronounced, triggering a 2.9-fold faster CFTR response, even after endogenous cAMP reduction by pretreatment of the cells with 1 μM indomethacin, prior to stimulation with 5 μM Fsk. Also noteworthy, the knockdown of SMURF1, which failed to produce a clear increase in wt-CFTR PM signal in the trafficking assay, produced a significant ($p < 0.01$) over twofold stimulation of the iodide influx rate in these cells (**Figure 3C**). Overall, interference with either of the three candidate proteins interfered with functional activity of wt-CFTR, but only GABARAP and NOS2 affected the clinically relevant rescued F508delCFTR, producing opposite functional outputs.

GABARAP Knockdown Increases the PM Stability of VX809-Rescued F508del-CFTR

Because the absolute increment of VX-809-rescued F508del-CFTR at the cell surface exceeded that computed for its trafficking efficiency upon downregulation of GABARAP, we asked whether the observed increase in both CFTR PM abundance and ion transport would rather reflect an improved stability of the rescued channels at the PM. To test this, we used the previously described thermal shift assay (Loureiro et al., 2015). This assay employs the mCherry-Flag-F508del-CFTR CFBE cell line used for the trafficking assay but with a different experimental procedure. First, F508del-CFTR is rescued with VX-809 and then stabilized at the cell surface by incubating the cells at 30°C for 24 h. Next, cells are returned to 37°C for 4 h, which destabilizes the rescued mutant channels causing their endocytic removal from the cell surface, unless the tested co-treatment procedure is able to delay or prevent CFTR internalization. Cells are then stained as before and analyzed by confocal microscopy. Images of the cell surface are used to quantify the fluorescence signal corresponding to the amount of CFTR at the membrane (**Figure 4A**; see Materials and methods). We used treatment with HGF as a positive control, since this growth factor was previously shown to induce the retention of VX-809-rescued F508del CFTR at the cell surface (Moniz et al., 2013; Matos et al., 2018). Indeed, co-treatment with HGF not only increased the overall PM abundance of CFTR at 30°C, as it was able to promote the surface retention of ~80% of the rescued protein, upon switching to 37°C (**Figure 4B** and **C**), corresponding to ~70% of the wt protein at this temperature

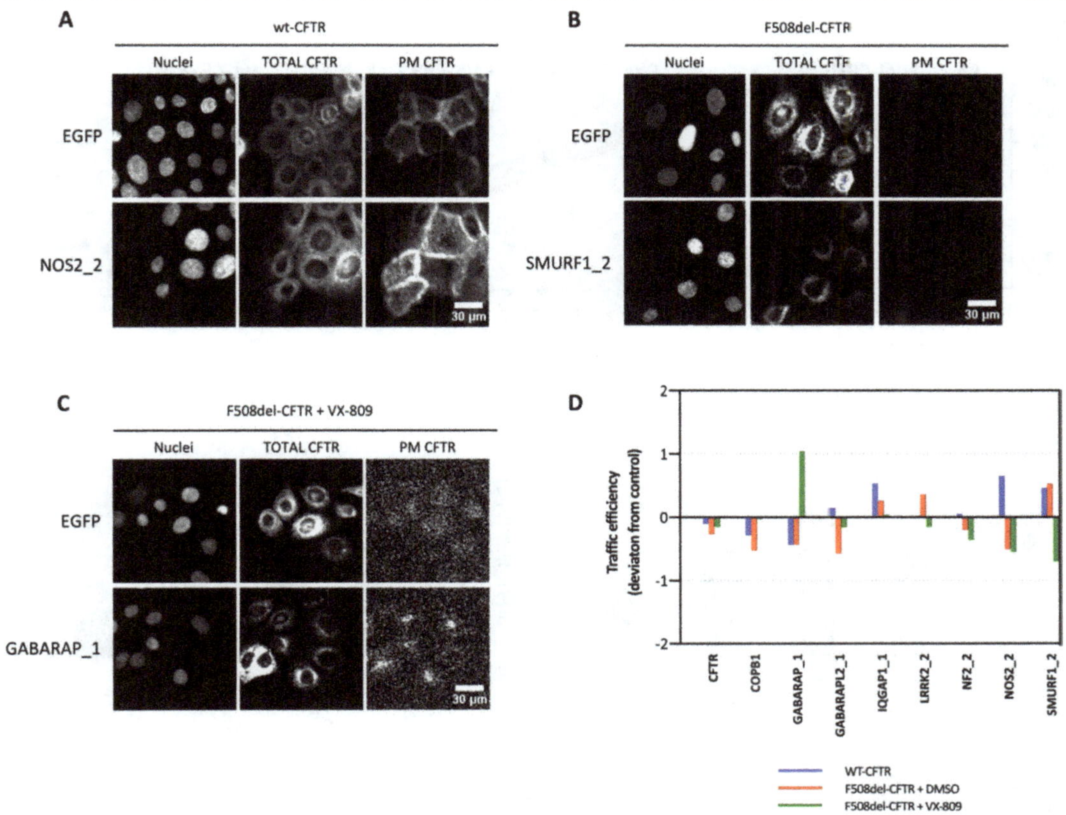

FIGURE 2 | CFTR trafficking upon knock-down of the possible hits. CFBE cell lines expressing mCherry-Flag-wt-, mCherry-Flag-F508del-, and mCherry-Flag-F508del-CFTR treated with VX-809 (3 µM for 48 h) under the control of a doxycycline-inducible promoter were transfected with siRNAs targeting CUL3, GABARAP, GABARAPL1, GABARAPL2, ILK, IQGAP1, LRRK2, NF2, NOS2, SMURF1, and UBASH3B. NT (non-treated cells) and COPB1 and EGFP (no-target siRNA) siRNA were used as controls. **(A–C)** Representative images for the three cell lines and one target for each cell line. PM CFTR image contrast was optimized after quantification to allow visualization of detected signal differences. **(D)** The CFTR traffic efficiency is obtained with the ratio PM/total CFTR with PM CFTR assessed by Flag staining (Cy5 fluorescence) and the amount of total CFTR with the mCherry signal. Data are shown as the deviation score as detailed in Formula 2, where positive values correspond to traffic efficiencies larger than the negative control (siRNA against EGFP) and negative values correspond to traffic efficiencies lower than the negative control, *n* = 3.

(**Figure 4C**). Importantly, the knockdown of GABARAP also partially prevented the internalization of rescued F508del-CFTR (**Figure 4B** and **C**). Albeit having a more moderate effect than HGF, the absence of GABARAP caused the retention of ~46% of the rescued protein at the cell surface at 37°C (~25% of wt-CFTR), which when compared to the ~30% control cells (siLUC; ~17% of wt-CFTR) reflects a ~1.5-fold increase in surface protein stability, in agreement with the observed extent of functional rescue.

DISCUSSION

In this work, we identified novel candidate proteins that are involved in the regulation of CFTR membrane traffic and/or its retention at the PM. The results were obtained based on experimental data from independent proteomic studies conducted in the host lab, namely, on PM CFTR levels following phosphorylation by SYK or the activation of EPAC1- or RAC1-mediated signaling. Subsequently,

TABLE 4 | Deviation score (DS)-based analysis of CFTR traffic efficiency for wt- or F508del-CFTR (incubated with either DMSO or VX-809) following the siRNA-mediated hit protein knockdown.

siRNA	$\langle DS_{wt} \rangle$	$\langle DS_{F508del} \rangle$	$\langle DS_{F508del+VX\text{-}809} \rangle$	$\Sigma \lvert \langle DS_i \rangle \rvert$	*p*
GABARAP_1	−0.433	−0.431	1.049	1.912	**0.013**
GABARAPL2_1	0.151	−0.570	−0.153	0.875	0.449
IQGAP1_1	0.536	0.264	0.044	0.844	0.479
LRRK2_2	0.031	0.364	−0.146	0.540	0.794
NF2_1	−0.701	0.319	−0.761	1.781	**0.023**
NOS2_2	0.650	−0.501	−0.549	1.701	**0.031**
SMURF1_2	0.463	0.533	−0.398	1.693	**0.032**

DS_i (i corresponding to wt-, F508del-, or F508del-CFTR+ VX-809) informs on the siRNA capacity to influence the traffic efficiency of a particular CFTR type. The sum of the three DS mean absolute values ($\Sigma \lvert \langle DS_i \rangle \rvert$) constitutes a global measure of the siRNA effect. Statistical significance (p) of these effects were calculated using a random permutation test (see Materials and Methods for details). Values highlighted in bold when significant.

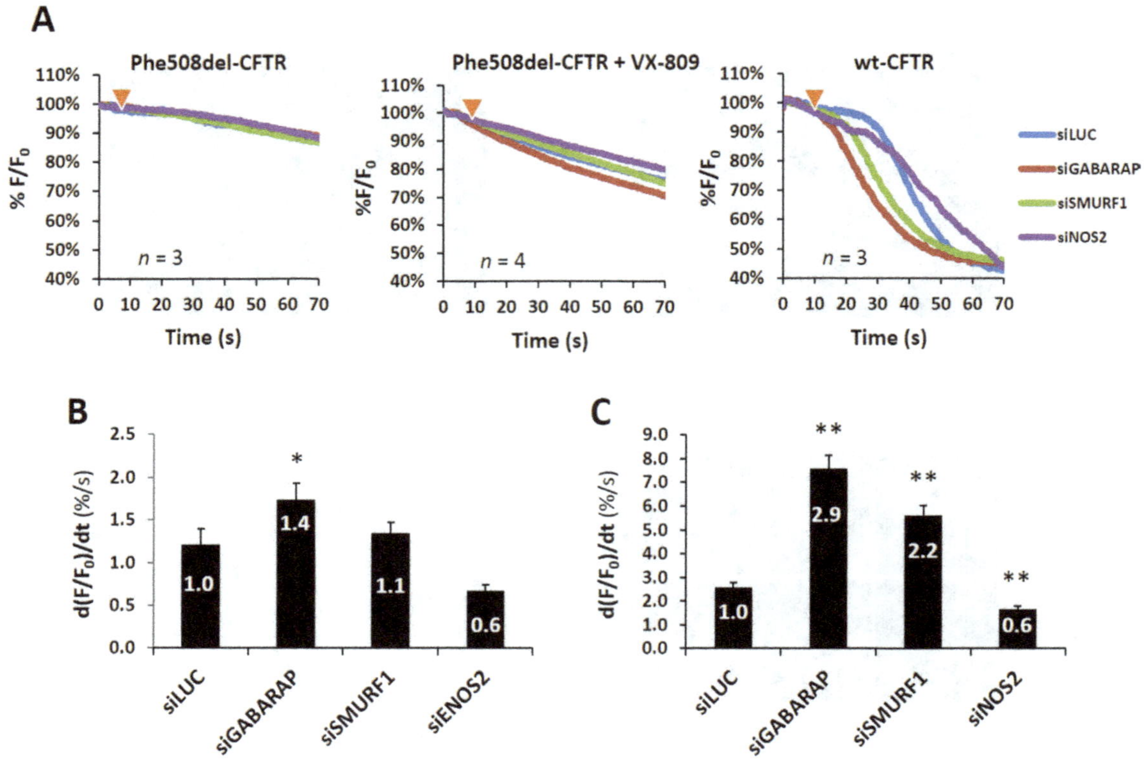

FIGURE 3 | Knockdown of selected candidate proteins influences wt- and F508del-CFTR function. **(A)** Representative fluorescence decay curves of the iodide influx assay. Wt- or F508del-CFBE cells stably expressing the HS-YFP sensor were transfected and treated for 48 h, as indicated. Fluorescence microscopy images were acquired continuously, first for 10 s (baseline) and then for 60 s after the rapid (≤1 s) addition of isosmotic buffer, containing 100 mM iodide together with either 5 μM Fsk (wt-CFTR cells) or 5 μM Fsk plus 20 μM Gen (F508del-CFTR cells). **(B)** Iodide influx rates from VX-809-treated (3 μM, 48 h) F508del-CFTR cells, transfected with the indicated siRNAs. The average fluorescence decay was fitted to an exponential decay function to derive the maximal slope [$d(F/F_0)/dt$, at $t = 0$] that is proportional to the initial influx of I⁻ into the cells. **(C)** Iodide influx rates, calculated as in **(B)**, for wt-CFTR CFBE cells, transfected as indicated. Data are means ± SEM of three independent assays. *$p < 0.05$; **$p < 0.01$.

the resulting interactomes were explored by computational network biology to identify novel protein nodes, never described before to interact with or regulate CFTR.

Recently, several authors have proposed network analysis methods to find novel proteins in common (or mediating the interactions) between two related network modules (Silberberg et al., 2017; Garcia-Vaquero et al., 2018). These candidate proteins may contribute to the common phenotypes associated with both modules. Here, we considered the different sets of CFTR interactors as network modules that have in common their potential role in regulating CFTR stability at the PM. To seek for novel proteins in common between these modules, we selected proteins specifically enriched in direct neighbors from at least two of the CFTR interactor sets. An analogous strategy has been successfully employed to expand the composition of disease-associated network modules (Ghiassian et al., 2015). This method requires candidates to have known direct interactions with module members, so it is limited by the completeness and accuracy of the accessed interaction databases. Our analysis is restricted to physical protein interactions, which will also limit our ability to find candidates regulating CFTR stability through indirect mechanisms such as expression regulation.

Besides the enrichment in protein localization and modification processes, the list of candidate proteins identified 12 (AHSA1, BAG3, COPS5, HDAC6, HSP90AB1, HSP90B1, HSPA5, LGLALS3BP, PABPC1, RACK1, USP19, and YBX1) out of 25 recently reviewed putative CFTR-interacting targets for restoring CFTR biogenesis and function identified through proteomic approaches (Lim et al., 2017). Both observations support the validity of our approach.

Among the novel protein nodes identified, the proteins encoded by the *GABARAP*, *NOS2*, and *SMURF1* genes were functionally validated in the physiologically relevant bronchio-epithelial cell line CFBE. For this, the expression of the endogenous proteins was depleted by RNA interference and the effect on PM localization and function of CFTR was analyzed.

NOS2 encodes the inducible isoform of nitric oxide synthase (NOS), which is expressed maximally following an inflammatory stimulus and produces relatively large micromolar quantities of NO. While macrophages and neutrophils express higher levels of iNOS in the lung, it can also be expressed by bronchial epithelial cells. NOS2 expression in these cells is upregulated by lipopolysaccharide (LPS) and by proinflammatory cytokines, such as interleukin-1, tumor necrosis factor alpha, and gamma interferon (Ermert et al., 2002). Expression of iNOS appears to be nearly absent in bronchial cells from CF patients (Meng et al., 1998; Thomas et al., 2000; Dotsch et al., 2002) and may be caused by abnormalities in the signaling system that normally causes its induction, such as cytokine receptors, second messengers, or transcription factors (Meng et al., 1998; Satitsri et al., 2016). Given the apparent negative

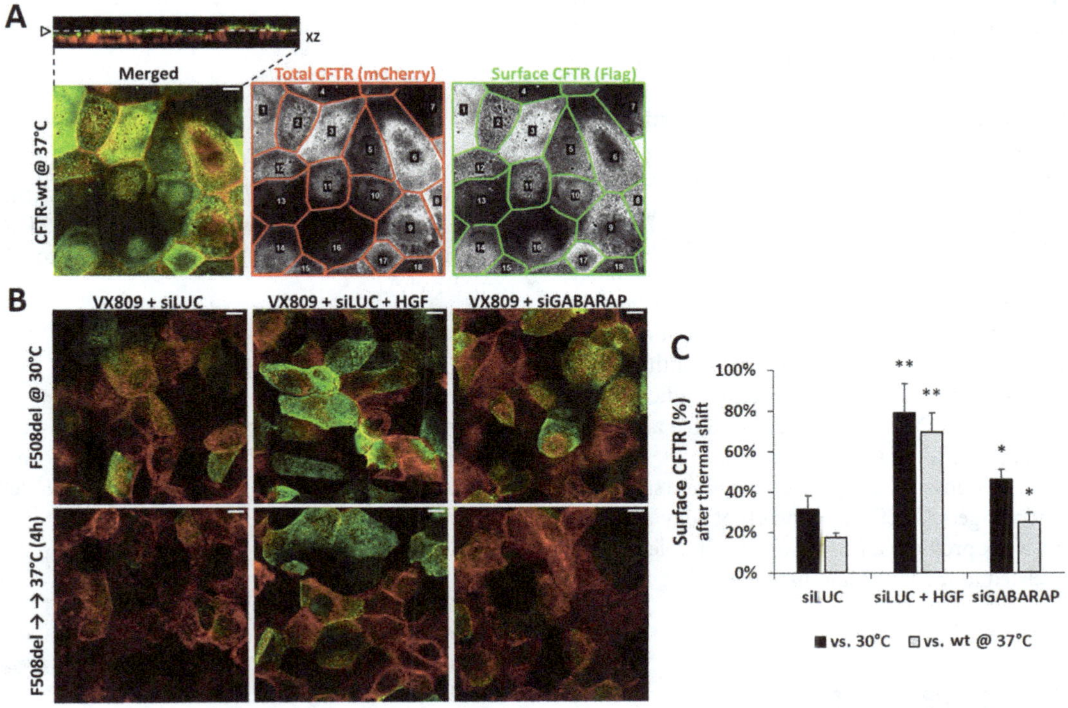

FIGURE 4 | GABARAP downregulation increases rescued F508del-CFTR PM abundance. **(A)** Confocal images of Dox-induced, mCherry-Flag-wt-CFTR expressing CFBE cells. Images are of double-labeled non-permeabilized cells, where mCherry fluorescence is proportional to the total amount of CFTR and Alexa Fluor 488 fluorescence is proportional to the amount of CFTR present at the cell surface. A 0.2-μm Z-stack of 1-Airy confocal images was acquired (top left inset) to select the best *XY* plane to analyze the CFTR protein at the cell surface. ImageJ software (NIH) was used to delimit each single cell as individual ROIs (regions of interest) to allow measurement of mCherry (red lined lattice) and Alexa488 (green lined lattice) fluorescence signal intensities. **(B)** Confocal images, obtained as in (A) of Dox-induced, VX-809-treated (3 μM, 48 h) mCherry-Flag-F508del-CFTR CFBE cells, transfected with either siLUC or siGABARAP and co-treated with 50 ng/ml HGF, when indicated. Cells were first pre-incubated for 24 h at 30°C to stabilize PM rescued F508del-CFTR and then moved to 37°C for 4 h to allow destabilization and internalization of the recued protein, unless otherwise prevented by the treatment conditions. White bars correspond to 10 μm. **(C)** Analysis of single-cell fluorescence signals in three independent experiments. Data presented refer to mean values ±SEM of three independent assays. CFTR at the surface was estimated by the ratio of Flag/mCherry signals in all conditions and expressed as percentage of surface F508del-CFTR at 30°C (siLUC, black bars) or surface wt-CFTR at 37°C (gray bars). $^{*}p < 0.05$; $^{**}p < 0.01$.

functional effect on both wt and VX-809-rescued F508del-CFTR observed here upon iNOS downregulation, our results suggest that, besides an improved resistance to microbial infection, any therapeutic approach that increased iNOS production in the airways might further benefit CF patients by stimulating residual CFTR function. This has, however, to be further investigated since, in a previous study, micromolar concentrations of NO were shown to inhibit forskolin-stimulated cAMP production by adenylyl cyclase and cAMP-dependent Cl^- transport and fluid secretion mediated by CFTR (Spirli et al., 2003).

SMURF1 functions as an E3 ubiquitin ligase protein and has been shown previously to regulate endocytosis of other membrane proteins such as the bone morphogenetic protein type II receptor (BMPR), related to pulmonary arterial hypertension. Blockage of SMURF1 ubiquitin ligase activity increased cell surface expression of BMPR (Murakami and Etlinger, 2019). Here, we observed that depletion of SMURF1 produced a twofold stimulation of the iodide influx rate in CFTR wt cells but did not promote any significant rescue of F508del-CFTR to the PM. Moreover, while endogenous cAMP depletion by pretreatment with indomethacin delayed the response to Fsk in control wt-CFTR CFBE cells, this effect was much less pronounced upon SMURF1 knockdown. This is suggestive that the knockdown of these proteins can have an effect not only in CFTR's PM abundance but also on its gating efficiency. Such an effect might nevertheless have therapeutic potential for class III to V CFTR mutations.

Similar effects were also observed upon knockdown of the GABA receptor-associated protein GABARAP, which belongs to the Atg8 family of ubiquitin-like proteins that are involved in the regulation of autophagy. GABARAP proteins associate with the membrane of the autophagosome through conjugation of phosphatidylethanolamine (Ichimura et al., 2000) and are primary drivers of autophagy working upstream of LC3 proteins and operate mainly at the late stages of autophagy driving the fusion of autophagosomes to lysosomes (Nguyen et al., 2016). Our results show that knockdown of GABARAP increased the temperature-dependent stability and function at the PM of F508del-CFTR after correction with VX-809. Furthermore, depletion of GABARAP also increased wt-CFTR function and, similar to SMURF1 knockdown, its response to Fsk stimulation after pretreatment with indomethacin. Since we observed no detectable impact of GABARAP downregulation on wt-CFTR traffic, it is possible that GABARAP may function by stabilizing the molecular machinery required to anchor and activate CFTR at the PM, thus increasing its gating efficiency. While the high levels of wt-CFTR at the surface may have led to an underestimation of fluorescence signals at the cell surface, the PM stabilizing effects observed with VX-809-rescued F508del-CFTR seem to support a functional potentiation hypothesis. In this case, interference with GABARAP activity may also prove beneficial for class III to class V CFTR mutations.

The identification of novel regulators of CFTR levels at the PM has important biomedical implications. The pharmacological rescue of mutant CFTR folding or gating improves symptoms in CF patients (Zhang et al., 2016); however, a truly relevant clinical benefit appears to require the targeting of additional cellular processes: the trafficking of CFTR as well as its retention at the PM (Farinha and Matos, 2016). The proteins identified here suggest that the cellular processes of membrane traffic, protein stabilization at the PM, and NO signaling are suitable targets for novel therapeutic approaches in CF.

Besides providing new insights into CFTR biology and suggesting possible therapeutic targets in CF, the network biology approach delineated in this work provides a framework applicable to other human diseases related to the traffic and function of PM transport proteins.

AUTHOR CONTRIBUTIONS

CL, JS, and AM conducted the experiments. PJ, CF, and PM designed the experimental studies. FP provided the network analysis. PJ, CF, PM, and FP analyzed the data and wrote the manuscript.

FUNDING

This work was supported by FCT, Portugal, through center grant UID/MULTI/04046/2019 to BioISI and the BioSys PhD program PD65-2012 (fellowships SFRH/BD/52488/2014, SFRH/BD/106084/2015, and SFRH/BD/52490/2014 to CL, JS, and AM, respectively).

ACKNOWLEDGMENTS

We would like to acknowledge technical support by the high-throughput imaging facility of BioISI and thank Prof. Margarida Amaral for providing the CFBE cells expressing mCherry-Flag-CFTR.

SUPPLEMENTARY MATERIAL

FIGURE S1 | qPCR assessment of siRNA efficiency in CFBE cells for the targeted transcript, $^{*}p < 0.05$.

TABLE S1 | Specific common neighbours of CFTR interactor sets.

TABLE S2 | Enriched biological processes in the list of strong mediator proteins.

REFERENCES

Almaca, J., Dahimene, S., Appel, N., Conrad, C., Kunzelmann, K., Pepperkok, R., et al. (2011). Functional genomics assays to study CFTR traffic and ENaC function. *Methods Mol. Biol.* 742, 249–264. doi: 10.1007/978-1-61779-120-8_15

Alonso-Lopez, D., Gutierrez, M. A., Lopes, K. P., Prieto, C., Santamaria, R., and De Las Rivas, J. (2016). APID interactomes: providing proteome-based interactomes with controlled quality for multiple species and derived networks. *Nucleic Acids Res.* 44, W529–535. doi: 10.1093/nar/gkw363

Amaral, M. D. (2005). Processing of CFTR: traversing the cellular maze—How much CFTR needs to go through to avoid cystic fibrosis? *Pediatr. Pulmonol.* 39, 479–491. doi: 10.1002/ppul.20168

Bos, J. L. (2006). Epac proteins: multi-purpose cAMP targets. *Trends Biochem. Sci.* 31, 680–686. doi: 10.1016/j.tibs.2006.10.002

Botelho, H. M., Uliyakina, I., Awatade, N. T., Proenca, M. C., Tischer, C., Sirianant, L., et al. (2015). Protein traffic disorders: an effective high-throughput fluorescence microscopy pipeline for drug discovery. *Sci. Rep.* 5, 9038. doi: 10.1038/srep09038

Carpenter, A. E., Jones, T. R., Lamprecht, M. R., Clarke, C., Kang, I. H., Friman, O., et al. (2006). CellProfiler: image analysis software for identifying and quantifying cell phenotypes. *Genome Biol.* 7, R100. doi: 10.1186/gb-2006-7-10-r100

Csardi, G. N., and Nepusz, T. (2006). The igraph software package for complex network research. *InterJournal Complex Syst.* 1695, 1–9.

Dalemans, W., Barbry, P., Champigny, G., Jallat, S., Dott, K., Dreyer, D., et al. (1991). Altered chloride ion channel kinetics associated with the delta F508 cystic fibrosis mutation. *Nature* 354, 526–528. doi: 10.1038/354526a0

Dotsch, J., Puls, J., Klimek, T., and Rascher, W. (2002). Reduction of neuronal and inducible nitric oxide synthase gene expression in patients with cystic fibrosis. *Eur. Arch. Otorhinolaryngol.* 259, 222–226. doi: 10.1007/s00405-001-0436-8

Ermert, M., Ruppert, C., Gunther, A., Duncker, H. R., Seeger, W., and Ermert, L. (2002). Cell-specific nitric oxide synthase-isoenzyme expression and regulation in response to endotoxin in intact rat lungs. *Lab. Invest.* 82, 425–441. doi: 10.1038/labinvest.3780436

Farinha, C., and Amaral, M. (2005). Most F508del-CFTR is targeted to degradation at an early folding checkpoint and independently of calnexin. *Mol. Cell. Biol.* 25, 5242–5252. doi: 10.1128/MCB.25.12.5242-5252.2005

Farinha, C. M., and Canato, S. (2017). From the endoplasmic reticulum to the plasma membrane: mechanisms of CFTR folding and trafficking. *Cell. Mol. Life Sci.* 74, 39–55. doi: 10.1007/s00018-016-2387-7

Farinha, C. M., and Matos, P. (2016). Repairing the basic defect in cystic fibrosis—One approach is not enough. *FEBS J.* 283, 246–264. doi: 10.1111/febs.13531

Farinha, C. M., Matos, P., and Amaral, M. D. (2013). Control of CFTR membrane trafficking: not just from the ER to the Golgi. *FEBS J.* 280, 4396–4406. doi: 10.1111/febs.12392

Galietta, L. J., Haggie, P. M., and Verkman, A. S. (2001). Green fluorescent protein-based halide indicators with improved chloride and iodide affinities. *FEBS Lett.* 499, 220–224. doi: 10.1016/S0014-5793(01)02561-3

Garcia-Vaquero, M. L., Gama-Carvalho, M., Rivas, J. L., and Pinto, F. R. (2018). Searching the overlap between network modules with specific betweeness (S2B) and its application to cross-disease analysis. *Sci. Rep.* 8, 11555. doi: 10.1038/s41598-018-29990-7

Ghiassian, S. D., Menche, J., and Barabasi, A. L. (2015). A DIseAse MOdule Detection (DIAMOnD) algorithm derived from a systematic analysis of connectivity patterns of disease proteins in the human interactome. *PLoS Comput. Biol.* 11, e1004120. doi: 10.1371/journal.pcbi.1004120

Guerra, L., Fanelli, T., Favia, M., Riccardi, S. M., Busco, G., Cardone, R. A., et al. (2005). Na+/H+ exchanger regulatory factor isoform 1 overexpression modulates cystic fibrosis transmembrane conductance regulator (CFTR) expression and activity in human airway 16HBE14o- cells and rescues DeltaF508 CFTR functional expression in cystic fibrosis cells. *J. Biol. Chem.* 280, 40925–40933. doi: 10.1074/jbc.M505103200

Guggino, W. B., and Stanton, B. A. (2006). New insights into cystic fibrosis:

molecular switches that regulate CFTR. *Nat. Rev. Mol. Cell Biol.* 7, 426–436. doi: 10.1038/nrm1949

Huang Da, W., Sherman, B. T., and Lempicki, R. A. (2009a). Bioinformatics enrichment tools: paths toward the comprehensive functional analysis of large gene lists. *Nucleic Acids Res.* 37, 1–13. doi: 10.1093/nar/gkn923

Huang Da, W., Sherman, B. T., and Lempicki, R. A. (2009b). Systematic and integrative analysis of large gene lists using DAVID bioinformatics resources. *Nat. Protoc.* 4, 44–57. doi: 10.1038/nprot.2008.211

Ichimura, Y., Kirisako, T., Takao, T., Satomi, Y., Shimonishi, Y., Ishihara, N., et al. (2000). A ubiquitin-like system mediates protein lipidation. *Nature* 408, 488–492. doi: 10.1038/35044114

Jensen, T. J., Loo, M. A., Pind, S., Williams, D. B., Goldberg, A. L., and Riordan, J. R. (1995). Multiple proteolytic systems, including the proteasome, contribute to CFTR processing. *Cell* 83, 129–135. doi: 10.1016/0092-8674(95)90241-4

Lim, S. H., Legere, E. A., Snider, J., and Stagljar, I. (2017). Recent progress in CFTR interactome mapping and its importance for cystic fibrosis. *Front. Pharmacol.* 8, 997. doi: 10.3389/fphar.2017.00997

Lobo, M. J., Amaral, M. D., Zaccolo, M., and Farinha, C. M. (2016). EPAC1 activation by cAMP stabilizes CFTR at the membrane by promoting its interaction with NHERF1. *J. Cell Sci.* 129, 2599–2612. doi: 10.1242/jcs.185629

Loureiro, C. A., Matos, A. M., Dias-Alves, A., Pereira, J. F., Uliyakina, I., Barros, P., et al. (2015). A molecular switch in the scaffold NHERF1 enables misfolded CFTR to evade the peripheral quality control checkpoint. *Sci. Signal* 8, ra48. doi: 10.1126/scisignal.aaa1580

Luz, S., Cihil, K. M., Brautigan, D. L., Amaral, M. D., Farinha, C. M., and Swiatecka-Urban, A. (2014). LMTK2-mediated phosphorylation regulates CFTR endocytosis in human airway epithelial cells. *J. Biol. Chem.* 289, 15080–15093. doi: 10.1074/jbc.M114.563742

Luz, S., Kongsuphol, P., Mendes, A. I., Romeiras, F., Sousa, M., Schreiber, R., et al. (2011). Contribution of casein kinase 2 and spleen tyrosine kinase to CFTR trafficking and protein kinase A-induced activity. *Mol. Cell. Biol.* 31, 4392–4404. doi: 10.1128/MCB.05517-11

Matos, A. M., Gomes-Duarte, A., Faria, M., Barros, P., Jordan, P., Amaral, M. D., et al. (2018). Prolonged co-treatment with HGF sustains epithelial integrity and improves pharmacological rescue of Phe508del-CFTR. *Sci. Rep.* 8, 13026. doi: 10.1038/s41598-018-31514-2

Matos, P., Oliveira, C., Velho, S., Goncalves, V., Da Costa, L. T., Moyer, M. P., et al. (2008). B-Raf(V600E) cooperates with alternative spliced Rac1b to sustain colorectal cancer cell survival. *Gastroenterology* 135, 899–906. doi: 10.1053/j.gastro.2008.05.052

Mendes, A. I., Matos, P., Moniz, S., Luz, S., Amaral, M. D., Farinha, C. M., et al. (2011). Antagonistic regulation of cystic fibrosis transmembrane conductance regulator cell surface expression by protein kinases WNK4 and spleen tyrosine kinase. *Mol. Cell. Biol.* 31, 4076–4086. doi: 10.1128/MCB.05152-11

Meng, Q. H., Springall, D. R., Bishop, A. E., Morgan, K., Evans, T. J., Habib, S., et al. (1998). Lack of inducible nitric oxide synthase in bronchial epithelium: a possible mechanism of susceptibility to infection in cystic fibrosis. *J. Pathol.* 184, 323–331. doi: 10.1002/(SICI)1096-9896(199803)184:3<323::AID-PATH2>3.0.CO;2-2

Moniz, S., Sousa, M., Moraes, B. J., Mendes, A. I., Palma, M., Barreto, C., et al. (2013). HGF stimulation of Rac1 signaling enhances pharmacological correction of the most prevalent cystic fibrosis mutant F508del-CFTR. *ACS Chem. Biol.* 8, 432–442. doi: 10.1021/cb300484r

Murakami, K., and Etlinger, J. D. (2019). Role of SMURF1 ubiquitin ligase in BMP receptor trafficking and signaling. *Cell. Signal.* 54, 139–149. doi: 10.1016/j.cellsig.2018.10.015

Nguyen, T. N., Padman, B. S., Usher, J., Oorschot, V., Ramm, G., and Lazarou, M. (2016). Atg8 family LC3/GABARAP proteins are crucial for autophagosome-lysosome fusion but not autophagosome formation during PINK1/Parkin mitophagy and starvation. *J. Cell Biol.* 215, 857–874. doi: 10.1083/jcb.201607039

Okiyoneda, T., Barriere, H., Bagdany, M., Rabeh, W. M., Du, K., Hohfeld, J., et al. (2010). Peripheral protein quality control removes unfolded CFTR from the plasma membrane. *Science* 329, 805–810. doi: 10.1126/science.1191542

Pankow, S., Bamberger, C., Calzolari, D., Martinez-Bartolome, S., Lavallee-Adam, M., Balch, W. E., et al. (2015). F508 CFTR interactome remodelling promotes rescue of cystic fibrosis. *Nature* 528, 510–516. doi: 10.1038/nature15729

Riordan, J. R. (2008). CFTR function and prospects for therapy. *Annu. Rev. Biochem.* 77, 701–726. doi: 10.1146/annurev.biochem.75.103004.142532

Rolland, T., Tasan, M., Charloteaux, B., Pevzner, S. J., Zhong, Q., Sahni, N., et al. (2014). A proteome-scale map of the human interactome network. *Cell* 159, 1212–1226. doi: 10.1016/j.cell.2014.10.050

Rual, J. F., Venkatesan, K., Hao, T., Hirozane-Kishikawa, T., Dricot, A., Li, N., et al. (2005). Towards a proteome-scale map of the human protein–protein interaction network. *Nature* 437, 1173–1178. doi: 10.1038/nature04209

Satitsri, S., Pongkorpsakol, P., Srimanote, P., Chatsudthipong, V., and Muanprasat, C. (2016). Pathophysiological mechanisms of diarrhea caused by the *Vibrio cholerae* O1 El Tor variant: an *in vivo* study in mice. *Virulence* 7, 789–805. doi: 10.1080/21505594.2016.1192743

Schultz, B. D., Singh, A. K., Devor, D. C., and Bridges, R. J. (1999). Pharmacology of CFTR chloride channel activity. *Physiol. Rev.* 79, S109–S144. doi: 10.1152/physrev.1999.79.1.S109

Sharma, M., Pampinella, F., Nemes, C., Benharouga, M., So, J., Du, K., et al. (2004). Misfolding diverts CFTR from recycling to degradation: quality control at early endosomes. *J. Cell Biol.* 164, 923–933. doi: 10.1083/jcb.200312018

Silberberg, Y., Kupiec, M., and Sharan, R. (2017). GLADIATOR: a global approach for elucidating disease modules. *Genome Med.* 9, 48. doi: 10.1186/s13073-017-0435-z

Spirli, C., Fabris, L., Duner, E., Fiorotto, R., Ballardini, G., Roskams, T., et al. (2003). Cytokine-stimulated nitric oxide production inhibits adenylyl cyclase and cAMP-dependent secretion in cholangiocytes. *Gastroenterology* 124, 737–753. doi: 10.1053/gast.2003.50100

Swiatecka-Urban, A., Brown, A., Moreau-Marquis, S., Renuka, J., Coutermarsh, B., Barnaby, R., et al. (2005). The short apical membrane half-life of rescued {Delta}F508-cystic fibrosis transmembrane conductance regulator (CFTR) results from accelerated endocytosis of {Delta}F508-CFTR in polarized human airway epithelial cells. *J. Biol. Chem.* 280, 36762–36772. doi: 10.1074/jbc.M508944200

Thomas, S. R., Kharitonov, S. A., Scott, S. F., Hodson, M. E., and Barnes, P. J. (2000). Nasal and exhaled nitric oxide is reduced in adult patients with cystic fibrosis and does not correlate with cystic fibrosis genotype. *Chest* 117, 1085–1089. doi: 10.1378/chest.117.4.1085

Venkatesan, K., Rual, J. F., Vazquez, A., Stelzl, U., Lemmens, I., Hirozane-Kishikawa, T., et al. (2009). An empirical framework for binary interactome mapping. *Nat. Methods* 6, 83–90. doi: 10.1038/nmeth.1280

Wang, X., Venable, J., Lapointe, P., Hutt, D. M., Koulov, A. V., Coppinger, J., et al. (2006). Hsp90 cochaperone Aha1 downregulation rescues misfolding of CFTR in cystic fibrosis. *Cell* 127, 803–815. doi: 10.1016/j.cell.2006.09.043

Yang, X., Coulombe-Huntington, J., Kang, S., Sheynkman, G. M., Hao, T., Richardson, A., et al. (2016). Widespread expansion of protein interaction capabilities by alternative splicing. *Cell* 164, 805–817. doi: 10.1016/j.cell.2016.01.029

Yu, H., Tardivo, L., Tam, S., Weiner, E., Gebreab, F., Fan, C., et al. (2011). Next-generation sequencing to generate interactome datasets. *Nat. Methods* 8, 478–480. doi: 10.1038/nmeth.1597

Zhang, W., Zhang, X., Zhang, Y. H., Strokes, D. C., and Naren, A. P. (2016). Lumacaftor/ivacaftor combination for cystic fibrosis patients homozygous for Phe508del-CFTR. *Drugs Today* 52, 229–237. doi: 10.1358/dot.2016.52.4.2467205

4

Human Primary Epithelial Cell Models: Promising Tools in the Era of Cystic Fibrosis Personalized Medicine

Nikhil T. Awatade[1,2†], Sharon L. Wong[1,2†], Chris K. Hewson[1,2,3], Laura K. Fawcett[1,2,4], Anthony Kicic[5,6,7,8,9], Adam Jaffe[1,2,4] and Shafagh A. Waters[1,2]*

[1] Faculty of Medicine, School of Women's and Children's Health, University of New South Wales, Sydney, NSW, Australia, [2] Molecular and Integrative Cystic Fibrosis Research Centre (miCF_RC), School of Medical Sciences, Faculty of Medicine, University of New South Wales, Sydney, NSW, Australia, [3] School of Biotechnology and Biomolecular Sciences, University of New South Wales, Sydney, NSW, Australia, [4] Department of Respiratory Medicine, Sydney Children's Hospital, Sydney, NSW, Australia, [5] Centre for Child Health Research, Telethon Kids Institute, The University of Western Australia, Nedlands, WA, Australia, [6] Occupation and Environment, School of Public Health, Curtin University, Bentley, WA, Australia, [7] Faculty of Health and Medical Sciences, The University of Western Australia, Nedlands, WA, Australia, [8] Department of Respiratory and Sleep Medicine, Perth Children's Hospital, Nedlands, WA, Australia, [9] Centre for Cell Therapy and Regenerative Medicine, School of Medicine and Pharmacology, The University of Western Australia, Nedlands, WA, Australia

***Correspondence:**
Shafagh A. Waters
shafagh.waters@unsw.edu.au

[†] These authors have contributed equally to this work

Cystic fibrosis (CF) is an inherited disorder where individual disease etiology and response to therapeutic intervention is impacted by CF transmembrane regulator (CFTR) mutations and other genetic modifiers. CFTR regulates multiple mechanisms in a diverse range of epithelial tissues. In this Review, we consolidate the latest updates in the development of primary epithelial cellular model systems relevant for CF. We discuss conventional two-dimensional (2-D) airway epithelial cell cultures, the backbone of *in vitro* cellular models to date, as well as improved expansion protocols to overcome finite supply of the cellular source. We highlight a range of strategies for establishment of three dimensional (3-D) airway and intestinal organoid models and evaluate the limitations and potential improvements in each system, focusing on their application in CF. The *in vitro* CFTR functional assays in patient-derived organoids allow for preclinical pharmacotherapy screening to identify responsive patients. It is likely that organoids will be an invaluable preclinical tool to unravel disease mechanisms, design novel treatments, and enable clinicians to provide personalized management for patients with CF.

Keywords: cystic fibrosis, organoid, personalized medicine, CFTR, drug development, sweat chloride, CFTR modulator

INTRODUCTION

Cystic Fibrosis (CF; OMIM 219700) is the most common life-limiting, autosomal recessive monogenic disease in Caucasian populations (Riordan, 2008). It is caused by mutations in the gene encoding CF transmembrane conductance regulator (CFTR), an anion channel essential for regulating trans-epithelial secretion of chloride (Cl^-) and bicarbonate (HCO_3^-). The loss of CFTR function leads to abnormalities at the mucosal surfaces in multiple exocrine organs including the lungs, pancreas, liver, and intestine. Notably however, progressive lung disease and respiratory failure are the major cause of morbidity and mortality for most patients (Ratjen et al., 2015). While the regulatory role of CFTR in ion and fluid transport is widely known, the exact mechanism of its defect in the development of CF remains debatable. Two competing hypotheses attempt to explain CF pathogenesis; (1) the "high salt" hypothesis postulates that diminished trans-epithelial Cl^- conductance associated with CFTR dysfunction results in increased retention of salt at the mucosal surface, which negates the activity of antimicrobial peptides present in the epithelial apical secretions (Zabner et al., 1998; Wine, 1999); (2) the more favorable "low volume" hypothesis suggests the lack of epithelial sodium channel (ENaC) inhibition in the absence of CFTR function causes sodium (Na^+) hyper-absorption, with accompanying intracellular flux of Cl^- and water (Matsui et al., 1998; Wine, 1999). Mucus becomes dehydrated, viscous and sticky which then leads to decreased airway surface liquid (ASL) height, as well as mucus stasis and obstruction (Riordan, 2008). Irrespective of the mechanism of action, impaired mucociliary clearance in the lung and the innate inability to eradicate inhaled pathological agents are hallmarks of CF. Recurrent cycles of lung infection and exacerbations result in chronic inflammatory responses which then lead to structural lung damage, loss of lung function, and ultimately respiratory insufficiency (Ratjen et al., 2015).

Major advances in symptom management have been instrumental in delaying disease progression in CF. Administration of enzyme replacement therapy, nutritional support, mucolytic agents airway clearance techniques, and antibiotics for bacterial lung infection, along with early detection of disease (newborn screening, pathogen surveillance) has dramatically improved life expectancy in CF patients over the last 4 decades. The median age of death is now above 40 years (Keogh et al., 2018). Importantly, a class of small molecule compounds termed CFTR modulators were recently discovered. These compounds directly correct defective CFTR protein in CF patients and have now transformed the therapeutic landscape of CF in a precision-based fashion. The first part of this review outlines the current developments in CFTR modulators addressing the different dysfunctional CFTR mutation class and highlights the need for individualized strategies to restore their function.

The second part of this review discusses the evolving use of different epithelial cell models and reporter assays for assessing clinical response to CFTR-directed drugs on a personalized basis, and highlights the strengths and limitations of each application. This review also elaborates on the breakthrough discoveries of long-term cultures of patient-derived 3-dimentional (3-D) airway and rectal organoids. We also discuss their emerging use as *ex vivo* biomarkers and preclinical predictive tools for the disease.

CURRENT CFTR-BASED THERAPY WITH CFTR MODULATORS

More than 2,000 CFTR mutations have been identified so far and at least 336 of these are reported to lead to symptoms characteristic of CF (Cystic Fibrosis Mutations Database report 31 August 2018 (US CF Foundation, 2011). It is thus perceivable that a multi-pronged approach is required to target the different defective mechanisms that each CFTR mutation confers. For the past 15 years, high-throughput screening (HTS) has accelerated the process of drug discovery. To identify candidate CFTR modulators, hundreds of thousands of chemical compounds with diverse structures were screened and the potential of a compound to rescue or activate CFTR was tested in cellular-based assays (Pedemonte et al., 2005; Van Goor et al., 2006; Sutanto et al., 2018). The promising compounds, called "hits," underwent further medicinal and chemical optimization to improve potency and minimize potential off-target activities of the compounds. This process has led to successful identification of multiple compounds, some of which have moved forward to human clinical trials.

The different approaches targeted toward correcting each CFTR mutation class as well as the compounds currently tested in clinical trials are summarized in **Table 1**. CFTR-modulating compounds are classified into five main groups: read-through agents, correctors, potentiators, stabilizers, and amplifiers. Of these, two classes of modulators (potentiators and correctors) have gained regulatory approval to treat CF patients with specific CFTR mutations.

Potentiators

Potentiators were developed for CFTR mutant proteins that are expressed at the apical membrane of epithelial cells but are functionally impaired. HTS performed by Vertex pharmaceuticals involving 280,000 small molecule compounds led to the discovery of the potentiator VX-770 (Generic name: Ivacaftor; Trade name: Kalydeco) (Van Goor et al., 2010). Ivacaftor corrects the gating impairment of Class III mutations. Its use has now been extended beyond the most common Class III G551D-CFTR mutation, to additional Class III mutations, as well as CFTR mutations with conductance (Class IV−R117H) or biosynthesis (Class V−3,849 + 10 kb C>T) defects. In clinical studies of participants with G551D-CFTR mutations, the impact of Ivacaftor on CFTR was evidenced by normalization of sweat Cl^-, improved lung function (10% mean increase in FEV_1), reduced episodes of pulmonary exacerbations and improved body mass index (BMI) (Accurso et al., 2010; Ramsey et al., 2011; Davies et al., 2013).

Correctors

The potentiators' mode of action does not benefit the majority of the CF population who have the Class II F508del-CFTR mutation, as F508del-CFTR is degraded while transitioning

Abbreviations: 2-D, 2-Dimensional; 3-D, 3-Dimensional; ALI, Air-liquid interface; ASL, Airway surface liquid; BAL, Bronchoalveolar lavage; BEGM, Bronchial epithelial growth media; BMI, Body mass index; BMP, Bone morphogenic protein; CaCC, Calcium-activated chloride channels; CF, Cystic Fibrosis; CFTR, Cystic Fibrosis transmembrane conductance regulator; Cl^-, Chloride; CRCs, Conditionally reprogrammed cells; DMSO, Dimethyl sulfoxide; ECM, Extracellular matrix; ENaC, Epithelial sodium channel; FEV1, Forced expiratory volume—one second; FIS, Forskolin-induced swelling; FRT, Fischer rat thyroid; HAE, Human airway epithelial; HBE, Human bronchial epithelial; HCO_3^-, Bicarbonate; HNE, Human nasal epithelial; HTS, High-throughput screening; ICM, Intestinal current measurement; Na^+, Sodium; P#, Passage #; PTC, Premature termination codon; ROCK, Rho-associated protein kinase; TEER, Trans-epithelial electrical resistance; TGF-β, Transforming growth factor-beta.

TABLE 1 | CFTR mutation class and current modulator therapeutic approach.

Mutation class	Molecular defect	Type of mutation	Therapeutic approach	Approved or drugs in clinical trial	Mutation examples
IA~	No mRNA synthesis	Large deletions	Bypass therapies (Activate alternative Cl⁻ channels)	–	Dele2, 3(21 kb) 1717-1G->A 621+1G->T
IB~	Protein synthesis	Nonsense (PTC), Frame-shift, Splicing	Read-through compounds	Phase 2: QBW276, SPX-101 Phase 1: AZD5634, BI443651	G542X, W1282X
II	Trafficking	Missense	Correctors and potentiators	Approved: Orkambi, Symdeko Phase 3: VX-445#, VX-659# Phase 2: VX-152#, VX-440#, GLPG2222, GLPG2737, FDL169 Phase 1: PTI-801	F508del, R560T, A561E
III	Channel Gating	Missense	Potentiators	Approved: Ivacaftor Phase 2: VX-561, QBW251, GLPG1837, GLPG2451, GLPG3067 Phase 1: PTI-808	G551D, S1251N, G178R
IV	Conductance	Missense	Potentiators	Approved: Ivacaftor	R334W, R347P, R117H
V	Protein synthesis	Missense, Alternative splicing	Correctors, Potentiators, Antisense Oligonucleotides	Approved: Ivacaftor	3849+10kbC>T, 3272-26A>G, 2789+5G>A
VI	Reduced CFTR stability at PM	Missense, Frameshift	Stabilizers	–	120del23, N287Y, Q1412X

Compounds starting with VX are developed by Vertex Pharmaceuticals, GLPG by Galapagos NV and AbbVie, FDL, Flatley discovery lab; QBW, Novartis pharmaceuticals; PTI, Proteostasis therapeutics; SPX, Spyryx biosciences; AZD, AstraZeneca; BI, Boehringer ingelheim; Orkambi, VX-809+VX-770; Symdeko, VX-661+VX-770; Ivacaftor, VX-770; # Triple combination therapy with VX-661 and VX-770. PTC, Premature termination codons; PM, Plasma membrane; ~, classification is based on (Marson et al., 2016).

through the endoplasmic reticulum, with very little or no mutant protein reaching the apical membrane of epithelial cell. Effective rescue of the F508del mutation thus requires chaperones that can repair defective protein folding and rescue trafficking of the mature CFTR to the plasma membrane. VX-809 (Generic name: Lumacaftor; available as Lumacaftor-Ivacaftor combination therapy—Trade name Orkambi) restored F508del-CFTR channel activity to 15% of wild-type CFTR in *in vitro* preclinical testing performed in primary airway epithelial cells (Van Goor et al., 2012). This result led to Lumacaftor monotherapy clinical trials in CF patients homozygous for the F508del-CFTR mutation, where a significant improvement in sweat Cl^- concentrations were observed but lung function remained unchanged (Clancy et al., 2017). Considering that F508del channel gating defect, administration of Lumacaftor-Ivacaftor combination therapy was proposed as a solution that may augment correction of CFTR function to clinically significant levels.

Combination Therapy

Lumacaftor-Ivacaftor combination therapy increased CFTR activity at the plasma membrane *in vitro* (Van Goor et al., 2012). However, results from phase III trials in children and adults homozygous for the F508del-CFTR mutation showed that the combination therapy failed to produce the magnitude of clinical improvements observed with Ivacaftor. While a reduction in pulmonary exacerbations and improved BMI was observed, there was only a modest improvement in lung function (2–3%) (Boyle et al., 2014; Wainwright et al., 2015). In addition, CF patients receiving Lumacaftor-Ivacaftor combination therapy reported unwanted side effects such as dyspnoea, liver damage, and bronchospasm. Lumacaftor is also associated with significant drug-drug interactions which alter its pharmacokinetic profile and potentially hamper its therapeutic efficacy (Talamo Guevara and McColley, 2017). Tezacaftor is a new CFTR corrector with an improved pharmacokinetic profile, longer half-life and less drug-drug interactions compared to Lumacaftor. It has recently been approved as a combination therapy with Ivacaftor (Trade name: Symdeko/Symveki) for the treatment of patients homozygous for F508del mutation by the Food and Drug Administration (FDA) and European Medicines Agency. Phase III clinical trials data showed that improvement in lung function with Tezacaftor-Ivacaftor combination therapy was generally comparable or better than those observed in patients treated with Lumacaftor-Ivacaftor combination therapy (Rowe et al., 2017; Taylor-Cousar et al., 2017). It is notable however that while overall benefit was demonstrated, individual patient responses have been heterogeneous in the clinical trials of both Lumacaftor-Ivacaftor and Tezacaftor-Ivacaftor.

Theratyping

It is now known that patients display a spectrum of responses to CFTR-modulator drugs despite having the same CFTR mutation variant (Wainwright et al., 2015; Donaldson et al., 2018). This suggests that although the current classification system may be an important indicator for prognosis and disease severity in CF, it is inadequate for predicting how individual patients respond to therapy. Indeed, *in vitro* experimental studies have shown that contrary to findings in the Class II F508del-CFTR mutation, other Class II processing mutations such as N1303K, R560S, and G85E could not be rescued by Lumacaftor treatment (Awatade et al., 2015, 2018; Dekkers et al., 2016b; Lopes-Pacheco et al.,

2017). These results suggest that the underlying pathomechanism of each CFTR mutation is distinct and that individualized strategies to restore their function may be warranted.

To address this, CFTR mutations have been classified according to their response to modulator compounds. This approach termed "theratyping," groups together patients who harbor different CFTR mutations but respond to the same CFTR-directed compounds. It is clear that treatment regimens of the future will need to take into consideration the individual's genetic makeup and not just their CFTR mutations. A personalized approach will optimize patient's clinical outcomes by accounting for the specific genetic mutations of the individual patient.

TOWARD PERSONALIZED MODULATOR THERAPY

One of the major hurdles to the development of novel treatment regimens in CF is the bench-to-bedside translation of scientific knowledge. Many drugs that perform well in a laboratory setting fail to advance in clinical trials, largely due to inappropriate selection of *in vivo* and *in vitro* models for HTS. In the context of CF, animal models and immortalized epithelial cell lines do not fully portray patient-specific disease phenotypes. Animal models of CF have provided insights into disease pathophysiology. However, their generation is time consuming, expensive, and more importantly they poorly represent the full repertoire of disease manifestations in individual patients. For instance, mouse models of CF do not have lung disease and bacterial infections, attributed to the compensatory effect of a secondary Cl^- ion channel (Lavelle et al., 2016). On the other hand, immortalized epithelial cell lines derived from primary patient material have contributed tremendously to CF research, but not without limitations. Their generation from primary patient material is very inefficient. It involves extensive adaptation and selection to *in vitro* 2-D culture conditions, as only rare clones are able to expand and be maintained over many passages. Furthermore, these cell lines may have undergone substantial genetic changes and no longer retain features of the original parental cells. Drug development pipeline for new CFTR-directed compounds have relied heavily on unpolarized Fischer rat thyroid (FRT) epithelial cell lines. It is thus not surprising that this model has a higher propensity of false-positive and false-negative "hits" compared to that performed in primary human bronchial epithelial (HBE) cells.

PATIENT-DERIVED ORGANOTYPIC CELLULAR MODELS FOR PERSONALIZED MEDICINE

Although CF is a monogenic disease, the diverse mutation variants identified within the CFTR gene as well as the presence of modifier genes (known and unknown), warrants adoption of new technologies to extend research capabilities. There is a clear unmet need for a representative library of patient-specific epithelial cell models for disease modeling, preclinical testing of drug response, and biobanking for future drug discovery. The cell models can be derived from embryonic stem cells (ESCs), induced pluripotent stem cells (iPSCs), or tissue-resident adult stem cells. Whereas, ethical concerns pertaining the source of human ESC, limit their use in research, generation of CFTR gene corrected iPSC lines enable disease modeling, drug discovery and toxicology studies [reviewed in (Pollard and Pollard, 2018)]. In this Review, we focus on airway and intestine epithelium models derived from adult stem cells.

Human Airway Epithelial (HAE) Cells

The pulmonary epithelium is divided into three regions; upper (nasal and oral cavities), lower (trachea and primary bronchi), and distal small airway epithelia (alveolar). Persistent inflammation, bacterial colonization, and airway structural changes in CF occur in the lower respiratory tract. Primary HBE cells are therefore the gold standard for studying CF disease pathogenesis and evaluating CFTR functional response (Van Goor et al., 2006; Awatade et al., 2015). HBE cells can be isolated from biopsy samples, lung explants and cadavers. Explanted lung and post-mortem samples from individuals with CF provide high cell yield. However, the extensive damage to the tissue, particularly the epithelial cell layer, plus the presence of chronic microbial colonization present technical challenges to establishing successful *ex vivo* cultures. Acquisition of airway biopsies or brushings involves highly invasive procedures, while bronchoalveolar lavage (BAL) fluid and induced sputum samples usually do not provide sufficient cell counts to initiate culture. Therefore, supply of CF patient-derived HBE cells are often limited and hard to come by.

Human nasal epithelial (HNE) cells are increasingly used as surrogates for the lower airway epithelium in CF research (de Courcey et al., 2012; Brewington et al., 2018a). HNE cells demonstrate many characteristics common to HBE cells including the ability to form polarized, pseudostratified epithelium mimicking *in vivo* airways and the expression of ion channels such as CFTR. Their advantage is the lack of need for invasive procurement (Clarke et al., 2013). HNE cells are grown using the same culture media and protocol as for HBE cells.

Human Airway Epithelial (HAE) Cell Culture Models

Primary human airway epithelial cells are conventionally cultured as monolayers (2-D cultures). Expansion of epithelial cells is often necessary in the initial passages for biobanking purposes and to generate enough cell numbers needed to differentiate cells under air-liquid interface (ALI) conditions. HBE cells are most "*in vivo*" like when fully differentiated; they display a striking phenotypic resemblance to the lower airway epithelium. They form pseudostratified epithelium with mucociliary differentiation indicated by the presence of functional beating cilia and mucus secretion. They also exhibit characteristic epithelial barrier functions, including expression of cell junctional proteins and the development of robust trans-epithelial electrical resistance (TEER) values (Berube et al., 2010). The polarized, differentiated phenotype is critical for *in vitro* measurement of CFTR function as the protein is primarily expressed at the apical surface of ciliated cells. While ALI cultures accurately represent *in vivo* phenotypes, their wider use is deterred by limited propagation of cells in culture, attributed to squamous transformation and cellular senescence (Gentzsch et al., 2017). To date, three expansion methods have been used to extend the lifespan of cells and delay cellular senescence beyond that of the standard cultures.

Improved Cell Expansion Culture Methods

Conditionally reprogrammed cells (CRCs) are generated by co-culturing patient-derived airway epithelial cells with irradiated fibroblast feeder cells. Specialized conditioned media (termed F-Media) which contains Rho-associated protein kinase (ROCK) inhibitor, promotes serial passages of airway epithelial cells and enhances population doubling without compromising the characteristic epithelial cell morphology. Both ROCK inhibitor and the feeder layer are essential in maintaining the stem cell-like phenotype evident in CRCs (Reynolds et al., 2016; Martinovich et al., 2017). Their removal results in differentiated cell lines, with intact barrier function and the ability to polarize and form mucociliary epithelium. CFTR-mediated Cl^- transport in these cells is also preserved.

A modified CRCs protocol using BEGM, ROCK inhibitor and an irradiated feeder layer cultured in reduced oxygen concentration (2%) demonstrated some advantage over the standard CRCs. The modified CRCs could support airway epithelial cell growth up to passage 10 with robust formation of pseudostratified epithelium at the extended passage, although a modest decrease in CFTR-dependent Cl^- transport was observed. Meanwhile, reduced numbers of ciliated cells and goblet cells were observed in standard CRCs cultures at P10 and robust TEER could not be established (Peters-Hall et al., 2018).

A feeder-free culture protocol that relies on disruption of SMAD signaling pathway through inhibition of dual ligands, transforming growth factor-beta (TGF-β) and bone morphogenic protein (BMP), showed airway epithelial cells could be expanded up to 18–25 passages without loss of proliferative potential (Mou et al., 2016). Combined TGF-β/BMP inhibition led to basal cell hyperplasia with hyper-proliferative p63 cells (basal cell marker) and produced homogenous, tightly packed cells, resembling stem cell morphology. Epithelial cells expanded using dual SMAD inhibition method can undergo mucociliary differentiation up to P12 with preserved TEER although Na^+ currents and Cl^- conductance declined fairly rapidly after serial passage 6 (Mou et al., 2016).

Three-Dimensional Airway Spheroids and Organoids

Two-D cultures lack a third dimension, the scaffolding extracellular matrix (ECM), which establishes intercellular cues or network in the *in vivo* airway epithelium. Therefore, 3-D cell cultures are a major area of development, where cells are cultured in a matrix (such as matrigel) or are cultured in such a manner that they develop ECM-like scaffolds between them, thus mimicking the *in vivo* phenotype more faithfully. While cell-derived ECMs such as Matrigel have been most commonly used for development of organoids, their undefined components introduce inconsistency in replicating the native 3-D culture environment (Czerwinski and Spence, 2017). To overcome this challenge, new biomaterial systems, such as polymers and hydrogels are being developed [reviewed in (Dye et al., 2017)].

Different methods for generating organoids (or spheroids) from human lung cells have been described to date, each producing organoids with distinct definitive structure and cellular compositions. Barkauskas and colleagues have elegantly reviewed the different lung organoids (airway organoids inclusive) established from varying lung progenitor cell populations, including basal cells in the proximal airways, secretory club Clara cells in bronchioles and alveolar type II cells in the alveoli, as well as those from embryonic and iPSCs (Barkauskas et al., 2017). Given CFTR is primarily expressed at the apical surface of ciliated cells and recently discovered in the pulmonary ionocytes in tracheal epithelium (Montoro et al., 2018; Plasschaert et al., 2018), only airway organoids displaying proximal differentiation are discussed here in light of their relevance for measuring CFTR functional response (**Table 2**).

Three-Dimensional Airway Explant Spheroid (ECM—Free)

Airway spheroid cultures were first described in 1991 when nasal epithelial multicellular spheroids were generated from non-dissociated nasal epithelial sheets (Bridges et al., 1991). These explant spheroids were maintained in culture media (no matrigel) and were reported to form rapidly, within 2–5 days. Explant spheroids have an apical-membrane-out orientation; apical ciliated cells face the media bath and the basolateral membrane lines the fluid-filled lumen (Bridges et al., 1991). Pedersen and colleagues later found amiloride-sensitive Na^+ transport drives changes in the lumen size, suggesting nasal spheroids may be a useful model for ion/fluid transport studies and for investigating diseases associated with defective ion channels such as cystic fibrosis (Pedersen et al., 1999). Nasal spheroids were also responsive to forskolin stimulation (Guimbellot et al., 2017). As the CFTR-expressing apical side of nasal spheroids face outward, forskolin causes the outflow of fluid from the lumen to the exterior bath and the spheroids to shrink in size. This response was blunted in spheroids established from CF patients but could be partially rescued by CFTR modulators (Guimbellot et al., 2017). Notably, successful spheroids have also been established from bronchial brushings, although CFTR function was not tested in the study (Deslee et al., 2007). Interestingly, no evidence of cell proliferation was observed throughout the nasal spheroid formation process and the spheroids plateaued in size once fully formed. This suggests that the spheroids are self-organizing aggregates of terminally differentiated epithelial cells only (Castillon et al., 2002). While spheroids may be ready for *ex vivo* CFTR measurement rapidly, they are short-lived, lasting for up to 12 weeks only and biobanking for future drug screening is not possible (Guimbellot et al., 2017).

Three-Dimensional Spheroid From Airway Basal Progenitor Cells

Airway spheroids, both bronchial and nasal can also be derived from primary airway basal cells embedded in the

TABLE 2 | Comparison of three-dimensional organotypic airway epithelial culture methods.

	Respiratory—nasal and bronchial			
	Airway explant spheroid	**Airway basal cell spheroid**		**Long term expanding airway organoid**
		Method 1—Dome	**Method 2–25% layer**	
Cultures	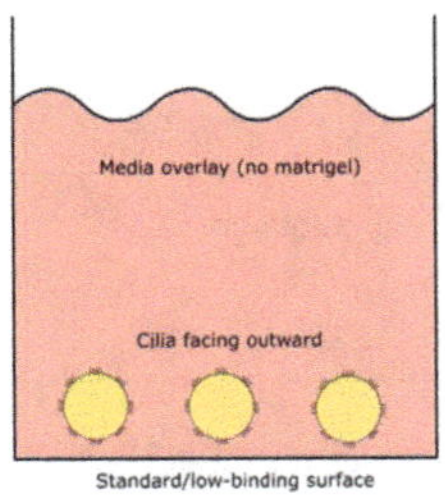	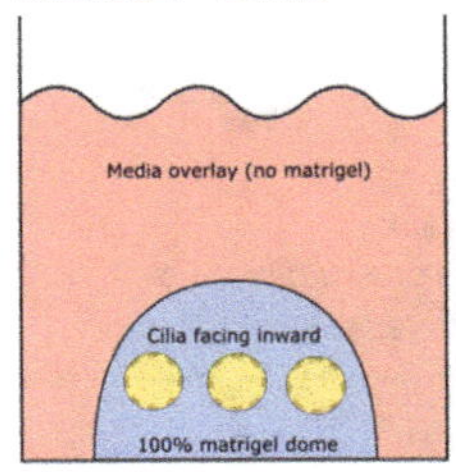	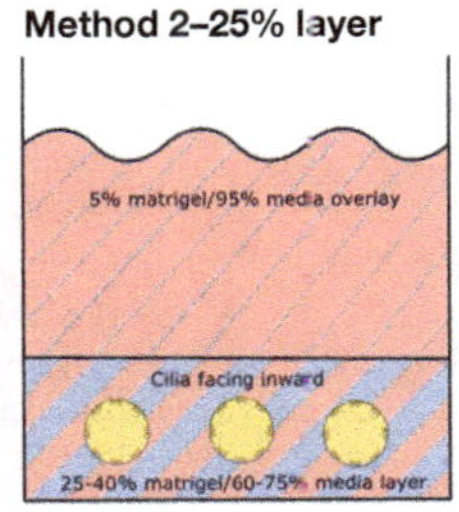	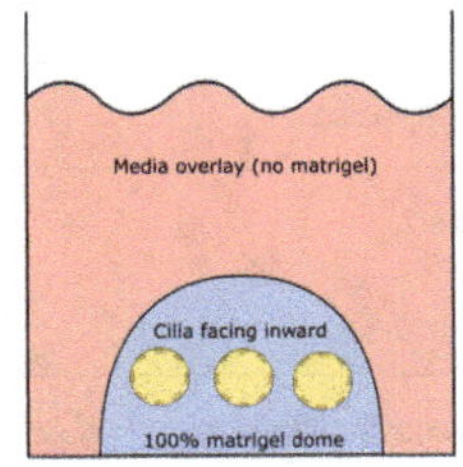
Cellular source	Freshly isolated non-dissociated airway epithelial sheets	Airway basal progenitor cells expanded as traditional primary cultures or conditionally reprogrammed cultures		Lung biopsies and cells from BAL fluid
Media	Standard, non-differentiating culture media e.g., BEGM	Differentiation media—same as those used for 2D ALI cultures		Media containing biochemical cues for self-renewal. Content: Advanced DMEM/F12 R-Spondin 1 Noggin FGF 7 FGF 10 A83-01 Y-27632 SB202190 B27 supplement N-Acetylcysteine Nicotinamide Glutamax
Require ECM (matrigel)	No	Yes		Yes
Constitute differentiated epithelium structure	Yes (*ex vivo*—already differentiated)	Yes (after 14–21 days culture)		Yes (duration to form not reported)
Orientation of apical ciliated side	Facing outwards (media)	Facing inwards (lumen)		Facing inwards (lumen)
Use of cultures	End-point experiments	End-point experiments		Can be passaged for on-going cultures (reported up to P18)
CFTR functional assay	Yes—spheroids shrink when CFTR is activated	Yes—spheroids swell when CFTR is activated		Yes—spheroids swell when CFTR is activated
Cryopreservation	No	No		Not reported
References	Bridges et al., 1991 Pedersen et al., 1999 Deslee et al., 2007 Guimbellot et al., 2017	Danahay et al., 2015 Hild and Jaffe, 2016 Brewington et al., 2018c		Sachs et al., 2018 Zhou et al., 2018

2D, Two-dimensional; ALI, Air-liquid interphase; BAL, Bronchoalveolar lavage; BEGM, Bronchial epithelial cell growth media; ECM, Extracellular matrix; FGF, Fibroblast growth factor; TGF-β, Transforming growth factor-beta.

basement membrane matrix matrigel (Hild and Jaffe, 2016; Brewington et al., 2018c). Matrigel is fundamental for the formation of intact spheroids, with a lumen surrounded by a slightly thickened wall upon maturity (7–14 days) and a complete cell-apex-in morphology (Danahay et al., 2015; Brewington et al., 2018c). Different culture protocols using varying concentrations of matrigel have been reported; (1) cells are resuspended in 100% matrigel and seeded as spherical drops, then overlaid with ALI differentiation media; (2) cells are resuspended in 5% matrigel with ALI differentiation media and then layered over a denser 25–40% matrigel base layer which the cells sink into (Hild and Jaffe, 2016; Tan et al., 2017; Brewington et al., 2018c). Method 1 (100% matrigel) was reported to yield the best success, as the sinking method could result in formation of some spheroids with cell-apex-out morphology and disorganized cellular aggregates (Brewington et al., 2018b), likely due to incomplete embedding of cells in the denser matrigel base layer e.g., growing on top of

TABLE 3 | Comparison of human cell models relevant for CF therapeutic application.

Cell models	Established immortalized cell lines	Pulmonary				Gut		
		HBE		Nasal		Intestinal		
		Bronchial ALI	Bronchial organoid	Nasal ALI	Nasal organoid	Rectal biopsies	Rectal organoid	Organoid 2-D monolayer
Patient-specific	No	Yes	Yes	Yes	Yes	Yes	Yes	Yes
Tissue source	-	Lung explants Bronchial brushing/biopsies Bronchoalveolar lavage fluid		Nasal brushing/curettage		Rectal biopsies		
Invasiveness of sample acquisition	-	+++		+		++		
Easy-to-culture	- Flexible - Easy to manipulate	- Limited expansion and differentiation potential (decreases as a function of passage) - ALI cultures take 4 weeks to form pseudostratified epithelium -No standardized protocol available for airway organoids				- Long term expanding cultures - Long term expanding cultures -Established and standardized protocol for organoid -Monolayer in development phase		
Phenocopies CF lung	No (prone to artifact)	Yes (gold standard)	Yes	Yes	Yes	No	No	No
Phenocopies CF intestine	No	No	No	No	No	Yes	Yes	Yes
CFTR functional readout	- Ussing - Halide assay	- Ussing	- FIS	- Ussing	- FIS	ICM	- FIS/SLA	Ussing
Assay dynamic range	Large	Moderate	Moderate	Small	Small	Large	Large	Large
Biochemical/physiological readout	- CFTR western blotting	- CFTR western blotting - ASL -CBF	- CFTR western blotting	- CFTR western blotting	- CFTR western blotting		- CFTR western blotting	
Drug screening	- High-throughput - Hit-to-lead drug development	- Mid-throughput - Checkpoint before drugs enter clinical trial/use	Exploratory	Mid-throughput	Exploratory	Low-throughput	Mid-throughput	Exploratory
Predictive value	++	+++	Exploratory	Exploratory	Exploratory	++	++	Exploratory

+++, High; ++, Moderate; +, Low; 2-D, 2-Dimensional; ALI, Air-liquid interphase; ASL, Airway surface liquid; CBF, Cilia beating frequency; FIS, Forskolin-induced swelling; HBE, Human bronchial epithelial; ICM, Intestinal current measurement; SLA, Steady-state lumen area.

or at the interface of the denser matrigel base layer. For certain downstream applications such as live imaging (e.g., forskolin-induced swelling—see section The Cell Model of the Future), the sinking method confers an advantage because spheroids are suspended in the same plane and permit HTS. We also note that successful differentiated, pseudostratified spheroid formation has been reported from airway basal cells maintained in the standard BEGM media and those derived from conditionally reprogrammed culture (Hild and Jaffe, 2016; Brewington et al., 2018c). Airway basal cell spheroids have no self-renewal capacity and are used for end-point applications.

Three-Dimensional Airway Organoid—Long-Term Expanding

Long term expanding human airway organoids were first reported by Sachs et al. (Sachs et al., 2018). These organoids were established from lung biopsies or cells isolated from BAL fluid and then cultured in media containing biochemical cues for self-renewal such as R-spondin, Noggin, fibroblast growth factor (FGF) and TGF-β inhibitors. The established organoids comprised of a polarized, pseudostratified airway epithelium containing basal cells, ciliated cells, mucus-producing goblet cells, and secretory club (Clara) cells. The airway organoids are amenable to passaging by mechanical disruption every other week for at least a year, with no loss in proliferation reported up to P18. In addition, single cell suspensions dissociated from the indefinitely expanding airway organoids yield an improved 2-D ALI culture (Zhou et al., 2018). These cultures displayed full ALI differentiation by day 12–14 as opposed to 21–28 days for conventional cultures grown from 2-D basal cells (Zhou et al., 2018). Together, these findings suggest the possibility of expanding isolated primary lung epithelial cells in 3-D, given cells maintained under conditionally reprogrammed and dual SMAD inhibition culture conditions do not expand beyond P10 without reaching senescence (Mou et al., 2016; Gentzsch et al., 2017). The indefinite expansion of airway organoids also means in theory the availability of "endless" amounts of ready-to-use airway epithelial cells.

Human Intestinal Epithelial Cells

While work in CF research has primarily focused on primary airway epithelial cells (the gold standard), patient-derived intestinal epithelial cells also present an invaluable resource in characterizing the relationship between the CFTR gene mutation and the disease phenotype. More recently, they play an important role in the development of HTS strategies to elucidate novel drugs for the treatment of CF.

Intestinal Organoids

Compared to human airway tissue, colon tissue damage in CF patients is minimal and the rectal epithelium is accessible in a less invasive manner. The abundant expression of CFTR in the distal colon makes rectal biopsies an attractive cellular source for interrogating CFTR function (Hug et al., 2011). Assessment of intestinal current measurement (ICM) as a readout for CFTR activity has provided strong evidence for the diagnostic and prognostic utility of rectal biopsies (De Jonge et al., 2004; Hirtz et al., 2004; Mall et al., 2004; De Boeck et al., 2006; Taylor et al., 2009; Derichs et al., 2010; Sousa et al., 2012; Clancy et al., 2013; Cohen-Cymberknoh et al., 2013). ICM can be applied to biopsies collected from CF patients which are subsequently exposed to CFTR modulators, to assess the efficacy of treatment in a personalized manner. One concern is the possibility of reduced penetration of modulator drug into the biopsy tissues under *ex vivo* conditions. Other limitations to the use of rectal biopsies include the small number of biopsies collected (4–8 biopsies) and the need for all biopsies to be tested on collection day i.e., the biopsies cannot be preserved for further testing.

Emergence of intestinal organoids (or mini-guts) overcome these limitations by extending the use of rectal biopsies in cultures. Intestinal organoids can be grown from crypts isolated from freshly isolated rectal biopsies. Crypts are rich in $Lgr5^+$ stem cells which grow and differentiate into self-organizing, multicellular structures (Sato et al., 2009; Jung et al., 2011). These organoids contain all of the distinct intestinal cell types present in the *in vivo* epithelium (Leushacke and Barker, 2014). The growth and differentiation of $Lgr5^+$ stem cells into eventual closed epithelial structures with an internal lumen requires a fine balance of growth factors (R-spondin, EGF, Noggin, Wnt-3a), inhibitors of TGF-β and BMP signaling and the basement membrane matrix (matrigel). Intestinal organoids can be indefinitely cultured and remain genetically and phenotypically stable upon repeated passaging and long term culture (Ikpa et al., 2014). Capitalizing on the high expression of CFTR in rectal tissues and rapidly expanding stem cells, they make an attractive model for assessment of CFTR functional response in pharmacologic testing. They provide the added advantage to test combination of modulators without established safety profiles as part of pre-clinical evaluation in CF patients with rare CFTR genotype.

FORSKOLIN-INDUCED SWELLING ASSAY AS A PROXY FOR CFTR FUNCTION

The primary functional assay to assess CFTR activity in organoids, the forskolin-induced swelling (FIS) assay is CFTR dependent. This approach does not measure the net transepithelial ionic transport. Rather, forskolin is used to stimulate intracellular cAMP production which then activates CFTR at the plasma membrane. CFTR activation drives chloride and fluid flux to the organoid lumen (apical membrane facing inwards), causing rapid swelling of organoids with functional CFTR or those derived from non-CF subjects. This swelling effect is significantly reduced or absent in organoids derived from CF subjects who exhibit differing rates of FIS with different classes of CFTR mutations and also between individuals with the same CFTR mutation (Dekkers et al., 2013). There is accumulating evidence that the CFTR modulator-corrected FIS response is predictive of patient-specific clinical response, with close correlation observed between rescued swelling and improvement in lung function (measured by FEV1) and sweat chloride concentration (Dekkers et al., 2016a; Guimbellot et al., 2017; Brewington et al., 2018c). Intestinal organoids can be disrupted to single cells to generate 2-D-monolayers on porous membranes for electrophysiological studies. FIS was shown to positively correlate with forskolin-induced current in subject-matched organoid-derived monolayers, supporting the notion that CFTR-dependent fluid secretion in rectal organoids reflects CFTR-dependent ion transport (Zomer-van Ommen et al., 2018)

The FIS assay has been adapted for use in airway organoids but is much less well-characterized compared to rectal organoids (Guimbellot et al., 2017; Brewington et al., 2018c; McCarthy et al., 2018). Studies performed thus far, have involved cultures from small datasets of patients. Given the lack of standardized culture protocol for airway organoids, forskolin induces either swelling or shrinking of airway organoid depending on the orientation of CFTR-expressing apical epithelium (swelling for apical membrane facing inwards organoids and vice versa). Similar to rectal organoids, forskolin-induced changes in cross sectional area is dependent on the severity of CFTR genotypes, and could be altered with CFTR modulators. However, the changes are far smaller given the lower expression of CFTR in the airways compare to the intestine. It is noteworthy that only a single concentration of forskolin (10 μM) has been interrogated in airway organoids FIS, while a total of eight concentrations (0.008–5 μM) were used in rectal organoids (Dekkers et al., 2016a; Guimbellot et al., 2017; Brewington et al., 2018c). To detect CFTR rescue with adequate resolution and sensitivity, higher-powered objectives are used resulting in lower throughput application compared to rectal (Dekkers et al., 2016a; Guimbellot et al., 2017; Brewington et al., 2018c). Establishment of a broader assay dynamic range may facilitate higher throughput use of FIS in airway organoids. Although preliminary, favorable correlation between *in vitro* FIS response to clinical response FEV1, sweat chloride concentration and BMI have been reported (Brewington et al., 2018c; McCarthy et al., 2018).

THE CELL MODEL OF THE FUTURE

In this Review, we described the rapidly developing field of organoid models specific to CF. Organoids, with their close resemblance to the human organs most affected by CF disease, hold great appeal for translational research. The capacity to adapt these models for assays such as FIS is important for theratyping and for conferring decisions on personalized CFTR pharmacotherapy. This provides an almost immediate application of *in vitro* research findings in the clinical setting. Nonetheless, it is apparent that each model has respective strengths and limitations (**Table 3**). The question as to which model has the essential features for precision medicine in CF and best predicts the long-term clinical benefits of a drug remains. Is it sufficient to use just one model and if so which cell model is best?

Intestinal organoids are the most developed so far amongst the 3-D model systems and seemingly an easier model to establish. But how representative is the intestinal epithelium to its respiratory counterpart? There are clear physiological differences between the airway mucosal surface and the gut. First, alternative ion channels critical for solute and water transport in the airways such as ENaC and calcium-activated chloride channels (CaCC), are either absent or present in negligible amounts in the gut to be functional (Rajendran et al., 2018). A modified swelling assay showed airway but not rectal organoids swell upon addition of E_{act}, an activator of the alternative chloride channel TMEM16A (Sachs et al., 2018). Second, there is no mucociliary clearance in the gastrointestinal tract. These differences highlight the need for organoids of bronchial or nasal epithelial origin to provide a closer resemblance to the *in vivo* airways. It then seems logical that one will need to choose the most appropriate 3-D cell culture model for each specific application.

AUTHOR CONTRIBUTIONS

SAW, NTA, and SLW wrote the manuscript with critical input from CKH, LKF, AK and AJ.

FUNDING

SAW, NTA, and SLW are supported by Sydney Children's Hospitals Foundation (SCHF). AK holds a Rothwell Family Fellowship.

REFERENCES

Accurso, F. J., Rowe, S. M., Clancy, J. P., Boyle, M. P., Dunitz, J. M., Durie, P. R., et al. (2010). Effect of VX-770 in persons with cystic fibrosis and the G551D-CFTR mutation. *N. Engl. J. Med.* 363, 1991–2003. doi: 10.1056/NEJMoa0909825

Awatade, N. T., Ramalho, S., Silva, I. A. L., Felicio, V., Botelho, H. M., de Poel, E., et al. (2018). R560S: a class II CFTR mutation that is not rescued by current modulators. *J. Cyst. Fibros.* doi: 10.1016/j.jcf.2018.07.001. [Epub ahead of print].

Awatade, N. T., Uliyakina, I., Farinha, C. M., Clarke, L. A., Mendes, K., Sole, A., et al. (2015). Measurements of functional responses in human primary lung cells as a basis for personalized therapy for cystic fibrosis. *EBioMedicine* 2, 147–153. doi: 10.1016/j.ebiom.2014.12.005

Barkauskas, C. E., Chung, M. I., Fioret, B., Gao, X., Katsura, H., and Hogan, B. L. (2017). Lung organoids: current uses and future promise. *Development* 144, 986–997. doi: 10.1242/dev.140103

Berube, K., Prytherch, Z., Job, C., and Hughes, T. (2010). Human primary bronchial lung cell constructs: the new respiratory models. *Toxicology* 278, 311–318. doi: 10.1016/j.tox.2010.04.004

Boyle, M. P., Bell, S. C., Konstan, M. W., McColley, S. A., Rowe, S. M., Rietschel, E., et al. (2014). A CFTR corrector (lumacaftor) and a CFTR potentiator (ivacaftor) for treatment of patients with cystic fibrosis who have a phe508del CFTR mutation: a phase 2 randomised controlled trial. *Lancet Respir Med.* 2, 527–538. doi: 10.1016/s2213-2600(14)70132-8

Brewington, J. J., Filbrandt, E. T., LaRosa, F. J. III, Moncivaiz, J. D., Ostmann, A. J., Strecker, L. M., et al. (2018a). Brushed nasal epithelial cells are a surrogate for bronchial epithelial CFTR studies. *JCI Insight* 3:e99385. doi: 10.1172/jci.insight.99385

Brewington, J. J., Filbrandt, E. T., LaRosa, F. J. III, Moncivaiz, J. D., Ostmann, A. J., Strecker, L. M., et al. (2018b). Generation of human nasal epithelial cell spheroids for individualized cystic fibrosis transmembrane conductance regulator study. *J. Vis. Exp.* 11:e57492. doi: 10.3791/57492

Brewington, J. J., Filbrandt, E. T., LaRosa, F. J. III, Ostmann, A. J., Strecker, L. M., Szczesniak, R. D., et al. (2018c). Detection of CFTR function and modulation in primary human nasal cell spheroids. *J. Cyst. Fibros.* 17, 26–33. doi: 10.1016/j.jcf.2017.06.010

Bridges, M. A., Walker, D. C., Harris, R. A., Wilson, B. R., and Davidson, A. G. (1991). Cultured human nasal epithelial multicellular spheroids: polar cyst-like model tissues. *Biochem. Cell Biol.* 69, 102–108.

Castillon, N., Hinnrasky, J., Zahm, J. M., Kaplan, H., Bonnet, N., Corlieu, P., et al. (2002). Polarized expression of cystic fibrosis transmembrane conductance regulator and associated epithelial proteins during the regeneration of human airway surface epithelium in three-dimensional culture. *Lab. Invest.* 82, 989–998. doi: 10.1097/01.LAB.0000022221.88025.43

Clancy, J. P., Rowe, S. M., Accurso, F. J., Aitken, M. L., Amin, R. S., Ashlock, M. A., et al. (2017). Results of a phase IIa study of VX-809, an investigational CFTR corrector compound, in subjects with cystic fibrosis homozygous for the F508del-CFTR mutation. *Thorax* 67, 12–8. doi: 10.1136/thoraxjnl-2011-200393

Clancy, J. P., Szczesniak, R. D., Ashlock, M. A., Ernst, S. E., Fan, L., Hornick, D. B., et al. (2013). Multicenter intestinal current measurements in rectal biopsies from CF and non-CF subjects to monitor CFTR function. *PLoS ONE* 8:e73905. doi: 10.1371/journal.pone.0073905

Clarke, L. A., Sousa, L., Barreto, C., and Amaral, M. D. (2013). Changes in transcriptome of native nasal epithelium expressing F508del-CFTR and intersecting data from comparable studies. *Respir. Res.* 14:38. doi: 10.1186/1465-9921-14-38

Cohen-Cymberknoh, M., Yaakov, Y., Shoseyov, D., Shteyer, E., Schachar, E., Rivlin, J., et al. (2013). Evaluation of the intestinal current measurement method as a diagnostic test for cystic fibrosis. *Pediatr. Pulmonol.* 48, 229–235. doi: 10.1002/ppul.22586

Czerwinski, M., and Spence, J. R. (2017). Hacking the matrix. *Cell Stem Cell* 20, 9–10. doi: 10.1016/j.stem.2016.12.010

Danahay, H., Pessotti, A. D., Coote, J., Montgomery, B. E., Xia, D., Wilson, A., et al. (2015). Notch2 is required for inflammatory cytokine-driven goblet cell metaplasia in the lung. *Cell Rep.* 10, 239–252. doi: 10.1016/j.celrep.2014.12.017

Davies, J. C., Wainwright, C. E., Canny, G. J., Chilvers, M. A., Howenstine, M. S., Munck, A., et al. (2013). Efficacy and safety of ivacaftor in patients aged 6 to 11 years with cystic fibrosis with a G551D mutation. *Am. J. Respir. Crit. Care Med.* 187, 1219–1225. doi: 10.1164/rccm.201301-0153OC

De Boeck, K., Wilschanski, M., Castellani, C., Taylor, C., Cuppens, H., Dodge, J., et al. (2006). Cystic fibrosis: terminology and diagnostic algorithms. *Thorax* 61, 627–635. doi: 10.1136/thx.2005.043539

de Courcey, F., Zholos, A. V., Atherton-Watson, H., Williams, M. T., Canning, P., Danahay, H. L., et al. (2012). Development of primary human nasal epithelial cell cultures for the study of cystic fibrosis pathophysiology. *Am. J. Physiol. Cell Physiol.* 303:C1173–C1179. doi: 10.1152/ajpcell.00384.2011

De Jonge, H. R., Ballmann, M., Veeze, H., Bronsveld, I., Stanke, F., Tummler, B., et al. (2004). *Ex vivo* CF diagnosis by intestinal current measurements (ICM) in small aperture, circulating Ussing chambers. *J. Cyst. Fibros.* 3(Suppl. 2):159–63. doi: 10.1016/j.jcf.2004.05.034

Dekkers, J. F., Berkers, G., Kruisselbrink, E., Vonk, A., de Jonge, H. R., Janssens, H. M., et al. (2016a). Characterizing responses to CFTR-modulating drugs using rectal organoids derived from subjects with cystic fibrosis. *Sci. Transl. Med.* 8:344ra384. doi: 10.1126/scitranslmed.aad8278

Dekkers, J. F., Gogorza Gondra, R. A., Kruisselbrink, E., Vonk, A. M., Janssens, H. M., de Winter-de Groot, K. M., et al. (2016b). Optimal correction of distinct CFTR folding mutants in rectal cystic fibrosis organoids. *Eur. Respir. J.* 48, 451–458. doi: 10.1183/13993003.01192-2015

Dekkers, J. F., Wiegerinck, C. L., de Jonge, H. R., Bronsveld, I., Janssens, H. M., de Winter-de Groot, K. M., et al. (2013). A functional CFTR assay using primary cystic fibrosis intestinal organoids. *Nat. Med.* 19, 939–945. doi: 10.1038/nm.3201

Derichs, N., Sanz, J., Von Kanel, T., Stolpe, C., Zapf, A., Tummler, B., et al. (2010). Intestinal current measurement for diagnostic classification of patients with questionable cystic fibrosis: validation and reference data. *Thorax* 65, 594–599. doi: 10.1136/thx.2009.125088

Deslee, G., Dury, S., Perotin, J. M., Al Alam, D., Vitry, F., Boxio, R., et al. (2007). Bronchial epithelial spheroids: an alternative culture model to investigate epithelium inflammation-mediated COPD. *Respir. Res.* 8:86. doi: 10.1186/1465-9921-8-86

Donaldson, S. H., Pilewski, J. M., Griese, M., Cooke, J., Viswanathan, L., Tullis, E., et al. (2018). Tezacaftor/ivacaftor in subjects with cystic fibrosis and F508del/F508del-CFTR or F508del/G551D-CFTR. *Am. J. Respir. Crit. Care Med.* 197, 214–224. doi: 10.1164/rccm.201704-0717OC

Dye, B. R., Kasputis, T., Spence, J. R., and Shea, L. D. (2017). Take a deep breath and digest the material: organoids and biomaterials of the respiratory and digestive systems. *MRS Commun.* 7, 502–514. doi: 10.1557/mrc.2017.61

Gentzsch, M., Boyles, S. E., Cheluvaraju, C., Chaudhry, I. G., Quinney, N. L., Cho, C., et al. (2017). Pharmacological rescue of conditionally reprogrammed cystic fibrosis bronchial epithelial cells. *Am. J. Respir. Cell Mol. Biol.* 56, 568–574. doi: 10.1165/rcmb.2016-0276MA

Guimbellot, J. S., Leach, J. M., Chaudhry, I. G., Quinney, N. L., Boyles, S. E., Chua, M., et al. (2017). Nasospheroids permit measurements of CFTR-dependent fluid transport. *JCI Insight* 2:e95734. doi: 10.1172/jci.insight.95734

Hild, M., and Jaffe, A. B. (2016). Production of 3-D airway organoids from primary human airway basal cells and their use in high-throughput screening. *Curr. Protoc. Stem Cell Biol.* 37:Ie.9.1–Ie.9.15. doi: 10.1002/cpsc.1

Hirtz, S., Gonska, T., Seydewitz, H. H., Thomas, J., Greiner, P., Kuehr, J., et al. (2004). CFTR Cl- channel function in native human colon correlates with the genotype and phenotype in cystic fibrosis. *Gastroenterology* 127, 1085–1095. doi: 10.1053/j.gastro.2004.07.006

Hug, M. J., Derichs, N., Bronsveld, I., and Clancy, J. P. (2011). Measurement of ion transport function in rectal biopsies. *Methods Mol. Biol.* 741, 87–107. doi: 10.1007/978-1-61779-117-8_7

Ikpa, P. T., Bijvelds, M. J., and de Jonge, H. R. (2014). Cystic fibrosis: toward personalized therapies. *Int. J. Biochem. Cell Biol.* 52, 192–200. doi: 10.1016/j.biocel.2014.02.008

Jung, P., Sato, T., Merlos-Suárez, A., Barriga, F. M., Iglesias, M., Rossell, D., et al. (2011). Isolation and *in vitro* expansion of human colonic stem cells. *Nat. Med.* 17:1225. doi: 10.1038/nm.2470

Keogh, R. H., Szczesniak, R., Taylor-Robinson, D., and Bilton, D. (2018). Up-to-date and projected estimates of survival for people with cystic fibrosis using baseline characteristics: a longitudinal study using UK patient registry data. *J. Cyst. Fibrosis* 17, 218–27. doi: 10.1016/j.jcf.2017.11.019

Lavelle, G. M., White, M. M., Browne, N., McElvaney, N. G., and Reeves, E. P. (2016). Animal models of cystic fibrosis pathology: phenotypic parallels and divergences. *Biomed Res. Int.* 2016:5258727. doi: 10.1155/2016/5258727

Leushacke, M., and Barker, N. (2014). *Ex vivo* culture of the intestinal epithelium: strategies and applications. *Gut* 63, 1345–1354. doi: 10.1136/gutjnl-2014-307204

Lopes-Pacheco, M., Boinot, C., Sabirzhanova, I., Rapino, D., and Cebotaru, L. (2017). Combination of correctors rescues CFTR transmembrane-domain mutants by mitigating their interactions with proteostasis. *Cell. Physiol. Biochem.* 41, 2194–2210. doi: 10.1159/000475578

Mall, M., Grubb, B. R., Harkema, J. R., O'Neal, W. K., and Boucher, R. C. (2004). Increased airway epithelial Na– absorption produces cystic fibrosis-like lung disease in mice. *Nat. Med.* 10, 487–493. doi: 10.1038/nm1028

Marson, F. A. L., Bertuzzo, C. S., and Ribeiro, J. D. (2016). Classification of CFTR mutation classes. *Lancet Respir. Med.* 4:e37–e38. doi: 10.1016/s2213-2600(16)30188-6

Martinovich, K. M., Iosifidis, T., Buckley, A. G., Looi, K., Ling, K. M., Sutanto, E. N., et al. (2017). Conditionally reprogrammed primary airway epithelial cells maintain morphology, lineage and disease specific functional characteristics. *Sci. Rep.* 7:17971. doi: 10.1038/s41598-017-17952-4

Matsui, H., Grubb, B. R., Tarran, R., Randell, S. H., Gatzy, J. T., Davis, C. W., et al. Evidence for periciliary liquid layer depletion, not abnormal ion composition, in the pathogenesis of cystic fibrosis airways disease. *Cell* (1998) 95, 1005–1015.

McCarthy, C., Brewington, J. J., Harkness, B., Clancy, J. P., and Trapnell, B. C. (2018). Personalised CFTR pharmacotherapeutic response testing and therapy of cystic fibrosis. *Eur. Respir. J.* 51:1702457. doi: 10.1183/13993003.02457-2017

Montoro, D. T., Haber, A. L., Biton, M., Vinarsky, V., Lin, B., Birket, S. E., et al. (2018). A revised airway epithelial hierarchy includes CFTR-expressing ionocytes. *Nature* 560, 319–324. doi: 10.1038/s41586-018-0393-7

Mou, H., Vinarsky, V., Tata, P. R., Brazauskas, K., Choi, S. H., Crooke, A. K., et al. (2016). Dual SMAD signaling inhibition enables long-term expansion of diverse epithelial basal cells. *Cell Stem Cell* 19, 217–31. doi: 10.1016/j.stem.2016.05.012

Pedemonte, N., Lukacs, G. L., Du, K., Caci, E., Zegarra-Moran, O., Galietta, L. J., et al. (2005). Small-molecule correctors of defective DeltaF508-CFTR cellular processing identified by high-throughput screening. *J. Clin. Invest.* 115, 2564–2571. doi: 10.1172/jci24898

Pedersen, P. S., Frederiksen, O., Holstein-Rathlou, N. H., Larsen, P. L., and Qvortrup, K. (1999). Ion transport in epithelial spheroids derived from human airway cells. *Am. J. Physiol.* 276(1 Pt 1):L75–L80.

Peters-Hall, J. R., Coquelin, M. L., Torres, M. J., LaRanger, R., Alabi, B. R., Sho, S., et al. (2018). Long-term culture and cloning of primary human bronchial basal cells that maintain multipotent differentiation capacity and CFTR channel function. *Am. J. Physiol. Lung Cell. Mol. Physiol.* 315, 313–327. doi: 10.1152/ajplung.00355.2017

Plasschaert, L. W., Zilionis, R., Choo-Wing, R., Savova, V., Knehr, J., Roma, G., et al. (2018). A single-cell atlas of the airway epithelium reveals the CFTR-rich pulmonary ionocyte. *Nature* 560, 377–381. doi: 10.1038/s41586-018-0394-6

Pollard, B. S., and Pollard, H. B. (2018). Induced pluripotent stem cells for treating cystic fibrosis: state of the science. *Pediatr. Pulmonol.* 53:S12–S29. doi: 10.1002/ppul.24118

Rajendran, V. M., Schulzke, J.-D., and Seidler, U. E. (2018). "Chapter 58—Ion channels of the gastrointestinal epithelial cells A2-said," in *Physiology of the Gastrointestinal Tract, 6th Edn.*, eds J. D. K. M. Hamid, F. K. Ghishan, J. L. Merchant, and J. D. Wood (Irvine, CA: Academic Press), 1363–1404.

Ramsey, B. W., Davies, J., McElvaney, N. G., Tullis, E., Bell, S. C., Drevínek, P., et al. (2011). A CFTR potentiator in patients with cystic fibrosis and the G551D mutation. *N. Engl. J. Med.* 365, 1663–1672. doi: 10.1056/NEJMoa1105185

Ratjen, F., Bell, S. C., Rowe, S. M., Goss, C. H., Quittner, A. L., and Bush, A. (2015). Cystic fibrosis. *Nat. Rev. Dis. Primers* 1:15010. doi: 10.1038/nrdp.2015.10

Reynolds, S. D., Rios, C., Wesolowska-Andersen, A., Zhuang, Y., Pinter, M., Happoldt, C., et al. (2016). Airway progenitor clone formation is enhanced by Y-27632-dependent changes in the transcriptome. *Am. J. Respir. Cell Mol. Biol.* 55, 323–336. doi: 10.1165/rcmb.2015-0274MA

Riordan, J. R. (2008). CFTR function and prospects for therapy. *Annu. Rev. Biochem.* 77, 701–26. doi: 10.1146/annurev.biochem.75.103004.142532

Rowe, S. M., Daines, C., Ringshausen, F. C., Kerem, E., Wilson, J., Tullis, E., et al. (2017). Tezacaftor-ivacaftor in residual-function heterozygotes with cystic fibrosis. *N. Engl. J. Med.* 377, 2024–2035. doi: 10.1056/NEJMoa1709847

Sachs, N., Zomer-van Ommen, D. D., Papaspyropoulos, A., Heo, I., Bottinger, L., Klay, D., et al. (2018). Long-term expanding human airway organoids for disease modelling. *bioRxiv [Preprint].* doi: 10.1101/318444

Sato, T., Vries, R. G., Snippert, H. J., van de Wetering, M., Barker, N., Stange, D. E., et al. (2009). Single Lgr5 stem cells build crypt–villus structures *in vitro* without a mesenchymal niche. *Nature* 459:262. doi: 10.1038/nature 07935

Sousa, M., Servidoni, M. F., Vinagre, A. M., Ramalho, A. S., Bonadia, L. C., Felicio, V., et al. (2012). Measurements of CFTR-mediated Cl- secretion in human rectal biopsies constitute a robust biomarker for Cystic Fibrosis diagnosis and prognosis. *PLoS ONE* 7:e47708. doi: 10.1371/journal.pone.0047708

Sutanto, E. N., Scaffidi, A., Garratt, L. W., Looi, K., Foo, C. J., Tessari, M. A., et al. (2018). Assessment of p.Phe508del-CFTR functional restoration in pediatric primary cystic fibrosis airway epithelial cells. *PLoS ONE* 13:e0191618. doi: 10.1371/journal.pone.0191618

Talamo Guevara, M., and McColley, S. A. (2017). The safety of lumacaftor and ivacaftor for the treatment of cystic fibrosis. *Expert. Opin. Drug Saf.* 16, 1305–1311. doi: 10.1080/14740338.2017.1372419

Tan, Q., Choi, K. M., Sicard, D., and Tschumperlin, D. J. (2017). Human airway organoid engineering as a step toward lung regeneration and disease modeling. *Biomaterials* 113, 118–132. doi: 10.1016/j.biomaterials.2016. 10.046

Taylor, C. J., Hardcastle, J., and Southern, K. W. (2009). Physiological measurements confirming the diagnosis of cystic fibrosis: the sweat test and measurements of transepithelial potential difference. *Paediatr. Respir. Rev.* 10, 220–226. doi: 10.1016/j.prrv.2009.05.002

Taylor-Cousar, J. L., Munck, A., McKone, E. F., van der Ent, C. K., Moeller, A., Simard, C., et al. (2017). Tezacaftor-ivacaftor in patients with cystic fibrosis homozygous for Phe508del. *N. Engl. J. Med.* 377, 2013–2023. doi: 10.1056/NEJMoa1709846

US CF Foundation, JHU, and The Hosptial for Sick Children (2011). *The Clinical and Functional TRanslation of CFTR (CFTR2).* Available online at: http://cftr2.org

Van Goor, F., Hadida, S., Grootenhuis, P. D., Burton, B., Cao, D., Neuberger, T., et al. (2010). Rescue of CF airway epithelial cell function *in vitro* by a CFTR potentiator, VX-770. *Proc. Natl. Acad. Sci. U. S. A.* (2009) 106, 18825–18830. doi: 10.1073/pnas.0904709106

Van Goor, F., Hadida, S., Grootenhuis, P. D., Burton, B., Stack, J. H., Straley, K. S., et al. (2012). Correction of the F508del-CFTR protein processing defect *in vitro* by the investigational drug VX-809. *Proc. Natl. Acad. Sci. U. S. A.* (2011) 108, 18843–18848. doi: 10.1073/pnas.1105787108

Van Goor, F., Straley, K. S., Cao, D., Gonzalez, J., Hadida, S., Hazlewood, A., et al. (2006). Rescue of DeltaF508-CFTR trafficking and gating in human cystic fibrosis airway primary cultures by small molecules. *Am. J. Physiol. Lung Cell. Mol. Physiol.* 290:L1117–L1130. doi: 10.1152/ajplung.00169.2005

Wainwright, C. E., Elborn, J. S., Ramsey, B. W., Marigowda, G., Huang, X., Cipolli, M., et al. (2015). Lumacaftor-ivacaftor in patients with cystic fibrosis homozygous for Phe508del CFTR. *N. Engl. J. Med.* 373, 220–231. doi: 10.1056/NEJMoa1409547

Wine, J. J. (1999). The genesis of cystic fibrosis lung disease. *J. Clin. Investig.* 103, 309–12. doi: 10.1172/JCI6222

Zabner, J., Smith, J. J., Karp, P. H., Widdicombe, J. H., and Welsh, M. J. (1998). Loss of CFTR chloride channels alters salt absorption by cystic fibrosis airway epithelia *in vitro*. *Mol. Cell* 2, 397–403.

Zhou, J., Li, C., Sachs, N., Chiu, M. C., Wong, B. H., Chu, H., et al. (2018). Differentiated human airway organoids to assess infectivity of emerging influenza virus. *Proc. Natl. Acad. Sci. U.S.A.* 115, 6822–6827. doi: 10.1073/pnas.1806308115

Zomer-van Ommen, D. D., de Poel, E., Kruisselbrink, E., Oppelaar, H., Vonk, A. M., Janssens, H. M., et al. (2018). Comparison of *ex vivo* and *in vitro* intestinal cystic fibrosis models to measure CFTR-dependent ion channel activity. *J. Cyst. Fibros.* 17, 316–24. doi: 10.1016/j.jcf.2018.02.007

5

Variable Responses to CFTR Correctors *in vitro*: Estimating the Design Effect in Precision Medicine

Elizabeth Matthes[1,2], Julie Goepp[1,2], Carolina Martini[1,2], Jiajie Shan[1,2†], Jie Liao[1,2], David Y. Thomas[2,3] and John W. Hanrahan[1,2,4*]

[1] Department of Physiology, McGill University, Montréal, QC, Canada, [2] Cystic Fibrosis Translational Research Centre, McGill University, Montréal, QC, Canada, [3] Department of Biochemistry, McGill University, Montréal, QC, Canada, [4] Research Institute of the McGill University Health Centre, McGill University, Montréal, QC, Canada

****Correspondence:***
John W. Hanrahan
john.hanrahan@mcgill.ca

†Present address:
Jiajie Shan,
School of Medicine, South China University of Technology, Guangzhou University, Guangzhou, China

Interest in precision medicine has grown in recent years due to the variable clinical benefit provided by some medications, their cost, and by new opportunities to tailor therapies to individual patients. In cystic fibrosis it may soon be possible to test several corrector drugs that improve the folding and functional expression of mutant cystic fibrosis transmembrane conductance regulator (CFTR) prospectively using cells from a patient to find the one that is best for that individual. Patient-to-patient variation in cell culture responses to correctors and the reproducibility of those responses has not been studied quantitatively. We measured the functional correction provided by lumacaftor (VX-809) using bronchial epithelial cells from 20 patients homozygous for the F508del-CFTR mutation. Significant differences were observed between individuals, supporting the utility of prospective testing. However, when correction of F508del-CFTR was measured repeatedly using cell aliquots from the same individuals, a design effect was observed that would impact statistical tests of significance. The results suggest that the sample size obtained from power calculations should be increased to compensate for group sampling when CFTR corrector drugs are compared *in vitro* for precision medicine.

Keywords: precision medicine, cystic fibrosis, correctors, lumacaftor, Orkambi, group sampling, design effect, power calculations

INTRODUCTION

Cystic fibrosis (CF) is a relatively common orphan disease caused by loss-of-function mutations in the gene encoding CFTR (cystic fibrosis transmembrane conductance regulator), a tightly regulated anion channel (Riordan, 2008). CFTR mediates secretion across many epithelia in the body and is required for efficient mucociliary clearance of inhaled pathogens from the lungs (Ratjen et al., 2015). CF modulators such as lumacaftor (VX-809) that partially correct the misfolding and/or potentiate the activity of mutant CFTR channels are available and more are in the pipeline, however, they are expensive and their clinical benefit varies between individuals (Boyle et al., 2014;

Hanrahan et al., 2017). With precision medicine one could potentially test multiple drugs on cells from a patient to identify the one that is most efficacious for that individual.

Although CF seems ideally suited for applying the precision medicine approach (Amaral, 2015; Martiniano et al., 2016; Burgener and Moss, 2018; Cholon and Gentzsch, 2018), some practical issues remain to be addressed. Foremost among these is whether differences in functional correction measured using primary cultured cells from different patients are statistically significant. This is obviously essential if prospective testing *in vitro* is to be useful for making prescribing decisions. The variable clinical benefit provided by Orkambi® is well known (Boyle et al., 2014), however, it remains unclear if similar variability exists at the level of epithelial cells and persists in cell culture. If cells from different patients vary in their response to drugs and the responses correlate with clinical benefit, a practical question arises as to how many assays would be needed to conclude that one corrector is more effective than another for that individual. The causes of variability are not yet understood therefore it is not possible to develop a statistical model capable of predicting responses to a drug. Nevertheless, methods for collecting and analyzing data are needed if efficacy in cell-based assays is to be useful for precision medicine.

Assays of CFTR function that utilize different cell types have been developed and could potentially be used to test the drug responsiveness of individual patients. Rescue of the mutant CFTR can be assayed directly by measuring Cl^- transport across tissue samples or primary cell cultures using electrophysiology (Van Goor et al., 2011; Brewington et al., 2018). CFTR function can also be assayed indirectly by measuring net fluid transport across intestinal organoids prepared from rectal biopsies (Dekkers et al., 2013, 2016) or airway epithelial spheroids prepared from cells that are obtained by brushing or curettage of the nasal or bronchial mucosa (Guimbellot et al., 2017; McCarthy et al., 2018). Induced pluripotent stem cells (iPSCs) may be useful if they can be made to differentiate fully and recapitulate variable drug responses between patients having the same CFTR genotype, which may depend on both genetic and epigenetic factors. Correlations have recently been reported when assaying CFTR function in the nasal epithelium *in vivo* and in cultured cells from patients with different CFTR mutations (Pranke et al., 2017). Similar responses have also been observed in nasal and bronchial epithelial cultures (Pranke et al., 2017; Brewington et al., 2018). Importantly, for seven patients homozygous for F508del-CFTR there was a correlation between mean functional rescue in nasal cell cultures and the clinical response to Orkambi measured as % FEV1 (% predicted forced expiratory volume in 1 s) (Pranke et al., 2017).

In this paper we start by quantifying variability in functional correction amongst patients having the same genotype (F508del-CFTR/F508del-CFTR) using well differentiated bronchial epithelial cell cultures. Then we explore the reproducibility of correction by repeatedly testing samples from large pools of cells from two individuals, analogous to sampling the airway *in vivo*. We observe a design effect caused by group sampling that needs to be considered when testing the statistical significance of differences in correction.

MATERIALS AND METHODS

Cells

Primary human bronchial epithelial (HBE) cells were obtained from the Primary Airway Cell Biobank at the McGill CF Translational Research centre (CFTRc) and cultured at the air liquid interface as described previously (Fulcher et al., 2005; Robert et al., 2007). Briefly, lung tissue from patients undergoing lung transplantation was obtained from the Biobank of respiratory tissues at the Centre Hospitalier de l'Université de Montréal and Institut de recherche cliniques de Montréal. Informed, written consent was obtained and all procedures were approved by the Institutional Review Board of McGill University (#A08-M70-14B) and followed Canadian Institutes of Health Research guidelines. Cells were isolated from bronchial tissue by enzyme digestion and cultured in bronchial epithelial growth medium (BEGM) on type I collagen-coated plastic flasks (Vitrogen 100, PureCol; Advanced BioMatrix), then trypsinized, counted, and used immediately for experiments (**Figures 1D,F**) or cryopreserved in aliquots of 2 million cells and used within 18 months (**Figures 1F** and **2A,B**). Bronchial epithelial cell growth medium (BEGM) was used during cell isolation and initial culture of the cells (i.e., passage 0, P0). BEGM consists of Laboratory of Human Carcinogenesis (LHC) Basal Medium (Invitrogen) and ~20 supplements including bovine serum albumin (BSA) but not serum [see (Fulcher et al., 2005) for details]. Once cells had been thawed and seeded on porous supports they were cultured using air-liquid interface (ALI) medium to induce differentiation. The ALI medium was a 50:50 mixture of LHC Basal Medium and Dulbecco's modification of Eagle medium (D-MEM) with less added human epidermal growth factor (hEGF) but other supplements including BSA at similar levels to BEGM. Drug treatments were performed for 24 h in ALI medium without BSA or antibiotics.

Freshly isolated or thawed cells were seeded on collagen coated 6.5 mm Costar® 0.4 μm pore, polyester membrane inserts (Corning) and grown under submerged conditions for 4 days. The apical medium was then removed and cells were allowed to differentiate at the ALI for 4 weeks before use in correction assays. Isolation and growth media were supplemented with antibiotics that were selected based on recent patient microbiology reports. Only penicillin and streptomycin were added to ALI cultures. Cells were used at first passage (P1), and comparisons between patients used recently isolated cells that had not been frozen. Repeated sampling of two patients was performed using cells from large isolates that had been cryopreserved in aliquots of 2 million cells (Fulcher et al., 2005; Robert et al., 2010). Mature cultures were pseudostratified and appeared highly differentiated with ciliated, goblet and basal cells (**Figure 1A**).

Corrector Treatment and CFTR Functional Assays

When comparing different patients, three well differentiated monolayers were pretreated for 24 h at 37°C with vehicle (0.1% DMSO dimethyl sulfoxide) and three were pretreated

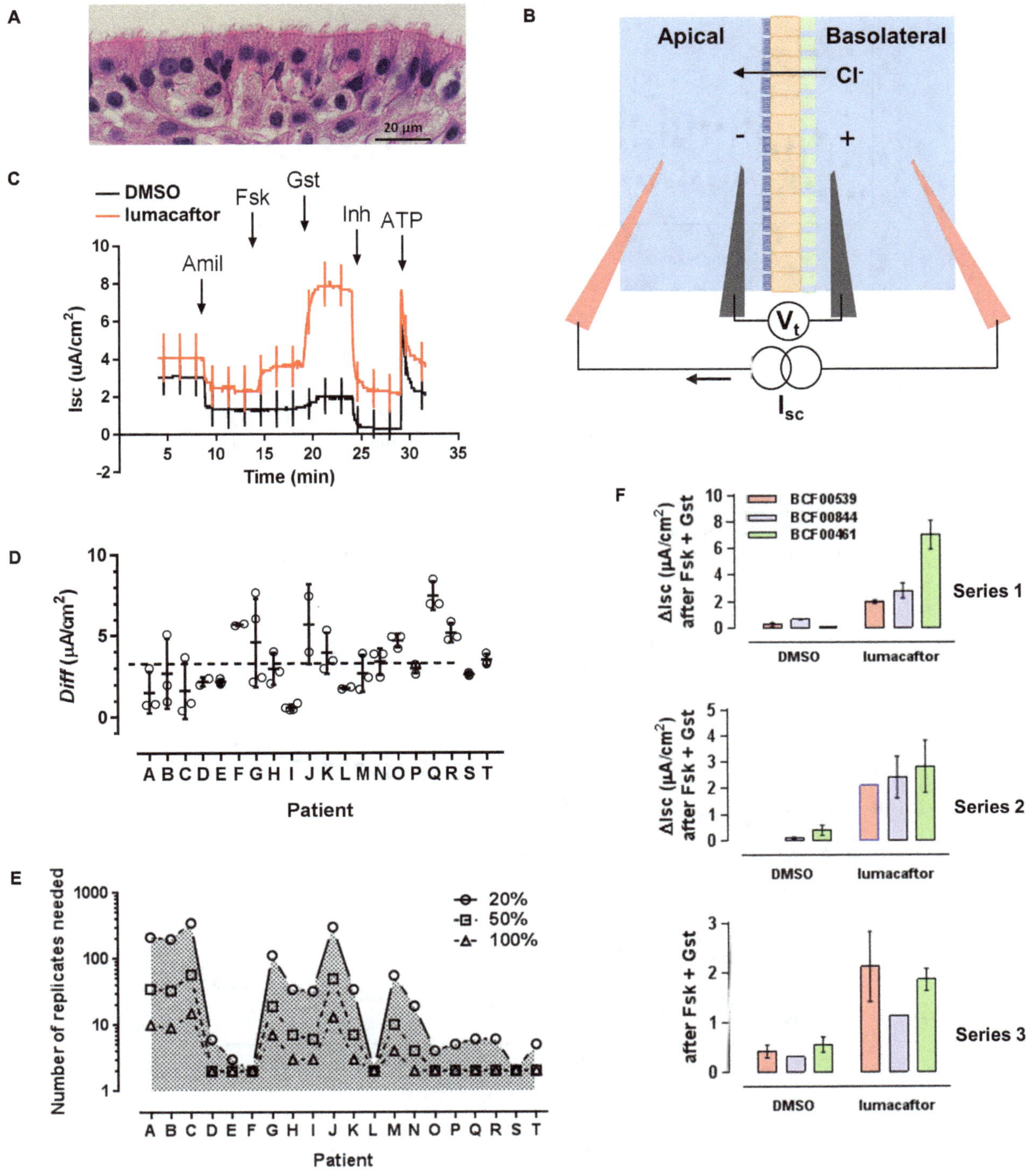

FIGURE 1 | An assay for testing F508del-CFTR corrector drugs. **(A)** Well differentiated primary human bronchial epithelial (HBE) cells cultured at the air-liquid interface. **(B)** Electrophysiological measurement of CFTR function as short-circuit current (I_{sc}), the current needed to clamp the transepithelial voltage (V_t) at 0 mV. Epithelial cells (orange) cultured on a porous support (green) are mounted in modified Ussing chambers. A basolateral-to-apical Cl^- gradient is imposed to generate a secretory flux through rescued mutant CFTR channels. **(C)** Representative recordings of cells pretreated for 24 h with DMSO (vehicle) or lumacaftor (corrector), then exposed sequentially to Na^+ channel blocker amiloride (10 μM Amil, apical), forskolin (10 μM Fsk, bilateral, activator), genistein (50 μM Gst, apical, potentiator), $CFTR_{inh}$-172 (10 μM Inh, apical, CFTR inhibitor), and ATP (10 μM, apical, purinergic agonist to stimulate Ca^{2+}-activated Cl^- channels as a positive control for viability). Current deflections show responses to brief voltage steps to +/−1 mV to monitor transepithelial resistance. **(D)** Response of cells from 20 patients to lumacaftor shown as the difference (*Diff*) in ΔI_{sc} stimulated by forskolin + genistein when cells were pretreated with lumacaftor or DMSO. (means +/− s.d., $n = 3$ for each condition). **(E)** Predicted number of replicates needed to detect a 20, 50, and 100% change in correction, calculated for each patient. **(F)** Three series of assays performed independently on the same three patients under identical conditions. In each series, cells from the same patients were exposed in triplicate to vehicle (DMSO) or corrector (lumacaftor).

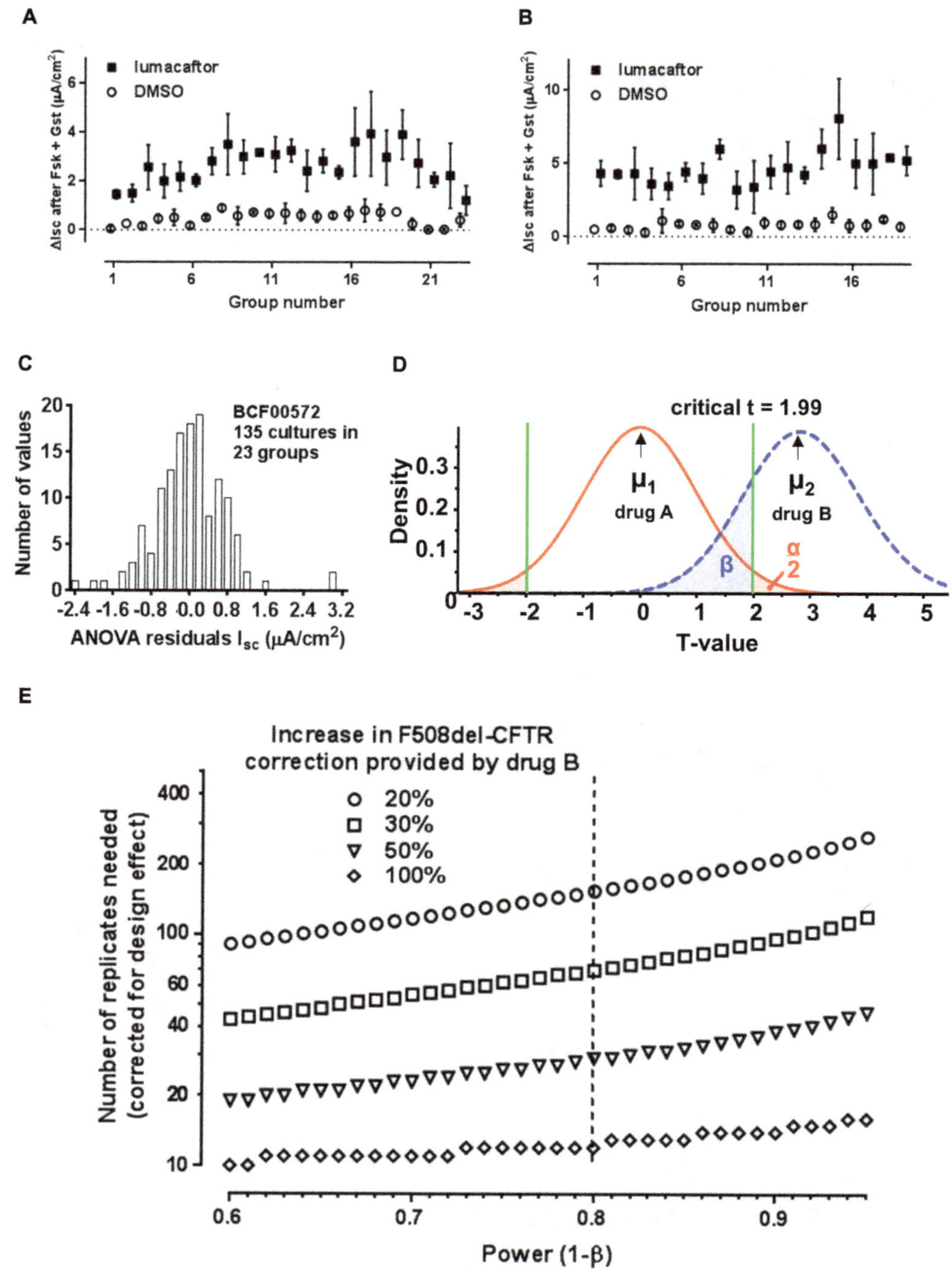

FIGURE 2 | Impact of group sampling when comparing two correctors. **(A)** Simulation of group sampling by measuring F508del-CFTR functional correction in aliquots of the same cell population (patient BCF00572). Response to forskolin + genistein after treatment with vehicle (open circles) or corrector (closed squares) in 23 groups of 3–9 cultures (technical replicates). **(B)** Same as panel **A** but with cells from patient BCF00710. **(C)** Distribution of the residuals from one-way random effects ANOVA of lumacaftor treated cell cultures from patient BCF00572. **(D)** Predicted *t*-distributions for two correctors, where hypothetical drug B gives a mean F508del-CFTR correction μ_2 that is 20% higher than corrector A (μ_1). The calculations assume $\alpha = 0.05$, $\beta = 0.8$, mean response to forskolin + genistein after pretreatment with corrector A = 3.3 $\mu A/cm^2$, and s.d. = 1.0 $\mu A/cm^2$ for both drugs. **(E)** Number of replicates needed to detect a significant change in correction by drug B compared to drug A, assuming there is a real improvement of 20, 30, 50, or 100%, after compensation for the design effect due to group sampling. The number of replicates is shown for power 0.60–0.95 (i.e., probability of a false negative of 0.4–0.05).

with lumacaftor (1 μM; Selleck Chemicals, Houston, TX, United States) and the same final concentration of DMSO. The six monolayers were then mounted in modified Ussing chambers and short-circuit current (I_{sc} in $\mu A\ cm^{-2}$) was measured to assay CFTR function in all six cultures simultaneously (**Figure 1B**). Transepithelial voltage was clamped at 0 mV except for 2 s bipolar pulses to ±1 mV at 100 s intervals to monitor transepithelial resistance. A basolateral-to-apical NaCl chloride gradient was imposed to increase the signal-to-noise of the current response; apical (in mM): 1.2 NaCl, 115 Na-gluconate, 25 $NaHCO_3$, 1.2 $MgCl_2$, 4 $CaCl_2$, 2.4 KH_2PO_4, 1.24 K_2HPO_4, 10 Glucose; basolateral (in mM): 115 NaCl, 25 $NaHCO_3$, 1.2 MgCl, 1.2 $CaCl_2$, 2.4 KH_2PO_4, 1.24 K_2HPO_4, 10 Glucose. After the short-circuit current had stabilized (typically 2–3 min), Fsk (10 μM) was added to both sides to raise intracellular cAMP. This was followed by sequential additions of the potentiator genistein (Gst, 50 μM), the CFTR inhibitor $CFTR_{inh}$-172 (10 μM) and the purinergic agonist ATP (100 μM) to the apical side to stimulate Ca^{2+}-activated Cl^- channels as a positive control and to confirm cell viability (Matthes et al., 2016). Potentiation by 50 μM genistein was similar to that produced by 0.1 μM ivorcaftor (VX-770 or Kalydeco®) and was used because it was more easily washed from the chambers. The stimulation of I_{sc} (taken as the increase from the steady-state baseline level before adding forskolin to the maximum current after genistein addition; ΔI_{sc}) was used to measure of F508del-CFTR functional expression (**Figure 1C**). Assays using CF mouse intestine were performed as described previously (Robert et al., 2010). Rotterdam delF508/delF508–CFTR mice ($Cftr^{tm1\ Eur}$), FVB inbred, 14–17 weeks old, 24–30 g) were used (van Doorninck et al., 1995; Scholte et al., 2004). All procedures followed Canadian Institutes of Health Research guidelines and were approved by the faculty Animal Care Committee at McGill University (#2012-7119). The ileum was stripped of muscle and mounted in mini-Ussing chambers (Physiological Instruments, San Diego, CA, United States). Tissues were bathed with William's E–Glutamax (x1; Gibco) supplemented with insulin (10 μg/ml) and dexamethasone (20 μg/ml). Short-circuit current and resistance were measured before and after sequential additions of forskolin (10 μM) and genistein (50 μM) to the apical side. After steady-state stimulation these were washed from the chambers and lumacaftor or vehicle (0.1% DMSO) was added for 4 h. Forskolin and genistein were then re-assayed and the difference between the I_{sc} responses before and after exposure to lumacaftor or vehicle (which served as a time control) were used as a measure of correction. Reagents were from Sigma unless otherwise indicated.

Statistics

Results are expressed as the mean ± S.E.M. of n observations. F508del-CFTR correction was displayed as *Diff* (the difference between maximum I_{sc} response to forskolin + genistein when cells were pretreated with lumacaftor vs. DMSO

$$Diff = \Delta Isc_{\ treated} - \overline{\Delta Isc}_{\ ctrl} \tag{1}$$

Although the same number of cultures was exposed to drug and to vehicle, the measurements were unpaired and all three DMSO controls were equally applicable to each drug-treated culture. *Diff* was calculated and plotted for clarity to show correction but was not used in statistical tests, which were based on the raw data collected under each condition.

The impact of group sampling was determined as the intraclass correlation coefficient (ICC, also called intracluster correlation coefficient or "rho" ρ) the ratio of the variance between groups to the sum of variances between and within groups (Donner and Klar, 2000; Killip et al., 2004). ρ can range from 0 when there is no effect of group sampling to 1 when the replicates within groups are perfectly consistent and variation is entirely between groups. The results of ANOVA were then used to determine $\rho(\Delta Isc_{\ treated})$ as:

$$\rho = \frac{MS_B - MS_W}{MS_B + (n_o - 1)MS_W} \tag{2}$$

where MS_B and MS_W are the mean squares between and within groups, respectively, and η_o is the average number of replicates per group calculated as:

$$\frac{\begin{array}{l}(\text{total \# of replicates} \\ \quad - \text{sum of the squared \# of replicates in each group} \\ \quad /\text{total \# of replicates})\end{array}}{\text{total \# of groups} - 1} \tag{3}$$

Residuals for 22 of the 23 group samples passed the Kolmogorov-Smirnov normality test with α = 0.05 using GraphPad Prism v. 6.04 (GraphPad Software, La Jolla, CA, United States)[1]. When the more stringent D'Agostino-Pearson K^2 omnibus test (D'agostino et al., 1990) was applied to groups having $n \geq 9$ (the minimum needed) they passed the normality test. When residuals for samples from all groups were pooled there was deviation from normality due to positive kurtosis, however, the distribution was symmetric and well fitted by a Gaussian curve (r^2 = 0.9944) after excluding two bins as outliers (**Figure 2C**). The robustness of ANOVA when there are moderate departures from normality (Motulsky, 2014) suggests the ANOVA results are valid. The standard deviation of the I_{sc} response to drug $(\Delta Isc_{\ treated})$ was used in the program G*Power v3.9.1.2 when estimating the number of replicates needed to determine if lumacaftor causes significant correction for each of the 20 patients and for different effect sizes (Faul et al., 2007).

RESULTS

Cystic fibrosis bronchial epithelial cells from all 20 patients were more strongly stimulated by forskolin + genistein after 24 h pretreatment lumacaftor (**Figure 1D**). The average stimulation after treatment with lumacaftor was 11.4% that measured in non-CF cells expressing wild-type CFTR (pooled data from 11 non-CF donors). This is similar to a previous report in which cells from seven patients that had been cultured in medium supplemented with Ultroser G and assayed acutely using a different potentiator (Van Goor et al., 2011).

The I_{sc} responses were ~15-fold more variable after drug pretreatment than after pretreatment with vehicle. The variation was quantified using a mixed, two-way analysis of variance (ANOVA) of all data in both groups (i.e., baseline I_{sc} and

[1] www.graphpad.com

maximum I_{sc} after stimulation by forskolin + genistein). Most (51.0%) of the variability was associated with the effect of drug pretreatment while 19.3% could be attributed to patients and 11.9% was explained by interaction between these factors; i.e., patient-to-patient differences in the response to lumacaftor (parameter of interest for precision medicine). Despite the small sample size, the null hypothesis that cells from different patients respond similarly to lumacaftor could be rejected with $P = 0.0001$. This is consistent with a previous study using a linear random effects model in which most variability in the response to lumacaftor was due to inter-patient rather than intra-patient variability (Pranke et al., 2017). Our power calculations to estimate the number of replicates needed for lumacaftor responses to reach statistical significance for a given effect size (i.e., increase of 20, 50, or 100%) yielded variable results when based on triplicate assays (**Figure 1E**) suggesting a larger sample size is needed to reliably estimate the standard deviation. Nevertheless, the results provide support for precision medicine in CF in that they show significant variability in drug responses between airway epithelial cells cultured from different individuals.

To assess the reproducibility of F508del-CFTR correction we compared the stimulation by forskolin + genistein on 3 successive weeks using different ALI cultures. The cells were prepared from different patients, cryopreserved and then thawed at 1 week intervals and cultured under identical conditions for 1 month for assays. Cells from one patient responded similarly to forskolin + genistein after pretreatment with lumacaftor in all three sets of experiments. However, ΔI_{sc} was more variable when cells from the other two patients (**Figure 1F**).

To explore this variability further we simulated *in vivo* sampling by dividing a pool of 170 million HBE cells from one patient into aliquots of 2 million. Each aliquot was considered a group sample from the airway surface epithelium to mimic repeated collection of small samples *in vivo* by bronchial brushing, but under well controlled conditions. Multiple ALI cultures were prepared using 23 randomly chosen aliquots (2–18 cultures per aliquot) and the ΔI_{sc} response to forskolin + genistein was measured using equal numbers of vehicle- and lumacaftor-treated replicates from each aliquot. Cells that had been treated with lumacaftor were always more responsive to forskolin + genistein than DMSO controls as expected (**Figure 2A**). One-way random effects ANOVA of ΔI_{sc} revealed significant variation between the groups ($P < 0.0001$), despite coming from the same original pool of cells.

Since prospective testing for the response to a CF drug will likely involve analyzing small cell samples *in vitro*, we examined the statistical consequences of such group sampling on correction. We calculated the intraclass correlation coefficient (ICC, also called ρ rho), which is the ratio of the variance between groups to the sum of the variances between and within groups. This was done when correction by lumacaftor was assayed repeatedly using 135 cultures from one patient (BCF00572). On average, each group consisted of $\eta_o = 5.86$ replicates and had $\rho = 0.377$, yielding a design effect $[1 + \rho(\eta_o - 1)] = 2.83$. ICC was somewhat higher for vehicle-treated cells ($\rho = 0.4466$), in agreement with the lower variability of DMSO controls in **Figure 2A**.

To determine if the design effect is observed generally when assaying F508del correction we analyzed cells from a second patient (BCF00710). We selected 19 aliquots of cells (2 million cells each) at random from a pool of 280 million cells, cultured them at the ALI for 1 month, and assayed their stimulation by forskolin + genistein with and without lumacaftor pretreatment as before (**Figure 2B**). In this experiment there were $\eta_o = 4.34$ replicates per lumacaftor treatment group and equation (2) yielded $\rho = 0.2816$ and a design effect of 1.94. Plotting the residuals from a one-way random effects ANOVA of all data from lumacaftor-treated cultures from patient BCF00572 gave a bell-shaped frequency distribution that showed positive kurtosis but only moderate deviation from normality, supporting the validity of ANOVA (**Figure 2C**). In summary, the results from both patients indicate that variability of drug responses measured using group samples underestimates the true variation in the original population. Correcting for the design effect is necessary when comparing drug responses *in vitro* for precision medicine; two- to three-fold more replicates than estimated by regular power calculations are needed to draw conclusions based on two-tailed *t*-tests.

With this in mind we asked "How many replicates are needed to conclude that corrector B is more effective than corrector A using cells from one individual that have been collected and cultured *in vitro*?" To answer this we assumed a typical stimulation by forskolin + genistein after pretreatment with corrector A (lumacaftor; $\Delta I_{sc} = 3.3\ \mu A/cm^2$, s.d. = $0.962\ \mu A/cm^2$; the mean from 20 patients studied under our conditions). This response was compared to that generated by hypothetical "corrector B," which was assumed to have the same variance as lumacaftor. We set $\alpha = 0.05$ (probability of Type I error or false positive when testing the null hypothesis H_o that correctors A and B have the same efficacy) and $\beta = 0.2$ (probability of a Type II error or false negative, corresponding to a statistical power of $1-\beta = 0.8$; see **Figure 2D**). The number of replicates needed was then calculated as a function of power when corrector B would provide a real improvement in F508del-CFTR correction that is 20, 30, 50, or 100% higher than corrector A. Replicates were assumed to be independent samples, then the predicted number of replicates was then multiplied by 2.83 to correct for the effect of group sampling (**Figure 2E**).

The results indicate that if hypothetical corrector B has twice the efficacy of corrector A (i.e., increases F508del-CFTR rescue by 100%), 12 replicates from a group sample would be sufficient to conclude there is a significant difference between correctors. However, more replicates are needed if the real change in efficacy is less dramatic, e.g., 153 when corrector B increases F508del-CFTR function by only 20%.

DISCUSSION

The present results demonstrate statistically significant variation in responses to lumacaftor when assayed using cultured cells from different patients. Variable corrector responses have been observed previously (Van Goor et al., 2011; Eckford et al., 2014) and were analyzed for homozygous F508del CFTR patients in one study (Pranke et al., 2017), however, the implications for comparing efficacies of different drugs have not been explored. We also found considerable variability between cell samples from the same patient and explored its consequences when distinguishing between correctors. Prospective drug testing *in vitro* will likely begin with the collection of a small sample of epithelial cells from the patient. We used bronchial epithelial cells, however, similar results would be expected when small numbers of epithelial cells are harvested from the nasal or bronchial mucosa or by rectal biopsy. Since group samples have reduced standard deviation compared to the original epithelial cell population, they are expected to cause underestimation of the sample size needed for statistical testing, although this estimate can be corrected by determining the design effect.

Air-liquid interface cultures are considered to be the "gold standard" for testing CFTR modulators and have been accepted by the FDA when evaluating new drug applications (Durmowicz et al., 2018). Using this model to assay samples from a single large population of airway cells we estimated the design effect to range between 2 and 3. The sources of variability between group samples and replicates within groups are unknown and may reflect heterogeneity in the cell isolate and/or subtle differences during differentiation in prolonged culture. Cells were handled identically according to detailed standard operating procedures, nevertheless we cannot exclude slight variations in cell viability after thawing that could affect seeding density, or volume when the cells were fed with fresh medium. Cells were treated with corrector for 24 h in our study, however, lumacaftor is hydrophobic and longer exposures (48–72 h) are expected to increase its uptake and might reduce variability. The efficacy of Orkambi appears to be limited mainly by the modest efficacy of lumacaftor, therefore we have focussed on it in this study and pretreated cells only with lumacaftor. Simultaneous exposure to another drug such as ivacaftor could increase variability since variances add, although it will be important to test prolonged exposure to ivacaftor at clinically-relevant, low nanomolar free concentrations to avoid adverse effects on CFTR functional rescue by lumacaftor (Matthes et al., 2016). When multiple corrector drugs become available for CF they may be compared *in vitro* for precision medicine on the assumption that more functional expression *in vitro* will correlate with better symptoms *in vivo*. Such a correlation is observed between mean responses of multiple homozygous F508del-CFTR patients to Orkambi *in vivo* and nasal epithelial cultures from the same patients treated with ivorcaftor + lumacaftor (Pranke et al., 2017). Those results are also consistent with the ability of ivorcaftor alone to increase Cl^- conductance in cells expressing G551D-CFTR but not F508del-CFTR (Van Goor et al., 2009) and to improve lung function in patients with G551D (Accurso et al., 2010) but not in F508del homozygotes (Flume et al., 2012). Why correction varies between patients with the same CFTR genotype remains uncertain. Variation in genetic background (i.e., genes other than CFTR) may contribute since genome wide association studies have identified several genes that can modify CF disease severity (Cutting et al., 1990; Wright et al., 2011; Sun et al., 2012; Blackman et al., 2013; Corvol et al., 2015). Epigenetic variation caused by exposure to environmental factors could also contribute to variable corrector responses *in vitro*. Measuring correction *in vitro* probably excludes some off-target drug effects, however, the underlying genetic and epigenetic factors that affect F508del-CFTR expression, folding and trafficking may persist.

We were interested to compare the variability of correction in cells from patients and in F508del-CFTR homozygous mice (van Doorninck et al., 1995; Wilke et al., 2011). The genomes and epigenomes of CF mice are expected to be more similar than humans because they are inbred and housed under identical conditions. We examined correction in the ileum because the CF phenotype is stronger in the intestine than in the lung in mice. In preliminary experiments we isolated small pieces of ileum from CF mice (*Cftr*$^{tm1\ Eur}$) (van Doorninck et al., 1995) in quadruplicate and measured the forskolin-stimulated ΔI_{sc} after exposing tissues to DMSO or lumacaftor for 4 h *ex vivo* as described previously (Robert et al., 2010). Mixed, two-way ANOVA showed that the variability of F508del-CFTR correction was less in inbred mice than in patients. The interaction term (i.e., variability in drug response between individuals) accounted for ~6.5% of the variance in mouse intestinal assays vs. 11.9% in HBE cultures from patients but was still significant ($P < 0.0001$). We believe this variation reflects the health of the mice or the condition of tissues after dissection, but cannot exclude that genetic and/or epigenetic variations persist in the mice despite inbreeding and the same environment.

The application of personalized medicine in CF has a bright future, however, the predictive value of *in vitro* assays remains to be established when there are alternative drugs and multiple patients carrying the same mutation. The present results indicate that patient-to-patient differences in F508del-CFTR correction can be assayed using airway cell cultures, however, a design effect due to group sampling needs to be compensated by increasing the number of replicates. Hopefully, CF correctors and corrector combinations will continue improving until they become so effective for all patients that precision medicine is no longer necessary (Hanrahan et al., 2017).

AUTHOR CONTRIBUTIONS

JH, EM, and DT: conceptualization. EM, JG, CM, JS, JL, and JH: investigation, and validation. JH: writing—original draft. JH, EM, JG, CM, and DT: writing—review and editing. JH and DT: funding acquisition. JG, CM, JL, and EM: resources.

FUNDING

This work was supported by grants from the Canadian Institutes of Health Research to JH (MOP-287879) and DT (MOP-119341) and from Cystic Fibrosis Canada to the Primary Airway Cell Biobank (PACB) at McGill (2997).

ACKNOWLEDGMENTS

We thank Dr. Andrea Benedetti (McGill University) for helpful discussions and Dr. Vanessa Dumeaux (Concordia University) for comments on the manuscript. We also thank the Biobank of respiratory tissues at the Centre Hospitalier de l'Université de Montréal and Institut de Recherche Cliniques de Montréal (Respiratory Health Network of Fonds de Recherche du Québec-Santé) for providing lung samples. We are grateful to Dr. Bob Scholte, Dr. Hugo de Jonge, and Dr. Martina Wilke (Erasmus MC, Rotterdam, Netherlands) for providing F508del-CFTR mice (*Cftr*$^{tm1\ Eur}$) and a protocol for assaying correction in mouse intestine.

REFERENCES

Accurso, F. J., Rowe, S. M., Clancy, J. P., Boyle, M. P., Dunitz, J. M., Durie, P. R., et al. (2010). Effect of VX-770 in persons with cystic fibrosis and the G551D-CFTR mutation. *N. Engl. J. Med.* 363, 1991–2003. doi: 10.1056/NEJMoa0909825

Amaral, M. D. (2015). Novel personalized therapies for cystic fibrosis: treating the basic defect in all patients. *J. Intern. Med.* 277, 155–166. doi: 10.1111/joim.12314

Blackman, S. M., Commander, C. W., Watson, C., Arcara, K., Strug, L. J., Stonebraker, J. R., et al. (2013). Genome-wide association studies for type 2 diabetes and Cfrd reveal common risk loci. *Pediatr. Pulmonol.* 48, 263–264.

Boyle, M. P., Bell, S. C., Konstan, M. W., Mccolley, S. A., Rowe, S. M., Rietschel, E., et al. (2014). A CFTR corrector (lumacaftor) and a CFTR potentiator (ivacaftor) for treatment of patients with cystic fibrosis who have a phe508del CFTR mutation: a phase 2 randomised controlled trial. *Lancet Respir. Med.* 2, 527–538. doi: 10.1016/S2213-2600(14)70132-8

Brewington, J. J., Filbrandt, E. T., Larosa, F. J. III, Moncivaiz, J. D., Ostmann, A. J., Strecker, L. M., et al. (2018). Brushed nasal epithelial cells are a surrogate for bronchial epithelial CFTR studies. *JCI Insight* 3:98699. doi: 10.1172/jci.insight.99385

Burgener, E. B., and Moss, R. B. (2018). Cystic fibrosis transmembrane conductance regulator modulators: precision medicine in cystic fibrosis. *Curr. Opin. Pediatr.* 30, 372–377. doi: 10.1097/MOP.0000000000000627

Cholon, D. M., and Gentzsch, M. (2018). Recent progress in translational cystic fibrosis research using precision medicine strategies. *J. Cyst. Fibros.* 17, S52–S60. doi: 10.1016/j.jcf.2017.09.005

Corvol, H., Blackman, S. M., Boelle, P. Y., Gallins, P. J., Pace, R. G., Stonebraker, J. R., et al. (2015). Genome-wide association meta-analysis identifies five modifier loci of lung disease severity in cystic fibrosis. *Nat. Commun.* 6:8382. doi: 10.1038/ncomms9382

Cutting, G. R., Kasch, L. M., Rosenstein, B. J., Zielenski, J., Tsui, L. C., Antonarakis, S. E., et al. (1990). A cluster of cystic fibrosis mutations in the first nucleotide-binding fold of the cystic fibrosis conductance regulator protein. *Nature* 346, 366–368. doi: 10.1038/346366a0

D'agostino, R. B., Belanger, A., and D'agostin, R. B. J. (1990). A suggestion for using powerful and informative tests of normality. *Am. Stat.* 44, 316–321.

Dekkers, J. F., Berkers, G., Kruisselbrink, E., Vonk, A., De Jonge, H. R., Janssens, H. M., et al. (2016). Characterizing responses to CFTR-modulating drugs using rectal organoids derived from subjects with cystic fibrosis. *Sci. Transl. Med.* 8:344ra384. doi: 10.1126/scitranslmed.aad8278

Dekkers, J. F., Wiegerinck, C. L., De Jonge, H. R., Bronsveld, I., Janssens, H. M., De Winter-De Groot, K. M., et al. (2013). A functional CFTR assay using primary cystic fibrosis intestinal organoids. *Nat. Med.* 19, 939–945. doi: 10.1038/nm.3201

Donner, A., and Klar, N. (2000). *Design and Analysis of Cluster Randomization Trials in Health Research.* Oxford: Oxford University Press Inc.

Durmowicz, A. G., Lim, R., Rogers, H., Rosebraugh, C. J., and Chowdhury, B. A. (2018). The U.S. food and drug administration's experience with ivacaftor in cystic fibrosis. establishing efficacy using *in vitro* data in lieu of a clinical trial. *Ann. Am. Thorac. Soc.* 15, 1–2. doi: 10.1513/AnnalsATS.201708-668PS

Eckford, P. D., Ramjeesingh, M., Molinski, S., Pasyk, S., Dekkers, J. F., Li, C., et al. (2014). VX-809 and related corrector compounds exhibit secondary activity stabilizing active F508del-CFTR after its partial rescue to the cell surface. *Chem. Biol.* 21, 666–678. doi: 10.1016/j.chembiol.2014.02.021

Faul, F., Erdfelder, E., Lang, A. G., and Buchner, A. (2007). G*Power 3: a flexible statistical power analysis program for the social, behavioral, and biomedical sciences. *Behav. Res. Methods* 39, 175–191. doi: 10.3758/BF03193146

Flume, P. A., Liou, T. G., Borowitz, D. S., Li, H., Yen, K., Ordonez, C. L., et al. (2012). Ivacaftor in subjects with cystic fibrosis who are homozygous for the F508del-CFTR mutation. *Chest* 142, 718–724. doi: 10.1378/chest.11-2672

Fulcher, M. L., Gabriel, S., Burns, K. A., Yankaskas, J. R., and Randell, S. H. (2005). "Well-differentiated human airway epithelial cell cultures," in *Human Cell Culture Protocols*, 2nd Edn, ed. J. Picot (New York, NY: Humana Press), 183–206.

Guimbellot, J. S., Leach, J. M., Chaudhry, I. G., Quinney, N. L., Boyles, S. E., Chua, M., et al. (2017). Nasospheroids permit measurements of CFTR-dependent fluid transport. *JCI Insight* 2:95734. doi: 10.1172/jci.insight.95734

Hanrahan, J. W., Matthes, E., Carlile, G., and Thomas, D. Y. (2017). Corrector combination therapies for F508del-CFTR. *Curr. Opin. Pharmacol.* 34, 105–111. doi: 10.1016/j.coph.2017.09.016

Killip, S., Mahfoud, Z., and Pearce, K. (2004). What is an intracluster correlation coefficient? Crucial concepts for primary care researchers. *Ann. Fam. Med.* 2, 204–208. doi: 10.1370/afm.141

Martiniano, S. L., Sagel, S. D., and Zemanick, E. T. (2016). Cystic fibrosis: a model system for precision medicine. *Curr. Opin. Pediatr.* 28, 312–317. doi: 10.1097/MOP.0000000000000351

Matthes, E., Goepp, J., Carlile, G. W., Luo, Y., Dejgaard, K., Billet, A., et al. (2016). Low free drug concentration prevents inhibition of F508del CFTR functional expression by the potentiator VX-770 (ivacaftor). *Br. J. Pharmacol.* 173, 459–470. doi: 10.1111/bph.13365

McCarthy, C., Brewington, J. J., Harkness, B., Clancy, J. P., and Trapnell, B. C. (2018). Personalised CFTR pharmacotherapeutic response testing and therapy of cystic fibrosis. *Eur. Respir. J.* 51:1702457. doi: 10.1183/13993003.02457-2017

Motulsky, H. J. (2014). *Intuitive Biostatistics. A Non-Mathematical Guide to Statistical Thinking.* New York, NY: Oxford University Press Inc.

Pranke, I. M., Hatton, A., Simonin, J., Jais, J. P., Le Pimpec-Barthes, F., Carsin, A., et al. (2017). Correction of CFTR function in nasal epithelial cells from cystic fibrosis patients predicts improvement of respiratory function by CFTR modulators. *Sci. Rep.* 7:7375. doi: 10.1038/s41598-017-07504-1

Ratjen, F., Bell, S. C., Rowe, S. M., Goss, C. H., Quittner, A. L., and Bush, A. (2015). Cystic fibrosis. *Nat. Rev. Dis. Primers* 1:15010. doi: 10.1038/nrdp.2015.10

Riordan, J. R. (2008). CFTR function and prospects for therapy. *Annu. Rev. Biochem.* 77, 701–726. doi: 10.1146/annurev.biochem.75.103004.142532

Robert, R., Carlile, G. W., Liao, J., Balghi, H., Lesimple, P., Liu, N., et al. (2010). Correction of the Delta phe508 cystic fibrosis transmembrane conductance regulator trafficking defect by the bioavailable compound glafenine. *Mol. Pharmacol.* 77, 922–930. doi: 10.1124/mol.109.062679

Robert, R., Carlile, G. W., Pavel, C., Liu, N., Anjos, S. M., Liao, J., et al. (2007). Structural analogue of sildenafil identified as a novel corrector of the F508del-CFTR trafficking defect. *Mol. Pharmacol.* 73, 478–489. doi: 10.1124/mol.107.040725

Scholte, B. J., Davidson, D. J., Wilke, M., and De Jonge, H. R. (2004). Animal models of cystic fibrosis. *J. Cyst. Fibros.* 3, 183–190. doi: 10.1016/j.jcf.2004.05.039

Sun, L., Rommens, J. M., Corvol, H., Li, W., Li, X., Chiang, T. A., et al. (2012). Multiple apical plasma membrane constituents are associated with susceptibility to meconium ileus in individuals with cystic fibrosis. *Nat. Genet.* 44, 562–569. doi: 10.1038/ng.2221

van Doorninck, J. H., French, P. J., Verbeek, E., Peters, R. H., Morreau, H., Bijman, J., et al. (1995). A mouse model for the cystic fibrosis delta F508 mutation. *EMBO J.* 14, 4403–4411. doi: 10.1002/j.1460-2075.1995.tb00119.x

Van Goor, F., Hadida, S., Grootenhuis, P. D., Burton, B., Cao, D., Neuberger, T., et al. (2009). Rescue of CF airway epithelial cell function *in vitro* by a CFTR potentiator, VX-770. *Proc. Natl. Acad. Sci. U.S.A.* 106, 18825–18830. doi: 10.1073/pnas.0904709106

Van Goor, F., Hadida, S., Grootenhuis, P. D., Burton, B., Stack, J. H., Straley, K. S., et al. (2011). Correction of the F508del-CFTR protein processing defect *in vitro* by the investigational drug VX-809. *Proc. Natl. Acad. Sci. U.S.A.* 108, 18843–18848. doi: 10.1073/pnas.1105787108

Wilke, M., Buijs-Offerman, R. M , Aarbiou, J., Colledge, W. H., Sheppard, D. N., Touqui, L., et al. (2011). Mouse models of cystic fibrosis: phenotypic analysis and research applications. *J. Cyst. Fibros* 10(Suppl. 2), S152–S171. doi: 10.1016/S1569-1993(11)60020-9

Wright, F. A., Strug, L. J., Doshi, V. K., Commander, C. W., Blackman, S. M., Sun, L., et al. (2011). Genome-wide association and linkage identify modifier loci of lung disease severity in cystic fibrosis at 11p13 and 20q13.2. *Nat. Genet.* 43, 539–546. doi: 10.1038/ng.838

6

Identification and Characterization of Novel CFTR Potentiators

*Maarten Gees[1†], Sara Musch[1†], Steven Van der Plas[1], Anne-Sophie Wesse[1], Ann Vandevelde[1], Katleen Verdonck[1], Oscar Mammoliti[1], Tzyh-Chang Hwang[2], Kathleen Sonck[1], Pieter Stouten[1], Andrew M. Swensen[3], Mia Jans[1], Jan Van der Schueren[1], Luc Nelles[1], Martin Andrews[1] and Katja Conrath[1]**

[1] Galapagos NV, Mechelen, Belgium, [2] Department of Medical Pharmacology and Physiology, University of Missouri, Columbia, MO, United States, [3] AbbVie, North Chicago, IL, United States

***Correspondence:**
Katja Conrath
katja.conrath@glpg.com

† These authors have contributed equally to this work

There is still a high unmet need for the treatment of most patients with cystic fibrosis (CF). The identification and development of new Cystic Fibrosis Transmembrane conductance Regulator (CFTR) modulators is necessary to achieve higher clinical benefit in patients. In this report we describe the characterization of novel potentiators. From a small screening campaign on F508del CFTR, hits were developed leading to the identification of pre-clinical candidates GLPG1837 and GLPG2451, each derived from a distinct chemical series. Both drug candidates enhance WT CFTR activity as well as low temperature or corrector rescued F508del CFTR, and are able to improve channel activity on a series of Class III, IV CFTR mutants. The observed activities in YFP halide assays translated well to primary cells derived from CF lungs when measured using Trans-epithelial clamp circuit (TECC). Both potentiators improve F508del CFTR channel opening in a similar manner, increasing the open time and reducing the closed time of the channel. When evaluating the potentiators in a chronic setting on corrected F508del CFTR, no reduction of channel activity in presence of potentiator was observed. The current work identifies and characterizes novel CFTR potentiators GLPG1837 and GLPG2451, which may offer new therapeutic options for CF patients.

Keywords: CF, CFTR, potentiator, bronchial epithelial cells, electrophysiology

INTRODUCTION

Cystic fibrosis (CF) is the most common genetic (autosomal recessive) disease in Caucasians, with an estimated 80,000 CF diagnosed cases worldwide (Lubamba et al., 2012; Hanrahan et al., 2013; Merk and Schubert-Zsilavecz, 2013; De Boeck et al., 2014). Current strategies for treatment of CF patients can be broadly divided into two main categories: agents that target downstream effects of Cystic Fibrosis Transmembrane conductance Regulator (CFTR) dysfunction (i.e., symptomatic treatment) and agents that target the root cause of the disease, i.e., CFTR modulators which address the absent or dysfunctional CFTR in epithelial membranes. The treatments in the latter category are further classified as either correctors, which increase the levels of CFTR present on the cell surface, or potentiators which enhance the function of CFTR channels, There are three approved CFTR modulator treatments available for CF patients, namely the potentiator Ivacaftor (Kalydeco®) or VX770, the corrector Lumacaftor or VX809 and the corrector Tezacaftor or VX661, The Ivacaftor/Lumacaftor combination therapy (Orkambi®) or the Ivacaftor/Tezacaftor combination therapy (Symedeko®) are available for the treatment of patients homozygous for the F508del CFTR mutation. However, these treatments result in only minor benefit to these patients (Wainwright et al., 2015; Taylor-Cousar et al., 2017) and thus there is a demand for improved combinations to further improve clinical benefit for CF patients with the F508del mutation.

Potentiators can only function if CFTR is already present at the cell membrane, and work by increasing the opening probability (Po) of CFTR (Moran, 2010). VX770 is a potentiator which improves the channel opening of CFTR mutants with gating or conductance defects (class III and IV mutations, respectively) such as G551D (Van Goor et al., 2009; Yu et al., 2012; Jih and Hwang, 2013) and R117H (Yu et al., 2016). Overall, these two classes of mutations that could benefit from VX770 represent approximately 8–10% of the total patient population. Clinical trials indeed showed significant benefit in these patient populations with VX770 including an improvement of lung function by 10.6% (Ramsey et al., 2011; Hadida et al., 2014). The availability of additional potentiator molecules with improved potency, efficacy, and safety could provide further benefit to that provided by VX770.

Here we describe the characterization of two chemically distinct clinical candidate potentiators. This characterization was performed by evaluating their activity using higher throughput methodologies such as yellow fluorescent protein (YFP)-halide assays, low throughput patch clamp assays and more clinically relevant assays using primary cells derived from CF patients.

MATERIALS AND METHODS

Cell Cultures

CFBe41o- cells were cultured in Eagle's minimal essential medium (MEM) (Life Technologies) supplemented with 10% fetal bovine serum (FBS), 1% penicillin/streptomycin, 1% L-glutamine and 500 μg/ml hygromycin B. The cells were grown on culture flasks coated with 0.01% bovine serum albumin (BSA) (Sigma), 30 μg/ml Purecol (Nutacon), and 0.001% human fibronectin (Sigma). A CFBe41o- cell line stably expressing F508del CFTR harboring an HRP-tag in the 4th extracellular loop was obtained from Professor Gergely Lukacs (Department of Physiology, McGill University, Montreal, Canada) (Veit et al., 2012). Cells were grown in MEM supplemented with 10% FBS, 1% L-glutamine (Life Technologies), 10 mM HEPES (Life Technologies), 200 μg/ml geneticin (Life Technologies) and 3 μg/ml puromycin (Sigma) on culture flasks coated as for CFBe41o-. HEK293 cells were cultured in uncoated flasks using Dulbecco's Modified Eagle Medium (DMEM) (Life Technologies) supplemented with 10% FBS and 1% penicillin/streptomycin. CHO cells were cultured in DMEM containing 10% FBS.

Human Bronchial Epithelial (HBE) Cell Culture

Bronchial epithelial cells isolated from transplanted lungs from wild-type (WT), CF patients homozygous for the F508del mutation or heterozygous G551D/F508del or R334W/F508del patients, were obtained from McGill University (Montreal, Canada) and University of North Carolina (Chapel Hill, NC, United States). Cells were isolated from lungs obtained from donors undergoing a planned transplantation. These primary cells were cultured directly on type IV collagen-coated polycarbonate Transwell supports with a diameter of 6.5 mm and pore size of 0.4 μm (Costar, #3397) for 18–25 days in air liquid (ali) interface essentially as previously described (Fulcher et al., 2005).

Yellow Fluorescent Protein (YFP) Halide Assay (CFBE, Low Temperature Corrected)

CFBe41o- cells were plated in black 384-well microplates at a density of 1,500 cells per well. After 24 h, cells were transduced with adenoviruses containing F508del CFTR and YFP (H148Q/I152L/) F47L using a multiplicity of infection of 30 infectious units per cell for each adenovirus. The next day, for the low temperature corrected assay, cells were incubated at 27°C for 24 h, for the chemically corrected assay cells were treated with corrector for 24 h at 37°C. On the day of analysis, cells were washed five times with Dulbecco's Phosphate-Buffered Saline (DPBS) containing Ca^{2+} and Mg^{2+} (Life Technologies) using a Microplate Washer (BioTek). Then, cells were treated with 10 μM forskolin and the desired concentration of potentiator in a volume of 30 μl and the plates were incubated at room temperature for 10 min, a timepoint optimized in previous experiments showing good window (positive control/negative control > 2) and signal to background ratio. The YFP fluorescence was recorded for 2 min, starting immediately before addition of 30 μl NaI buffer (375 mM NaI, 7.5 mM KI, 1.76 mM KH_2PO_4, 10.1 mM Na_2HPO_4, 13.75 mM glucose) to the wells, using a FDSS/μCell (Hamamatsu) fluorescence reader with a 480 nm excitation filter and a 540 nm emission filter. The capacity of potentiators to increase CFTR channel function was expressed as 1-[fluorescence 36 s after NaI addition (F)/fluorescence before NaI addition (F0)], a timepoint optimized previously, resulting in an optimal signal window. Data was normalized using the formula: normalized response = 100* (absolute response – negative control response)/(VX770 response – negative response) as such, VX770 response corresponds to 100. For Dose-response experiments, data was fitted using a 4 parameter hill function of the form Response = Bottom + (Top-Bottom)/(1 + 10^((LogEC50-concentration)*HillSlope)) to determine EC_{50} values.

YFP Halide Assay (HEK293)

HEK293 cells were transfected with 10–80 ng of plasmid encoding G551D, G178R, G1349D, S549N, R117H, R334W, or wild type CFTR and 20 ng of plasmid encoding YFP (H148Q/I152L/F47L) using jetPEI (Polyplus transfection). Directly after transfection, cells were seeded in black 96-well plates coated with Poly-D-lysine at a density of 70,000 cells per well. The next day, cells were incubated at 27°C for 24 h, for low temperature correction. When evaluating in a chronic setting, the potentiator concentration range was also added to the cells for 24 h. After this incubation period, cells were washed twice with

DPBS with Ca^{2+} and Mg^{2+}. Subsequently, cells were treated with 10 μM forskolin and the desired concentration of potentiator in a volume of 40 μl and incubated at room temperature for 10 min, a timepoint optimized in previous experiments resulting in a good window (positive control/negative control > 2) and signal to background ratio. YFP fluorescence was measured using an EnVision plate reader (PerkinElmer). The signal was recorded for 7 s, starting just before injection of 110 μl NaI buffer (137 mM NaI, 2.7 mM KI, 1.7 mM KH_2PO_4, 10.1 mM Na_2HPO_4, 5 mM D-glucose) into the well with a speed of 150 μl/s, resulting in a final volume of 150 μl. The excitation wavelength was 485 nm and the emission wavelength 530 nm. The capacity of potentiators to increase CFTR channel function was expressed as 1-[fluorescence 7 s after NaI addition (F)/fluorescence before NaI addition (F0)]. Data was normalized using the formula: normalized response = 100* (absolute response – negative control response)/(VX770 response – negative response) as such, VX770 response corresponds to 100. For Dose-response experiments, data was fitted using a 4 parameter hill function of the form Response = Bottom + (Top-Bottom)/(1 + 10^((LogEC50-concentration)*HillSlope)) to determine EC_{50} values.

Cell Surface Expression Assay

CFBE41o$^-$ TetON cells expressing HRP tagged F508del-CFTR (Veit et al., 2012) were seeded at a density of 4,000 cells per well in white 384-well plates (Greiner). Medium containing 500 ng/ml doxycycline was used to induce expression of the F508del-CFTR–HRP construct. After 3 days, cells were treated with corrector and/or potentiator compounds and transferred to an incubator at 33°C. On day 4, cells were washed 5 times with PBS containing Ca^{2+} and Mg^{2+} using a Bio-Tek plate washer and incubated with a chemiluminescent HRP substrate (SuperSignal West Pico Chemiluminescent Substrate, Thermo Scientific) for 15 min. Chemiluminescence was measured using an Envision plate reader (Perkin Elmer).

TECC Experiments

Trans-epithelial clamp circuit (TECC) recordings were performed using the TECC instrument developed and sold by EP Design (Bertem, Belgium). During the recording, the epithelial cells were bathed in a NaCl-Ringer solution (120 mM NaCl, 20 mM HEPES, 1.2 mM $CaCl_2$, 1.2 mM $MgCl_2$, 0.8 mM KH_2PO_4, 0.8 mM K_2HPO_4, 5 mM glucose, pH 7.4) on both the basolateral (640 μl) and the apical side (160 μl) and kept at 37°C. Apical amiloride was used to inhibit the endogenous ENaC currents (100 μM) while forskolin (10 μM) was applied on both the apical and basolateral sides to stimulate CFTR. All triggers and compounds used during the experiment were first dissolved in DMSO to a 1000 X concentrated solution, just prior to treatment a 10 X stock was prepared in the NaCl-Ringer solution which was used for addition of the correct concentration of trigger and or compound during the experiment. When using the F508del CFTR mutant, VX809 (3 μM) or GLPG2222 (1 μM) corrector was added on the basolateral side for 24 h to partially rescue F508del CFTR before adding the potentiator. For chronic experiments, the potentiator range was also added to the cells for 24 h and reapplied in the NaCl-ringer buffer prior to the electrophysiological recording. Measurements were done during a 20 min timeframe with recordings every 2 min. The transepithelial potential (PD) and transepithelial resistance (R_t) were measured in an open circuit and transformed to I_{eq} using Ohm's law. The increase in I_{eq} (Δ I_{eq}) was used as a measure for the increased CFTR activity. EC_{50} values were generated by measuring impact of different concentrations of compound on I_{eq} in primary cells. For this purpose each transwell was treated with a different compound concentration. CFTRInh-172 was used at 10 μM to assess the specificity of the response. Each compound concentration was tested in duplicate or triplicate and standard error of mean (SEM) was calculated except for R334W/F508del which was single replicate but had a large concentration range showing a clear concentration-responsive effect. Data was fitted using a 3 parameter hill function of the form Response = Bottom + (Top-Bottom)/(1 + 10^((LogEC50-concentration))) to determine EC_{50} values.

Patch-Clamp Electrophysiological Recording

A more complete description of the patch-clamp methodology can be found in a recent publication (Lin et al., 2016). Briefly, CHO (Chinese Hamster Ovary) cells were transiently transfected with pcDNA plasmids containing various CFTR constructs and pEGFP-C3. After transfection, cells were trypsinized and plated onto 35 mm tissue culture dishes dispersed with sterilized glass chips. Electrophysiological experiments were performed 3–7 days following transfection.

Patch-clamp experiments were performed at room temperature with an EPC-9 patch clamp amplifier (HEKA Instruments, Holliston, MA, United States). Recording microelectrodes were made from borosilicate capillary glass with a two-stage pipette puller (Narishige, Tokyo, Japan). The pipette tip was polished with a home-made microforge before use. The pipette solution contained (in mM) 140 NMDG (*N*-methyl-d-glucamine)-Cl (Fisher Biotec), 2 $MgCl_2$ (Fisher Biotec, Perth, Australia), 5 $CaCl_2$ (Fisher Biotec), and 10 HEPES (Fisher Biotec), pH 7.4, with NMDG (see Lin et al., 2016 for details). The pipette resistance when filled with the regular pipette solution was 3–5 MΩ. Once the tip of the pipette and the cell membrane established GΩ resistance, the electrode was quickly pulled away from the cell to form an inside-out patch, where the cytosolic side of the membrane was exposed to the perfusion solution. Cells were perfused with a bath solution having (in mM) 145 NaCl (Fisher Biotec), 5 KCl (Fisher Biotec), 2 $MgCl_2$, 1 $CaCl_2$, 5 glucose (Fisher Biotec), 5 HEPES, and 20 sucrose (Fisher Biotec), pH 7.4, with NaOH (Fisher Biotec). After establishing an inside-out configuration, the patch was perfused with a standard perfusion solution (i.e., intracellular solution) containing (in mM) 150 NMDG-Cl, 2 $MgCl_2$, 10 EGTA (Fisher Biotec), and 8 Tris (Fisher Biotec), pH 7.4, with NMDG (see Lin et al., 2016 for details) containing the catalytic subunit of protein kinase A (PKA) and 2 mM ATP. Once the phosphorylation-dependent

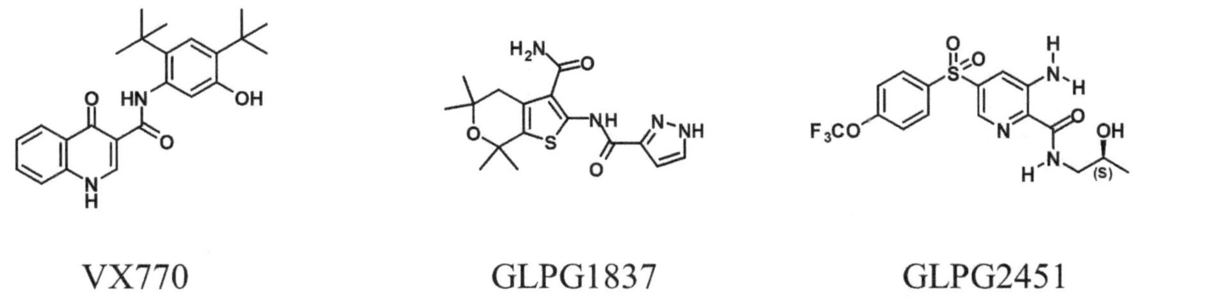

FIGURE 1 | Structure of VX770, GLPG1837, and GLPG2451.

activation of CFTR reached a plateau, 3 μM GLPG1837 or 10 μM GLPG2451 was applied in the continuous presence of 2 mM ATP until a steady state was attained.

Microscopic kinetic analysis was performed with a program provided by Dr. László Csanády (Semmelweis University, Budapest, Hungary) (Csanády, 2000). Experiments were performed 4-5 times and averages and SEM were calculated. The resulting Po values and single-channel kinetic parameters were compared with paired *t*-test (Excel, Microsoft); $P < 0.05$ is considered statistically significant.

RESULTS

Small compound libraries, selected on the basis of molecular shape and electrostatic similarity to known potentiators and correctors, were screened for their ability to improve channel activity of low temperature rescued F508del CFTR using a YFP halide based assay. Several hits were identified including several series of structurally related compounds. Two of these series were selected for further medicinal chemistry efforts and optimization, resulting in the molecules GLPG1837 (described by Van der Plas et al., 2018) and GLPG2451. The chemical structures of both molecules and VX770 as comparator are represented in **Figure 1**.

Both molecules effectively potentiate low temperature rescued F508del CFTR with an EC_{50} of 11.1 ± 3.6 nM (n = 10) and 3.5 ± 0.2 nM (n = 31) for GLPG2451 and GLPG1837 (a representation of the YFP quenching with time in the assay is represented in **Supplementary Figure 1**), respectively. Evaluation in a cell surface expression assay (Veit et al., 2014) shows that both molecules are not able to increase F508del CFTR levels at the plasma membrane and as such show no corrector activity (**Figure 2**).

Characterization of Novel Potentiators on Class III Mutations Using YFP Halide Assay

Both compounds were characterized for their ability to increase channel open probability of various gating defective CFTR mutants. **Figure 3**, represents a comparison of the potency and activity of VX770, GLPG1837, and GLPG2451 on various Class III CFTR mutations. A concentration-dependent increase in activity of G178R, S549N, G551D, and R117H CFTR was observed in the YFP halide assay. In this setting, GLPG1837 shows both a higher potency and a higher efficacy on all mutants tested when compared to VX770. The extent of the increased efficacy varies between the different mutations, 154% for G178R, 137% for S549N, 260% for G551D and 120% for R117H. The behavior of GLPG2451 is slightly different, being more potent on F508del CFTR when compared to VX770, but having similar potency on the other CFTR mutants evaluated. At saturation, the maximal ion channel activity is not as high as that seen for GLPG1837, but is similar to or higher than for VX770 (106% for G178R, 109% for S549N, 171% for G551D and 105% for R117H).

Characterization Using Patient Derived Bronchial Epithelial Cells

Compound activity was then tested in a more physiologically relevant system, i.e., primary bronchial epithelial cells derived from CF patients. The effect on the function of VX809 (3 μM) corrected F508del/F508del CFTR was determined using

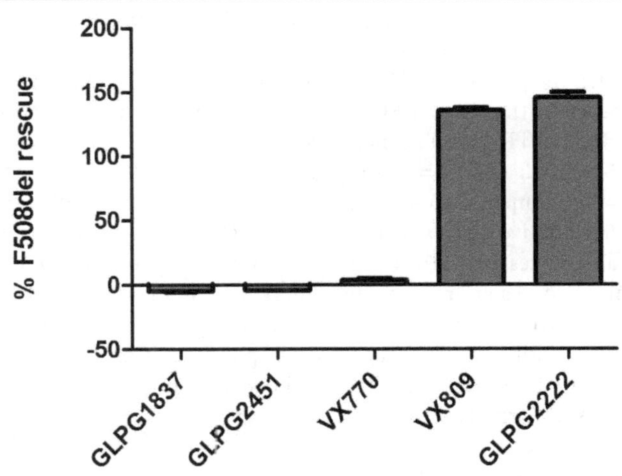

FIGURE 2 | Cell Surface Expression assay: Rescue of HRP-tagged F508del CFTR in CFBe41O- cells was evaluated in presence of (from left to right), 10 μM GLPG1837, GLPG2451, VX770, VX809, or GLPG2222. Percent of cell surface rescue of F508del CFTR was calculated using an internal reference compound 15 (derived from same chemical series as GLPG2222). (n between 1 and 155 for different samples).

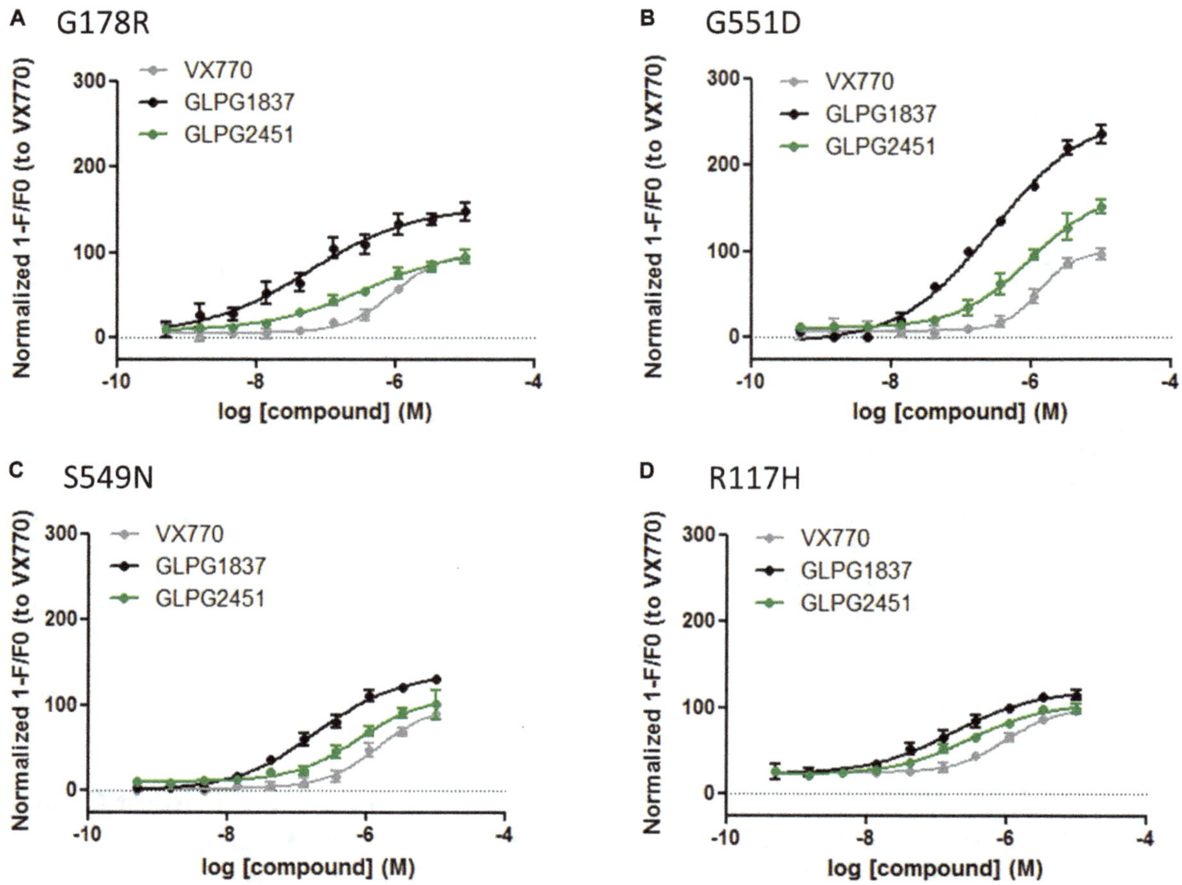

FIGURE 3 | YFP-Halide assay on HEK cells expressing different CFTR mutants: Effect of a concentration range of GLPG1837, GLPG2451, or VX770 on **(A)** G178R CFTR, **(B)** G551D CFTR, **(C)** S549N CFTR, **(D)** R117H CFTR. 10 μM Forskolin was used for channel activation. The measured YFP fluorescence quenching was normalized to VX770 response (*n* between 2 and 8 for each concentration tested).

an electrophysiological readout (TECC) and the data were compared to the data generated in the YFP halide assay. This showed the potency on VX809 corrected F508del/F508del HBEs to be lower (i.e., higher EC_{50}) than on low temperature rescued F508del CFTR in a YFP halide assay [46.6 ± 14.2 nM (n = 6) vs. 3.5 ± 0.2 nM (n = 31) for GLPG1837 and 68.9 ± 25.7 nM (n = 4) compared to 11.1 ± 3.6 nM (n = 10) for GLPG2451 (representative curves in **Figure 4A**)]. This could be the result of differences in the cell background or assay sensitivity but could also result from subtle differences in the structures of low temperature corrected and chemically corrected F508del CFTR resulting in different compound potencies. Consistent with the latter interpretation, VX770 showed a similar potency in both assay formats implying it is not simply an assay difference and that these novel potentiators may act in a mechanistically different manner to VX770 (80.7 ± 21.7 nM (n = 7) (TECC) compared to 126.2 ± 10.9 nM (n = 56) (YFP halide assay), data not shown). To further understand this difference, a YFP halide assay was developed using a GLPG2222-like compound (1 μM) to chemically correct F508del CFTR which allows to determine the potency of the novel potentiators in a setting more similar to the HBE setting. In this case, the potency of both GLPG1837 and GLPG2451 corresponded closely to the potency obtained on chemically corrected F508del HBE cells (**Supplementary Figure 2**), suggesting that the potentiators can differentiate between chemical and temperature corrected F508del CFTR while this is not the case for VX770. Evaluation of low temperature corrected F508del HBE cells was not feasible.

The data in HBE cells were generated by simultaneous addition of potentiators and forskolin, to activate CFTR channels, a protocol referred to as "acute setting." We also tested the compounds ability to potentiate F508del CFTR when incubated with the cells 24 h prior to the addition of forskolin, a setting called "chronic." Under "chronic" conditions the potency of GLPG1837 and GLPG2451 improved ~6 fold as compared to the "acute" setting (representative curves in **Figure 4B**).

As performed in the YFP halide assay, the effect of GLPG1837 and GLPG2451 on different gating defects was then investigated by TECC using G551D/F508del and R334W/F508del bronchial epithelial cells derived from CF patients.

On G551D/F508del cells, GLPG1837 had an EC_{50} value of 159 nM and an efficacy level of 173% of that of VX770. GLPG2451 had an EC_{50} value of 675 nM and an efficacy level

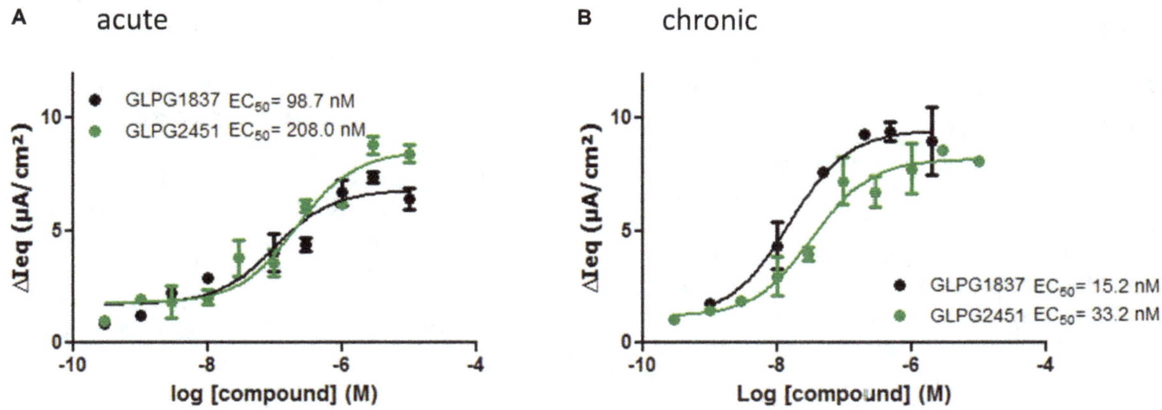

FIGURE 4 | TECC assay on F508del/F508del HBEs: effect of a concentration range of GLPG1837, GLPG2451 on GLPG2222 corrected F508del CFTR. **(A)** Potentiators were added to the cells in "acute" setting, correctors were added 24 h prior to electrophysiological recording. **(B)** Corrector GLPG2222 and a concentration range of the potentiators were added to the cells 24 h prior to electrophysiological recording ("chronic" setting). Data represented is net current obtained from the combined FSK and potentiator treatment (tested in duplicate for each concentration, single F508del/F508del HBE donor shown).

of 147% of that of VX770 (**Figures 5A,B**). The R334W/F508del mutant has residual activity, but improved channel activity can be obtained by addition of a potentiator. In this setting a potency similar to that for corrected F508del CFTR was found (EC_{50} value of 40.7 and 40.3 nM for GLPG1837 and GLPG2451, respectively) again with a higher channel opening

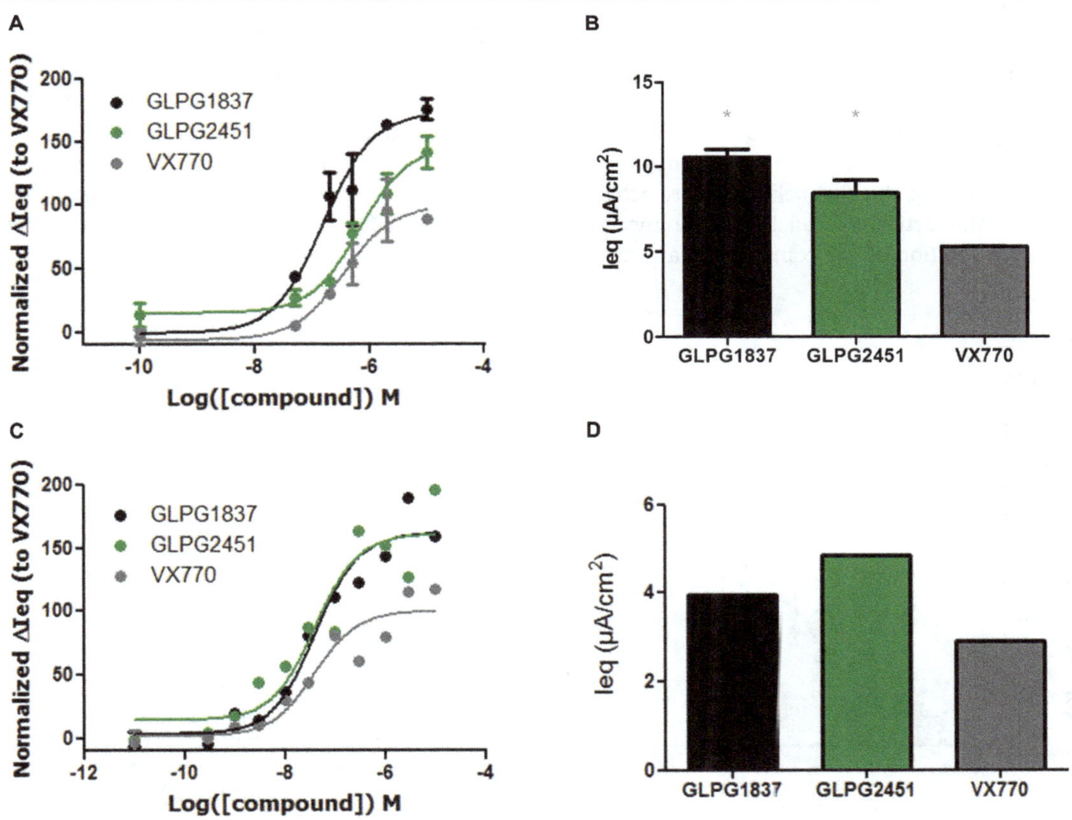

FIGURE 5 | Effect of a concentration range or maximal efficacy at 3 μM of GLPG1837, GLPG2451, and VX770 on G551D/F508del **(A,B)** and R334W/F508del **(C,D)** primary human bronchial epithelial cells. (n = 2 for each tested concentration in G551D/F508del, n = 1 for each tested concentration in R334W/F508del), data in **(A,C)** was normalized to VX770. * denotes a P < 0.05 compared to VX770 treatment. **(A)** Contains data for VX770 and GLPG1837 adapted with permission from Van der Plas et al. (2018).

when compared to VX770 (162% for GLPG1837 and 161% for GLPG2451) (**Figures 5C,D**).

GLPG1837 and GLPG2451 Activation of Wild Type (WT) CFTR

Potentiators influence the open probability of CFTR and are expected to interact directly with CFTR. It has been demonstrated by Yu et al. (2012) that VX770 is able to improve Cl-current carried by WT CFTR. We investigated whether GLPG1837 and GLPG2451 could also improve WT CFTR channel activity. For this, a YFP halide assay was set up using WT CFTR and the assay was optimized to have maximal sensitivity by transfecting with low amounts of WT CFTR plasmid to avoid saturation of the YFP quenching signal. Upon activation of WT CFTR with 10 μM forskolin, GLPG1837 and GLPG2451 were able to increase the open probability with a potency of 103.5 and 79.7 nM, respectively, which is slightly weaker than their potency on F508del CFTR (**Figure 6A**). In primary cells derived from a WT CFTR donor, EC_{50} values of 88.0 and 102.5 nM after activation with 0.1 μM forskolin were found for GLPG1837 and GLPG2451, respectively, similar to the observations in the YFP halide assay (**Figure 6B**).

GLPG1837 and GLPG2451 Improve CFTR Channel Function

The impact of GLPG1837 and GLPG2451 on the CFTR channel activity was further investigated with the patch-clamp technique using WT and/or F508del CFTR. Inside-out patches were excised from cells transiently expressing WT or F508del CFTR, and application of the compounds was found to result in reversible potentiation of the activity of the channels when pre-activated with PKA and ATP. This activation can be seen immediately (within seconds) after addition of the compounds (an example using GLPG2451 is shown in **Supplementary Figure 3**). For WT CFTR, the Po before potentiator stimulation was 0.39 ± 0.04 (with τ = 0.97 ± 0.34 s and τ_c = 1.35 ± 0.27 s, n = 5), in the presence of 3 μM GLPG1837 the Po increased to 0.78 ± 0.04 (n = 5) with open time (τ_o) and closed time (τ_c) constants of 1.48 ± 0.41 s and 0.29 ± 0.03 s, respectively, a result comparable to those seen with VX770 (Jih and Hwang, 2013). For F508del, the Po was also dramatically increased to 0.55 ± 0.05 (n = 5) with τ_o = 3.29 ± 0.82 s and τ_c = 2.18 ± 0.52 s with GLPG1837 (Pre-potentiator Po was 0.04 ± 0.01 with τ_o = 1.16 ± 0.15 s and τ_c = 17.86 ± 1.90 s). Addition of GLPG2451 to F508del CFTR resulted in an increase in Po to 0.57 ± 0.05 (n = 4) with τ_o = 5.05 ± 1.82 s and τ_c = 4.44 ± 2.23 s (Pre-potentiator Po was 0.05 ± 0.01 with τ_o = 2.14 ± 0.86 s and τ_c = 47.88 ± 20.41 s) (**Figure 7**). When determining the channel opening probability impact on F508del CFTR, GLPG1837, and GLPG2451 both behave in a manner comparable to that of VX770, i.e., reducing the closed time and increasing the open time of the channel resulting in a net increase in Po to the comparable level. As there is always an uncertainty regarding the number of functional channels in the patch, the estimated Po should be considered as a maximal value.

Are GLPG1837 and GLPG2451 Additive to Other Potentiators?

A next question we wanted to address is whether the novel potentiators would be able to increase further the CFTR activity when combined with each other or VX770. Whilst using the YFP halide assay to look into additivity/synergy seemed straightforward, none of the combinations resulted in higher CFTR (WT of F508del) activity when compared to the single components (data not shown). The absence of

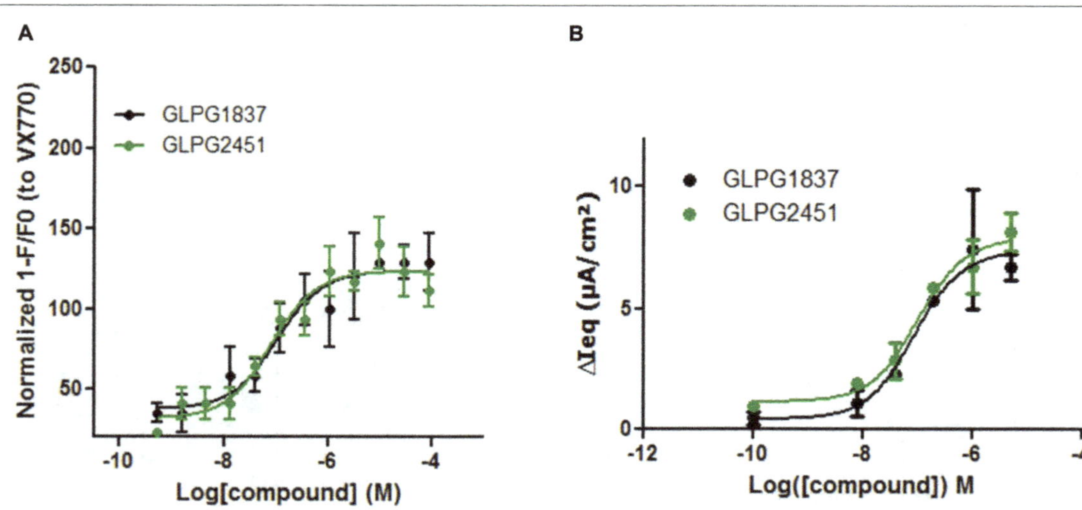

FIGURE 6 | Effect of a concentration range of GLPG1837, GLPG2451 on WT CFTR activity. **(A)** Effect of GLPG1837, GLPG2451 on WT CFTR using a YFP halide assay in HEK293 cells. Data is normalized to the response observed for VX770 set at 100% and each condition was tested in triplicate. **(B)** Effect of GLPG1837 and GLPG2451 on WT CFTR expressed by primary human bronchial epithelial cells (tested in duplicate for each concentration, potentiator response is shown after FSK treatment).

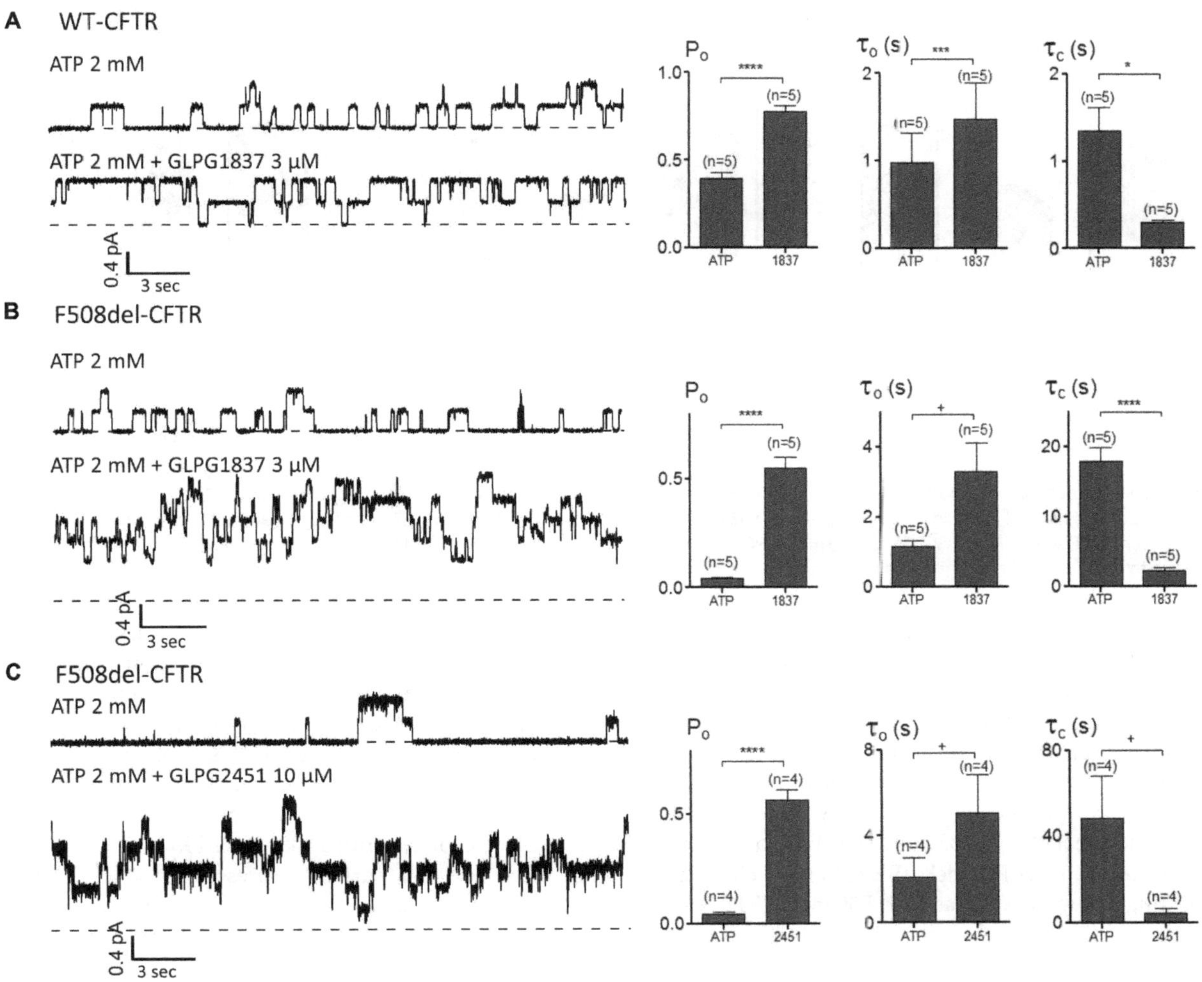

FIGURE 7 | Patch clamp studies on excised patches using CHO cells showing the effect of GLPG1837 on **(A)** WT (Po, τ_O, and τ_C), **(B)** F508del (Po, τ_O, and τ_C) and of GLPG2451 on **(C)** F508del (Po, τ_O, and τ_C) CFTR. The statistical analysis of single-channel kinetic parameters was described in Materials and Methods, every condition was tested at least 4 times. *$P < 0.05$; ***$P < 0.005$; ****$P < 0.001$; $^{+}P > 0.05$.

any additional effect on CFTR activity could be due to both potentiators having the same binding site, as molecules are then competing to bind CFTR or due to the dynamic window of the YFP halide assay which might not allow us to see further increase in CFTR activity. Since the maximal effect on WT or F508del CFTR with different potentiators was similar, but different in the case of G551D, it was decided to evaluate potentiator effects on G551D CFTR using the YFP halide assay (**Figure 8**). The experiments showed that GLPG2451 and GLPG1837 failed to show any additive effect, suggesting that both compounds either bind in the same area or are hampering each other's binding (**Figure 8C**). The two potentiators also did not show any additive effect to VX770 (**Figures 8A,B**). A possible limitation to this assay is that a Po of 1 could be reached and therefore no additivity would be observed. However, single channel patch clamp suggests that a Po of only 0.78 ± 0.04 is reached for WT CFTR and 0.55 ± 0.05 for F508del (**Figure 7**). While single channel studies on G551D CFTR were unsuccessful due to the low Po, it is highly unlikely that it would be reaching 1 when treated with either GLPG1837 or GLPG2451. Secondly, it could be that the signal in the assay itself reaches saturation, resulting in an apparent lack of additivity; we therefore performed similar experiments at a lower FSK concentration of 0.3 μM (data not shown). While these experiments resulted in a reduced assay window with higher variability, the data support a similar conclusion as presented with the higher forskolin concentration. In the case of GLPG1837, these data support the observations from Yeh et al. (2017) which suggested GLPG1837 and VX770 may share the same binding site.

GLPG1837 and GLPG2451 Have a Greatly Reduced Detrimental Effect on Surface Expression of Corrected F508del CFTR After Chronic Exposure

Recently, several groups published data on the potential inhibitory effect of chronically exposed VX770 on VX809

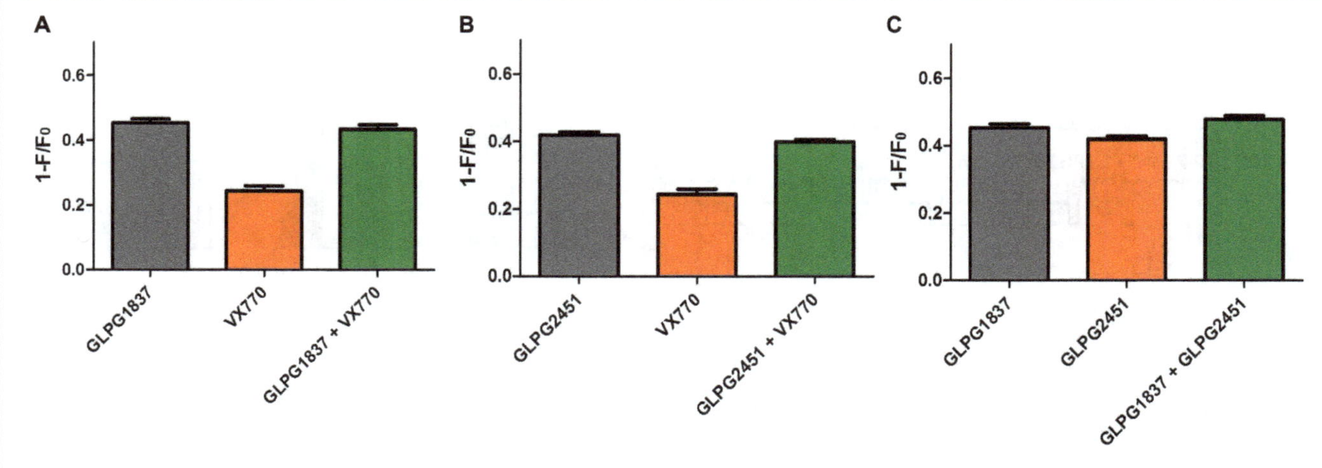

FIGURE 8 | Evaluation of additivity of potentiators on G551D CFTR in a YFP-Halide assay using HEK cells. **(A)** Effect of 90 μM GLPG1837, 10 μM VX770 and combination of both using 1 μM forskolin for channel activiation. **(B)** Effect of 90 μM GLPG2451, 10 μM VX770 and combination of both using 1 μM forskolin for channel activation. **(C)** Effect of 90 μM GLPG1837, 90 μM GLPG2451 and combination of both using 1 μM forskolin for channel activiation. $n = 9$ for each condition.

corrected F508del CFTR leading to reduced amounts of corrected VX809 F508del CFTR on the plasma membrane (Cholon et al., 2014; Veit et al., 2014; Avramescu et al., 2017). The translation to clinical efficacy of these observations at the concentrations evaluated is improbable, however not all types of potentiators show this effect under similar conditions (Veit et al., 2014). We thus included this analysis here. Addition of 10 μM of either GLPG1837, GLPG2451, or VX770 to VX809 corrected F508del/F508del HBE cells in a "chronic" and "acute" setting shows a decrease in F508del CFTR channel activity using VX770 in "chronic" setting, but this negative drug-drug interaction was not observed for GLPG2451 and GLPG1837 in similar experimental conditions (**Figure 9A**). A concentration range of the three potentiators was also evaluated in the cell surface expression assay using F508del CFTR tagged with HRP. F508del CFTR was first partially rescued with VX809 and co-incubated with various concentrations of potentiators. After 24 h co-incubation, the amount of rescued F508del CFTR present at the plasma membrane was determined by measuring the horseradish peroxidase activity. **Figure 9B** shows concentration-dependence of these potentiators on surface expression of F508del CFTR. While VX770 reduces the level of cell surface expressed F508del CFTR at all concentrations tested, a higher concentration of GLPG2451 or GLPG1837 is required to see this detrimental effect. In addition, between GLPG2451 and GLPG1837, GLPG1837 appears to be slightly more potent in decreasing the effect of corrector VX809.

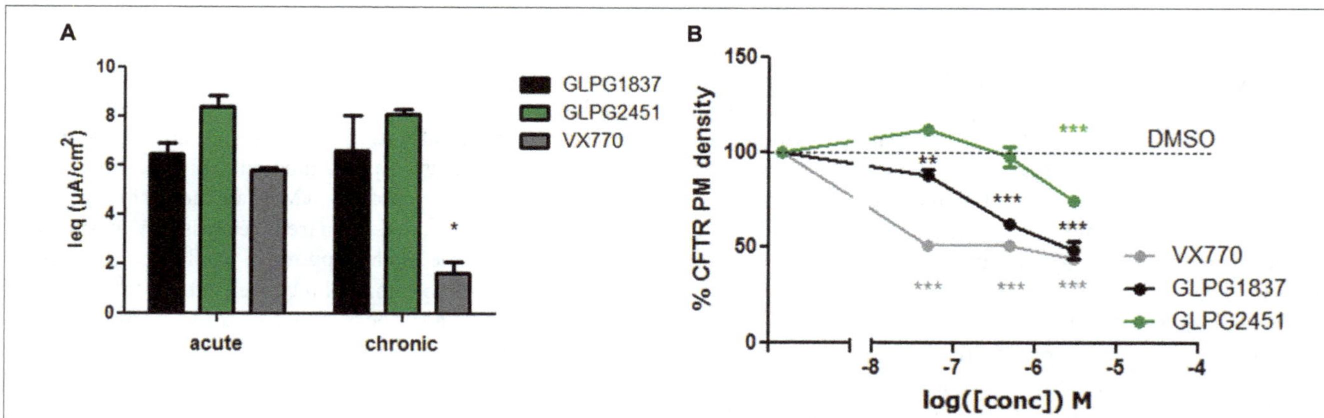

FIGURE 9 | Treatment of F508del CFTR expressing cells corrected with VX809 or GLPG2222 with potentiator in acute or chronic setting. **(A)** Activity of F508del CFTR in primary HBE cells treated for 24 h with 3 μM corrector VX809 (for evaluation with VX770) or 0.15 μM GLPG2222 (in combination with GLPG1837 or GLPG2451). Potentiators were added at 10 μM together with the corrector ("chronic") or just prior to the electrophysiological recording ("acute"). $N = 3$ for each condition, * denotes a $P < 0.05$ compared to similar compound treatment in the acute condition. **(B)** Rescue of HRP-tagged F508del CFTR in CFBe41O- cells treated for 24 h with 10 μM VX809 in combination with a concentration range of VX770, GLPG1837, or GLPG2451. Data was normalized to cells treated with VX809 only. In black, results for GLPG1837 are shown, in green, results for GLPG2451 and in gray results for VX770 ($n > 2$ for each point). $^{**}P < 0.01$; $^{***}P < 0.005$ compared to the control condition without compound treatment.

DISCUSSION

There are currently three approved CFTR modulator treatments available for cystic fibrosis patients, namely Ivacaftor, Orkambi and Symdeko. Of these, Ivacaftor (VX770) is a potentiator which improves the channel function for CFTR mutants with a gating or a conductance defect (Van Goor et al., 2009; Yu et al., 2012). In a clinical trial for patients carrying the G551D mutation, Ivacaftor improved the lung function by 10.6% (Ramsey et al., 2011). Orkambi and Symdeko on the other hand are combination therapies containing VX770 and VX809 or VX661, respectively, and are used for the treatment of patients homozygous for the F508del CFTR mutation. These later treatments show only minor benefit to the patients (Wainwright et al., 2015). Thus, there is a demand for the identification and development of novel correctors and potentiators, or more potent combinations of CFTR modulators for more effective therapy for CF patients with the F508del mutation.

This paper described the characterization of two chemically distinct potentiators GLPG1837 and GLPG2451 which have recently been identified (Van der Plas et al., 2018). Whilst other potentiators with interesting biological activities (absence of detrimental effect on the surface expression of corrected F508del CFTR and good efficacy on G551D CFTR) have recently been reported (Phuan et al., 2015; Park et al., 2016), these are not suitable for clinical development.

Both GLPG1837 and GLPG2451 are able to potentiate F508del, and some of the Class III and IV mutant CFTR. The pharmacological effects measured with YFP halide assays were found to correlate well to the results from more physiologically relevant assays using patient derived primary cells. In the case of F508del CFTR, the potency observed in the YFP halide assay on low temperature rescued CFTR was higher compared to chemical rescued F508del CFTR in both YFP halide and primary HBE cells. This difference was not observed for VX770 used in the same assay settings, suggesting that the novel potentiators may act on CFTR by a different binding mechanism. However, patch clamp data on F508del CFTR showed both GLPG1837 and GLPG2451 enhance the open probability by prolonging the open time and reducing the closed time, similar to that measured in a similar setting for VX770 (Jih and Hwang, 2013). The extent of activation of, e.g., G551D observed with GLPG1837 and GLPG2451 was higher compared to that seen with VX770 supporting a potentially different mechanism of action for the potentiators. Yeh et al. (2017) reported that GLPG1837 induced a 27.5-fold increase of macroscopic G551D CFTR current in comparison to a 10-fold increase by VX770 described in Jih and Hwang (2013). This increase in macroscopic current on G551D is in line with the observed higher channel activity observed in G551D/F508del bronchial epithelial cells in TECC.

We investigated whether both potentiators could act additively to each other or to other potentiators. On F508del CFTR, no further increase in CFTR was observed after addition of any second potentiator to GLPG1837 or GLPG2451. These data suggest that the potentiators cannot bind at the same time to F508del CFTR, or if they do, no further activation of the channel is possible. Yeh et al. (2017) suggested GLPG1837 and VX770 both bind to a similar epitope on CFTR using the patch clamp technique. Since for all potentiators a similar maximal signal is observed when using WT or F508del CFTR, use of these constructs does not allow for the assessment of whether they compete for a similar binding site.

On G551D CFTR, however, several of the potentiators yielded a different maximal quenching rate and therefore we investigated possible interactions between potentiators. GLPG1837 and GLPG2451 didn't show any additive effect to each other nor to VX770, suggesting that the potentiators compete for the same binding site or binding of one hampers binding of the other.

All these data demonstrate that the interactions between potentiators and the channel are complex and additional experiments including structural as well as mechanistic studies would be needed to better understand the binding site and mode of action of these potentiators.

Recently, two groups published data on the potential inhibitory effect of chronically dosed VX770 on VX809 corrected F508del CFTR leading to reduced levels of VX809 corrected F508del CFTR at the plasma membrane (Cholon et al., 2014; Veit et al., 2014; Avramescu et al., 2017). The clinical impact of this observation remains, however, unknown. In this study; the impact of chronic incubation of GLPG1837, GLPG2451, or VX770 together with VX809 was assessed in two different types of assays. When adding a high concentration of potentiator (10 μM) together with VX809 in primary bronchial epithelial cells derived from a F508del/F508del homozygous patient, the detrimental effect of VX770 on VX809 rescued F508del CFTR was observed, comparable to the data presented previously by Cholon et al. (2014). In the same setting, both GLPG1837 and GLPG2451 did not show this effect. Similar effects of VX770 were noted when looking into the effect of the potentiators using a cell surface expression assay as described by Veit et al. (2014). In the same assay, GLPG1837 also showed some reduction of partial rescued F508del CFTR but with a concentration response curve shifted to the right when compared to VX770. GLPG2451 on the other hand showed a minor effect on F508del CFTR rescued protein only at the highest concentration evaluated. These data show that there is a difference in sensitivity toward the negative effect of potentiators on partial rescued F508del CFTR, depending on the assay format used. Overall, GLPG1837 and GLPG2451 reduce membrane density of VX809 rescued F508del CFTR to a lesser extent than VX770 but to a slightly higher extent compared to the potentiator P5 described by Veit et al. (2014).

Based on the more desirable properties of GLPG1837 and GLPG2451 as potentiators, further testing was performed to determine suitability for use in the clinic. GLPG1837 was evaluated in humans and was well tolerated in healthy volunteers, with single doses up to 2,000 mg and 14 days dosing up to 800 mg (Vanhoutte et al., 2015). Similarly, GLPG2451 was evaluated in humans and was well tolerated in healthy volunteers (Brearley et al., 2017). These data supported progression of GLPG1837 and GLPG2451 into Phase 2 studies. Two studies have been designed based on the *in vitro* characteristics of GLPG1837 on Class III CFTR mutants. GLPG1837 has been dosed in patients harboring a G551D or S1251N CFTR mutation. A phase 1b study evaluating the triple combination of GLPG2451, GLPG2222, and GLPG2737 in F508del CF patients is currently ongoing.

In summary, having additional therapeutic options available is of high interest to the CF community. Here, we have characterized two CFTR potentiators with distinct chemical structures GLPG1837 and GLPG2451, the hallmark of which is their higher efficacy for promoting Class III mutant channel gating in comparison to VX770. Having these molecules available to the CF field will enable a better understanding of the molecular mechanism of defects associated with different CFTR variants. Moreover, further testing and optimization of these may pave the way for the development of additional treatment regimens for patients with CF.

AUTHOR CONTRIBUTIONS

MG, SM, KC and JVdS conceptualized the data. MG, SM, SVdP, A-SW, KV, AV, KS, OM, T-CH, PS, AS, MJ, LN, and MA investigated the data. KC wrote the original draft. MG, SM, and MA wrote, reviewed, and edited the manuscript. MG, SM, and KC visualized the data.

ACKNOWLEDGMENTS

We would like to acknowledge Niels Foolen, Moussa El-Abdellati for technical assistance.

REFERENCES

Avramescu, R. G., Kai, Y., Xu, H., Bidaud-Meynard, A., Schnúr, A., Frenkiel, S., et al. (2017). Mutation-specific downregulation of CFTR2 variants by gating potentiators. *Hum. Mol. Genet.* 26, 4873–4885. doi: 10.1093/hmg/ddx367

Brearley, C., Gesson, C., Kanters, D., Cock, P., Conrath, K., Corveleyn, S., et al. (2017). *Safety, Tolerability and Pharmacokinetics of a Novel CFTR Potentiator GLPG2451 with and Without a Novel CFTR Corrector GLPG2222 in Healthy Volunteers.* Available at: http://www.glpg.com/docs/view/59fc5e55eaea7-en

Cholon, D. M., Quinney, N. L., Fulcher, M. L., Esther, C. R., Das, J., Dokholyan, N. V., et al. (2014). Potentiator ivacaftor abrogates pharmacological correction of F508 CFTR in cystic fibrosis. *Sci. Transl. Med.* 6:246ra96. doi: 10.1126/scitranslmed.3008680

Csanády, L. (2000). Rapid kinetic analysis of multichannel records by a simultaneous fit to all dwell-time histograms. *Biophys. J.* 78, 785–799. doi: 10.1016/S0006-3495(00)76636-7

De Boeck, K., Zolin, A., Cuppens, H., Olesen, H. V. V., and Viviani, L. (2014). The relative frequency of CFTR mutation classes in European patients with cystic fibrosis. *J. Cyst. Fibros.* 13, 403–409. doi: 10.1016/j.jcf.2013.12.003

Fulcher, M. L., Gabriel, S., Burns, K. A., Yankaskas, J. R., and Randell, S. H. (2005). Well-differentiated human airway epithelial cell cultures. *Methods Mol. Med.* 107, 183–206.

Hadida, S., Van Goor, F., Zhou, J., Arumugam, V., McCartney, J., Hazlewood, A., et al. (2014). Discovery of N -(2,4-Di- tert -butyl-5-hydroxyphenyl)-4-oxo-1,4-dihydroquinoline-3-carboxamide (VX-770, Ivacaftor), a potent and orally bioavailable CFTR potentiator. *J. Med. Chem.* 57, 9776–9795. doi: 10.1021/jm5012808

Hanrahan, J. W., Sampson, H. M., and Thomas, D. Y. (2013). Novel pharmacological strategies to treat cystic fibrosis. *Trends Pharmacol. Sci.* 34, 119–125. doi: 10.1016/j.tips.2012.11.006

Jih, K.-Y., and Hwang, T.-C. (2013). Vx-770 potentiates CFTR function by promoting decoupling between the gating cycle and ATP hydrolysis cycle. *Proc. Natl. Acad. Sci. U.S.A.* 110, 4404–4409. doi: 10.1073/pnas.1215982110

Lin, W.-Y., Sohma, Y., and Hwang, T.-C. (2016). Synergistic potentiation of cystic fibrosis transmembrane conductance regulator gating by two chemically distinct potentiators, ivacaftor (VX-770) and 5-Nitro-2-(3-Phenylpropylamino) benzoate. *Mol. Pharmacol.* 90, 275–285. doi: 10.1124/mol.116.104570

Lubamba, B., Dhooghe, B., Noel, S., and Leal, T. (2012). Cystic fibrosis: insight into CFTR pathophysiology and pharmacotherapy. *Clin. Biochem.* 45, 1132–1144. doi: 10.1016/j.clinbiochem.2012.05.034

Merk, D., and Schubert-Zsilavecz, M. (2013). Repairing mutated proteins–development of small molecules targeting defects in the cystic fibrosis transmembrane conductance regulator. *Expert Opin. Drug Discov.* 8, 691–708. doi: 10.1517/17460441.2013.788495

Moran, O. (2010). Model of the cAMP activation of chloride transport by CFTR channel and the mechanism of potentiators. *J. Theor. Biol.* 262, 73–79. doi: 10.1016/j.jtbi.2009.08.032

Park, J., Khloya, P., Seo, Y., Kumar, S., Lee, H. K., Jeon, D.-K., et al. (2016). Potentiation of ΔF508- and G551D-CFTR-mediated Cl- current by novel hydroxypyrazolines. *PLoS One* 11:e0149131. doi: 10.1371/journal.pone.0149131

Phuan, P.-W., Veit, G., Tan, J. A., Finkbeiner, W. E., Lukacs, G. L., and Verkman, A. S. (2015). Potentiators of defective F508-CFTR gating that do not interfere with corrector action. *Mol. Pharmacol.* 88, 791–799. doi: 10.1124/mol.115.099689

Ramsey, B. W., Davies, J., McElvaney, N. G., Tullis, E., Bell, S. C., Døevínek, P., et al. (2011). A CFTR potentiator in patients with cystic fibrosis and the G551D mutation. *N. Engl. J. Med.* 365, 1663–1672. doi: 10.1056/NEJMoa1105185

Taylor-Cousar, J. L., Munck, A., McKone, E. F., van der Ent, C. K., Moeller, A., Simard, C., et al. (2017). Tezacaftor–ivacaftor in patients with cystic fibrosis homozygous for phe508del. *N. Engl. J. Med.* 377, 2013–2023. doi: 10.1056/NEJMoa1709846

Van der Plas, S. E., Kelgtermans, H., De Munck, T., Martina, S. L. X., Dropsit, S., Quinton, E., et al. (2018). Discovery of *N*-(3-Carbamoyl-5,5,7,7-tetramethyl-5,7-dihydro-4*H*-thieno[2,3-c]pyran-2-yl)-l*H*-pyrazole-5-carboxamide (GLPG1837), a novel potentiator which can open class iii mutant cystic fibrosis transmembrane conductance regulator (CFTR) channels to a high. *J. Med. Chem.* 61, 1425–1435. doi: 10.1021/acs.jmedchem.7b01288

Van Goor, F., Hadida, S., Grootenhuis, P. D. J., Burton, B., Cao, D., Neuberger, T., et al. (2009). Rescue of CF airway epithelial cell function *in vitro* by a CFTR potentiator, VX-770. *Proc. Natl. Acad. Sci. U.S.A.* 106, 18825–18830. doi: 10.1073/pnas.0904709106

Vanhoutte, F., Gouy, M., Haazen, W., Kanters, D., De Beckker, G., Geller, D., et al. (2015). "Safety, tolerability and pharmacokinetics of a novel CFTR potentiator GLPG1837 in healthy volunteers," in *Poster Presented at North American Cystic Fibrosis Conference (NACFS)*, Phoenix, AZ.

Veit, G., Avramescu, R. G., Perdomo, D., Phuan, P.-W., Bagdany, M., Apaja, P. M., et al. (2014). Some gating potentiators, including VX-770, diminish F508-CFTR functional expression. *Sci. Transl. Med* 6:246ra97. doi: 10.1126/scitranslmed.3008889

Veit, G., Bossard, F., Goepp, J., Verkman, A. S., Galietta, L. J. V., Hanrahan, J. W., et al. (2012). Proinflammatory cytokine secretion is suppressed by TMEM16A or CFTR channel activity in human cystic fibrosis bronchial epithelia. *Mol. Biol. Cell* 23, 4188–4202. doi: 10.1091/mbc.e12-06-0424

Wainwright, C. E., Elborn, J. S., Ramsey, B. W., Marigowda, G., Huang, X., Cipolli, M., et al. (2015). Lumacaftor–Ivacaftor in patients with cystic fibrosis homozygous for Phe508del CFTR. *N. Engl. J. Med.* 373, 220–231. doi: 10.1056/NEJMoa1409547

Yeh, H.-I., Sohma, Y., Conrath, K., and Hwang, T.-C. (2017). A common mechanism for CFTR potentiators. *J. Gen. Physiol.* 149, 1105–1118. doi: 10.1085/jgp.201711886

Yu, H., Burton, B., Huang, C.-J., Worley, J., Cao, D., Johnson, J. P., et al. (2012). Ivacaftor potentiation of multiple CFTR channels with gating mutations. *J. Cyst. Fibros.* 11, 237–245. doi: 10.1016/j.jcf.2011.12.005

Yu, Y.-C., Sohma, Y., and Hwang, T.-C. (2016). On the mechanism of gating defects caused by the R117H mutation in cystic fibrosis transmembrane conductance regulator. *J. Physiol.* 594, 3227–3244. doi: 10.1113/JP271723

7

Emerging microRNA Therapeutic Approaches for Cystic Fibrosis

Pauline Bardin[1], Florence Sonneville[1], Harriet Corvol[1,2] and Olivier Tabary[1]*

[1] *INSERM UMR-S938, Centre de Recherche Saint Antoine, Faculté des Sciences, Sorbonne Université, Paris, France,*
[2] *Paediatric Respiratory Department, Hôpital Trousseau, Assistance Publique – Hôpitaux de Paris, Paris, France*

***Correspondence:**
Olivier Tabary
olivier.tabary@inserm.fr

Cystic fibrosis (CF) is caused by mutations in the cystic fibrosis transmembrane conductance regulator *(CFTR)* gene and remains the most common life-shortening diseases affecting the exocrine organs. The absence of this channel results in an imbalance of ion concentrations across the cell membrane and results in more abnormal secretion and mucus plugging in the gastrointestinal tract and in the lungs of CF patients. The direct introduction of fully functional CFTR by gene therapy has long been pursued as a therapeutical option to restore CFTR function independent of the specific CFTR mutation, but the different clinical trials failed to propose persuasive evidence of this strategy. The last ten years has led to the development of new pharmacotherapies which can activate CFTR function in a mutation-specific manner. Although approximately 2,000 different disease-associated mutations have been identified, a single codon deletion, F508del, is by far the most common and is present on at least one allele in approximately 70% of the patients in CF populations. This strategy is limited by chemistry, the knowledge on CFTR and the heterogenicity of the patients. New research efforts in CF aim to develop other therapeutical approaches to combine different strategies. Targeting RNA appears as a new and an important opportunity to modulate dysregulated biological processes. Abnormal miRNA activity has been linked to numerous diseases, and over the last decade, the critical role of miRNA in regulating biological processes has fostered interest in how miRNA binds to and interacts explicitly with the target protein. Herein, this review describes the different strategies to identify dysregulated miRNA opens up a new concept and new opportunities to correct CFTR deficiency. This review describes therapeutic applications of antisense techniques currently under investigation in CF.

Keywords: cystic fibrosis, miRNA, therapy, oligonucleotides, CFTR (Cystic Fibrosis Transmembrane conductance Regulator), ANO 1 channel

INTRODUCTION

Cystic fibrosis (CF) is the most common lethal genetic disease in the Caucasian population. Since the gene responsible for the disease was identified in 1989 (Riordan et al., 1989), numerous discoveries have led to an improvement in patients' longevity and quality of life. It is a complex disease, and many advances are still needed to understand the mechanisms of the pathology, to cure patients.

Cystic fibrosis affects about 70,000 people worldwide (in the homozygous or heterozygous composite state). It is induced by the recessive mutation of the gene that encodes a chloride channel called CFTR for Cystic Fibrosis Transmembrane conductance Regulator (Riordan et al., 1989).

The *CFTR* gene is located on the long arm of chromosome 7 (7q31) and encoded for the CFTR protein composed of 1,480 amino acids and belongs to the family of ABC transporters (ATP-binding cassette transporters) whose central role is the active transport of various substrates, such as amino acids, peptides, proteins, and ions through the plasma membrane. The CFTR protein participates directly in the regulation of the transport of chloride ions at the cell membrane, as well as in the transport of bicarbonate ions, which are involved in the regulation of the pH of the airway surface liquid covering the pulmonary epithelium (Jun et al., 2016).

From a pathophysiological point of view, mutations cause alterations in the tissues or organs integrating the exocrine glands, such as the skin, pancreas, lungs, intestines, and reproductive systems. Currently, the leading cause of morbidity and mortality is related to damage to the lungs. They are characterized by an accumulation of thick, viscous mucus, recurrent infections, and chronic inflammation, causing an impairment of mucociliary clearance. Inflammation could appear before any infection; the secondary infection would only exacerbate the uncontrollable inflammation (Jacquot et al., 2008). In the long term, these various symptoms lead to the deterioration of the pulmonary epithelium with, as a result, repair mechanisms being activated at the root of the appearance of areas of epithelial rearrangement. Alongside the peeling and remodeling of the epithelium, subepithelial fibrosis develops, leading to impaired respiratory function.

To date, more than 2,000 mutations of the CFTR gene have been identified, the most common (found in nearly 70% of patients) being the F508del mutation of the protein (deletion of a phenylalanine at position 508). These mutations are divided into six classes according to their degree of severity in CF disease and the mechanism that disrupts CFTR function and induced a tremendous phenotypic variability of CF patients (Corvol et al., 2016). CFTR mutation classes were created according to their consequences on CFTR function mutations interfering with protein synthesis (class I), mutations affecting protein maturation (class II), mutations altering channel regulation (class III), mutations affecting chloride conductance (class IV), mutations reducing the level of normally functioning CFTR at the apical membrane (class V), and mutations decreasing the stability of CFTR present at the plasma membrane (class VI) (Fanen et al., 2014). The high number of these mutations and their effects on the functionality of the protein make an unique therapeutic approach complicated[1].

CYSTIC FIBROSIS AND THERAPEUTIC APPROACHES

At the moment, there is no cure for CF. The increase in life expectancy observed in recent years is in fact mainly due to better management of the disease with symptomatic treatments (physical therapy, mucolytic agents, anti-inflammatories, and antibiotics). New pharmacological therapeutic approaches (Vertex Pharmaceuticals) have been proposed to patients for less than a decade. They help to restore the defective protein to the cell membrane (correctors) and/or to potentiate its activity (potentiators). The first small molecule that has demonstrated efficacy is ivacaftor. Preclinical and different clinical studies have shown that ivacaftor corrects CFTR-mediated chloride transport in most class III mutations, class IV mutations, and some other residual function mutations (Bessonova et al., 2018). A subsequent series of clinical trials have shown that ivacaftor has a high level of efficacy in class III mutations, particularly in patients with G551D (Gly551Asp) mutation even in very young children (Rosenfeld et al., 2018). In all clinical studies, compared with placebo, treatment with ivacaftor improved lung function (FEV1) by around 10%, reduced sweat chloride concentration by around 50 mmol/L, improved quality of life, and reduced the frequency of pulmonary exacerbations. The second small molecule strategy has been to target patients who are homozygous for the F508del mutation with a combination of a corrector drug to restore trafficking of CFTR and a potentiator to make it functional even if the activity of the channel remained low. The different clinical trials have demonstrated an improvement of 2.8 to 3.3% in FEV1 read out, that reflect a small effect for a high cost that induces a debate in the different national institute for health (Gulland, 2016). Due to the heterogeneity of the mutations that affect the *CFTR* gene from patient to patient (Veit et al., 2016), these treatments are not applicable to everyone and therefore have a highly variable benefit, depending on the class mutation (Gulland, 2016). Unfortunately, at present, there is no treatment that would treat all patients and in particular patients with a class I mutation. These drug classes, however, are a frame of reference in the field, and new molecules based on the same strategy are still under development. However, other strategies are proposed at the same time. They improve mucociliary clearance, decrease inflammation or fight infection[2]. One of the new therapeutic strategies proposed in the literature is based on the stimulation of an alternative pathway to that involving CFTR for the transfer of chloride ions, such as that induced by the chloride channel ANO1 (Anoctamin-1, also called TMEM16A [transmembrane protein 16A]) (Caputo et al., 2008; Schroeder et al., 2008; Yang et al., 2008; Sonneville et al., 2017), which could also participate in the activation of CFTR in the cell membrane (Benedetto et al., 2017). Another proposed emerging approach is based on modulating the expression of the microRNAs that regulate target RNAs such as CFTR.

miRNAs: CFTR AND OTHER ASSOCIATED CHANNEL PROTEINS

MicroRNAs (miRNAs) are defined as small, non-coding, 21–23 nucleotide endogenous RNAs able of suppressing the expression of their target genes. miRNAs can be classified on their genomic location and gene structure, and in the miRBase database, more than 28,000 miRNAs are referenced (Kozomara and Griffiths-Jones, 2014). Almost half of the known

[1] www.genet.sickkids.on.ca/cftr

[2] https://www.cff.org/Trials/Pipeline

miRNA genes are located in intergenic regions. Intronic miRNA, are located in the introns of annotated genes, including both coding and non-coding genes. Intergenic and intronic miRNAs gene may exist as a single gene or a cluster of genes under the control of their own promoters. Mixed miRNA are found overlapping across an exon and an intron of non-coding genes (Wang and Cai, 2017; **Figure 1**).

They participate in the regulation of many cellular processes, and the impairment of their expression may be associated with some pathologies (Foster et al., 2013). miRNAs are produced by transcription and maturation of their mRNA, ultimately with the release of a mature miRNA that will be incorporated into a ribonucleoprotein complex called miRISC (miRNA-induced silencing complex; **Figure 2**). Traditionally, the regulation exerted by miRNAs on their target gene is specific, through the pairing of the mature miRNA with the 3′-UTR sequence of the target mRNA, called miRNA response element (MRE) (**Figure 3**). The activity of the miRNAs depends on a long sequence of only 6 nucleotides (the "seed" sequence). An MRE motif can, therefore, be found on different mRNAs, and a mRNA can contain a repetition of the same MRE motif or other motifs. miRNAs play a dominant role in the complex multiple-gene expression regulation networks (Sonneville et al., 2015). When talking about a therapeutic approach, it is essential to take into account the emergence of isomiR, the 3′ and 5′ sequence variants of canonical miRNAs, as well as the wrong annotations that can be found in the database. The data collected by sequencing also need to be systematically verified, as described previously for isomiR-34/449, involved in ciliogenesis (Mercey et al., 2017). Today, it is estimated that more than 60% of the genes encoding a protein are regulated by miRNAs (Friedman et al., 2009). Modulating the activity of a single miRNA as a result of the inhibition of its function or overexpression can thereby have a significant biological impact.

Many studies have focused on the potentially regulatory miRNAs of *CFTR* expression in CF. Gillen et al. (2011) were the first to identify miRNAs related to CFTR activity, several of them directly regulated its expression by binding to the 3′-UTR end of its mRNA. The regulation of *CFTR* mRNA expression differs according to the cell type being studied: it is, in fact, tissue-specific, and time-dependent, which makes the development of miRNA-targeting therapies meant to restore the function of CFTR complicated (**Table 1**). Thus, Viart et al. (2015) showed that *CFTR* regulation was different before and after birth, confirming previous results CFTR channel is strongly expressed but it falls after birth at the pulmonary level (Marcorelles et al., 2007). In fact, miR-101 negatively regulates *CFTR* expression in adult lung cell lines, but it has no effect on fetal bronchial epithelial cells. It, therefore, seems to play a crucial role, which evolves over time (Viart et al., 2015). The combination of this miRNA with miR-494 makes it possible to remarkably suppress the expression of CFTR in human renal embryos. *In silico* analyzes have shown that these two miRNAs can target genes concomitantly and thus influence the severity of CF patients' pathology (Megiorni et al., 2011). The direct link between miRNA and *CFTR* has subsequently been confirmed by other teams who have shown that miR-145, miR-223, and miR-494, alone or together synergistically, directly regulate *CFTR* expression. This is also the case for miR-509-3p and miR-494, which induce stronger repression of its expression (Oglesby et al., 2013; Ramachandran et al., 2013). In addition to being able to interact directly with *CFTR*, some miRNAs can also act on intermediate actors of its biosynthesis, such as the transcription factor *SIN3A* (SIN3 transcription regulator family member A), repressed by miR-138 (Ramachandran et al., 2012; **Table 1**). They showed that the overexpression of miR-138 contributes to increase the expression and the number of CFTR channels on the cell surface of secretory epithelia but also the activity of the channel, in healthy subjects and CF patient with F508del mutations even if the mutated channel is less active than the wild-type. All these results were mainly performed on mutated F508del CFTR protein and should be also performed on other class mutations. The implication of miRNAs in CFTR expression is also controlled by the highly variable, and compelling information on phenotypic variability and lack of genotype-phenotype correlation among patients with the same mutation in the CFTR gene. Thus, three polymorphisms have been identified in the miR-99b/let-7e/miR-125a cluster that modulates the expression of these miRNAs and may be associated with patient phenotypes (Endale Ahanda et al., 2015). In addition, polymorphisms present in the 3′-UTR region of CFTR mediate the binding of miR-509-3p and cause a decrease in CFTR expression (Amato et al., 2013).

Expression of miRNAs can also regulate the expression of other channels or others proteins whose activity is modulated by CFTR (**Table 2**), such as the cotransporter NKCC1 ($Na^+-K^+-2Cl^-$-cotransport protein) (Gillen et al., 2011) or the sodium channel ENaC (epithelial sodium channel) by miR-183, which is able to target the three subunit of ENaC (Kim et al., 2017). Recently, an increase in the expression of miR-9 was at the root of a decrease in expression of the chloride channel, ANO1, which modulated mucus hydration and chloride efflux activity (Sonneville et al., 2017).

miRNAs: OBSTRUCTION, INFECTION, AND INFLAMMATION

In recent years, studies showing the involvement of miRNAs in the regulation of other targets involved in various aspects of the pathology, such as inflammation, airway obstruction or infection, have opened up new ways of investigation. In fact, miRNAs are able to modulate the expression of genes involved in airway obstruction and the production of mucus, such as miR-146a modulating *MUC5AC*, which encodes one of the main pulmonary mucins implicated in the obstruction of the airway. The data highlight a negative feedback role for miR-146a in the control of MUC5AC production from airway epithelial cells stimulated by neutrophil elastase, which may be associated with the inactivation of MAP kinase and NF-κB signaling, the primary pathways implicated in CF airway inflammation (Zhong et al., 2011). The expression of miR-101 in the airways is therefore increased in the lungs of patients with CF, with an airway obstruction characterized by low levels of

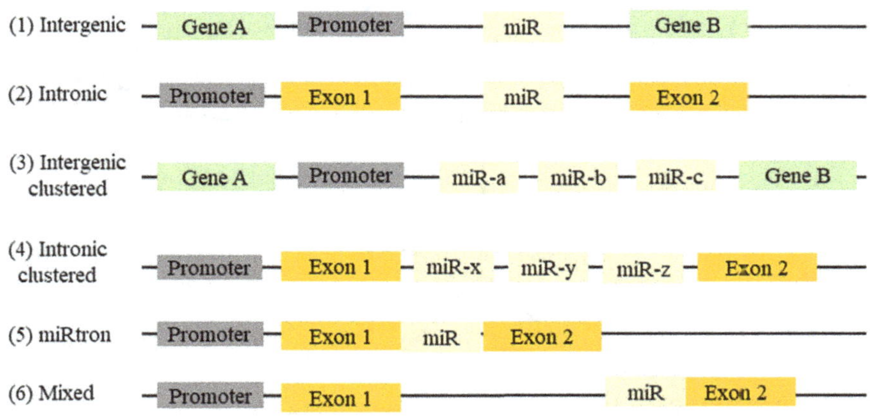

FIGURE 1 | Location of miRNAs gene in the genome: (1) miRNAs can be found between two genes (intergenic) or (2) in a gene (intronic). (3) They may be present in a single miRNA gene or (4) in a cluster of miRNA genes. (5) Sometimes intronic miRNAs may exist between two exons (miRtron) or (6) overlapping an exon and an intron of non-coding genes (mixed).

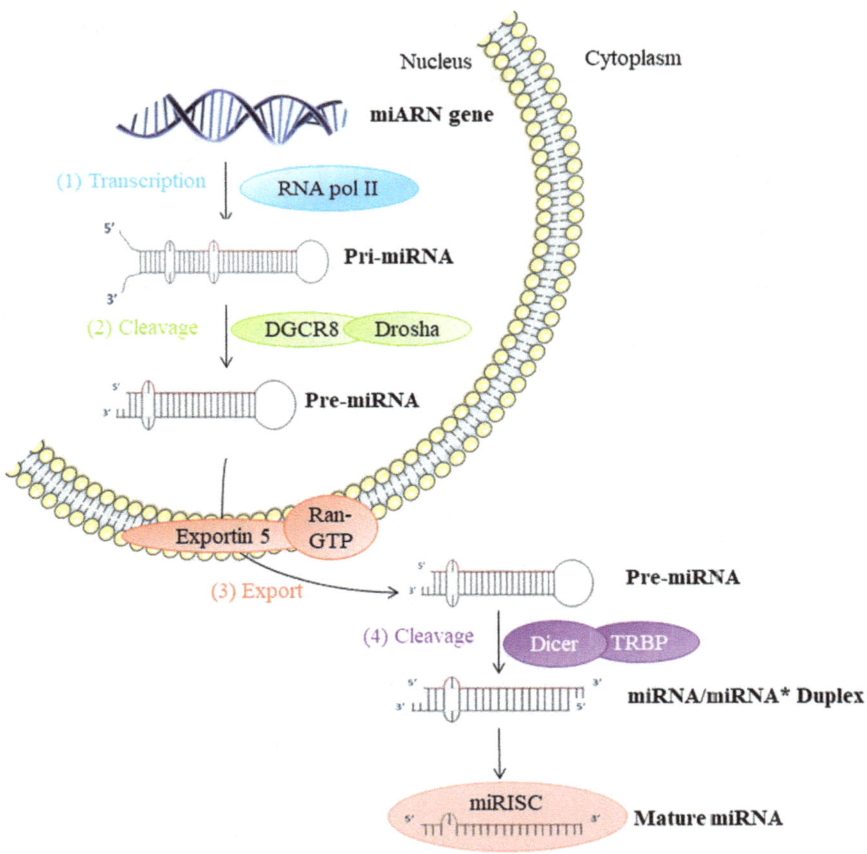

FIGURE 2 | Biosynthesis of miRNAs: (1) The biosynthesis begins in the nucleus by transcription of miRNA genes by RNA polymerase II (Pol II). (2) Long transcripts, pri-miRNA, are cleaved by Drosha and DGCR8 protein creating pre-miRNA with hairpin structure. (3) Exportin 5 transfers pre-miRNA into the cytoplasm. (4) Pre-miRNA is cleaved by Dicer into miRNA duplex in mature single-strand miRNA form. This miRNA mature form is incorporated into a miRISC ribonucleoprotein complex. This complex can then act directly on the mRNA in the cell where it is synthesized or out of the cell.

CFTR (Hassan et al., 2012) expression. miRNA expression is also influenced by external factors, like pathogenic bacteria, such as *Haemophilus influenza, Staphylococcus aureus,* or *Pseudomonas aeruginosa* (Oglesby et al., 2013; Ramachandran et al., 2013). The presence of pathogens in the light of CF airway surface epithelium contributes to modulate miR expression and consequently CFTR

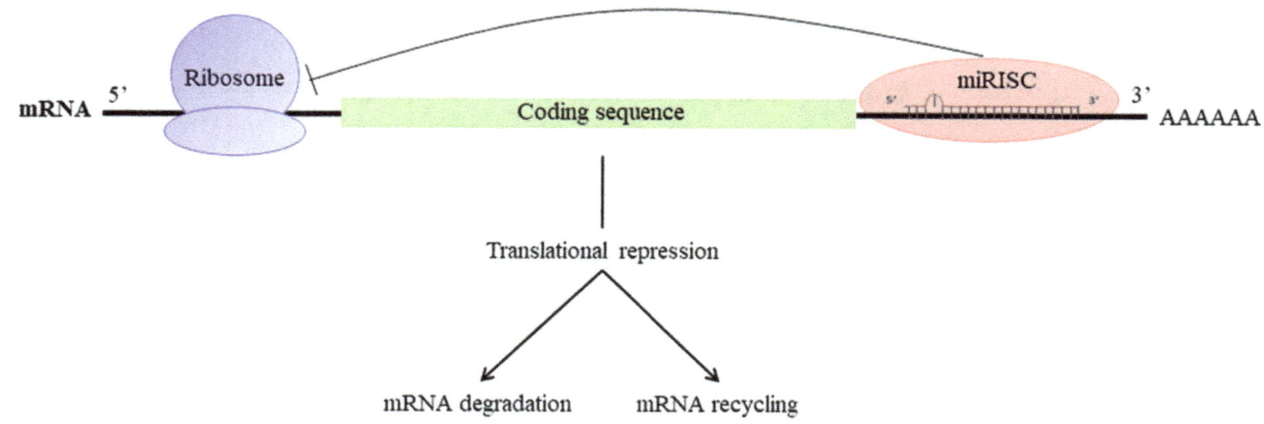

FIGURE 3 | Mechanism of action of miRNAs: miRISC complex attenuates mRNA translation and leads to the destabilization of mRNA by deadenylation and/or inhibition of translation.

TABLE 1 | Table showing deregulated miRNAs targeting directly or indirectly CFTR in the context of cystic fibrosis.

Target	miRNA	Models	Reference	Year
CFTR mRNA	miR-494, miR-384, miR-376b, miR-1246, miR-145, miR-331-3p et miR-939	Caco-2	Gillen et al., 2011	2011
	miR-600, miR-494, miR-384, miR-1290, miR-1246, miR-145, miR-1827, miR-331-3p et miR-939	PANC-1		
	miR-600, miR-494, miR-607 et miR-384	16HBE14o-		
	miR-101, miR-494	HEK293	Megiorni et al., 2011	
	miR-101, miR-144	16HBE14o-	Hassan et al., 2012	2012
	miR-145, miR-223, miR-494	Bronchial brushing, 16HBE14o-, CFBE41o-, HEK293	Oglesby et al., 2013	2013
	miR-509-3p, miR-494	Differentiated primary cell cultures, Calu-3	Ramachandran et al., 2013	
	miR-145, miR-384, miR-101, miR-600	A549	Viart et al., 2015	2015
	miR-505, miR-943, miR-377, miR-384, miR-101, miR-600	Beas-2B		
	miR-600	HBEpiC		
	groupe miR-17-92	Human macrophages	Tazi et al., 2016	2016
	miR-145-5p	Calu-3	Fabbri et al., 2017	2017
	miR-200b	Calu-3, 16HBE14o-	Bartoszewska et al., 2017	
	miR-145	CF and non-CF differentiated primary cell cultures	Lutful Kabir et al., 2017	
CFTR mRNA through SIN3A mRNA	miR-138	Differentiated primary cell cultures, Calu-3, HEK293, HeLa	Ramachandran et al., 2012	2012

expression. In an infectious diseases context (e.g., in the presence of *P. aeruginosa*), miR-93 expression, which is decreased, is associated with stabilization of IL-8 mRNA, thereby contributing to the maintenance of the inflammatory state. Altogether, the different works highlighted some complexes regulation and needed further investigation (Fabbri et al., 2014).

In the airways, inflammatory processes controlled by NF-κB are also partially regulated by miRNAs. The miR-199a-3p expression in the airway, which is decreased in CF context, is associated with an NF-κB hyperactivation. In fact, miR-199a-3p directly regulates IKKβ, which acts on the NF-κB signaling pathway and therefore on IL-8 secretion, the main cytokine dysregulated in the airways of CF patients (Bardin et al., 2018). Moreover, miR-509-3p, miR-494, and miR-126 directly target NF-κB and have shown that CFTR expression and function decreases when NF-κB is functional (McKiernan et al., 2013; Ramachandran et al., 2013). The two miR-93 and miR-17 regulate the production of IL-8 in bronchial epithelial cells (Fabbri et al., 2014; Oglesby et al., 2015). Bhattacharyya et al. (2011) therefore showed that miR-155 expression was

TABLE 2 | Table showing deregulated miRNAs direct/indirect targeting others targets in the context of cystic fibrosis.

miRNA	Target	Models	Reference	Year
miR-126	TOM1 Target of Myb1 Membrane Trafficking Protein	Bronchial brushing, 16HBE14o-, CFBE41o-, HEK293	Oglesby et al., 2010	2010
miR-155	SHIP1 (indirect: IL-8) SH-2 containing inositol 5′ polyphosphatase 1	IB-3, S9	Bhattacharyya et al., 2011	2011
miR-101, miR-1246, miR-494 et miR-384	SLC12A2 Solute Carrier family 12 Member 2	PANC-1	Gillen et al., 2011	
miR-449	Notch1 Notch homolog 1	Differentiated primary cell cultures	Marcet et al., 2011	
miR-146a	MUC5AC Mucin 5 AC	16HBE14o-	Zhong et al., 2011	
miR-145	SMAD3 Mothers Against Decapentaplegic homolog 3	Nasal epithelium cells, HEK293	Megiorni et al., 2013	2013
miR-31	IRF1 (indirect: Cathepsin 5) Interferon Regulatory Factor 1	Differentiated primary cell cultures	Weldon et al., 2014	2014
miR-93	IL-8 Interleukin 8	IB3-1, CuFi-1, NuLi-1	Fabbri et al., 2014	
miR-17	IL-8	Bronchial brushing, 16HBE14o-, CFBE41o-, HEK293	Oglesby et al., 2015	2015
miR-221	ATF6 Activating Transcription Factor 6			
miR-199a-5p	CAV1 Caveolin 1	Human and murine macrophages from lungs	Zhang et al., 2015	
miR-155	RPTOR Regulatory Associated Protein of mTOR complex	IB3-1, S9	Tsuchiya et al., 2016	2016
miR-199a-5p	TβRII TGF beta receptor II	Stellar hepatic cells	Chen et al., 2016	
miR-1343	TGF-β receptor	A549, 16HBE14o-, Caco-2	Stolzenburg et al., 2016	
miR-145	TGF-β Transforming growth factor beta	Primary cells from CF and non-CF patients	Lutful Kabir et al., 2017	
miR-183	SCNN1α,β,γ Sodium Channel Epithelial 1 alpha, beta, gamma subunit	CFBE41o-	Kim et al., 2017	2017
miR-9	ANO1 Anoctamin 1 (TMEM16A)	16HBE14o-, CFBE41o-	Sonneville et al., 2017	
miR-199a-3p	IKKβ Inhibitor of Kappa light polypeptide gene enhancer in beta cells, kinase beta	CFBE41o-	Bardin et al., 2018	2018

associated with CFTR activity. This miRNA can directly regulate SHIP1 (SH-2 containing inositol 5′ polyphosphatase 1) and indirectly alter the expression of IL-8 through activation of the signaling pathway involving PI3K/Akt (phosphatidylinositol-3 kinase/protein kinase B) and inhibition of the MAPKs (mitogen-activated protein kinases) (Bhattacharyya et al., 2011). The origin of the deregulation of miR-155 expression in CF cells is mediated by TTP (tristetraprolin) and KSRP (KH-type splicing regulatory protein) known to regulate miRNA biogenesis. The origin of this miRNAs dysregulation needs to be assessed. Some miRNAs may participate in the remodeling of the pulmonary epithelium and have a significant role in the development of the pathophysiology of the disease. Expression of miR-449 in the respiratory epithelium is essential to inducing direct inhibition of the Notch pathway and modulation of that involving the small GTPases, two events necessary for the production of motile cilia the beating of which allows mucus to be evacuated (Marcet et al., 2011; Chevalier et al., 2015). The remodeling of the pulmonary epithelium can also be caused by deregulation of TGF-β (transforming growth factor-beta) pathway, both in the expression of its receptors (TGF-βR1 and R2), and in signaling intermediates such as RPTOR (regulatory associated of mTOR complex 1) resulting in increased fibrosis and CTGF (connective tissue growth factor) or SMAD proteins, respectively through miR-1343, miR-155 and miR-145, thereby affecting fibrotic markers, cell migration and epithelial-mesenchymal transition (Stolzenburg et al., 2016; Tsuchiya et al., 2016; Fabbri et al., 2017). The deregulation of miR-31 in the airways of patients with CF contributes to pulmonary inflammation by increasing the activity of cathepsin 5, which causes antimicrobial proteins to deteriorate (Weldon et al., 2014). As for miR-221, it controls the transcription factor *ATF6* (activating transcription factor 6), which is involved in inflammation caused by endoplasmic reticulum stress (Oglesby et al., 2015). At last, miR-199a-5p regulates caveolin 1 (CAV1), a protein involved in the resolution of inflammation processes, targeting the PI3K/Akt/CAV1 axis (Zhang et al., 2015) and the TGF-β pathway (Lino Cardenas et al., 2013). Furthermore, it has been shown that Celecoxib, which modulates the Akt/miR-199a-5p/CAV1 axis, improves pulmonary hyper-inflammation caused by macrophages in patients.

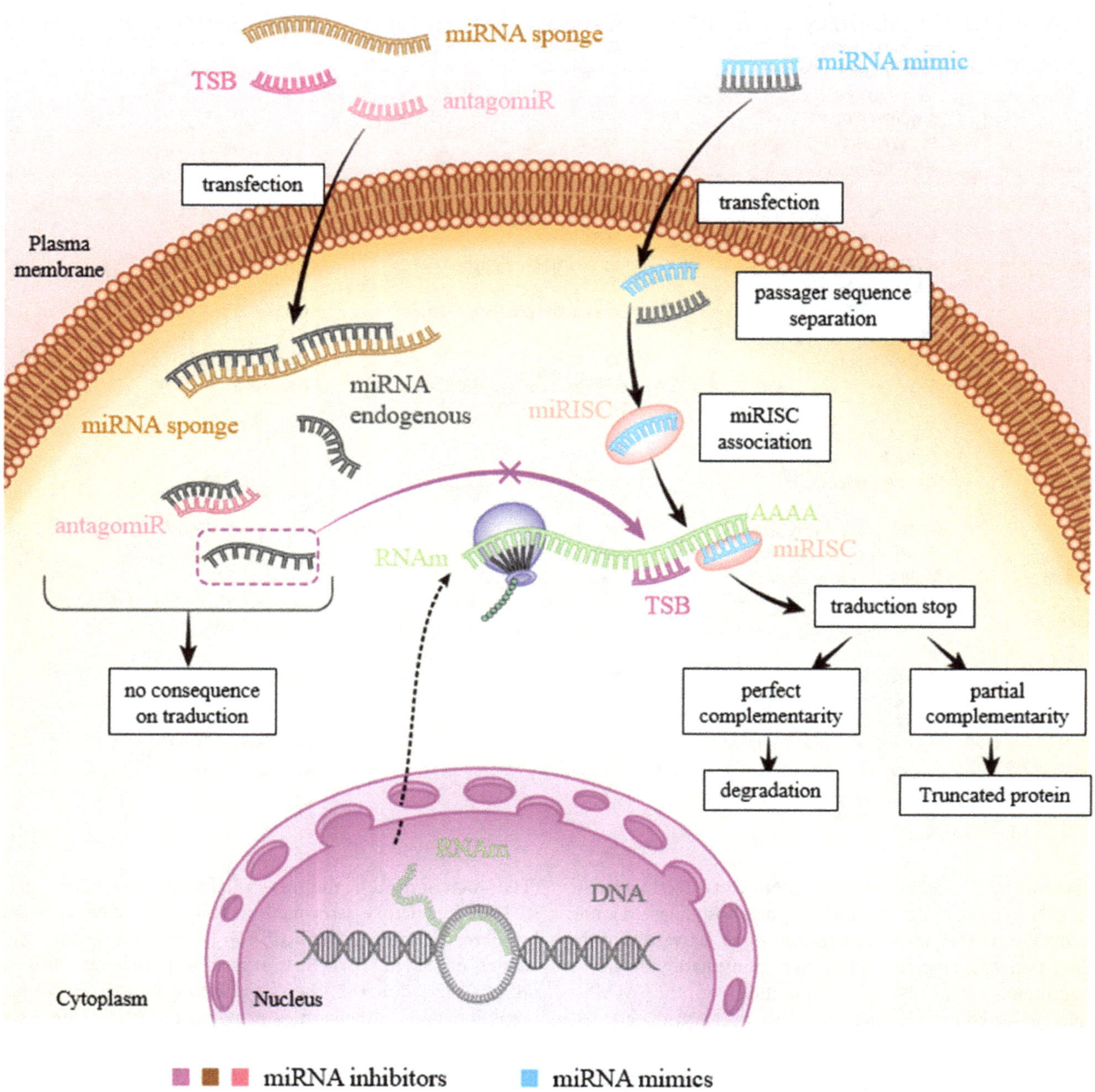

FIGURE 4 | Figure showing the various approaches to inhibit or mimic a miRNA. In physiological condition: the miRNA will bind to the 3′-UTR of its target to inhibit translation resulting to RNA degradation and/or mRNA recycling. To inhibit a miR action, there are three possibilities: transfection of (1) miRNA inhibitor (antagomiR): the miRNA inhibitor binds to the latter by complementarity and prevents its action on its target; (2) TSB: the TSB specifically binds to the 3′-UTR of the target mRNA at the miRNA binding site, the miRNA can then no longer attach to it and exert its action; and (3) mRNA sponge: the miRNA is saturated by the miRNA sponge which contains many miRNA complementary sequences, the miRNA can then no longer attach itself to its target. To increase the expression of a miR, transfection of a mimic of this miR is sufficient to inhibit translation of mRNA.

miRNAs: THERAPEUTIC STRATEGIES

MicroRNAs (miRNAs) are now considered as potential therapeutic targets. Two approaches have been followed for developing therapies based on their use: antagonists also called antisense oligonucleotides (ASOs) including inhibitors, miR sponges and target site blocker [TSB]) and miRNA mimics (**Figure 4**).

miRNA mimics are RNAs mimicking endogenous molecules and helping amplify their function. They are used to restore a loss of function. The purpose of this so-called "miRNA replacement therapy" approach is to reintroduce miRNAs whose expression is reduced in a pathological context. The proof of concept of this miRNA replacement therapy has been demonstrated with the use of miRNA tumor suppressors that stimulate anti-oncogenic signaling pathways and lead to the eradication of tumor cells (Wiggins et al., 2010). Let-7 and miR-34 mimics are currently in the clinical development phase to target a broad spectrum of tumors. The first molecule aimed at increasing the expression of miR-34 through the use of a mimic (MRX34) entered phase I clinical trials in 2013, as part of studies on multiple solid tumors (Bouchie, 2013). The main limitation of this approach is the difficulty formulating the mimic for its delivery to the target cells. One of the existing strategies to remedy, this is their coupling to nanoparticles. In the clinical trial using MRX34, the mimic is encapsulated in a liposome delivery system to facilitate its uptake by the target cells (Bouchie, 2013). An alternative approach uses delivery through miRNA expression vectors using adenovirus infection as previously described in a cancer therapy approach (Kota and Balasubramanian, 2010).

As for miRNA antagonists, they are used to inhibit endogenous miRNAs that show a-gain-of function in a pathological context. These therapies are similar to using siRNA (small interfering RNA), even through the regulatory systems involved are different. The miRNA antagonist or antagomiR (also called antimiR) binds to the mature miRNA targets with a powerful affinity. The duplex thus formed will then deteriorate. The main disadvantage of this type of therapy is that a miRNA can regulate the expression of several genes. Inhibition of a miRNA, which is nonspecific for a particular gene, can thus result in many side effects (**Figure 4**). TSB are antisense oligonucleotides designed to bind perfectly to the region of the 3′-UTR complementary to the miRNA.

Recent developments on miRNAs have accelerated the evolution of methods and chemical modifications that make it possible to inhibit miRNAs in a stable manner, and to optimize their delivery. These are locked nucleic acids (LNA), peptide nucleic acids (PNA), phosphorothioate groups, miRNA sponges and nanoparticles (McKiernan et al., 2013; Nguyen and Chang, 2017). Phosphorothioate oligonucleotides increase the resistance to 3′-exonuclease hydrolysis and bind more promiscuously and with higher affinity to proteins than antisense oligonucleotides with phosphodiester linkages, which are present in natural DNA and RNA (Gilar et al., 1998; Crooke et al., 2017).

The base constituting the LNA is a nucleic acid analog in which the ribose ring is chemically modified with through the introduction of a methylene bridge. This chemical modification provides the molecule with great thermodynamic stability and prevents its deterioration by nucleases by reinforcing its affinity for its target (Lindow and Kauppinen, 2012).

miRNA sponges are constructs, or RNAs, which have several binding sites for a miRNA of interest, which makes it possible to limit its availability and therefore its action on associated targets (**Figure 4**). In melanoma, TYRP1 (tyrosinase-related protein 1) RNA acts like a sponge which, when associated with miR-16, limits its tumor suppressor activity. Inhibition of the targets with a binding blocker allows miR-16 to act on its target RAB17 and prevents cell proliferation (Gilot et al., 2017). This type of approach using the properties of miRNA sponges and LNA could be considered for therapeutic purposes.

The primary route of administration for oligonucleotides for systemic applications is by parenteral injection, including intravenous (IV) or subcutaneous injection (SCI). Following systemic administration, phosphorothioate-modified single-stranded ASOs rapidly transfer from the blood into tissues (minutes to hours). Following SC administration, ASOs are rapidly absorbed from the injection site into the circulation with peak plasma concentrations consistently reached within 3 to 4 h, followed by a much slower terminal elimination phase (half-life of up to several weeks). Cell uptake is predominantly mediated by endocytosis. The substitution of one non-bridging oxygen with the more hydrophobic sulfur atom, as phosphorothioate, increases both plasma stability and plasma protein binding and thus, ultimately, tissue bioavailability (Yu et al., 2013).

Pharmacokinetic properties of ASOs are similar across species and gender that facilitate drug development (Yu et al., 2007). In the case with all second-generation ASOs and for all animal species evaluated, ASOs distributes broadly into most tissues with the exception of the central nervous system after systemic administration. The major systemic tissues of distribution include liver, kidney, bone marrow, adipocytes (cell body but not lipid fraction), and lymph nodes (Geary et al., 2015). Once intracellular, ASOs exhibit long half-lives (2–4 weeks) and prolonged activity in suppressing or altering expression of their target RNA. Few data are available about the oral route of administration, because this strategy requires profound modification of the formulation for the delivery. An *in vivo* study have compared IV and oral administration of an ASO and demonstrated that the tissue distribution profile was similar following both routes of administration, with highest concentrations observed in the kidney followed by the liver, lymph nodes and spleen (Raoof et al., 2004). In the case of CF, inhaled ASOs could be considered because the lung remains the primary target and to dismissed side effects but we currently have no setback on this approach, which has only been carried out by two teams targeting chloride ion channels with modified activity in CF (Crosby et al., 2017; Sonneville et al., 2017).

The first clinical antagonist developed in clinical studies, miravirsen (SPC3649), is an antimiR-122, which targets and sequesters liver-specific miR-122. MiR-122 binds to the 5′-UTR of the hepatitis C virus (HCV) mRNA that it stabilizes, causing the virus to accumulate. Miravirsen has the advantage of being coupled to an LNA base (making it resistant to nucleases) and having phosphorothioate linkages. Miravirsen was initially tested in mice and African green monkeys (Elmen et al., 2008). Its action was then studied in chimpanzees chronically infected with HCV, and a prolonged decrease in viral replication, without any evidence of viral resistance or side effects, was observed in the treated animals. In 2011–2012, a phase IIa study was conducted in patients with chronic hepatitis C who received five SCIs per week of miravirsen for a period of 29 days. This clinical study showed a prolonged, dose-dependent decrease in viral RNA levels and cholesterol levels and a change in the expression of about 100 genes in the liver. Viral RNA levels became undetectable in five patients, with, however, a rebound in the virus's expression in some of them (van der Ree et al., 2014). The variability of responses observed in patients suggests, however, that viral and/or host factors would influence response to treatment with miravirsen. Recently, a 5′-UTR C3U nucleotide change in HCV mRNA was demonstrated in patients who had a viral replication rebound (Ottosen et al., 2015). This mutant C3U is, in fact, insensitive to miravirsen. It would, therefore, make the virus independent of miR-122; the virus would then use an alternative mechanism to stabilize and replicate itself. The decrease in plasma levels of miR-122 in patients is still observed two months after the last injection of miravirsen, most likely due to the long half-life of miravirsen in tissues (about 30 days) (Matthes et al., 2016). Two pharmaceutical companies (*Roche* and *Regulus Therapeutics*) are currently involved in clinical trials to treat the HCV using antimiR-122.

In the case of CF, a team used TSBs which, by binding to the 3′-UTR of CFTR mRNA, prevents the binding of miR-101 and miR-145. The transfection of these molecules into the bronchial epithelial cells of patients with CF leads to an increase in CFTR expression and activity, suggesting that these TSBs could be used therapeutically (Viart et al., 2015). Other targets are being considered, like the protein ANO1 which, like CFTR, is involved in the secretion of chloride ions, pH regulation and the fluidity of airway surface liquid (Ruffin et al., 2013; Jun et al., 2016). It has shown that a TSB specifically preventing the binding of a miRNA (miR-9) on the 3′-UTR of the mRNA of the alternative chloride channel ANO1, made it possible, in *in vitro* and *in vivo* models, to increase its expression, and also its chloride activity, and cell migration, as well as mucociliary clearance independently of intracellular calcium concentration (Sonneville et al., 2017). The restoration of these parameters, deregulated at a physiological level, makes it possible to now propose the TSB ANO1 as a potential therapeutic target in the context of CF. Each patient would be able to benefit from this type of approach leading to the activation of a chloride secretion independent of CFTR. In this study, the TSB ANO1 was administered to animals intranasally, if this molecule were to be used in humans, its mode of administration would need to be determined. Inhalation seems to be the most appropriate method since these patients often have lung damage. Tissue-specific, it has less systemic exposure, reducing the risk of side effects. However, the patients' lungs have barriers, such as airways that are obstructed by mucus, that can make administration difficult. The passage of TSBs through the mucus therefore still needs to be studied.

CONCLUSION

Despite the improved care and recent progress in the identification of new therapies the predicted median survival of CF patients still remains in the low 40-years range in developed countries. New therapies and new strategies, alone or in combination with established therapies, are needed to prolong survival and improve the quality of life for all CF patients. The potential for modulating gene expression by the use of antisense oligonucleotides has become increasingly interesting in recent years, but safe delivery, long-term efficacy and side effects of prolonged treatment still need to be assessed. Advances in chemistry and molecular biology have provided the basis to develop antisense oligodeoxynucleotides and improve their selectivity, stability, and specificity of action. The antisense oligonucleotide drug platform is a really new approach for drug discovery, but basic science must be improved notably in understanding the molecular mechanisms that regulate CFTR and other chloride channels. Therapies targeting CFTR increase with ASO should be limited because channel increase will not necessarily induce increased activity especially for class III to VI mutations. The ease of delivery of modified antisense oligonucleotides seems to be linked with a lack of any major adverse side effects, making antisense oligonucleotides suitable candidates as a potential treatment for CF diseases.

AUTHOR CONTRIBUTIONS

PB, FS, and OT wrote the manuscript. PB, FS, HC, and OT participated in the design of this manuscript.

FUNDING

This research group was funded by grants from Inserm, Sorbonne University, sciences faculty (UPMC Paris 06) and the French non-profit organization "Vaincre la Mucoviscidose." PB received a Ph.D. fellowship from the "Ministère de l'Enseignement Supérieur et de la Recherche" in France. FS obtained a grant from the SATT Lutech and "Vaincre la Mucoviscidose."

REFERENCES

Amato, F., Seia, M., Giordano, S., Elce, A., Zarrilli, F., Castaldo, G., et al. (2013). Gene mutation in microRNA target sites of CFTR gene: a novel pathogenetic mechanism in cystic fibrosis? *PLoS One* 8:e60448. doi: 10.1371/journal.pone.0060448

Bardin, P., Marchal-Duval, E., Sonneville, F., Blouquit-Laye, S., Rousselet, N., Le Rouzic, P., et al. (2018). Small RNA and transcriptome sequencing reveal the role of miR-199a-3p in inflammatory processes in cystic fibrosis airways. *J. Pathol.* 245, 410–420. doi: 10.1002/path.5095

Bartoszewska, S., Kamysz, W., Jakiela, B., Sanak, M., Kroliczewski, J., Bebok, Z., et al. (2017). miR-200b downregulates CFTR during hypoxia in human lung epithelial cells. *Cell. Mol. Biol. Lett.* 22:23. doi: 10.1186/s11658-017-0054-0

Benedetto, R., Ousingsawat, J., Wanitchakool, P., Zhang, Y., Holtzman, M. J., Amaral, M., et al. (2017). Epithelial chloride transport by CFTR Requires TMEM16A. *Sci. Rep.* 7:12397. doi: 10.1038/s41598-017-10910-0

Bessonova, L., Volkova, N., Higgins, M., Bengtsson, L., Tian, S., Simard, C., et al. (2018). Data from the US and UK cystic fibrosis registries support disease modification by CFTR modulation with ivacaftor. *Thorax* 73, 731–740. doi: 10.1136/thoraxjnl-2017-210394

Bhattacharyya, S., Balakathiresan, N. S., Dalgard, C., Gutti, U., Armistead, D., Jozwik, C., et al. (2011). Elevated miR-155 promotes inflammation in cystic fibrosis by driving hyperexpression of interleukin-8. *J. Biol. Chem.* 286, 11604–11615. doi: 10.1074/jbc.M110.198390

Bouchie, A. (2013). First microRNA mimic enters clinic. *Nat. Biotechnol.* 31:577. doi: 10.1038/nbt0713-577

Caputo, A., Caci, E., Ferrera, L., Pedemonte, N., Barsanti, C., Sondo, E., et al. (2008). TMEM16A, a membrane protein associated with calcium-dependent chloride channel activity. *Science* 322, 590–594. doi: 10.1126/science.1163518

Chen, L., Chen, R., Velazquez, V. M., and Brigstock, D. R. (2016). Fibrogenic signaling is suppressed in hepatic stellate cells through targeting of connective tissue growth factor (CCN2) by cellular or exosomal MicroRNA-199a-5p. *Am. J. Pathol.* 186, 2921–2933. doi: 10.1016/j.ajpath.2016.07.011

Chevalier, B., Adamiok, A., Mercey, O., Revinski, D. R., Zaragosi, L. E., Pasini, A., et al. (2015). miR-34/449 control apical actin network formation during multiciliogenesis through small GTPase pathways. *Nat. Commun.* 6:8386. doi: 10.1038/ncomms9386

Corvol, H., Thompson, K. E., Tabary, O., le Rouzic, P., and Guillot, L. (2016). Translating the genetics of cystic fibrosis to personalized medicine. *Transl. Res.* 168, 40–49. doi: 10.1016/j.trsl.2015.04.008

Crooke, S. T., Wang, S., Vickers, T. A., Shen, W., and Liang, X. H. (2017). Cellular uptake and trafficking of antisense oligonucleotides. *Nat. Biotechnol.* 35, 230–237. doi: 10.1038/nbt.3779

Crosby, J. R., Zhao, C., Jiang, C., Bai, D., Katz, M., Greenlee, S., et al. (2017). Inhaled ENaC antisense oligonucleotide ameliorates cystic fibrosis-like lung disease in mice. *J. Cyst. Fibros* 16, 671–680. doi: 10.1016/j.jcf.2017.05.003

Elmen, J., Lindow, M., Schutz, S., Lawrence, M., Petri, A., Obad, S., et al. (2008). LNA-mediated microRNA silencing in non-human primates. *Nature* 452, 896–899. doi: 10.1038/nature06783

Endale Ahanda, M.-L., Bienvenu, T., Sermet-Gaudelus, I., Mazzolini, L., Edelman, A., Zoorob, R., et al. (2015). The hsa-miR-125a/hsa-let-7e/hsa-miR-99b cluster is potentially implicated in cystic fibrosis pathogenesis. *J. Cyst. Fibros* 14, 571–579. doi: 10.1016/j.jcf.2015.02.011

Fabbri, E., Borgatti, M., Montagner, G., Bianchi, N., Finotti, A., Lampronti, I., et al. (2014). Expression of miR-93 and IL-8 during *Pseudomonas aeruginosa* mediated induction of Pro-Inflammatory responses. *Am. J. Respir. Cell Mol. Biol.* 50, 1144–1155. doi: 10.1165/rcmb.2013-0160OC

Fabbri, E., Tamanini, A., Jakova, T., Gasparello, J., Manicardi, A., Corradini, R., et al. (2017). A peptide nucleic acid against MicroRNA miR-145-5p enhances the expression of the cystic fibrosis transmembrane conductance regulator (CFTR) in Calu-3 cells. *Molecules* 23:E71. doi: 10.3390/molecules23010071

Fanen, P., Wohlhuter-Haddad, A., and Hinzpeter, A. (2014). Genetics of cystic fibrosis: CFTR mutation classifications toward genotype-based CF therapies. *Int. J. Biochem. Cell Biol.* 52, 94–102. doi: 10.1016/j.biocel.2014.02.023

Foster, P. S., Plank, M., Collison, A., Tay, H. L., Kaiko, G. E., Li, J., et al. (2013). The emerging role of microRNAs in regulating immune and inflammatory responses in the lung. *Immunol. Rev.* 253, 198–215. doi: 10.1111/imr.12058

Friedman, R. C., Farh, K. K., Burge, C. B., and Bartel, D. P. (2009). Most mammalian mRNAs are conserved targets of microRNAs. *Genome Res.* 19, 92–105. doi: 10.1101/gr.082701.108

Geary, R. S., Norris, D., Yu, R., and Bennett, C. F. (2015). Pharmacokinetics, biodistribution and cell uptake of antisense oligonucleotides. *Adv. Drug Deliv. Rev.* 87, 46–51. doi: 10.1016/j.addr.2015.01.008

Gilar, M., Belenky, A., Budman, Y., Smisek, D. L., and Cohen, A. S. (1998). Study of phosphorothioate-modified oligonucleotide resistance to 3′-exonuclease using capillary electrophoresis. *J. Chromatogr. B Biomed. Sci. Appl.* 714, 13–20.

Gillen, A. E., Gosalia, N., Leir, S. H., and Harris, A. (2011). MicroRNA regulation of expression of the cystic fibrosis transmembrane conductance regulator gene. *Biochem. J.* 438, 25–32. doi: 10.1042/BJ20110672

Gilot, D., Migault, M., Bachelot, L., Journe, F., Rogiers, A., Donnou-Fournet, E., et al. (2017). A non-coding function of TYRP1 mRNA promotes melanoma growth. *Nat. Cell Biol.* 19, 1348–1357. doi: 10.1038/ncb3623

Gulland, A. (2016). Cystic fibrosis drug is not cost effective, says NICE. *BMJ* 353:i3409. doi: 10.1136/bmj.i3409

Hassan, F., Nuovo, G. J., Crawford, M., Boyaka, P. N., Kirkby, S., Nana-Sinkam, S. P., et al. (2012). MiR-101 and miR-144 regulate the expression of the CFTR chloride channel in the lung. *PLoS One* 7:e50837. doi: 10.1371/journal.pone.0050837

Jacquot, J., Tabary, O., and Clement, A. (2008). Hyperinflammation in airways of cystic fibrosis patients: what's new? *Expert Rev. Mol. Diagn.* 8, 359–363.

Jun, I., Cheng, M. H., Sim, E., Jung, J., Suh, B. L., Kim, Y., et al. (2016). Pore dilatation increases the bicarbonate permeability of CFTR, ANO1 and glycine receptor anion channels. *J. Physiol.* 594, 2929–2955. doi: 10.1113/JP271311

Kim, K., Hung, R. J., and Perrimon, N. (2017). miR-263a regulates ENaC to maintain osmotic and intestinal stem cell homeostasis in *Drosophila*. *Dev. Cell* 40, 23–36. doi: 10.1016/j.devcel.2016.11.023

Kota, S. K., and Balasubramanian, S. (2010). Cancer therapy via modulation of micro RNA levels: a promising future. *Drug Discov. Today* 15, 733–740. doi: 10.1016/j.drudis.2010.07.003

Kozomara, A., and Griffiths-Jones, S. (2014). miRBase: annotating high confidence microRNAs using deep sequencing data. *Nucleic Acids Res.* 42, D68–D73. doi: 10.1093/nar/gkt1181

Lindow, M., and Kauppinen, S. (2012). Discovering the first microRNA-targeted drug. *J. Cell Biol.* 199, 407–412. doi: 10.1083/jcb.201208082

Lino Cardenas, C. L., Henaoui, I. S., Courcot, E., Roderburg, C., Cauffiez, C., Aubert, S., et al. (2013). miR-199a-5p Is upregulated during fibrogenic response to tissue injury and mediates TGFbeta-induced lung fibroblast activation by targeting caveolin-1. *PLoS Genet.* 9:e1003291. doi: 10.1371/journal.pgen.1003291

Lutful Kabir, F., Ambalavanan, N., Liu, G., Li, P., Solomon, G. M., Lal, C. V., et al. (2017). microRNA-145 antagonism reverses TGF-beta inhibition of F508del CFTR correction in airway epithelia. *Am. J. Respir. Crit. Care Med.* 197, 632–643. doi: 10.1164/rccm.201704-0732OC

Marcet, B., Chevalier, B., Luxardi, G., Coraux, C., Zaragosi, L. E., Cibois, M., et al. (2011). Control of vertebrate multiciliogenesis by miR-449 through direct repression of the Delta/Notch pathway. *Nat. Cell Biol.* 13, 693–699. doi: 10.1038/ncb2241

Marcorelles, P., Montier, T., Gillet, D., Lagarde, N., and Ferec, C. (2007). Evolution of CFTR protein distribution in lung tissue from normal and CF human fetuses. *Pediatr. Pulmonol.* 42, 1032–1040.

Matthes, E., Goepp, J., Carlile, G. W., Luo, Y., Dejgaard, K., Billet, A., et al. (2016). Low free drug concentration prevents inhibition of F508del CFTR functional expression by the potentiator VX-770 (ivacaftor). *Br. J. Pharmacol.* 173, 459–470. doi: 10.1111/bph.13365

McKiernan, P., Cunningham, O., Greene, C., and Cryan, S. (2013). Targeting miRNA-based medicines to cystic fibrosis airway epithelial cells using nanotechnology. *Int. J. Nanomed.* 8, 3907–3915. doi: 10.2147/IJN.S47551

Megiorni, F., Cialfi, S., Cimino, G., De Biase, R. V., Dominici, C., Quattrucci, S., et al. (2013). Elevated levels of miR-145 correlate with SMAD3 down-regulation in Cystic Fibrosis patients. *J. Cyst. Fibros* 12, 797–802. doi: 10.1016/j.jcf.2013.03.007

Megiorni, F., Cialfi, S., Dominici, C., Quattrucci, S., and Pizzuti, A. (2011). Synergistic post-transcriptional regulation of the Cystic Fibrosis Transmembrane conductance Regulator (CFTR) by miR-101 and miR-494 specific binding. *PLoS One* 6:e26601. doi: 10.1371/journal.pone.0026601

Mercey, O., Popa, A., Cavard, A., Paquet, A., Chevalier, B., Pons, N., et al. (2017). Characterizing isomiR variants within the microRNA-34/449 family. *FEBS Lett.* 591, 693–705. doi: 10.1002/1873-3468.12595

Nguyen, D. D., and Chang, S. (2017). Development of novel therapeutic agents by inhibition of oncogenic microRNAs. *Int. J. Mol. Sci.* 19:E65. doi: 10.3390/ijms19010065

Oglesby, I. K., Bray, I. M., Chotirmall, S. H., Stallings, R. L., O'Neill, S. J., McElvaney, N. G., et al. (2010). miR-126 is downregulated in cystic fibrosis airway epithelial cells and regulates TOM1 expression. *J. Immunol.* 184, 1702–1709. doi: 10.4049/jimmunol.0902669

Oglesby, I. K., Chotirmall, S. H., McElvaney, N. G., and Greene, C. M. (2013). Regulation of cystic fibrosis transmembrane conductance regulator by MicroRNA-145, -223, and -494 is altered in DeltaF508 cystic fibrosis airway epithelium. *J. Immunol.* 190, 3354–3362. doi: 10.4049/jimmunol.1202960

Oglesby, I. K., Vencken, S. F., Agrawal, R., Gaughan, K., Molloy, K., Higgins, G., et al. (2015). miR-17 overexpression in cystic fibrosis airway epithelial cells decreases interleukin-8 production. *Eur. Respir. J.* 46, 1350–1360. doi: 10.1183/09031936.00163414

Ottosen, S., Parsley, T. B., Yang, L., Zeh, K., van Doorn, L. J., van der Veer, E., et al. (2015). In vitro antiviral activity and preclinical and clinical resistance profile of miravirsen, a novel anti-hepatitis C virus therapeutic targeting the human factor miR-122. *Antimicrob. Agents Chemother.* 59, 599–608. doi: 10.1128/AAC.04220-14

Ramachandran, S., Karp, P. H., Jiang, P., Ostedgaard, L. S., Walz, A. E., Fisher, J. T., et al. (2012). A microRNA network regulates expression and biosynthesis of wild-type and DeltaF508 mutant cystic fibrosis transmembrane conductance regulator. *Proc. Natl. Acad. Sci. U.S.A.* 109, 13362–13367. doi: 10.1073/pnas.1210906109

Ramachandran, S., Karp, P. H., Osterhaus, S. R., Jiang, P., Wohlford-Lenane, C., Lennox, K. A., et al. (2013). Post-Transcriptional regulation of cystic fibrosis transmembrane conductance regulator expression and function by MicroRNAs. *Am. J. Respir. Cell Mol. Biol.* 49, 544–551. doi: 10.1165/rcmb.2012-0430OC

Raoof, A. A., Chiu, P., Ramtoola, Z., Cumming, I. K., Teng, C., Weinbach, S. P., et al. (2004). Oral bioavailability and multiple dose tolerability of an antisense oligonucleotide tablet formulated with sodium caprate. *J. Pharm. Sci.* 93, 1431–1439. doi: 10.1002/jps.20051

Riordan, J. R., Rommens, J. M., Kerem, B., Alon, N., Rozmahel, R., Grzelczak, Z., et al. (1989). Identification of the cystic fibrosis gene: cloning and characterization of complementary DNA. *Science* 245, 1066–1073.

Rosenfeld, M., Wainwright, C. E., Higgins, M., Wang, L. T., McKee, C., Campbell, D., et al. (2018). Ivacaftor treatment of cystic fibrosis in children aged 12 to < 24 months and with a CFTR gating mutation (ARRIVAL): a phase 3 single-arm study. *Lancet Respir. Med.* 6, 545–553. doi: 10.1016/S2213-2600(18)30202-9

Ruffin, M., Voland, M., Marie, S., Bonora, M., Blanchard, E., Blouquit-Laye, S., et al. (2013). Anoctamin 1 dysregulation alters bronchial epithelial repair in cystic fibrosis. *Biochim. Biophys. Acta* 1832, 2340–2351. doi: 10.1016/j.bbadis.2013.09.012

Schroeder, B. C., Cheng, T., Jan, Y. N., and Jan, L. Y. (2008). Expression cloning of TMEM16A as a calcium-activated chloride channel subunit. *Cell* 134, 1019–1029. doi: 10.1016/j.cell.2008.09.003

Sonneville, F., Ruffin, M., Coraux, C., Rousselet, N., Rouzic, P. L., Blouquit-Laye, S., et al. (2017). MicroRNA-9 downregulates the ANO1 chloride channel and contributes to cystic fibrosis lung pathology. *Nat. Commun.* 8:710. doi: 10.1038/s41467-017-00813-z

Sonneville, F., Ruffin, M., Guillot, L., Rousselet, N., Le Rouzic, P., Corvol, H., et al. (2015). New insights about miRNAs in cystic fibrosis. *Am. J. Pathol.* 185, 897–908. doi: 10.1016/j.ajpath.2014.12.022

Stolzenburg, L. R., Wachtel, S., Dang, H., and Harris, A. (2016). miR-1343 attenuates pathways of fibrosis by targeting the TGF-beta receptors. *Biochem. J.* 473, 245–256. doi: 10.1042/BJ20150821

Tazi, M. F., Dakhlallah, D. A., Caution, K., Gerber, M. M., Chang, S. W., Khalil, H., et al. (2016). Elevated Mirc1/Mir17-92 cluster expression negatively regulates autophagy and CFTR (cystic fibrosis transmembrane conductance regulator) function in CF macrophages. *Autophagy* 12, 2026–2037. doi: 10.1080/15548627.2016.1217370

Tsuchiya, M., Kalurupalle, S., Kumar, P., Ghoshal, S., Zhang, Y., Lehrmann, E., et al. (2016). RPTOR, a novel target of miR-155, elicits a fibrotic phenotype of cystic fibrosis lung epithelium by upregulating CTGF. *RNA Biol.* 13, 837–847. doi: 10.1080/15476286.2016.1197484

van der Ree, M. H., van der Meer, A. J., de Bruijne, J., Maan, R., van Vliet, A., Welzel, T. M., et al. (2014). Long-term safety and efficacy of microRNA-targeted therapy in chronic hepatitis C patients. *Antiviral Res.* 111, 53–59. doi: 10.1016/j.antiviral.2014.08.015

Veit, G., Avramescu, R. G., Chiang, A. N., Houck, S. A., Cai, Z., Peters, K. W., et al. (2016). From CFTR biology toward combinatorial pharmacotherapy: expanded classification of cystic fibrosis mutations. *Mol. Biol. Cell* 27, 424–433. doi: 10.1091/mbc.E14-04-0935

Viart, V., Bergougnoux, A., Bonini, J., Varilh, J., Chiron, R., Tabary, O., et al. (2015). Transcription factors and miRNAs that regulate fetal to adult CFTR expression change are new targets for cystic fibrosis. *Eur. Respir. J.* 45, 116–128. doi: 10.1183/09031936.00113214

Wang, H., and Cai, J. (2017). The role of microRNAs in heart failure. *Biochim. Biophys. Acta* 1863, 2019–2030. doi: 10.1016/j.bbadis.2016.11.034

Weldon, S., McNally, P., McAuley, D. F., Oglesby, I. K., Wohlford-Lenane, C. L., Bartlett, J. A., et al. (2014). miR-31 dysregulation in cystic fibrosis airways contributes to increased pulmonary cathepsin S production. *Am. J. Respir. Crit. Care Med.* 190, 165–174. doi: 10.1164/rccm.201311-1986OC

Wiggins, J. F., Ruffino, L., Kelnar, K., Omotola, M., Patrawala, L., Brown, D., et al. (2010). Development of a lung cancer therapeutic based on the tumor suppressor microRNA-34. *Cancer Res.* 70, 5923–5930. doi: 10.1158/0008-5472.CAN-100655

Yang, Y. D., Cho, H., Koo, J. Y., Tak, M. H., Cho, Y., Shim, W. S., et al. (2008). TMEM16A confers receptor-activated calcium-dependent chloride conductance. *Nature* 455, 1210–1215. doi: 10.1038/nature07313

Yu, R. Z., Grundy, J. S., and Geary, R. S. (2013). Clinical pharmacokinetics of second generation antisense oligonucleotides. *Expert Opin. Drug Metab. Toxicol.* 9, 169–182. doi: 10.1517/17425255.2013.737320

Yu, R. Z., Kim, T. W., Hong, A., Watanabe, T. A., Gaus, H. J., and Geary, R. S. (2007). Cross-species pharmacokinetic comparison from mouse to man of a second-generation antisense oligonucleotide, ISIS 301012, targeting human apolipoprotein B-100. *Drug Metab. Dispos.* 35, 460–468. doi: 10.1124/dmd.106.012401

Zhang, P. X., Cheng, J., Zou, S., D'Souza, A. D., Koff, J. L., Lu, J., et al. (2015). Pharmacological modulation of the AKT/microRNA-199a-5p/CAV1 pathway ameliorates cystic fibrosis lung hyper-inflammation. *Nat. Commun.* 6:6221. doi: 10.1038/ncomms7221

Zhong, T., Perelman, J. M., Kolosov, V. P., and Zhou, X. D. (2011). MiR-146a negatively regulates neutrophil elastase-induced MUC5AC secretion from 16HBE human bronchial epithelial cells. *Mol. Cell. Biochem.* 358, 249–255. doi: 10.1007/s11010-011-0975-2

8

Role of the SLC26A9 Chloride Channel as Disease Modifier and Potential Therapeutic Target in Cystic Fibrosis

*Anita Balázs[1,2,3] and Marcus A. Mall[1,2,3]**

[1] Department of Pediatric Pulmonology, Immunology and Intensive Care Medicine, Charité – Universitätsmedizin Berlin, Berlin, Germany, [2] Berlin Institute of Health, Berlin, Germany, [3] German Center for Lung Research, Giessen, Germany

***Correspondence:**
Marcus A. Mall
marcus.mall@charite.de

The solute carrier family 26, member 9 (SLC26A9) is an epithelial chloride channel that is expressed in several organs affected in patients with cystic fibrosis (CF) including the lungs, the pancreas, and the intestine. Emerging evidence suggests SLC26A9 as a modulator of wild-type and mutant CFTR function, and as a potential alternative target to circumvent the basic ion transport defect caused by deficient CFTR-mediated chloride transport in CF. In this review, we summarize *in vitro* studies that revealed multifaceted molecular and functional interactions between SLC26A9 and CFTR that may be implicated in normal transepithelial chloride secretion in health, as well as impaired chloride/fluid transport in CF. Further, we focus on recent genetic association studies and investigations utilizing genetically modified mouse models that identified SLC26A9 as a disease modifier and supported an important role of this alternative chloride channel in the pathophysiology of several organ manifestations in CF, as well as other chronic lung diseases such as asthma and non-CF bronchiectasis. Collectively, these findings and the overlapping endogenous expression with CFTR suggest SLC26A9 an attractive novel therapeutic target that may be exploited to restore epithelial chloride secretion in patients with CF irrespective of their *CFTR* genotype. In addition, pharmacological activation of SLC26A9 may help to augment the effect of CFTR modulator therapies in patients with CF carrying responsive mutations such as the most common disease-causing mutation F508del-CFTR. However, future research and development including the identification of compounds that activate SLC26A9-mediated chloride transport are needed to explore this alternative chloride channel as a therapeutic target in CF and potentially other muco-obstructive lung diseases.

Keywords: cystic fibrosis, epithelial ion transport, chloride channels, SLC26A9, pharmacology

INTRODUCTION

Cystic fibrosis (CF) is a severe life-shortening multiorgan disease caused by mutations in the gene encoding the CF transmembrane conductance regulator (CFTR) chloride channel, which plays a fundamental role in salt and fluid transport across the surfaces and ducts of many epithelial organs including the lungs, pancreas, and gastro-intestinal tract. In patients with CF, CFTR dysfunction results in impaired epithelial ion and water transport that leads to a characteristic multi-organ pathology (Mall and Hartl, 2014). More, than 2000 *CFTR* variants have been identified in CF patients, with F508del being the most common accounting for 70% of all CF mutations (Sosnay et al., 2013). Disease-causing mutations may lead to various molecular defects in CFTR protein production, processing, channel function, and stability at the plasma membrane (Welsh and Smith, 1993; Mall and Hartl, 2014). Drug development efforts aiming to restore CFTR function have yielded mutation specific pharmacotherapies that are now available for a subgroup of patients with CF (Gentzsch and Mall, 2018). These include the CFTR potentiator compound ivacaftor (VX-770) that can improve channel activity in CFTR gating mutations present in ~5% of CF patients and the combination of ivacaftor with the CFTR corrector compound lumacaftor (VX-809) that has been approved for F508del homozygous patients (Ratjen et al., 2017). The large number of disease-causing variants and the variability of biological effects of CFTR mutations and their responsiveness to CFTR modulator therapies argues that targeting an alternative chloride channel may be an attractive therapeutic strategy in CF (Li et al., 2017). Emerging evidence suggests that the alternative chloride channel SLC26A9 is a modulator of CFTR function and a potential candidate to circumvent the primary ion transport defect in several organs affected by CF including the lungs, the pancreas, and the gastro-intestinal tract independent of the *CFTR* genotype (Li et al., 2017; Gentzsch and Mall, 2018). In this review, we summarize the basic physiological and pharmacological properties of SLC26A9, outline its regulation and molecular interaction with CFTR, detail the role of SLC26A9 as a disease modifier in CF and potentially in other diseases, and finally discuss the impact of these discoveries on future research that is needed to explore this alternative chloride channel as a potential therapeutic target in the clinical arena.

PHYSIOLOGY, PHARMACOLOGY, AND REGULATION OF SLC26A9

SLC26A9 is a member of the solute-linked carrier 26 (SLC26) anion transporter family that functions uniquely as a chloride channel with minimal conductance to bicarbonate (Dorwart et al., 2007; Loriol et al., 2008). SLC26A9 is mainly expressed in epithelial cells of the respiratory tract, stomach, duodenum, ileum, and the pancreas, while transcripts were also detected in the salivary gland, kidney, brain, heart, prostate, testis, ovary, and skin (Lohi et al., 2002; Xu et al., 2005; Chang et al., 2009b; Lee et al., 2015; Liu et al., 2015; Consortium, 2017). SLC26 members share a conserved structural organization: N-terminally the SLC26/sulphate permease transmembrane domain and C-terminally the cytoplasmic sulphate transporter and anti-sigma factor antagonist (STAS) domain (Geertsma et al., 2015). The STAS domain plays a role in membrane targeting, interaction with scaffolding proteins and other ion channels (detailed later). Furthermore, structural variants in the STAS domain were reported to associate with diseases linked to SLC26 transporters (Sharma et al., 2011). SLC26A9 also has a type-I PDZ-binding domain at the C-terminus (T-A-L), which may promote vesicular trafficking or assembly of macromolecular complexes as seen in other SLC26 members (Lohi et al., 2003; Rossmann et al., 2005). The human SLC26A9 transcript is alternatively spliced, such that inclusion of an exon results in a 96 amino acid extension at the C-terminus (isoform 2). The shorter splice form of 791 residues was designated as canonical isoform, which was also mainly used in heterologous expression systems; however, the isoform-ratio in specific tissues has not yet been elucidated. Similarly to the glycosylation pattern of CFTR, SLC26A9 also displays both core- and complex N-glycosylated forms, which may be important for plasma membrane targeting or function (Li J. et al., 2014; Salomon et al., 2016; Thomson et al., 2016; Bertrand et al., 2017).

The function of SLC26A9 has been widely investigated in heterologous expression systems. Whole-cell patch clamp studies showed that SLC26A9 is a constitutively active chloride channel displaying linear current–voltage characteristics (Dorwart et al., 2007; Loriol et al., 2008; Bertrand et al., 2009; Avella et al., 2011b; Salomon et al., 2016), while the current amplitude was not affected by cAMP stimulation or increase in intracellular Ca^{2+} (Bertrand et al., 2009; Salomon et al., 2016). Interestingly, SLC26A9-expressing epithelial monolayers studied in Ussing chambers displayed constitutive and forskolin stimulated chloride currents, which may be attributed to the enhanced transepithelial electrochemical gradient generated by activation of basolateral potassium channels by cAMP/PKA signaling (Mall et al., 2000; Salomon et al., 2016). Moreover, studies in primary human bronchial epithelial (HBE) cells elegantly demonstrated the presence of a SLC26A9-mediated transepithelial chloride conductance, which contributed to basal and to cAMP/PKA stimulated chloride currents (Bertrand et al., 2009, 2017). These finding support that SLC26A9 could provide an alternative pathway for chloride secretion that may compensate for CFTR dysfunction in CF epithelia. In addition, several studies suggested that SLC26A9 also functions as a chloride-bicarbonate exchanger (Xu et al., 2005; Chang et al., 2009b; Demitrack et al., 2010) and sodium transporter (Chang et al., 2009b). However, the contribution of SLC26A9 to epithelial bicarbonate and sodium transport is not completely understood (see discussion at stomach) and it is possible that transport modes depend on the cell and tissue context.

In the absence of sensitive and specific antibodies for immunolocalization studies, investigations of SLC26A9 largely relied on pharmacological tools. Multiple compounds were found to inhibit SLC26A9 at various potency and selectivity. Highly effective inhibitors include several non-selective chloride channel blockers, such as flufenamic acid, niflumic acid, GlyH-101, and 5-Nitro-2-(3-phenylpropylamino)benzoic acid (NPPB), while anion-exchanger inhibitor 4,4′-Diisothiocyanatostilbene-2,2′-disulfonic acid (DIDS) only partially inhibited SLC26A9 (Dorwart et al., 2007; Loriol et al., 2008; Salomon et al., 2016). On the other hand, SLC26A9 is not sensitive to diphenylamine-2-carboxylic acid (DPC), glibenclamide or CFTRinh172, which makes differentiation from CFTR-mediated chloride currents possible (Loriol et al., 2008; Bertrand et al., 2009;

Salomon et al., 2016). Despite the lack of highly selective inhibitors, this characteristic "pharmacological fingerprint" enabled investigation of SLC26A9-mediated chloride secretion in primary epithelial cultures and native tissues (Anagnostopoulou et al., 2012; Bertrand et al., 2017).

The constitutive channel activity suggests that SLC26A9-mediated chloride secretion is controlled by the insertion and stability of SLC26A9 channels in the plasma membrane. Previous studies demonstrated that SLC26A9 cell surface expression is influenced by WNK (with no lysine [K]) kinases that have been implicated in the regulation of cell volume homeostasis and ion transport processes in epithelial cells (Dorwart et al., 2007; Salomon et al., 2016). WNK kinases uniquely function as intracellular chloride and/or osmolality sensors that activate downstream kinases serine/threonine-protein kinase 39 (SPAK) and oxidative stress-responsive 1 protein (OSR1), which can directly modulate ion transporters by phosphorylation (Alessi et al., 2014; Bazúa-Valenti et al., 2015). Furthermore, WNKs can also act as scaffolds that recruit other proteins that regulate the activity or plasma membrane abundance of ion channels (Rodan and Jenny, 2017). This kinase-independent function of WNKs has been demonstrated to affect plasma membrane trafficking of SLC26A9, as well as CFTR, by mechanisms that may involve lysosomal targeting or endosomal sorting (Dorwart et al., 2007; He et al., 2007; Yang et al., 2007; Zhou et al., 2010).

Notably, there is a large overlap in the expression pattern of SLC26A9 and CFTR in epithelial tissues and emerging evidence suggests a complex, multifaceted interaction between the two channels, both under physiological and pathophysiological conditions. First, there is a functional interaction between the two channels mediated by the STAS domain of SLC26A9 and the R domain of CFTR. Although an inhibitory relationship has also been suggested (Chang et al., 2009a), the nature of this molecular interaction is likely stimulatory, as SLC26A9 contributes to cAMP-stimulated chloride currents in HBE cells and co-expression of CFTR with SLC26A9 results in larger chloride currents than expression of CFTR alone (Loriol et al., 2008; Avella et al., 2011b). Interestingly, the cellular background and level of differentiation may be important determinants of this functional interaction between SLC26A9 and CFTR, as suggested by a study that showed a different behavior in human embryonic kidney (HEK293) cells compared to polarized airway epithelial cells (Ousingsawat et al., 2012). Of note, opposite functional interactions between CFTR and SLC26A9 were also reported in two heterologous expression studies that both used HEK cells (Bertrand et al., 2009; Ousingsawat et al., 2012). While these conflicting results are more difficult to reconcile, we speculate that the observed differences in CFTR/SLC26A9 interactions may be related to differences in the cellular background of the HEK cell clones used in the different laboratories.

Biochemical and functional studies of two other SLC26 family members, SLC26A6 and SLC26A3, showed that following cAMP-dependent stimulation, the phosphorylated R domain can bind to STAS domain, which leads to mutual activation of both CFTR and SLC26 transporters (Ko et al., 2004). Coding mutations located in the STAS domain of SLC26A9 may disrupt this stimulatory interaction, as demonstrated by functional analysis of variant L683P (Avella et al., 2011a). Interestingly, STAS domain variant V622L and domain adjacent variant V744M decreased chloride currents of SLC26A9, which could be partially attributed to decreased plasma membrane expression (Chen et al., 2012). Although no disease-association has been reported for the variants above, these studies demonstrate the role of SLC26A9 STAS domain in protein expression, channel function, and stimulation of CFTR currents.

Second, a recent study demonstrated a physical interaction between SLC26A9 and CFTR, which is mediated by PDZ proteins that facilitate trafficking and stabilization of both proteins at the cell surface (Bertrand et al., 2017). As shown by co-localization studies, this interaction is not restricted to the plasma membrane suggesting a common regulatory mechanism along the secretory pathway (Avella et al., 2011b; Bertrand et al., 2017). SLC26A9 shows affinity to a number of PDZ proteins, such as Na^+/H^+ exchanger-3 regulatory factor 1 (NHERF1) and CFTR-associated ligand (CAL), which display antagonistic effects in CFTR trafficking (Bertrand et al., 2017). CAL, also known as GOPC (Golgi-associated PDZ and coiled-coil motif-containing protein) facilitates ubiquitination and lysosomal degradation of CFTR, as well as endoplasmic reticulum (ER)-associated degradation of F508del-CFTR, whereas NHERF1 tethers CFTR to the plasma membrane thus promoting its cell surface expression (Cheng and Guggino, 2013; Bergbower et al., 2018). Moreover, F508del-CFTR could be rescued by NHERF1 overexpression or CAL silencing (Wolde et al., 2007; Castellani et al., 2012). Constitutive SLC26A9-mediated chloride secretion is diminished in human bronchial epithelium from CF donors carrying F508del-CFTR and recent evidence suggests a PDZ-domain sensitive, CAL-dependent underlying mechanism (Bertrand et al., 2009, 2017). Due to proteasomal degradation of F508del-CFTR, association of CAL with SLC26A9 increases, which in turn hampers its forward trafficking. Furthermore, restoration of F508del-CFTR by the small molecule CFTR corrector compound VX-809 increased CFTR as well as SLC26A9 cell surface expression indicating that rescue of intracellular processing of CFTR has a positive influence on SLC26A9 membrane targeting. Consistent with this notion, SLC26A9-mediated chloride currents were not affected by co-expression with the CFTR gating mutation G551D, which is inserted into the plasma membrane, but has impaired CFTR chloride channel regulation (Bertrand et al., 2017).

Third, numerous genetic association studies and investigations utilizing genetically modified mouse models supported an important role of SLC26A9 in the pathophysiology of several organ manifestations in CF, as well as other chronic lung diseases such as asthma and non-CF bronchiectasis (Anagnostopoulou et al., 2012; Sun et al., 2012; Bakouh et al., 2013; Blackman et al., 2013; Miller et al., 2015; Strug et al., 2016). The results of these studies are consistent with an important role of SLC26A9 as a disease modifier in CF and potentially other

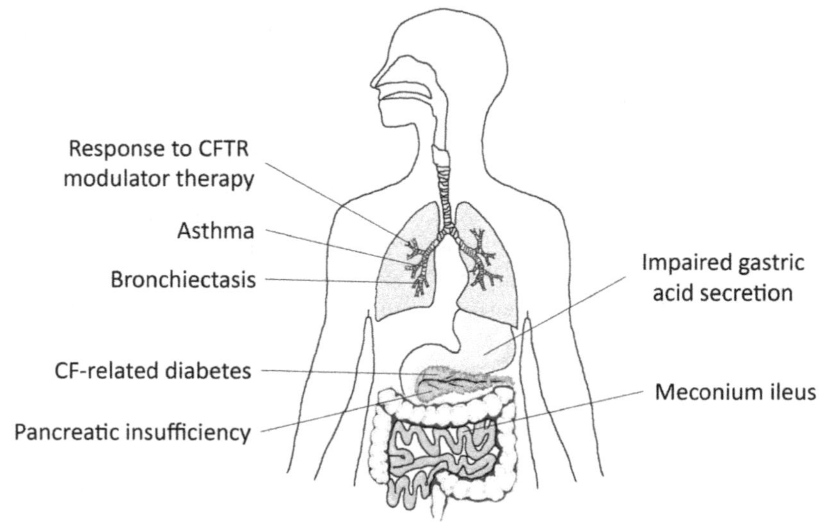

FIGURE 1 | SLC26A9 is a modifier of disease severity in multiple organs affected by CF. Graphical summary depicting associations of variants in *SLC26A9* with exocrine pancreatic insufficiency, CF-related diabetes mellitus (CFRD) and meconium ileus, and emerging data supporting a role of SLC26A9 as modifier of response to CFTR modulator therapy in patients with CF. Beyond CF, SLC26A9 has been implicated in the pathogenesis of asthma, diffuse bronchiectasis (DB), and impaired gastric acid secretion.

muco-obstructive lung diseases and are discussed in more detail below (**Figure 1**).

SLC26A9 CHLORIDE CHANNEL AS A DISEASE MODIFIER IN CF

Lung

Muco-obstructive lung disease remains the major cause of morbidity and mortality in patients with CF. The basic CF ion transport defect causes airway surface dehydration, impaired mucociliary clearance and mucus obstruction, which triggers chronic inflammation and infection, and ultimately leads to progressive lung damage (Button et al., 2016). There is a large heterogeneity in lung disease severity among CF patients, which is influenced by genetic and environmental factors. It is estimated that ~50% of the genetically determined variability can be attributed to the CFTR genotype and the other ~50% to CF modifier genes (Cutting, 2015). In an effort to identify genetic determinants of CF lung disease, genome-wide association studies (GWAS) were performed in large CF patient cohorts (Wright et al., 2011; Corvol et al., 2015). These studies revealed a number of loci and candidate genes that may influence lung function, but initially, these investigations did not find association with SLC26A9. However, more recently, SLC26A9 was reported as a modifier of lung function and response to CFTR modulator therapy in patients carrying the CFTR gating mutation G551D (Strug et al., 2016). In a cohort of over 1,700 F508del homozygous CF patients and 70 patients with at least one G551D allele the authors examined the effect of SLC26A9 SNP rs7512462, which was previously reported to associate with CF related diabetes, pancreatic insufficiency and meconium ileus. The minor C allele of rs7512462 positively influenced lung function in G551D CF patients, but had no effect in F508del homozygotes. Furthermore, improvement of lung function, as determined from FEV1 response to therapy with the small molecule CFTR potentiator ivacaftor (VX-770) was markedly higher in patients carrying at least one protective C allele. This study also assessed the effect of rs7512462 in primary HBE cultures from F508del homozygous CF patients and found that rescue of cAMP-stimulated currents in cultures pretreated with lumacaftor (VX-809) increased with each additional C allele (Strug et al., 2016). In the presence of an *in vitro* modulatory effect, the lack of SLC26A9 association with lung function in F508del homozygous patients is difficult to reconcile. One explanation may entail the F508del dependent trafficking defect of SLC26A9 and the necessity of CFTR plasma membrane targeting for SLC26A9 function discussed above (Bertrand et al., 2017). On the other hand, age-dependent expression may also be involved. Interestingly, a recent study in a Brazilian cohort of 188 CF patients revealed association of rs7512462 with several outcome measures of pulmonary function (Pereira et al., 2017). Taken together, these data support that SLC26A9 is a modulator of response to CFTR targeted therapies, which in the future may help predict patient outcomes and optimize tailored treatment regimens for individual patients with CF.

Idiopathic diffuse bronchiectasis (DB) is a chronic lung disease involving airway mucus obstruction, recurrent infections, airway inflammation, and remodeling that resembles CF lung disease in many aspects (Bergougnoux et al., 2015). Interestingly, a previous study reported rare loss-of-function SLC26A9 mutations in patients with DB suggesting that SLC26A9 may be implicated in disease pathogenesis. In a study comparing 147 patients with DB, 78 patients with CF and 50 healthy controls, exon sequencing of SLC26A9 revealed coding variants R575Y and V486I in two DB patients (Bakouh et al., 2013). Functional analysis showed that both mutations abolished chloride currents and that R575Y located in the STAS domain also interfered with the stimulatory interaction with CFTR.

Further insights on the importance of SLC26A9 in airway epithelial chloride secretion, airway surface hydration, and mucus clearance came from studies in mice with allergic airway disease. In a murine model of allergic asthma, it was shown that type 2 airway inflammation induced SLC26A9-mediated Cl^- secretion, which prevented airway mucus plugging in presence of mucus hypersecretion (Anagnostopoulou et al., 2010, 2012). In the absence of allergic airway inflammation, *Slc26a9*-deficient (*Slc26a9*$^{-/-}$) mice displayed normal lung morphology and no differences in epithelial ion transport when compared to wild-type mice. However, in the presence of allergic inflammation *Slc26a9*$^{-/-}$ mice lacked upregulation of chloride secretion and mucus hypersecretion led to airway mucus plugging. Furthermore, three SNPs at 3′ UTR of SLC26A9 were identified that were associated with a risk for childhood asthma, with an odds ratio of 1.48. Functional investigations revealed that one of these non-coding variants altered a putative micro-RNA response element in the 3′ UTR of SLC26A9 and lead to micro-RNA mediated translational repression *in vitro*, indicating that decreased SLC26A9 protein expression may be the underlying mechanism for disease association (Anagnostopoulou et al., 2012).

Stomach

Investigations in the stomach revealed an essential role of SLC26A9 in the regulation of gastric acid secretion. In the gastric mucosa SLC26A9 is expressed in the surface epithelial cells and in the parietal cells of the deep gastric gland. *Slc26a9*$^{-/-}$ mice displayed structural and ultrastructural changes, such as distended gastric glands, hypoplasia of parietal cells, and loss of tubulovesicular system inside the parietal cells (Xu et al., 2008). Furthermore, H-K-ATPase expression was decreased. *Slc26a9*$^{-/-}$ mice had complete achlorhydria, which could be explained by the absence of transmucosal chloride secretion and/or the role of Slc26a9 in the maintenance and maturation of the secretory pathway that regulates the H-K-ATPase trafficking. Alternatively, Slc26a9 could also promote gastric bicarbonate secretion and regulation of luminal pH to protect against injury by gastric acid (Xu et al., 2005; Demitrack et al., 2010). It is currently debated how SLC26A9 could contribute to bicarbonate secretion. One possibility would be that SLC26A9-mediated chloride secretion is paralleled by chloride-bicarbonate exchange via apical anion exchangers, similarly to the proposed model of pancreatic fluid secretion, where CFTR works tandem with anion exchangers to secrete bicarbonate (Stewart et al., 2009). The second possibility is that SLC26A9 itself can operate as an anion exchanger, which was supported by two studies on gastric epithelium (Xu et al., 2005; Demitrack et al., 2010), however, most heterologous expression data suggest that SLC26A9 functions as an ion channel with minimal bicarbonate conductance. Third, the channel conductance to bicarbonate could also be modulated, similarly to the regulation of CFTR bicarbonate permeability by WNK1-OSR1/SPAK pathway (Park et al., 2010). Notably, SLC26A9 expression was upregulated in *Helicobacter pylori* infection, as well as upon chronic gastritis induced by interleukin-11 in mice, indicating that SLC26A9 is a key player in gastric mucosal defense under pathological conditions (Henriksnäs et al., 2006; Howlett et al., 2012).

Intestine

Obstruction of the ileum due to highly viscous and sticky bowel content, also known as meconium ileus, affects ~15% of newborns with CF. Sibling and twin studies demonstrated a high heritability for this disease phenotype and a number of genetic studies reported association of SLC26A9 with meconium ileus (Blackman et al., 2006; Sun et al., 2012; Li W. et al., 2014; Miller et al., 2015). SLC26A9 expression decreases along the GI tract with relatively high levels in the stomach, medium levels in the proximal duodenum, low levels in the ileum and no detectable expression in the colon, whereas CFTR shows an inverse pattern with low expression in the stomach and high levels in the duodenum, small intestine and colon (Liu et al., 2015). *Cftr*-deficient (*Cftr*$^{-/-}$) mice show a severe meconium ileus-like intestinal phenotype characterized by severe intestinal plugging. When *Cftr*$^{-/-}$ mice were crossbred with *Slc26a9*$^{-/-}$ mice, mortality highly increased, indicating that SLC26A9-mediated anion secretion ameliorates meconium ileus (Liu et al., 2015). *Slc26a9*$^{-/-}$ mice also failed to elicit duodenal bicarbonate secretion in response to acid load, which may signify the physiological role of SLC26A9 to neutralize gastric acid in the duodenum (Singh et al., 2013).

Pancreas

Exocrine pancreatic insufficiency (PI) in CF is present from early life in nearly all patients with severe CFTR genotypes. CFTR is expressed in the pancreatic ductal epithelium and regulates the secretion of an alkaline, bicarbonate rich pancreatic fluid that washes out digestive enzymes produced by acinar cells. CFTR dysfunction leads to an acidic, low volume, protein rich secretion that can slow down or even block the outflow of zymogens from the ductal tree (Kopelman et al., 1988). Early histopathological changes include dilatation of ducts filled with inspissated zymogen material and destruction of acinar cells (Tucker et al., 2003). In advanced stages, fibrotic and adipose tissue replaces acinar mass and destroys Langerhans-islands (Gibson-Corley et al., 2016). PI shows a strong, but incomplete correlation with CF genotype and CFTR chloride channel function, while SLC26A9 can largely explain the remainder of genetic variability (Cystic Fibrosis Genotype-Phenotype Consortium, 1993; Hirtz et al., 2004; Li W. et al., 2014; Miller et al., 2015). These studies found correlation between circulating levels of immunoreactive trypsinogen (IRT), an early biomarker for exocrine damage, and SLC26A9 SNPs that also associated with meconium ileus and CF-related diabetes mellitus (CFRD). The physiological function of SLC26A9 in the pancreas is largely unexplored. Emerging data suggest that SLC26A9 may enhance ductal anion transport and fluid secretion (Li et al., 2016). Impaired SLC26A9-mediated secretion may thus aggravate the defective ductal wash-out mechanism and ductal plugging in CF. Reduced fluid secretion and ductal

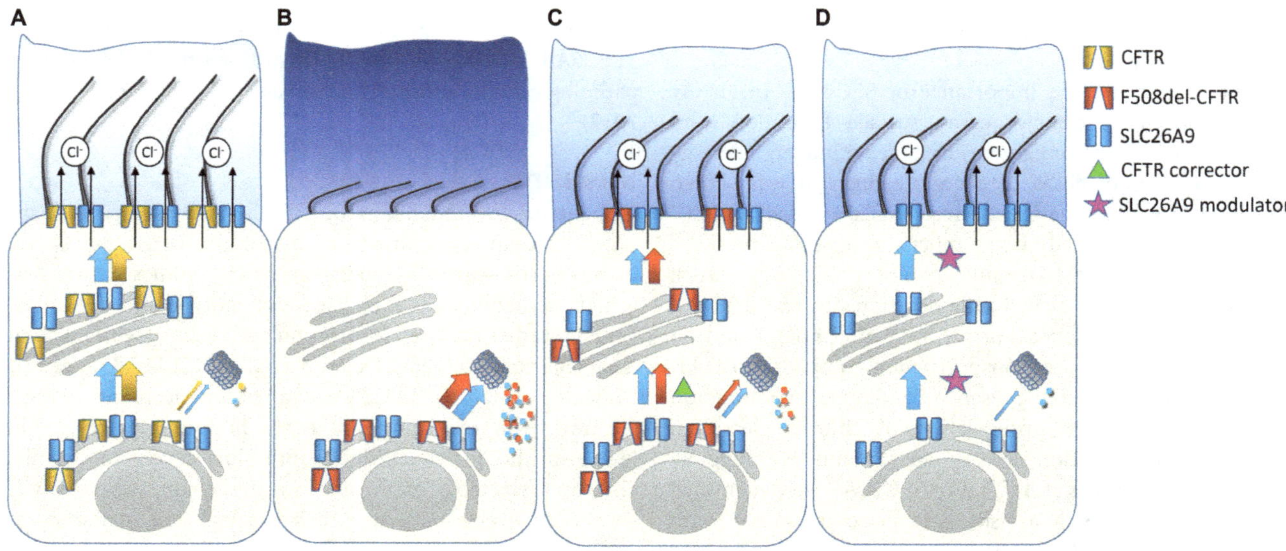

FIGURE 2 | Role SLC26A9 in healthy airways and as a therapeutic target in cystic fibrosis (CF). Healthy airway epithelia express SLC26A9 and CFTR that are co-trafficked from the ER to the plasma membrane, where SLC26A9 functions as a constitutive and CFTR as a cAMP/PKA-regulated chloride channel. Further, SLC26A9 and CFTR interact reciprocally to augment transepithelial chloride/fluid secretion essential to maintain proper airway surface hydration and effective mucociliary clearance **(A)**. In airway epithelial cells from patients with CF carrying the most common disease-causing mutation F508del-CFTR, impaired folding of F508del leads to its retention in the ER and degradation by the proteasome. The F508del trafficking defect also hampers co-trafficking of SLC26A9 and its insertion into the plasma membrane. Lack of SLC26A9 chloride channels may aggravate deficient chloride secretion in CF **(B)**. Pharmacological rescue of F508del-CFTR trafficking with the CFTR corrector lumacaftor (VX-809) restores co-trafficking and insertion of SLC26A9 chloride channels into the apical plasma membrane **(C)**. Compounds that facilitate trafficking of SLC26A9 in the absence of CFTR may improve chloride secretion and airway surface hydration in all patients with CF regardless of the type of CFTR mutation. Alternatively, chloride secretion may also be facilitated by compounds that potentiate SLC26A9 channels that are present and/or newly trafficked to the plasma membrane **(D)**.

mucus obstruction are also present in chronic pancreatitis, a disease that shares many key pathogenic features with CF of the pancreas (Maléth et al., 2015; Balázs et al., 2018). It is conceivable that SLC26A9 may also act as a modifier in these disorders.

Pancreatic insufficiency confers a major risk for CFRD. CFRD is an age-dependent complication that affects 2% of children and 50% of adults with high heritability (Blackman et al., 2009; Moran et al., 2009). A GWAS identified major association of SLC26A9 variants with CFRD, with a hazards ratio of 1.47. Interestingly, meta-analysis of two GWAS studies in type II diabetes showed evidence for association with the same SLC26A9 SNPs, although the risk allele was different (Blackman et al., 2013). There are two prevailing hypotheses on CFRD development: one is that CFRD is driven by the exocrine damage that stresses endocrine cells and causes islet remodeling (Rotti et al., 2018). This is supported by a Mendelian randomization study utilizing a disease-associated SLC26A9 SNP, where a causal relationship between PI and CFRD risk was determined (Soave et al., 2014). Alternatively, loss of CFTR function might have a direct role in insulin secretion (Guo et al., 2014) and/or result in an intrinsic defect that impairs endocrine function before acinar damage occurs (Gibson-Corley et al., 2016). Given its function as chloride channel, it is possible that SLC26A9 may regulate membrane potential and insulin secretion in β-cells, however, there are no data available that support expression of SLC26A9 in the endocrine pancreas.

CONCLUSION AND FUTURE DIRECTIONS

In summary, SLC26A9 constitutes an alternative chloride channel that is implicated in coordinated ion and fluid secretion in various epithelial tissues affected in CF including the airways, the pancreas and the gastro-intestinal tract (Lohi et al., 2002; Dorwart et al., 2007; Bertrand et al., 2009). Demonstration of its role as a disease modifier, as well as overlapping expression of SLC26A9 and CFTR in several affected organs, suggest SLC26A9 as an attractive alternative therapeutic target to bypass the primary ion transport defect in CF (Sun et al., 2012; Blackman et al., 2013; Miller et al., 2015; Strug et al., 2016). In the airways, activation of SLC26A9-mediated chloride/fluid secretion is predicted to counteract airway surface dehydration that sets the stage for mucus plugging and mucociliary dysfunction and constitutes an important disease mechanism in CF lung disease (Mall and Hartl, 2014). Similarly, in the gastro-intestinal tract, activation of SLC26A9 chloride channels is expected to improve the hydration of intestinal surfaces and facilitate pancreatic fluid secretion thus counteracting important extra-pulmonary organ dysfunctions in CF. Therefore, SLC26A9 is an attractive target not only for the treatment of CF lung disease, but also for systemic therapy that may be beneficial for the prevention and/or treatment of several extrapulmonary disease manifestations including meconium ileus and distal intestinal obstruction syndrome (DIOS), exocrine pancreatic insufficiency and CFRD. Further, pharmacological activation of SLC26A9-mediated chloride/fluid secretion may also be beneficial in other muco-obstructive lung diseases and in chronic pancreatitis (Mall, 2016; Balázs et al., 2018). Importantly activation of an alternative chloride channel is expected to be beneficial for all patients with CF, irrespective of their *CFTR* genotype, including patients with non-sense or splicing mutations, where no CFTR protein is made, or other rare CFTR mutations that do not respond to emerging CFTR modulator therapies (Li et al., 2017). Given the reciprocal interaction with CFTR (**Figures 2A–C**), pharmacological activation of SLC26A9 may also augment functional rescue of mutant CFTR achieved by CFTR modulator therapies (Strug et al., 2016; Bertrand et al., 2017). However, to date, no compounds that activate SLC26A9 chloride channel function have been reported and the development of such SLC26A9 modulators remains a major challenge for further testing of these concepts in preclinical models and in the clinical arena. In this context, the negative impact of the common CFTR mutation F508del present on at least one allele in ~90% of CF patients on SLC26A9 trafficking indicates that an ideal SLC26A9 modulator compound should overcome this interaction and facilitate trafficking of SLC26A9 from the ER to the plasma membrane independent of CFTR co-trafficking (Strug et al., 2016; Bertrand et al., 2017; **Figure 2D**). In addition to compounds that facilitate SLC26A9 trafficking to increase the number of channels, SLC26A9-mediated chloride secretion may be augmented by compounds that enhance the open probability of the channel or its stability in the plasma membrane. Single channel recordings demonstrated SLC26A9 channels with open and closed states and a conductance of ~3.2 pS (Chang et al., 2009b) suggesting that it may be possible to increase the open probability by SLC26A9 potentiator compounds. Taking the development of CFTR modulators as a model for drug development, such SCL26A9 modulators may be identified by high-throughput screening of compound libraries in SLC26A9-expression epithelial cells (Gentzsch and Mall, 2018). In addition, a better understanding of SLC26A9 regulation in epithelial tissues, including its interaction network and signaling pathways, may help to explore SLC26A9 as a novel therapeutic target in CF and potentially other muco-obstructive lung diseases.

AUTHOR CONTRIBUTIONS

AB and MM conceived and designed the review, contributed to analysis and interpretation of published literature, and drafted the article and revised it critically for important intellectual content.

FUNDING

MM was supported in part by the German Federal Ministry of Education and Research (82DZL004A1) and a grant from the Einstein Foundation Berlin (EP-2017-393).

REFERENCES

Alessi, D. R., Zhang, J., Khanna, A., Hochdörfer, T., Shang, Y., and Kahle, K. T. (2014). The WNK-SPAK/OSR1 pathway: master regulator of cation-chloride cotransporters. *Sci. Signal.* 7:re3. doi: 10.1126/scisignal.2005365

Anagnostopoulou, P., Dai, L., Schatterny, J., Hirtz, S., Duerr, J., and Mall, M. A. (2010). Allergic airway inflammation induces a pro-secretory epithelial ion transport phenotype in mice. *Eur. Respir. J.* 36, 1436–1447. doi: 10.1183/09031936.00181209

Anagnostopoulou, P., Riederer, B., Duerr, J., Michel, S., Binia, A., Agrawal, R., et al. (2012). SLC26A9-mediated chloride secretion prevents mucus obstruction in airway inflammation. *J. Clin. Invest.* 122, 3629–3634. doi: 10.1172/JCI60429

Avella, M., Borgese, F., and Ehrenfeld, J. (2011a). Characterization of the L683P mutation of SLC26A9 in Xenopus oocytes. *Biochim. Biophys. Acta* 1810, 577–583. doi: 10.1016/j.bbagen.2011.03.012

Avella, M., Loriol, C., Boulukos, K., Borgese, F., and Ehrenfeld, J. (2011b). SLC26A9 stimulates CFTR expression and function in human bronchial cell lines. *J. Cell. Physiol.* 226, 212–223. doi: 10.1002/jcp.22328

Bakouh, N., Bienvenu, T., Thomas, A., Ehrenfeld, J., Liote, H., Roussel, D., et al. (2013). Characterization of SLC26A9 in patients with CF-like lung disease. *Hum. Mutat.* 34, 1404–1414. doi: 10.1002/humu.22382

Balázs, A., Balla, Z., Kui, B., Maléth, J., Rakonczay, Z., Duerr, J., et al. (2018). Ductal mucus obstruction and reduced fluid secretion are early defects in chronic pancreatitis. *Front. Physiol.* 9:632. doi: 10.3389/fphys.2018.00632

Bazúa-Valenti, S., Chávez-Canales, M., Rojas-Vega, L., González-Rodríguez, X., Vázquez, N., Rodríguez-Gama, A., et al. (2015). The effect of WNK4 on the Na+-Cl- cotransporter is modulated by intracellular chloride. *J. Am. Soc. Nephrol.* 26, 1781–1786. doi: 10.1681/ASN.2014050470

Bergbower, E., Boinot, C., Sabirzhanova, I., Guggino, W., and Cebotaru, L. (2018). The CFTR-associated ligand arrests the trafficking of the mutant ΔF508 CFTR channel in the ER contributing to cystic fibrosis. *Cell. Physiol. Biochem.* 45, 639–655. doi: 10.1159/000487120

Bergougnoux, A., Viart, V., Miro, J., Bommart, S., Molinari, N., des Georges, M., et al. (2015). Should diffuse bronchiectasis still be considered a CFTR-related disorder? *J. Cyst. Fibros.* 14, 646–653. doi: 10.1016/j.jcf.2015.02.012

Bertrand, C. A., Mitra, S., Mishra, S. K., Wang, X., Zhao, Y., Pilewski, J. M., et al. (2017). The CFTR trafficking mutation F508del inhibits the constitutive activity of SLC26A9. *Am. J. Physiol. Lung. Cell Mol. Physiol.* 312, L912–L925. doi: 10.1152/ajplung.00178.2016

Bertrand, C. A., Zhang, R., Pilewski, J. M., and Frizzell, R. A. (2009). SLC26A9 is a constitutively active, CFTR-regulated anion conductance in human bronchial epithelia. *J. Gen. Physiol.* 133, 421–438. doi: 10.1085/jgp.200810097

Blackman, S. M., Commander, C. W., Watson, C., Arcara, K. M., Strug, L. J., Stonebraker, J. R., et al. (2013). Genetic modifiers of cystic fibrosis-related diabetes. *Diabetes Metab. Res. Rev.* 62, 3627–3635. doi: 10.2337/db13-0510

Blackman, S. M., Deering-Brose, R., McWilliams, R., Naughton, K., Coleman, B., Lai, T., et al. (2006). Relative contribution of genetic and nongenetic modifiers to intestinal obstruction in cystic fibrosis. *Gastroenterology* 131, 1030–1039. doi: 10.1053/j.gastro.2006.07.016

Blackman, S. M., Hsu, S., Vanscoy, L. L., Collaco, J. M., Ritter, S. E., Naughton, K., et al. (2009). Genetic modifiers play a substantial role in diabetes complicating cystic fibrosis. *J. Clin. Endocrinol. Metab.* 94, 1302–1309. doi: 10.1210/jc.2008-2186

Button, B., Anderson, W. H., and Boucher, R. C. (2016). Mucus hyperconcentration as a unifying aspect of the chronic bronchitic phenotype. *Ann. Am. Thorac. Soc.* 13(Suppl. 2), S156–S162. doi: 10.1513/AnnalsATS.201507-455KV

Castellani, S., Guerra, L., Favia, M., Di Gioia, S., Casavola, V., and Conese, M. (2012). NHERF1 and CFTR restore tight junction organisation and function in cystic fibrosis airway epithelial cells: role of ezrin and the RhoA/ROCK pathway. *Lab. Invest.* 92, 1527–1540. doi: 10.1038/labinvest.2012.123

Chang, M.-H., Plata, C., Sindic, A., Ranatunga, W. K., Chen, A.-P., Zandi-Nejad, K., et al. (2009a). Slc26a9 is inhibited by the R-region of the cystic fibrosis transmembrane conductance regulator via the STAS domain. *J. Biol. Chem.* 284, 28306–28318. doi: 10.1074/jbc.M109.001669

Chang, M.-H., Plata, C., Zandi-Nejad, K., Sinđić, A., Sussman, C. R., Mercado, A., et al. (2009b). Slc26A9 - anion exchanger, channel and Na+ transporter. *J. Membr. Biol.* 228, 125–140. doi: 10.1007/s00232-009-9165-5

Chen, A.-P., Chang, M.-H., and Romero, M. F. (2012). Functional analysis of non-synonymous single nucleotide polymorphisms in human SLC26A9. *Hum. Mutat.* 33, 1275–1284. doi: 10.1002/humu.22107

Cheng, J., and Guggino, W. (2013). Ubiquitination and degradation of CFTR by the E3 ubiquitin ligase MARCH2 through its association with adaptor proteins CAL and STX6. *PLoS One* 8:e68001. doi: 10.1371/journal.pone.0068001

Consortium, G. (2017). Genetic effects on gene expression across human tissues. *Nature* 550, 204–213. doi: 10.1038/nature24277

Corvol, H., Blackman, S. M., Boëlle, P.-Y., Gallins, P. J., Pace, R. G., Stonebraker, J. R., et al. (2015). Genome-wide association meta-analysis identifies five modifier loci of lung disease severity in cystic fibrosis. *Nat. Commun.* 6:8382. doi: 10.1038/ncomms9382

Cutting, G. R. (2015). Cystic fibrosis genetics: from molecular understanding to clinical application. *Nat. Rev. Genet.* 16, 45–56. doi: 10.1038/nrg3849

Cystic Fibrosis Genotype-Phenotype Consortium (1993). Correlation between genotype and phenotype in patients with cystic fibrosis. *N. Engl. J. Med.* 329, 1308–1313. doi: 10.1056/NEJM199310283291804

Demitrack, E. S., Soleimani, M., and Montrose, M. H. (2010). Damage to the gastric epithelium activates cellular bicarbonate secretion via SLC26A9 Cl-/HCO3- exchange. *Am. J. Physiol. Gastrointest. Liver Physiol.* 299, G255–G264. doi: 10.1152/ajpgi.00037.2010

Dorwart, M. R., Shcheynikov, N., Wang, Y., Stippec, S., and Muallem, S. (2007). SLC26A9 is a Cl(-) channel regulated by the WNK kinases. *J. Physiol.* 584, 333–345. doi: 10.1113/jphysiol.2007.135855

Geertsma, E. R., Chang, Y.-N., Shaik, F. R., Neldner, Y., Pardon, E., Steyaert, J., et al. (2015). Structure of a prokaryotic fumarate transporter reveals the architecture of the SLC26 family. *Nat. Struct. Mol. Biol.* 22, 803–808. doi: 10.1038/nsmb.3091

Gentzsch, M., and Mall, M. A. (2018). Ion channel modulators in cystic fibrosis. *Chest* 154, 383–393. doi: 10.1016/j.chest.2018.04.036

Gibson-Corley, K. N., Meyerholz, D. K., and Engelhardt, J. F. (2016). Pancreatic pathophysiology in cystic fibrosis. *J. Pathol.* 238, 311–320. doi: 10.1002/path.4634

Guo, J. H., Chen, H., Ruan, Y. C., Zhang, X. L., Zhang, X. H., Fok, K. L., et al. (2014). Glucose-induced electrical activities and insulin secretion in pancreatic islet β-cells are modulated by CFTR. *Nat. Commun.* 5:4420. doi: 10.1038/ncomms5420

He, G., Wang, H.-R., Huang, S.-K., and Huang, C.-L. (2007). Intersectin links WNK kinases to endocytosis of ROMK1. *J. Clin. Invest.* 117, 1078–1087. doi: 10.1172/JCI30087

Henriksnäs, J., Phillipson, M., Storm, M., Engstrand, L., Soleimani, M., and Holm, L. (2006). Impaired mucus-bicarbonate barrier in Helicobacter pylori-infected mice. *Am. J. Physiol. Gastrointest. Liver Physiol.* 291, G396–G403. doi: 10.1152/ajpgi.00017.2006

Hirtz, S., Gonska, T., Seydewitz, H. H., Thomas, J., Greiner, P., Kuehr, J., et al. (2004). CFTR Cl- channel function in native human colon correlates with the genotype and phenotype in cystic fibrosis. *Gastroenterology* 127, 1085–1095. doi: 10.1053/j.gastro.2004.07.006

Howlett, M., Chalinor, H. V., Buzzelli, J. N., Nguyen, N., van Driel, I. R., Bell, K. M., et al. (2012). IL-11 is a parietal cell cytokine that induces atrophic gastritis. *Gut* 61, 1398–1409. doi: 10.1136/gutjnl-2011-300539

Ko, S. B. H., Zeng, W., Dorwart, M. R., Luo, X., Kim, K. H., Millen, L., et al. (2004). Gating of CFTR by the STAS domain of SLC26 transporters. *Nat. Cell Biol.* 6, 343–350. doi: 10.1038/ncb1115

Kopelman, H., Corey, M., Gaskin, K., Durie, P., Weizman, Z., and Forstner, G. (1988). Impaired chloride secretion, as well as bicarbonate secretion, underlies the fluid secretory defect in the cystic fibrosis pancreas. *Gastroenterology* 95, 349–355. doi: 10.1016/0016-5085(88)90490-8

Lee, H. J., Yoo, J. E., Namkung, W., Cho, H.-J., Kim, K., Kang, J. W., et al. (2015). Thick airway surface liquid volume and weak mucin expression in pendrin-deficient human airway epithelia. *Physiol. Rep.* 3:e12480. doi: 10.14814/phy2.12480

Li, H., Salomon, J. J., Sheppard, D. N., Mall, M. A., and Galietta, L. J. (2017). Bypassing CFTR dysfunction in cystic fibrosis with alternative pathways for anion transport. *Curr. Opin. Pharmacol.* 34, 91–97. doi: 10.1016/j.coph.2017.10.002

Li, J., Xia, F., and Reithmeier, R. A. F. (2014). N-glycosylation and topology of the human SLC26 family of anion transport membrane proteins. *Am. J. Physiol. Cell Physiol.* 306, C943–C960. doi: 10.1152/ajpcell.00030.2014

Li, T., Riederer, B., Liu, X., Pallagi, P., Singh, A. K., Soleimani, M., et al. (2016). Tu1491 loss of Slc26a9 anion transporter results in reduced pancreatic fluid secretion in young female mice. *Gastroenterology* 150:S915. doi: 10.1016/S0016-5085(16)33103-1

Li, W., Soave, D., Miller, M. R., Keenan, K., Lin, F., Gong, J., et al. (2014). Unraveling the complex genetic model for cystic fibrosis: pleiotropic effects of modifier genes on early cystic fibrosis-related morbidities. *Hum. Genet.* 133, 151–161. doi: 10.1007/s00439-013-1363-7

Liu, X., Li, T., Riederer, B., Lenzen, H., Ludolph, L., Yeruva, S., et al. (2015). Loss of Slc26a9 anion transporter alters intestinal electrolyte and HCO3- transport and reduces survival in CFTR-deficient mice. *Pflugers Arch.* 467, 1261–1275. doi: 10.1007/s00424-014-1543-x

Lohi, H., Kujala, M., Makela, S., Lehtonen, E., Kestila, M., Saarialho-Kere, U., et al. (2002). Functional characterization of three novel tissue-specific anion exchangers SLC26A7, -A8, and -A9. *J. Biol. Chem.* 277, 14246–14254. doi: 10.1074/jbc.M111802200

Lohi, H., Lamprecht, G., Markovich, D., Heil, A., Kujala, M., Seidler, U., et al. (2003). Isoforms of SLC26A6 mediate anion transport and have functional PDZ interaction domains. *Am. J. Physiol Cell Physiol.* 284, C769–C779. doi: 10.1152/ajpcell.00270.2002

Loriol, C., Dulong, S., Avella, M., Gabillat, N., Boulukos, K., Borgese, F., et al. (2008). Characterization of SLC26A9, facilitation of Cl(-) transport by bicarbonate. *Cell. Physiol. Biochem.* 22, 15–30. doi: 10.1159/000149780

Maléth, J., Balázs, A., Pallagi, P., Balla, Z., Kui, B., Katona, M., et al. (2015). Alcohol disrupts levels and function of the cystic fibrosis transmembrane conductance regulator to promote development of pancreatitis. *Gastroenterology* 148, 427–439.e16. doi: 10.1053/j.gastro.2014.11.002

Mall, M., Wissner, A., Schreiber, R., Kuehr, J., Seydewitz, H. H., Brandis, M., et al. (2000). Role of K(V)LQT1 in cyclic adenosine monophosphate-mediated Cl(-) secretion in human airway epithelia. *Am. J. Respir. Cell Mol. Biol.* 23, 283–289. doi: 10.1165/ajrcmb.23.3.4060

Mall, M. A. (2016). Unplugging mucus in cystic fibrosis and chronic obstructive pulmonary disease. *Ann. Am. Thorac. Soc.* 13(Suppl. 2), S177–S185. doi: 10.1513/AnnalsATS.201509-641KV

Mall, M. A., and Hartl, D. (2014). CFTR: cystic fibrosis and beyond. *Eur. Respir. J.* 44, 1042–1054. doi: 10.1183/09031936.00228013

Miller, M. R., Soave, D., Li, W., Gong, J., Pace, R. G., Boëlle, P.-Y., et al. (2015). Variants in solute carrier SLC26A9 modify prenatal exocrine pancreatic damage in cystic fibrosis. *J. Pediatr.* 166, 1152–1157.e6. doi: 10.1016/j.jpeds.2015.01.044

Moran, A., Dunitz, J., Nathan, B., Saeed, A., Holme, B., and Thomas, W. (2009). Cystic fibrosis–related diabetes: current trends in prevalence, incidence, and mortality. *Diabetes Care* 32, 1626–1631. doi: 10.2337/dc09-0586

Ousingsawat, J., Schreiber, R., and Kunzelmann, K. (2012). Differential contribution of SLC26A9 to Cl- conductance in polarized and non-polarized epithelial cells. *J. Cell. Physiol.* 227, 2323–2329. doi: 10.1002/jcp.22967

Park, H. W., Nam, J. H., Kim, J. Y., Namkung, W., Yoon, J. S., Lee, J.-S., et al. (2010). Dynamic regulation of CFTR bicarbonate permeability by [Cl-]i and its role in pancreatic bicarbonate secretion. *Gastroenterology* 139, 620–631. doi: 10.1053/j.gastro.2010.04.004

Pereira, S. V.-N., Ribeiro, J. D., Bertuzzo, C. S., and Marson, F. A. L. (2017). Association of clinical severity of cystic fibrosis with variants in the SLC gene family (SLC6A14, SLC26A9, SLC11A1 and SLC9A3). *Gene* 629, 117–126. doi: 10.1016/j.gene.2017.07.068

Ratjen, F., Hug, C., Marigowda, G., Tian, S., Huang, X., Stanojevic, S., et al. (2017). Efficacy and safety of lumacaftor and ivacaftor in patients aged 6-11 years with cystic fibrosis homozygous for F508del-CFTR: a randomised, placebo-controlled phase 3 trial. *Lancet Respir. Med.* 5, 557–567. doi: 10.1016/S2213-2600(17)30215-1

Rodan, A. R., and Jenny, A. (2017). WNK kinases in development and disease. *Curr. Top. Dev. Biol* 123, 1–47. doi: 10.1016/bs.ctdb.2016.08.004

Rossmann, H., Jacob, P., Baisch, S., Hassoun, R., Meier, J., Natour, D., et al. (2005). The CFTR associated protein CAP70 interacts with the Apical Cl-/HCO3- exchanger DRA in rabbit small intestinal mucosa. *Biochemistry* 44, 4477–4487. doi: 10.1021/bi048828b

Rotti, P. G., Xie, W., Poudel, A., Yi, Y., Sun, X., Tyler, S. R., et al. (2018). Pancreatic and islet remodeling in cystic fibrosis transmembrane conductance regulator (CFTR) knockout ferrets. *Am. J. Pathol.* 188, 876–890. doi: 10.1016/j.ajpath.2017.12.015

Salomon, J. J., Spahn, S., Wang, X., Füllekrug, J., Bertrand, C. A., and Mall, M. A. (2016). Generation and functional characterization of epithelial cells with stable expression of SLC26A9 Cl- channels. *Am. J. Physiol. Lung. Cell. Mol. Physiol.* 310, L593–L602. doi: 10.1152/ajplung.00321.2015

Sharma, A. K., Rigby, A. C., and Alper, S. L. (2011). STAS domain structure and function. *Cell. Physiol. Biochem.* 28, 407–422. doi: 10.1159/000335104

Singh, A. K., Liu, Y., Riederer, B., Engelhardt, R., Thakur, B. K., Soleimani, M., et al. (2013). Molecular transport machinery involved in orchestrating luminal acid-induced duodenal bicarbonate secretion *in vivo*. *J. Physiol.* 591, 5377–5391. doi: 10.1113/jphysiol.2013.254854

Soave, D., Miller, M. R., Keenan, K., Li, W., Gong, J., Ip, W., et al. (2014). Evidence for a causal relationship between early exocrine pancreatic disease and cystic fibrosis–related diabetes: a mendelian randomization study. *Diabetes Metab. Res. Rev.* 63, 2114–2119. doi: 10.2337/db13-1464

Sosnay, P. R., Siklosi, K. R., Van Goor, F., Kaniecki, K., Yu, H., Sharma, N., et al. (2013). Defining the disease liability of variants in the cystic fibrosis transmembrane conductance regulator gene. *Nat. Genet.* 45, 1160–1167. doi: 10.1038/ng.2745

Stewart, A. K., Yamamoto, A., Nakakuki, M., Kondo, T., Alper, S. L., and Ishiguro, H. (2009). Functional coupling of apical Cl-/HCO3- exchange with CFTR in stimulated HCO3- secretion by guinea pig interlobular pancreatic duct. *Am. J. Physiol. Gastrointest. Liver Physiol.* 296, G1307–G1317. doi: 10.1152/ajpgi.90697.2008

Strug, L. J., Gonska, T., He, G., Keenan, K., Ip, W., Boëlle, P.-Y., et al. (2016). Cystic fibrosis gene modifier SLC26A9 modulates airway response to CFTR-directed therapeutics. *Hum. Mol. Genet.* 25, 4590–4600. doi: 10.1093/hmg/ddw290

Sun, L., Rommens, J. M., Corvol, H., Li, W., Li, X., Chiang, T. A., et al. (2012). Multiple apical plasma membrane constituents are associated with susceptibility to meconium ileus in individuals with cystic fibrosis. *Nat. Genet.* 44, 562–569. doi: 10.1038/ng.2221

Thomson, R. B., Thomson, C. L., and Aronson, P. S. (2016). N-glycosylation critically regulates function of oxalate transporter SLC26A6. *Am. J. Physiol. Cell Physiol.* 311, C866–C873. doi: 10.1152/ajpcell.00171.2016

Tucker, J. A., Spock, A., Spicer, S. S., Shelburne, J. D., and Bradford, W. (2003). Inspissation of pancreatic zymogen material in cystic fibrosis. *Ultrastruct. Pathol.* 27, 323–335. doi: 10.1080/716100784

Welsh, M. J., and Smith, A. E. (1993). Molecular mechanisms of CFTR chloride channel dysfunction in cystic fibrosis. *Cell* 73, 1251–1254. doi: 10.1016/0092-8674(93)90353-R

Wolde, M., Fellows, A., Cheng, J., Kivenson, A., Coutermarsh, B., Talebian, L., et al. (2007). Targeting CAL as a negative regulator of ΔF508-CFTR cell-surface expression an rna interference and structure-based mutagenetic approaCH. *J. Biol. Chem.* 282, 8099–8109. doi: 10.1074/jbc.M611049200

Wright, F. A., Strug, L. J., Doshi, V. K., Commander, C. W., Blackman, S. M., Sun, L., et al. (2011). Genome-wide association and linkage identify modifier loci of lung disease severity in cystic fibrosis at 11p13 and 20q13.2. *Nat. Genet.* 43, 539–546. doi: 10.1038/ng.838

Xu, J., Henriksnäs, J., Barone, S., Witte, D., Shull, G. E., Forte, J. G., et al. (2005). SLC26A9 is expressed in gastric surface epithelial cells, mediates Cl-/HCO3- exchange, and is inhibited by NH4+. *Am. J. Physiol. Cell Physiol.* 289, C493–C505. doi: 10.1152/ajpcell.00030.2005

Xu, J., Song, P., Miller, M. L., Borgese, F., Barone, S., Riederer, B., et al. (2008). Deletion of the chloride transporter Slc26a9 causes loss of tubulovesicles in parietal cells and impairs acid secretion in the stomach. *Proc. Natl. Acad. Sci. U.S.A.* 105, 17955–17960. doi: 10.1073/pnas.0800616105

Yang, C.-L., Liu, X., Paliege, A., Zhu, X., Bachmann, S., Dawson, D. C., et al. (2007). WNK1 and WNK4 modulate CFTR activity. *Biochem. Biophys. Res. Commun.* 353, 535–540. doi: 10.1016/j.bbrc.2006.11.151

Zhou, B., Zhuang, J., Gu, D., Wang, H., Cebotaru, L., Guggino, W. B., et al. (2010). WNK4 enhances the degradation of NCC through a sortilin-mediated lysosomal pathway. *J. Am. Soc. Nephrol.* 21, 82–92. doi: 10.1681/ASN.2008121275

9

Adapting Proteostasis and Autophagy for Controlling the Pathogenesis of Cystic Fibrosis Lung Disease

Manish Bodas[1] and Neeraj Vij[2,3,4]*

[1] Department of Medicine, University of Oklahoma, Oklahoma City, OK, United States, [2] Department of Pediatric Pulmonary Medicine, Johns Hopkins University School of Medicine, Baltimore, MD, United States, [3] 4Dx Limited, Los Angeles, CA, United States, [4] VIJ Biotech LLC, Baltimore, MD, United States

***Correspondence:**
Neeraj Vij
nvij@vijbiotech.com;
nvij@jhmi.edu

Cystic fibrosis (CF), a fatal genetic disorder predominant in the Caucasian population, is caused by mutations in the cystic fibrosis transmembrane conductance regulator (*Cftr*) gene. The most common mutation is the deletion of phenylalanine from the position-508 (F508del-CFTR), resulting in a misfolded-CFTR protein, which is unable to fold, traffic and retain its plasma membrane (PM) localization. The resulting CFTR dysfunction, dysregulates variety of key cellular mechanisms such as chloride ion transport, airway surface liquid (ASL) homeostasis, mucociliary-clearance, inflammatory-oxidative signaling, and proteostasis that includes ubiquitin-proteasome system (UPS) and autophagy. A collective dysregulation of these key homoeostatic mechanisms contributes to the development of chronic obstructive cystic fibrosis lung disease, instead of the classical belief focused exclusively on ion-transport defect. Hence, therapeutic intervention(s) aimed at rescuing chronic CF lung disease needs to correct underlying defect that mediates homeostatic dysfunctions and not just chloride ion transport. Since targeting all the myriad defects individually could be quite challenging, it will be prudent to identify a process which controls almost all disease-promoting processes in the CF airways including underlying CFTR dysfunction. There is emerging experimental and clinical evidence that supports the notion that impaired cellular proteostasis and autophagy plays a central role in regulating pathogenesis of chronic CF lung disease. Thus, correcting the underlying proteostasis and autophagy defect in controlling CF pulmonary disease, primarily *via* correcting the protein processing defect of F508del-CFTR protein has emerged as a novel intervention strategy. Hence, we discuss here both the rationale and significant therapeutic utility of emerging proteostasis and autophagy modulating drugs/compounds in controlling chronic CF lung disease, where targeted delivery is a critical factor-influencing efficacy.

Keywords: proteostasis, autophagy, cystic fibrosis, CFTR, ROS, protein-misfolding

INTRODUCTION

Cystic fibrosis (CF) is one of the most common fatal autosomal recessive disorders (Zhang et al., 2018), with emerging treatment options that have prolonged survival but limited success in diminishing overall mortality. Specially, subjects with homozygous F508-del (phenylalanine-508) mutation that suffer from the most serious form of ailment, lack effective treatment options that can warrant cure or normal survival. Briefly, chronic airway disease is a major contributor of the morbidity and mortality in CF subjects (Cantin et al., 2015; Mall, 2016), and accessibility of several novel and more potent therapeutic options has allowed substantially improved survival. Majority of these therapeutic strategies are aimed at controlling symptomatic CF-lung disease, while some of the newer strategies are designed to target the primary or "root" cause of the disease, which is the mutation(s) in the cystic fibrosis transmembrane conductance regulator (*Cftr*) gene (Esposito et al., 2016; Hudock and Clancy, 2017; Maiuri et al., 2017; Zhang et al., 2018). There are about 1700 known mutations affecting the generation (Class I), structure (Class II) or channel function (Class III–V) of the CFTR protein, and about 88% of these comprise of mutations that cause the protein misfolding defects (Class II) (C.F. Foundation, 2018). People with these mutations on both the copies of their *Cftr* gene demonstrate the classical manifestations of CF lung disease, such as a thick and sticky mucus, mucin hypersecretion, elevated inflammatory-oxidative stress and/or persistent bacterial infections, which collectively result in severe airway obstruction (Bodas and Vij, 2010; Bodas et al., 2018a). Evidence from newer animal models of CF and some clinical data indicate that symptoms of lung disease are present at very early age, or even at birth, thus proposing the concept of congenital origin of CF lung disease (Stoltz et al., 2015). With progressing age, persistent exacerbations primarily caused by *Pseudomonas aeruginosa* (*Pa*) and the ensuing IL-8 mediated persistent neutrophilic inflammation are the hallmark of clinical CF lung disease and a major contributor to irreversible lung damage as well as CF-related fatalities (Bodas and Vij, 2010; Ferrari et al., 2017; Bodas et al., 2018a).

In general, all the cellular processes that work to maintain a robust protein repertoire in the cell are collectively called the proteostasis network (PN) (Klaips et al., 2018). This complex molecular system tightly regulates the fate of a protein inside the cell, starting from its synthesis, folding, and maintenance of the folded functional state, to transport (trafficking), and eventual degradation. A vast amount of cellular energy is utilized to maintain the protein degradation machinery to get rid of misfolded, damaged, non-functional or even functional proteins that are no longer required by the cells. The main protein degradation or cellular clearance mechanisms include the ubiquitin-proteasome system (UPS) and the "autophagy-lysosomal pathway" (Korovila et al., 2017). The primary difference between proteasome and autophagy mechanisms is the type of cargo they can process as their starting material. The proteasome can only process proteins, while large protein aggregates, lipids and even damaged organelles can be processed and degraded by the autophagy pathway. Recent evidence suggests a strong inter-relationship between the proteasome and autophagy pathways (Bustamante et al., 2018) and thus it is not surprising that any disturbance in any of these mechanisms can form the basis of accumulation of aberrant proteins eventually leading to severe pathological conditions such as those seen in aging-related neurodegenerative diseases (Daniele et al., 2018; Klaips et al., 2018), proteinopathies (Chaudhuri and Paul, 2006; Hidvegi et al., 2015; Hartl, 2017), and genetic or environmentally induced chronic respiratory diseases such as CF (Lukacs and Verkman, 2012; Fraser-Pitt and O'Neil, 2015) and COPD (Tran et al., 2015; Bodas and Vij, 2017; Bodas et al., 2017; Vij, 2017), respectively. The deletion of phenylalanine-508 (F508-del) is the most common (about 80%) *Cftr* gene mutation associated with CF, which results in a misfolded CFTR protein that is unable to reach the plasma membrane (PM) (Lukacs et al., 1993; De Stefano et al., 2014). This results in the absence of mature CFTR ion-channel on the PM, leading to CFTR dysfunction, classically described as a chloride ion transport defect (Welsh et al., 1993). In addition, there is substantial evidence supporting the critical role of membrane-resident CFTR in regulating innate and adaptive immune responses in CF (Teichgraber et al., 2008; Vij et al., 2009; Bodas and Vij, 2010; Grassme et al., 2017; Svedin et al., 2017). Furthermore, a burgeoning number of studies now ascertain the crucial role of mature CFTR in regulating important cellular homeostatic processes such as proteostasis and autophagy, with a common consensus that autophagy is potentially inherently defective in CF (Gomes-Alves et al., 2010; Luciani et al., 2010, 2011; Bodas et al., 2012; Valle and Vij, 2012; Villella et al., 2013a). The genesis of defective autophagy in CF seems to be an inherent defect, as primary CF cells have diminished levels of several autophagy proteins (Abdulrahman et al., 2011, 2013), although the precise mechanism(s) are still unclear. Some interesting studies indicate the possible contribution of micro RNA's (Tazi et al., 2016) and DNA methylation (Tazi and Amer, 2015), as both could regulate the expression of autophagy proteins in CF cells. Nonetheless, it is well documented that the absence of membrane CFTR leads to ROS-mediated SUMOylation of transglutaminase 2 (TG2), which prevents its ubiquitination and subsequent degradation by the proteasome, leading to its intracellular accumulation. This results in the crosslinking of Beclin-1 (BECN1), an important protein required for autophagosome formation, leading to defective autophagy, and accumulation of SQSTM1 (p62) (Luciani et al., 2010; Bodas et al., 2017), which favors aggregation of BECN1 and other autophagy related proteins into p62+HDAC6+ aggresome bodies (**Figure 1**). The misfolded F508del-CFTR is also sequestered into aggresome bodies, as the accumulation of p62 leads to inhibition of both protein (proteasome) and aggresome clearance. This aggresome trapping of F508del-CFTR prevents its proper trafficking to the PM that contributes to the initiation and progression of inflammatory-oxidative stress responses in the CF lungs (Luciani et al., 2010).

This suggests that future strategies for managing and treating CF will need to be focused on correcting the underlying proteostasis/autophagy impairment, mainly *via* rescuing F508del-CFTR to the PM, which would simultaneously control the inflammatory-oxidative stress response in the airways of CF subjects. Lately, proteostasis-modulators and autophagy-inducers have shown encouraging results in pre-clinical studies in correcting both the F508del-CFTR trafficking to the PM (CFTR-corrector) (De Stefano et al., 2014; Tosco et al., 2016; Vu et al., 2017; Hutt et al., 2018; Stincardini et al., 2018; Zhang et al., 2018), as well as dampening the inflammatory-oxidative stress responses (anti-oxidant/anti-inflammatory) (Romani et al., 2017; Stincardini et al., 2018), although these strategies were not very efficient in restoring other rare class II CFTR mutations

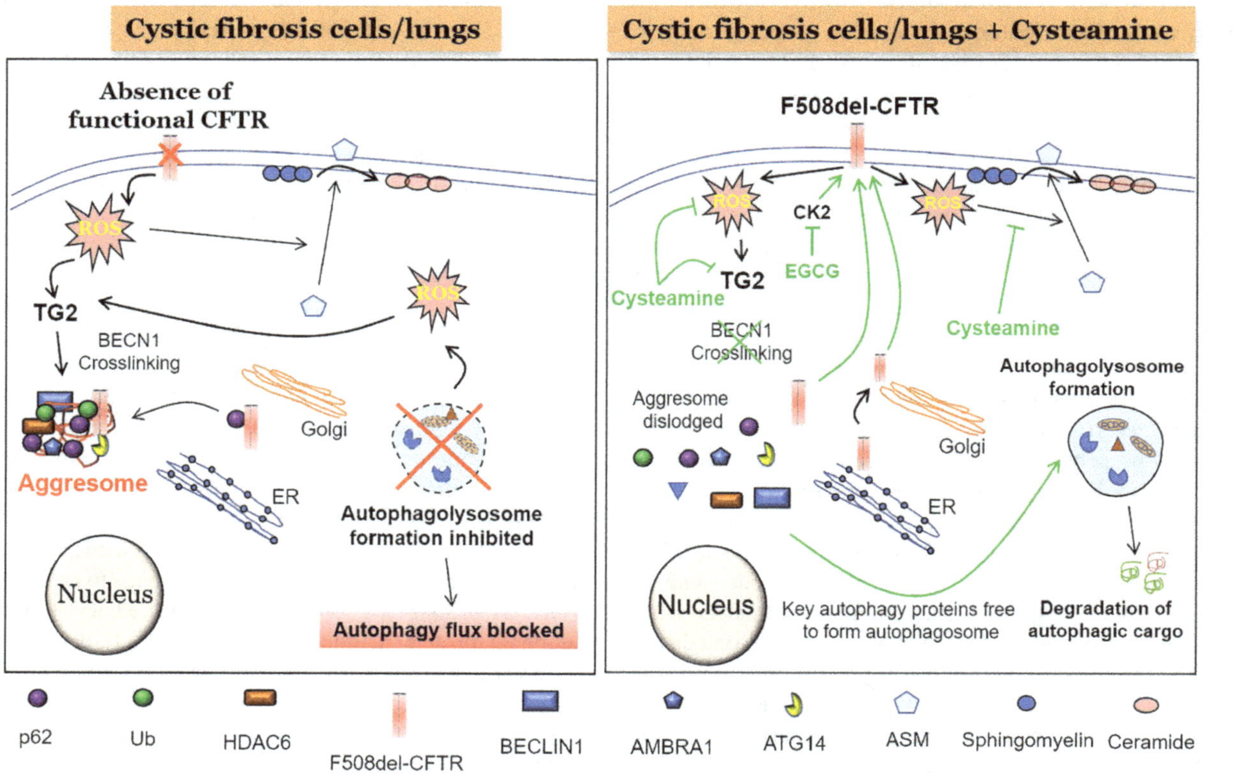

FIGURE 1 | Mechanism of cysteamine mediated autophagy induction and F508del-CFTR rescue. (Left panel) The absence of a functional CFTR at the plasma membrane (PM) leads to elevated reactive oxygen species (ROS) levels which cause activation of transglutaminase-2 (TG2). An active TG2 mediates cross-linking of crucial autophagy proteins such as Beclin1 (BECN1), ATG14, and AMBRA1 into Ub+/p62+/HDAC6+ aggresome bodies, render BECN1 and other autophagy proteins unavailable for the formation of autophagosome and thus blocking the subsequent autophagy flux process. Moreover, an accumulation of p62 could lead to aggresome sequestration of newly synthesized F508-delCFTR, thereby preventing its PM translocation. Additionally, accumulation of damaged mitochondria leads to more ROS production, further promoting TG2-mediated BECN1 crosslinking and autophagy inhibition. Further, the ROS mediated translocation of acid sphingomyelinase (ASM) from cytoplasm to PM, leads to increased conversion of sphingomyelin to ceramide, which is a deleterious sphingolipid implicated in CF pathogenesis. (Right Panel) The treatment of CF cells or mice with the autophagy inducing antioxidant drug, cysteamine, which is also an inhibitor of TG2, leads to prevention of BECN1 crosslinking. This results in dislodging of aggresome components resulting in availability of BECN1 and other key autophagy proteins to form the autophagosome, thus allowing the autophagy process to function and leading to the clearance of autophagic cargo. Moreover, decreased p62 levels due to a functional autophagy flux will possibly allow the newly synthesized F508-delCFTR to reach the PM and restore partial CFTR function, even though some of previously aggresome sequestered F508-delCFTR may be degraded by the active autophagy process. In addition to cysteamine, treatment with epigallocatechin-gallate (EGCG) at the time of cysteamine removal, potentiates the long-term stability of the PM-rescued F508-delCFTR, due to its inhibitory effect on protein kinase CK2, which would otherwise promote peripheral/PM degradation of F508-delCFTR. Additionally, a functional autophagy process means that the toxic aggregated proteins and other damaged organelles such as mitochondria are homeostatically degraded, thus decreasing overall ROS levels. Finally, cysteamine blocks the translocation of ASM from cytoplasm to the PM, thus reducing the conversion of sphingosine to ceramide, and preventing ceramide-mediated inflammatory-apoptotic signaling in CF cells and/or lungs.

(Awatade et al., 2018). Moreover, it is not known if rare CFTR mutations also lead to a autophagy defect, and thus many other CFTR modulators have been clinically tested to evaluate their efficacy in restoring the PM stability and function of different CFTR mutants (Lopes-Pacheco, 2016). This strategy is currently being developed as a personalized CF management plan and holds potential for CF patients with all classes of CFTR mutations (Lopes-Pacheco, 2016; Paranjape and Mogayzel, 2018). As an example, for people with the G551D mutation, the orally bioavailable potentiator drug, VX770, shows substantial promise as an inducer of mutant CFTR channel activity, and thus is FDA approved for clinical application in CF patients (Accurso et al., 2010). However, since about 80% of CF patients worldwide possesses the F508del-CFTR defect (Lopes-Pacheco, 2016), drugs that correct its PM trafficking, stability, and function have emerged as promising therapeutic pipeline for clinical validation in CF subjects. Since the single corrector drugs showed minimal clinical benefit, successful efforts have been made to develop combinatorial therapy for CF. In fact, several CFTR-corrector compounds have been clinically evaluated and few have even reached the CF patients in combination with CFTR-potentiator drugs Orkambi®, Symdeko® (Birault et al., 2013; Wainwright et al., 2015; Mayer, 2016), although their present costs are humongous (Mayer, 2016; Bulloch et al., 2017). Additionally, a recent study tested a triple combination of pharmacological chaperones (VX809+MCG1516A+RDR1) and demonstrated better CFTR functional correction than VX809 alone (Carlile et al., 2018), thus providing potentially promising future therapeutics for CF subjects. Similarly, another triple combination therapy was tested using VX-659-tezacaftor-ivacaftor (Davies et al., 2018), and is currently in Phase III clinical trials (Sala and Jain, 2018).

Another important aspect of current CF drugs is the challenge of drug-delivery and/or *in vivo* bioavailability due to the notoriously thick and sticky mucus layer (Brockman et al., 2017; Vij, 2017). Considerable pre-clinical research is ongoing to address these crucial issues, and there has been some success in designing novel drug-delivery systems that achieve targeted drug-delivery and long-term bioavailability in the CF lungs (Vij et al., 2010; Vij, 2011, 2017; van Rijt et al., 2014). Although scientists and clinicians have come a long way on significantly improving the median survival age of CF patients to reach adulthood (~40–50 years) (West and Flume, 2018), the disease is still incurable and numerous precious lives are lost at a very early age. Thus, continued basic and translational research is essential to develop a better armamentarium of preventive/therapeutic strategies to further improve patient survival and possibly find a cure to this life-restricting and life-taking genetic disease. The current perspective compiles some recent studies that have the potential to translate into emerging therapeutic strategies for CF subjects, with the focus on drugs/compounds that correct the underlying disease-promoting defect in proteostasis and autophagy, including the protein-processing defect in F508del-CFTR protein.

AUTOPHAGY INDUCERS AS EMERGING CF THERAPEUTICS

One of the foremost cellular proteostatic mechanism that regulates protein-processing is the catabolic autophagy process. There is a plethora of evidence in recent studies that a partial (in chronic obstructive pulmonary disease, COPD) (Cantin, 2016; Bodas et al., 2017; Vij, 2017; Shi et al., 2018) or complete loss (in CF) (Luciani et al., 2010; Cantin, 2016) of functional CFTR protein from the PM leads to reactive oxygen species (ROS)-mediated autophagy impairment. This results in the accumulation of misfolded CFTR in perinuclear aggresome bodies, which eventually promotes the development of the lung disease. In CF, the accumulation of misfolded F508del-CFTR leads to ROS mediated autophagy impairment that results in increased inflammatory-oxidative stress (Luciani et al., 2010) in the CF airways. Moreover, a non-functional CFTR also contributes to defective bacterial uptake, killing, and clearance (Brockman et al., 2017; Ferrari et al., 2017; Pehote et al., 2017; Shrestha et al., 2017), which contributes to persistent exacerbations and inflammation, eventually resulting in irreversible damage of the pulmonary architecture. Lately, some pre-clinical and clinical trials demonstrate the utility of autophagy inducing therapeutic compounds in controlling pathogenesis and progression of CF lung disease (Villella et al., 2013b; Junkins et al., 2014; Esposito et al., 2016; Romani et al., 2017; Stincardini et al., 2018), that have shown promise in Phase-I/II trials but none have hitherto reached the bedside yet (De Stefano et al., 2014; Devereux et al., 2015, 2016). As discussed before (Yang et al., 2013; Vu et al., 2017), some other autophagy inducing drugs are also tested as potential CF drug candidates but these may not reach the patients due to the high doses required for the treatment as well as an evidence of many off-target side effects (Yang et al., 2013; Vu et al., 2017). Thus, we highlight here the leading proteostasis/autophagy-modulating compounds/drugs, which can allow bedside translation as emerging CF drug candidates.

CYSTEAMINE: A MULTI-PRONGED DRUG FOR CF

Cysteamine is an FDA-approved drug for nephropathic cystinosis and has been very effectively used for over 25 years (Besouw et al., 2013; Fraser-Pitt et al., 2018). Chemically, cysteamine is an endogenously present, water soluble aminothiol, generated as a consequence of coenzyme A metabolism (Fraser-Pitt et al., 2018). It is commercially available as Cystagon® and Procysbi® and can be administered orally, although with well documented side effects (Cherqui, 2012; Veys et al., 2016). Over the years, cysteamine was introduced as a potential CF drug and henceforth several studies have been conducted to evaluate its efficacy in controlling CF lung disease (Besouw et al., 2013; Charrier et al., 2014; Devereux et al., 2015, 2016; Brockman et al., 2017; Shrestha et al., 2017). Mechanistically, cysteamine is a TG2 inhibitor, which dislodges the aggresome assembly, which is sequestering key autophagy proteins and F508del-CFTR, thereby restoring autophagy and decreasing p62 levels (**Figure 1**). This allows forward trafficking of misfolded F508del-CFTR to the Golgi and PM, thus reinstating its chloride channel function. Moreover, decreased p62 levels might also prevent sequestration of newly synthesized aggregation-prone F508del-CFTR protein (Luciani et al., 2010) into aggresome bodies, thus allowing its trafficking towards the PM. Additionally, knockdown of p62 also mimics the F508del-CFTR rescuing effect of cysteamine, thus confirming the crucial role of p62 in regulating the levels of F508del-CFTR on the PM. Recently, we demonstrated that cysteamine blocked translocation of acid sphingomyelinase (ASM) enzyme to the PM, thus blocking the conversion of sphingomyelin to ceramide, a pathogenic bioactive lipid implicated in CF lung disease (**Figure 1**; Bodas et al., 2018b). This study adds another novel mechanism of cysteamine action in controlling inflammatory-apoptotic signaling in CF lung disease, although further pre-clinical and clinical studies are warranted to verify these mechanisms. Nonetheless, it is encouraging that cysteamine is being developed as a delayed-release capsule form (Lynovex®) (Charrier et al., 2014) and has undergone preliminary clinical studies in CF subjects. A relatively recent small single arm, phase 1/2a open label study was conducted to evaluate the tolerance and pharmacokinetics of cysteamine in CF patients (Devereux et al., 2016). The results indicated that although some adverse reactions were observed in CF patients who were given oral cysteamine, these were similar to the side effects seen in cystinosis subjects (Devereux et al., 2016). Overall, cysteamine was well tolerated and entered the bronchial secretions at concentrations higher than plasma (Devereux et al., 2016). In addition, a recent promising study in mice and human CF subjects was conducted using cysteamine and epigallocatechin-gallate (EGCG) as a combinatorial drug strategy (Tosco et al., 2016). The beneficial effects of this approach were attributed to autophagy-induction mediated restoration of F508del-CFTR to the PM by cysteamine, followed by enhanced stability of the PM-resident CFTR protein via inhibition of protein kinase CK2, by EGCG. Intriguingly, we and others recently described that cysteamine can be utilized as a multi-pronged CF-drug candidate, as its abilities are not restricted to just correcting the CFTR-dependent chloride ion transport defect. In fact, cysteamine possesses a diverse repertoire of beneficial properties such as anti-oxidant (Bodas et al., 2016, 2018b; Govindaraju et al., 2017; Vij et al., 2018), anti-inflammatory (Ferrari et al., 2017), autophagy-inducer (Esposito et al., 2016; Tosco et al., 2016; Ferrari et al., 2017), bactericidal (Charrier et al., 2014; Ferrari et al., 2017; Shrestha et al., 2017), mucolytic and anti-biofilm (Charrier et al., 2014; Brockman et al., 2017), which are all necessary to control acute or recurring exacerbations and CF pulmonary disease progression. Even though cysteamine is a strong CF-drug candidate, it's utility is possibly restricted to patients with only the F508del-CFTR mutation, as it was not very effective in other types of CFTR mutations such as R560S-CFTR (Awatade et al., 2018) that warrants further evaluation. Moreover, in spite of all the beneficial properties, the main caveats in the use of cysteamine is its poor bioavailability and the requirement of a high dose which is difficult to achieve *in vivo* (Vu et al., 2017). Thus, novel attempts have been made to improve the bioavailability of cysteamine, as well as to decrease the effective dose, such as by conjugating it with a [3-fatty acid (docosahexaenoic acid, DHA)], which also has its own autophagy inducing properties via the AMPK pathway (Vu et al., 2017). This conjugate could effectively rescue F508del-CFTR to the PM at a substantially lower concentration, thus warranting its further evaluation in a clinical setting. In another report, nine "prodrugs" of -glutamyl-cysteamine were tested in cultured kidney cells, to overcome its major disadvantages (Frost et al., 2016). These prodrugs could undertake successful delivery of cysteamine into kidney epithelial cells with improved bioavailability and low toxicity (Frost et al., 2016). This approach seems promising and needs further evaluation in pre-clinical CF models.

We have previously demonstrated the utility of nanotechnology in the development of novel drug delivery systems aimed at sustained and targeted delivery to the CF airways (Vij et al., 2010; Vij, 2011, 2017; Brockman et al., 2017). Using a similar approach, we recently proposed the application of dendrimer technology in designing a novel drug-delivery system to improve cysteamine's bioavailability and specificity. We developed a dendrimer-cysteamine conjugate formulation (PAMAM-DEN^{CYS}), and tested its ability to induce trafficking of F508del-CFTR to the PM in CF cells (Brockman et al., 2017). Although this was an pre-clinical early stage investigation, we were able to demonstrate key therapeutic signatures such as rescue of F508del-CFTR from the aggresome bodies and it's trafficking to the PM, as well as control of *Pa* infection and growth, and mucolytic potential (Brockman et al., 2017). Therefore, this novel PAMAM-DEN^{CYS} conjugate has a potential for further development as an emerging CF therapeutic strategy, as it corrects the proteostasis and autophagy impairment, which is the central disease-promoting mechanism in pathogenesis of chronic CF lung disease.

GSNO AND GSNOR INHIBITORS

Another interesting strategy to correct the proteostasis and autophagy defect in CF is through nitric oxide (NO)-augmentation, which facilitates the rescue of misfolded F508del-CFTR protein to the PM. Some previous reports propose the use of NO-donors (such as S-nitrosoglutathione, GSNO) or the inhibitors of GSNO-reductase (GSNOR), in controlling airway inflammation in experimental allergic asthma (Blonder et al., 2014) and CF models (Zaman et al., 2006, 2014, 2016; Rafeeq and Murad, 2017). In the lungs, NO and its reservoir, GSNO, play a very crucial role in the maintaining airway smooth muscle tone and controlling inflammation (Que et al., 2009; Sun et al., 2011). The levels of GSNO are tightly regulated by GSNOR, the enzyme which degrades GSNO (Sun et al., 2011). In fact, GSNO levels are diminished, with a concomitant increase in GSNOR levels,

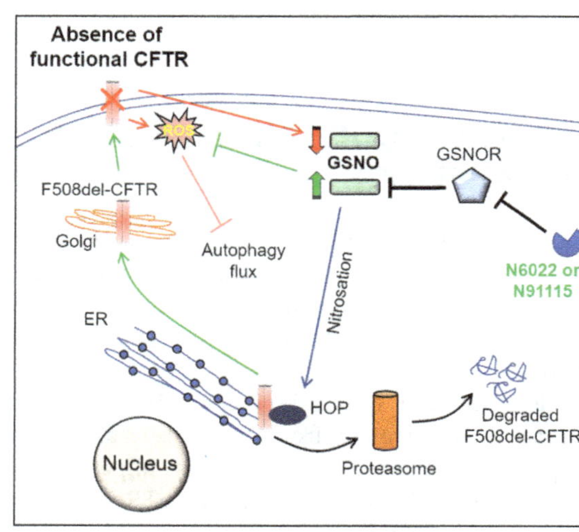

FIGURE 2 | Mechanisms of GSNOR-inhibitors mediated rescue of F508del-CFTR to the PM. Molecular chaperones such as Hsp70Hsp90 organizing protein (HOP) regulate CFTR biogenesis and proper trafficking to the PM. In the ER, association of HOP with F508del-CFTR leads to its degradation via the ER-associated proteasomal pathway. S-nitrosoglutathione (GSNO), a cellular nitric oxide (NO) donor, modulates the function of HOP by its S-nitrosation. In the absence of a functional CFTR, cellular GSNO levels are low, which results in decreased S-nitrosation of HOP, which promotes proteasome mediated degradation of F508del-CFTR. The cellular levels of GSNO are tightly regulated by the enzyme, GSNO-reductase (GSNOR), which mediates the catabolism of GSNO. Pharmacological inhibition of GSNOR using N6022 or N91115 increases GSNO levels that leads to increased S-nitrosation of HOP. It is believed that an increase in HOP S-nitrosation hampers its association with F508del-CFTR, thereby allowing the forward trafficking and maturation of F508del-CFTR. Moreover, recent studies from our group also indicate that GSNO augmentation using N6022 can control the elevated ROS levels and thus correct the ROS-mediated autophagy flux impairment in CF.

in both asthmatic and CF lungs (Que et al., 2009; Sun et al., 2011; Zaman et al., 2016), indicating that altered NO signaling contributes to asthma and CF pathogenesis. Mechanistically, the GSNO-mediated *S*-nitrosylation and subsequent degradation of Hsp70/Hsp90 organizing protein (HOP) favors the forward trafficking of CFTR to the PM (**Figure 2**; Odunuga et al., 2004; Marozkina et al., 2010). The findings that GSNO could increase the expression, maturation and function of both WT and F508del-CFTR in human bronchial epithelial cells led to clinical testing of a GSNOR-inhibitor, N91115 (Cavosonstat, Nivalis Therapeutics) (C.F. Foundation, 2015; Donaldson et al., 2017). The study reported that N91115 was well tolerated over a 28 day period, with no dose-limiting toxicities and no safety issues (Donaldson et al., 2017), albeit the study was discontinued in the Phase 2 stage as no improvement in lung function was observed in CF subjects. We recently reported that apart from its CFTR rescuing property, GSNO augmentation by using either GSNO or a GSNOR-inhibitor (N6022) effectively diminished CS-induced inflammatory-oxidative stress and also corrected the autophagy impairment (Bodas et al., 2017), thus targeting the underlying cause of CFTR dysfunction and resulting CF lung disease pathogenesis and progression. In fact, N6022 has been tested in clinical trials on CF patients with somewhat encouraging outcomes (C.F. Foundation, 2014; Rafeeq and Murad, 2017). The autophagy inducing property of GSNO or N6022 could be attributed to its rescue of CFTR to the PM (Zaman et al., 2016; Bodas et al., 2017), or other mechanisms such as its inhibitory effect on mTOR (Montagna et al., 2016), or its anti-oxidant function (Rauhala et al., 1998; Khan et al., 2011; Bodas et al., 2017). The *in vivo* application of N6022 could be restricted because of its low bioavailability, due to the presence of the highly polar imidazole group (Sun et al., 2011). Thus, GSNO-augmentation has the potential to be further tested in CF, where modifications in dosing and concurrent development of airway-delivery methodology can allow successful clinical outcomes.

POTENTIAL APPLICATION OF FISETIN AS A NUTRACEUTICAL FOR CF

A plant derived nutraceutical, Fisetin (3,3′,4′,7-tetra hydroxyflavone), demonstrates the potential to be a future CF drug candidate (Pal et al., 2016). Ongoing, experimental and clinical research is investigating the preventive and therapeutic properties of Fisetin in chronic inflammatory conditions (Pal et al., 2016), neurological diseases and various types of cancers (Pal et al., 2016). Previous studies have described Fisetin as a potent anti-oxidant (Khan et al., 2013; Pal et al., 2016; Govindaraju et al., 2017), anti-inflammatory (Khan et al., 2013; Pal et al., 2016), bactericidal (Pehote et al., 2017) and also an inhibitor of PI3K/AKT/mTOR signaling pathway (Adhami et al., 2012), which regulates key cellular processes including autophagy, and is discussed below in this article. In the context of inflammatory pulmonary diseases, Fisetin has demonstrated its therapeutic potential in murine models of allergic airway inflammation (Goh et al., 2012; Brown et al., 2016), and lipopolysaccharide (LPS) induced acute lung injury in rats, through its NFκB-targeted anti-inflammatory mechanism of action (Feng et al., 2016). Moreover, our recent report using cigarette smoke (CS)-extract and Pa model in murine macrophages, demonstrates the efficacy of Fisetin in correcting the CS-induced defect in bacterial clearance via transcription factor-EB (TFEB)-mediated autophagy-induction, and/or by restoring expression of mature (WT)-CFTR (Pehote et al., 2017). Additionally, similar to cysteamine, Fisetin also reveals direct bactericidal activity against Pa bacteria, a predominant CF-pathogen, by hitherto unknown mechanism(s) (Pehote et al., 2017). In another parallel study, using CS-exposure of retinal pigment epithelial cells (RPE) as an *in vitro* model of age-related macular degeneration (AMD), Fisetin successfully corrected the CS-induced autophagy-flux impairment and reduced the perinuclear accumulation of aggresome bodies, plausibly by controlling CS-induced ROS-activation (Govindaraju et al., 2017). Since CF lung disease is also characterized by chronic inflammatory-oxidative stress, persistent bacterial infections and autophagy impairment, proof of concept *in vitro* data warrants evaluation of the efficacy of Fisetin in pre-clinical CF-lung disease models. Although, it should be noted that similar to other promising autophagy-inducing drug candidates, the utility of Fisetin is hampered by its poor aqueous solubility (Bothiraja et al., 2014) and low oral bioavailability (Seguin et al., 2013), and thus attempts have been underway to improve its *in vivo* efficacy by the use of nanotechnology-based airway-delivery approaches (Ragelle et al., 2012; Kadari et al., 2017; Mehta et al., 2018).

A THYMIC PEPTIDE TO CORRECT THE BASIC CF-DEFECT

Recent studies have highlighted the potential of Thymosin α-1 (Tα1), a thymic peptide with broad immune-modulatory properties, in correcting the basic CF-defect, i.e., the restoration of misfolded F508del-CFTR to the PM (Romani et al., 2017; Garaci, 2018; Rubin, 2018; Stincardini et al., 2018). Mechanistically, activation of indoleamine 2, 3-dioxygenase (IDO1), and the resulting decrease in inflammation, along with autophagy-induction are proposed as the key means of Tα1-mediated F508del-CFTR rescue (Romani et al., 2017) (**Figure 3**). Tα1 was shown to rescue F508del-CFTR to the PM at a clinically achievable dose, and this was attributed to its activity as a proteostasis modulator. Tα1 act's on multiple steps of F508del-CFTR recycling such as the Rab GTPase's, the deubiquitinating enzyme USP36, and the ubiquitin-binding protein, p62, which is involved in the aggresome sequestration of F508del-CFTR (Romani et al., 2017). In Tα1 treated cells, the F508del-CFTR co-localized with Rab9, which is the marker of recycling endosome. Moreover, the co-localization of F508del-CFTR with Rab5 (early endosome marker) and Rab7 (late endosome marker) was diminished by Tα1 treatment. Thus, Tα1 reduces the endocytic recycling of F508del-CFTR into early endosomes and also prevents its transport into late endosomes and/or lysosomes, thereby promoting its forward recycling to the PM (Romani et al., 2017). Although Tα1 has a good clinical safety profile and is already available commercially as ZADAXIN® for the treatment

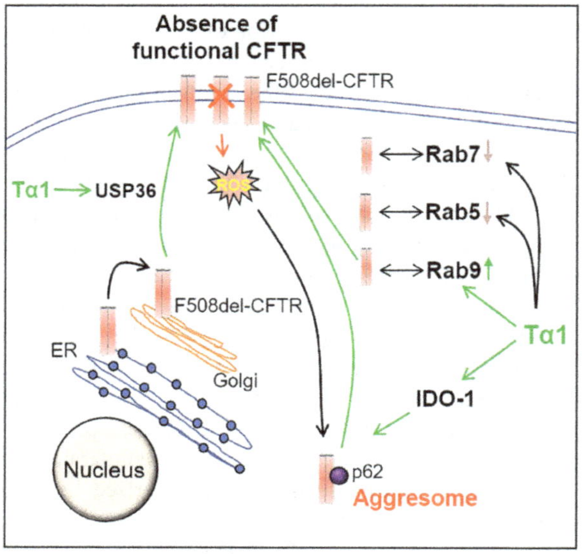

FIGURE 3 | Thymosin-α-1 acts on multiple-targets to rescue F508del-CFTR. Thymosin α-1 (Tα1) is a thymic peptide, which acts on multiple cellular pathways in the CFTR recycling and maturation process to restore the misfolded F508del-CFTR to the plasma membrane (PM). First, Tα1 can induce autophagy via activation of indoleamine 2, 3-dioxygenase (IDO-1), and reduction of p62 levels, thereby resulting in the rescue of F508del-CFTR to the PM. Additionally, Tα1 activates deubiquitinating enzyme USP36, which in turn prevents the ubiquitination and subsequent degradation of F508del-CFTR, thus improving its PM stability. Moreover, in Tα1 treated cells, F508del-CFTR is found to be associated with Rab9 GTPase (recycling endosome marker), which promotes recycling of F508del-CFTR to the PM. This happens in parallel to a decrease in co-localization of F508del-CFTR with Rab 5 (early endosome marker) and Rab7 (late endosome marker) GTPases, in Tα1 treated cells.

of several inflammatory and/or infectious diseases, such as viral infections, immunodeficiency diseases, HIV/AIDS and cancers (Romani et al., 2017), it remains to be investigated whether it possesses other important anti-CF attributes such as bactericidal and mucolytic. Moreover, some recent studies report that Tα1 failed to rescue CFTR in epithelial cells and primary bronchial epithelial cells from CF patients (Matthes et al., 2018; Tomati et al., 2018), although these effects may be due to the incorrect solvent used by these investigators (Garaci, 2018). Thus, the recent claims that Tα1 could be a potential "single-molecule" drug for preventing/treating chronic CF-lung disease seems to be a far shot that requires further in-depth studies in pre-clinical and clinical CF settings.

PI3K/AKT/mTOR INHIBITORS AS EMERGING CF DRUGS

The mammalian target of rapamycin (mTOR) is a member of the phosphatidylinositol 3-kinase (PI3K)-related kinase family of proteins that has long been implicated in regulating key cellular processes such as cell growth (Yu and Cui, 2016), survival (Yu and Cui, 2016), motility (Holroyd and Michie, 2018), metabolic pathways (Yu and Cui, 2016) and autophagy (Kim and Guan, 2015; Rabanal-Ruiz et al., 2017). The PI3K/AKT/mTOR signaling pathway is altered in several disease states such as cancer (Conciatori et al., 2018; Guri et al., 2018), immune system-related diseases (Guri et al., 2018; Jung et al., 2018), idiopathic pulmonary fibrosis (IPF) (Lawrence and Nho, 2018), COPD (Houssaini et al., 2018; Wang et al., 2018) and lymphangioleiomyomatosis (LAM) (Gao et al., 2018). Since mTOR is considered to be the master regulator of the autophagy pathway, its inhibitors have been investigated for their therapeutic potential in different types of cancers, and autophagy-induction is one of the proposed mechanisms of action (Saxton and Sabatini, 2017; Paquette et al., 2018). Moreover, in fibroblasts, higher than normal mTOR activity and the resulting autophagy-defect has been associated with pathogenesis of IPF (Lawrence and Nho, 2018), a fatal chronic restrictive lung disease. Additionally, elevated mTOR signaling mediated autophagy impairment was recently observed in lung cells and tissues isolated from COPD subjects, while the same conceptual evidence was also derived from transgenic mice with constitutive or conditional over-activation of mTOR (Houssaini et al., 2018). Interestingly, lung cell senescence and development of emphysema was found to be associated with elevated mTOR activity in these mice, as the effects could be ameliorated by rapamycin (an mTOR inhibitor) (Houssaini et al., 2018). It is also noteworthy that mTOR inhibition has been beneficial in the clearance of protein aggregates (aggresomes) in neurogenerative diseases (Heras-Sandoval et al., 2014), thus further confirming the crucial role of mTOR in regulating the autophagy process. Rapamycin mediated mTOR inhibition has been shown to reduce lung inflammatory responses in a CF mouse model (Abdulrahman et al., 2011), along with improved CFTR function (Luciani et al., 2011; Tazi and Amer, 2015). These studies confirmed that restoration of autophagy using Rapamycin, which is commercially available as Sirolimus, could benefit CF patients, although it has several limitations in clinical practice (Emoto et al., 2013; Li et al., 2014). Sirolimus has low oral bioavailability (Brattström C. et al., 2000), poor water solubility (Kim et al., 2011), a huge pharmacokinetic variability among patients (Emoto et al., 2013), adverse side effects (Bee et al., 2018), and off-target effects (Arriola et al., 2016; Lamming, 2016; Haeri et al., 2017), which are due to its inhibition of both mTORC1 and mTORC2 (Arriola et al., 2016). The primary side effects of sirolimus include hyperglycemia, hyperlipidemia, insulin resistance and increase in new onset of type 2 diabetes (Emoto et al., 2013; Bee et al., 2018). In a national cohort study, the lung function response to rapamycin treatment and its associated side effects in women with progressive lung disease due to LAM was investigated (Bee et al., 2018). It was observed that although side effects were common, but they were manageable over several years, and improvements in lung function were evident. Overall, a low dose rapamycin was associated with fewer side effects with no difference in the beneficial effects (Bee et al., 2018), thus warranting its further clinical evaluation in CF. Moreover, several studies have been conducted to devise ways to enhance the bioavailability and improve *in vivo* delivery of sirolimus (Kim et al., 2011; Haeri et al., 2017). Considering the central role of impaired-autophagy and resulting aggresome-pathology in CF, it seems worthwhile to test the efficacy of mTOR inhibitors in CF models. In accord with this idea, CFBE41o- cells demonstrated upregulated mTOR activity, and the resulting autophagy impairment was found to be associated with accumulation of F508del-CFTR into peri-nuclear aggresome bodies (Reilly et al., 2017). Moreover, the inhibition of PI3K/AKT/mTOR pathway by six different compounds enhanced CFTR-membrane stability and expression (Reilly et al., 2017). The study identified MK-2206 as the most potent CFTR rescuing compound, which functions through targeting Bcl-2-associated athanogene 3 (BAG3), a regulator of autophagy and aggresome clearance (Reilly et al., 2017). Thus, the efficacy of pharmacological PI3K/AKT/mTOR inhibitors warrants further evaluation as potential therapeutic candidates for chronic CF lung disease, based on their ability to rectify the disease-promoting proteostasis and autophagy defect, including the correction of underlying CFTR dysfunction.

HDAC INHIBITORS AS PROTEOSTASIS MODULATORS IN CF

Inhibition of histone deacetylases (HDAC) has been evaluated as a potential therapeutic strategy for several protein folding and other chronic inflammatory diseases such as neurodegenerative diseases (Benito et al., 2015; Rabal et al., 2016), chronic kidney disease (Liu and Zhuang, 2015), inflammatory bowel disease (Felice et al., 2015), cancer (Falkenberg and Johnstone, 2014; West and Johnstone, 2014; De Souza and Chatterji, 2015), graft-versus-host disease (Choi et al., 2014, 2017), rheumatoid arthritis (Oh et al., 2017) and CF (Hutt et al., 2010, 2011; Bodas et al., 2018a). Pharmacological studies of suberanilohydroxamic acid (SAHA, Vorinostat), a broad inhibitor of class I and II HDAC enzymes (Bubna, 2015), in different types of cancers indicate that SAHA is well tolerated and demonstrates good oral bioavailability (43%) (Kelly et al., 2005). Moreover, the major adverse effects of SAHA administration such as fatigue, diarrhea, dehydration, etc., where more prominent in the intravenous treatment route, rather than the oral treatment regime, and the more severe indications such as thrombocytopenia, were resolved upon discontinuation of treatment (O'Connor et al., 2006; Bubna, 2015). Additionally, SAHA is also an FDA approved drug for cutaneous T-cell lymphoma (Bubna, 2015). Thus, at least in patient-based studies targeting cancer, SAHA was safely administered over a prolonged period, with minimal toxicity and consistent anti-HDAC activity, thereby indicating its potential tolerance as a CF drug candidate. In CF, the pharmacological inhibition of HDACs, especially using SAHA seems encouraging as this provides twofold benefit of controlling the inflammation (Hull et al., 2016; Xu et al., 2017) and also function as a proteostasis regulator (Bouchecareilh et al., 2012; Han et al., 2015) to facilitate rescue and trafficking of F508del-CFTR to the PM (CFTR-corrector) (Bodas et al., 2018a). Indeed, we recently verified the potential utility of SAHA in rescuing the F508del-CFTR to the PM by delaying its degradation, thus confirming its potential as a CFTR-corrector (Bodas et al., 2018a). Additionally, SAHA treatment was also effective in controlling *Pa*-LPS induced inflammation and neutrophil activation in a pre-clinical CF murine model, which was possibly *via* induction of regulatory T cells (Bodas et al., 2018a). Intriguingly, this observation was CFTR-independent, as the inflammation quenching function of SAHA was evident even in *Cftr*$^{-/-}$ mice. This indicates that SAHA could provide a potential therapeutic benefit in CF irrespective of its ability to rescue mutant CFTR. An ostensibly contrasting study demonstrates the failure of SAHA to restore F508del-CFTR, albeit the cells and the dose of SAHA used in those reports are dissimilar to our studies, which possibly explains the disparity in the results (Bergougnoux et al., 2017). Moreover, in two other studies SAHA was able to increase forskolin-induced chloride secretion in cell lines expressing CFTR but failed to demonstrate the same effect in primary epithelial cells from CF patients (Sondo et al., 2011; Van Goor et al., 2011). Nonetheless, proteostasis regulators such as SAHA and specific HDAC 6/7 inhibitors, such as tubacin (Cebotaru et al., 2008) have been evaluated in rescuing misfolded F508del-CFTR from proteasomal degradation and aggresome-accumulation. Further pre-clinical studies are necessary to evaluate the therapeutic efficacy of specific HDAC inhibitors, which might be coupled with novel drug-delivery systems (Mohamed et al., 2012; Tran et al., 2014) to further enhance their *in vivo* efficacy and bioavailability in CF lungs.

Briefly, as a proof of concept in support of proposed strategy adapting proteostasis and autophagy for rescuing the CF lung disease, recent study demonstrates that VX-809 mediated CFTR rescue is proteostasis-dependent but autophagy-independent (Pesce et al., 2018), where potent autophagy augmentation will allow synergistic effects on both mutant-CFTR rescue and *other components* (Romani et al., 2017; Stincardini et al., 2018) of CF lung disease pathogenesis as discussed in detail above (De Stefano et al., 2014; Tosco et al., 2016; Vu et al., 2017; Hutt et al., 2018; Stincardini et al., 2018; Zhang et al., 2018). In this study investigators, attempted to augment autophagy using torin-1 (Pesce et al., 2018) but its effects are missed due to lack of serum-starvation and appropriate experimental conditions. Nonetheless, extensive body of experimental evidence from our group and other's suggest that adapting proteostasis and autophagy has significant potential in correcting the underlying causes of CF lung disease pathogenesis and will allow development of next generation of potent novel therapeutics as summarized below.

PERSPECTIVE

The absence of a functional membrane CFTR is the primary etiology of chronic lung disease development in CF patients, which progresses due to numerous pathological complications such as mucus-overproduction, elevated oxidative stress, chronic infections and sustained NFκB-mediated inflammation, eventually leading to early-life fatality, if left untreated. Although huge strides have been made in the development of novel "breakthrough" drug combinations such as Orkambi®, Symdeko® etc., to rectify the core CF-defect, their widespread therapeutic advantage has been restricted due to somewhat low efficacy in maintaining sustained CFTR-activation as well as controlling other components of CF lung disease such as chronic inflammatory-oxidative stress responses and exacerbations. Therefore, alternative therapeutic methodologies using novel drugs and/or drug-delivery systems need to be concurrently developed, which can fill the gap of an affordable yet potent and effective CF treatment strategy capable of rescuing overall CF lung disease. Since, significant experimental and pre-clinical evidence suggests the key central role of proteostasis and autophagy processes in regulating most of the disease-causing pathogenic features in the CF airways, this warrants further clinical evaluation and development of proteostasis and autophagy modulating drugs, as an emerging therapeutic approach for CF lung disease. Finally, since CF subjects possesses numerous types of CFTR mutations, genotyping of the patient before deciding on the proteostasis and autophagy modulating drug(s), will allow evaluating the therapeutic advantage for the patient as a part of emerging Precision Medicine Initiative.

AUTHOR CONTRIBUTIONS

Both authors contributed to the concept, framework and writing of the manuscript for publication.

ACKNOWLEDGMENTS

NV was supported by National Institutes of Health (NIH, R03HL09631 and CTSA UL RR025005ATIP), Flight Attendant Medical Research Institute (FAMRI, YCSA082131), and Cystic Fibrosis Foundation (CFF, R025-CR07 and VIJ07IO) grants to develop proteostasis/autophagy modulation therapeutic strategy and drug-delivery systems discussed in this publication.

REFERENCES

Abdulrahman, B. A., Khweek, A. A., Akhter, A., Caution, K., Kotrange, S., Abdelaziz, D. H., et al. (2011). Autophagy stimulation by rapamycin suppresses lung inflammation and infection by *Burkholderia cenocepacia* in a model of cystic fibrosis. *Autophagy* 7, 1359–1370. doi: 10.4161/auto.7.11.17660

Abdulrahman, B. A., Khweek, A. A., Akhter, A., Caution, K., Tazi, M., Hassan, H., et al. (2013). Depletion of the ubiquitin-binding adaptor molecule SQSTM1/p62 from macrophages harboring cftr ΔF508 mutation improves the delivery of *Burkholderia cenocepacia* to the autophagic machinery. *J. Biol. Chem.* 288, 2049–2058. doi: 10.1074/jbc.M112.411728

Accurso, F. J., Rowe, S. M., Clancy, J. P., Boyle, M. P., Dunitz, J. M., Durie, P. R., et al. (2010). Effect of VX-770 in persons with cystic fibrosis and the G551D-CFTR mutation. *N. Engl. J. Med.* 363, 1991–2003. doi: 10.1056/NEJMoa0909825

Adhami, V. M., Syed, D. N., Khan, N., and Mukhtar, H. (2012). Dietary flavonoid fisetin: a novel dual inhibitor of PI3K/Akt and mTOR for prostate cancer management. *Biochem. Pharmacol.* 84, 1277–1281. doi: 10.1016/j.bcp.2012.07.012

Arriola, S. I., Apelo, and Lamming, D. W. (2016). Rapamycin: an InhibiTOR of aging emerges from the soil of easter island. *J. Gerontol. A Biol. Sci. Med. Sci.* 71, 841–849. doi: 10.1093/gerona/glw090

Awatade, N. T., Ramalho, S., Silva, I. A. L., Felício, V., Botelho, H. M., de Poel, E., et al. (2018). R560S: a class II CFTR mutation that is not rescued by current modulators. *J. Cyst. Fibros* doi: 10.1016/j.jcf.2018.07.001 [Epub ahead of print].

Bee, J., Fuller, S., Miller, S., and Johnson, S. R. (2018). Lung function response and side effects to rapamycin for lymphangioleiomyomatosis: a prospective national cohort study. *Thorax* 73, 369–375. doi: 10.1136/thoraxjnl-2017-210872

Benito, E., Urbanke, H., Ramachandran, B., Barth, J., Halder, R., Awasthi, A., et al. (2015). HDAC inhibitor-dependent transcriptome and memory reinstatement in cognitive decline models. *J. Clin. Invest.* 125, 3572–3584. doi: 10.1172/JCI79942

Bergougnoux, A., Petit, A., Knabe, L., Bribes, E., Chiron, R., De Sario, A., et al. (2017). The HDAC inhibitor SAHA does not rescue CFTR membrane expression in cystic fibrosis. *Int. J. Biochem. Cell Biol.* 88, 124–132. doi: 10.1016/j.biocel.2017.05.002

Besouw, M., Masereeuw, R., van den Heuvel, L., and Levtchenko, E. (2013). Cysteamine: an old drug with new potential. *Drug Discov. Today* 18, 785–792. doi: 10.1016/j.drudis.2013.02.003

Birault, V., Solari, R., Hanrahan, J., and Thomas, D. Y. (2013). Correctors of the basic trafficking defect of the mutant F508del-CFTR that causes cystic fibrosis. *Curr. Opin. Chem. Biol.* 17, 353–360. doi: 10.1016/j.cbpa.2013.04.020

Blonder, J. P., Mutka, S. C., Sun, X., Qiu, J., Green, L. H., Mehra, N. K., et al. (2014). Pharmacologic inhibition of S-nitrosoglutathione reductase protects against experimental asthma in BALB/c mice through attenuation of both bronchoconstriction and inflammation. *BMC Pulm Med.* 14:3. doi: 10.1186/1471-2466-14-3

Bodas, M., Mazur, S., Min, T., and Vij, N. (2018a). Inhibition of histone-deacetylase activity rescues inflammatory cystic fibrosis lung disease by modulating innate and adaptive immune responses. *Respir. Res.* 19:2. doi: 10.1186/s12931-017-0705-8

Bodas, M., Pehote, G., Silverberg, D., Gulbins, E., and Vij, N. (2018b). Autophagy augmentation alleviates cigarette smoke-induced CFTR-dysfunction, ceramide-accumulation and COPD-emphysema pathogenesis. *Free Radic. Biol. Med.* doi: 10.1016/j.freeradbiomed.2018.11.023 [Epub ahead of print].

Bodas, M., Silverberg, D., Walworth, K., Brucia, K. A., and Vij, N. (2017). Augmentation of S-nitrosoglutathione (GSNO) controls cigarette-smoke induced inflammatory-oxidative stress and COPD-emphysema pathogenesis by restoring CFTR function. *Antioxid. Redox Signal.* 27, 433–451. doi: 10.1089/ars.2016.6895

Bodas, M., Van Westphal, C., Carpenter-Thompson, R., Mohanty, K. D., and Vij, N. (2016). Nicotine exposure induces bronchial epithelial cell apoptosis and senescence via ROS mediated autophagy-impairment. *Free Radic Biol. Med.* 97, 441–453. doi: 10.1016/j.freeradbiomed.2016.06.017

Bodas, M., Tran, I., and Vij, N. (2012). Therapeutic strategies to correct proteostasis-imbalance in chronic obstructive lung diseases. *Curr. Mol. Med.* 12, 807–814. doi: 10.2174/156652412801318809

Bodas, M., and Vij, N. (2010). The NF-kappaB signaling in cystic fibrosis lung disease: pathophysiology and therapeutic potential. *Discov. Med.* 9, 346–356.

Bodas, M., and Vij, N. (2017). Augmenting autophagy for prognosis based intervention of COPD-pathophysiology. *Respir Res.* 18:83. doi: 10.1186/s12931-017-0560-7

Bothiraja, C., Yojana, B. D., Pawar, A. P., Shaikh, K. S., and Thorat, U. H. (2014). Fisetin-loaded nanocochleates: formulation, characterisation, in vitro anticancer testing, bioavailability and biodistribution study. *Expert Opin. Drug Deliv.* 11, 17–29. doi: 10.1517/17425247.2013.860131

Bouchecareilh, M., Hutt, D. M., Szajner, P., Flotte, T. R., and Balch, W. E. (2012). Histone deacetylase inhibitor (HDACi) suberoylanilide hydroxamic acid (SAHA)-mediated correction of α1-antitrypsin deficiency. *J. Biol. Chem.* 287, 38265–38278. doi: 10.1074/jbc.M112.404707

Brattström, C., Säwe, J., Jansson, B., Lönnebo, A., Nordin, J., Zimmerman, J. J., et al. (2000). Pharmacokinetics and safety of single oral doses of sirolimus (rapamycin) in healthy male volunteers. *Ther. Drug Monit.* 22, 537–544. doi: 10.1097/00007691-200010000-00006

Brockman, S. M., Bodas, M., Silverberg, D., Sharma, A., and Vij, N. (2017). Dendrimer-based selective autophagy-induction rescues ΔF508-CFTR and inhibits *Pseudomonas aeruginosa* infection in cystic fibrosis. *PLoS One* 12:e0184793. doi: 10.1371/journal.pone.0184793

Brown, A., Danielsson, J., Townsend, E. A., Zhang, Y., Perez-Zoghbi, J. F., Emala, C. W., et al. (2016). Attenuation of airway smooth muscle contractility via flavonol-mediated inhibition of phospholipase-Cβ. *Am. J. Physiol. Lung Cell Mol. Physiol.* 310, L747–L758. doi: 10.1152/ajplung.00215.2015

Bubna, A. K. (2015). Vorinostat-an overview. *Ind. J. Dermatol.* 60:419. doi: 10.4103/0019-5154.160511

Bulloch, M. N., Hanna, C., and Giovane, R. (2017). Lumacaftor/ivacaftor, a novel agent for the treatment of cystic fibrosis patients who are homozygous for the F580del CFTR mutation. *Exp. Rev. Clin. Pharmacol.* 10, 1055–1072. doi: 10.1080/17512433.2017.1378094

Bustamante, H. A., González, A. E., Cerda-Troncoso, C., Shaughnessy, R., Otth, C., Soza, A., et al. (2018). Interplay between the autophagy-lysosomal pathway and the ubiquitin-proteasome system: a target for therapeutic development in Alzheimer's disease. *Front. Cell Neurosci.* 12:126. doi: 10.3389/fncel.2018.00126

Cantin, A. M. (2016). Cystic fibrosis transmembrane conductance regulator, implications in cystic fibrosis and chronic obstructive pulmonary disease. *Ann. Am. Thorac. Soc.* 13(Suppl. 2), S150–S155. doi: 10.1513/AnnalsATS.201509-588KV

Cantin, A. M., Hartl, D., Konstan, M. W., and Chmiel, J. F. (2015). Inflammation in cystic fibrosis lung disease: pathogenesis and therapy. *J. Cyst. Fibros* 14, 419–430. doi: 10.1016/j.jcf.2015.03.003

Carlile, G. W., Yang, Q., Matthes, E., Liao, J., Radinovic, S., Miyamoto, C., et al. (2018). A novel triple combination of pharmacological chaperones improves F508del-CFTR correction. *Sci. Rep.* 8:11404. doi: 10.1038/s41598-018-29276-y

Cebotaru, L., Vij, N., Ciobanu, I., Wright, J., Flotte, T., Guggino, W. B., et al. (2008). Cystic fibrosis transmembrane regulator missing the first four transmembrane segments increases wild type and DeltaF508 processing. *J. Biol. Chem.* 283, 21926–21933. doi: 10.1074/jbc.M709156200

C. F. Foundation. (2014). *Safety and Pharmacokinetic Study of N6022 in Subjects With Cystic Fibrosis Homozygous for the F508del-CFTR Mutation (SNO-1).* Available at: https://clinicaltrials.gov/ct2/show/results/NCT01746784

C. F. Foundation. (2018). *Types of CFTR Mutations.* https://www.cff.org/What-is-CF/Genetics/Types-of-CFTR-Mutations/

C. F. Foundation. (2015). *SNO4: Study of N91115 in People with Cystic Fibrosis Ages 18 and Older with Two Copies of F508del-CFTR Mutation (Nivalis N91115-2CF-03).* Available at: https://www.cff.org/Trials/Finder/details/388/SNO4-Study-of-N91115-in-people-with-cystic-fibrosis-ages-18-and-older-with-two-copies-of-F508del-CFTR-mutation

Charrier, C., Rodger, C., Robertson, J., Kowalczuk, A., Shand, N., Fraser-Pitt, D., et al. (2014). Cysteamine (Lynovex(R)), a novel mucoactive antimicrobial & antibiofilm agent for the treatment of cystic fibrosis. *Orphanet. J. Rare Dis.* 9:189. doi: 10.1186/s13023-014-0189-2

Chaudhuri, T. K., and Paul, S. (2006). Protein-misfolding diseases and chaperone-based therapeutic approaches. *FEBS J.* 273, 1331–1349. doi: 10.1111/j.1742-4658.2006.05181.x

Cherqui, S. (2012). Cysteamine therapy: a treatment for cystinosis, not a cure. *Kidney Int.* 81, 127–129. doi: 10.1038/ki.2011.301

Choi, S. W., Braun, T., Chang, L., Ferrara, J. L., Pawarode, A., Magenau, J. M., et al. (2014). Vorinostat plus tacrolimus and mycophenolate to prevent graft-versus-host disease after related-donor reduced-intensity conditioning allogeneic haemopoietic stem-cell transplantation: a phase 1/2 trial. *Lancet Oncol.* 15, 87–95. doi: 10.1016/S1470-2045(13)70512-6

Choi, S. W., Braun, T., Henig, I., Gatza, E., Magenau, J., Parkin, B., et al. (2017). Vorinostat plus tacrolimus/methotrexate to prevent GVHD after myeloablative conditioning, unrelated donor HC*Blood. T.* 130, 1760–1767. doi: 10.1182/blood-2017-06-790469

Conciatori, F., Bazzichetto, C., Falcone, I., Pilotto, S., Bria, E., Cognetti, F., et al. (2018). Role of mTOR signaling in tumor microenvironment: an overview. *Int. J. Mol. Sci.* 19:E2453. doi: 10.3390/ijms19082453

Daniele, S., Giacomelli, C., and Martini, C. (2018). Brain ageing and neurodegenerative disease: the role of cellular waste management. *Biochem. Pharmacol.* 158, 207–216. doi: 10.1016/j.bcp.2018.10.030

Davies, J. C., Moskowitz, S. M., Brown, C., Horsley, A., Mall, M. A., McKone, E. F., et al. (2018). VX-659-tezacaftor-ivacaftor in patients with cystic fibrosis and one or two Phe508del alleles. *N. Engl. J. Med.* 379, 1599–1611. doi: 10.1056/NEJMoa1807119

De Souza, C., and Chatterji, B. P. (2015). HDAC inhibitors as novel anti-cancer therapeutics. *Recent Pat Anticancer Drug Discov.* 10, 145–162. doi: 10.2174/1574892810666150317144511

De Stefano, D., Villella, V. R., Esposito, S., Tosco, A., Sepe, A., De Gregorio, F., et al. (2014). Restoration of CFTR function in patients with cystic fibrosis carrying the F508del-CFTR mutation. *Autophagy* 10, 2053–2074. doi: 10.4161/15548627.2014.973737

Devereux, G., Fraser-Pitt, D., Robertson, J., Devlin, E., Mercer, D and O'Neil, D., et al. (2015). Cysteamine as a future intervention in cystic fibrosis against current and emerging pathogens: a patient-based ex vivo study confirming its antimicrobial and mucoactive potential in sputum. *EBioMed.* 2, 1507–1512. doi: 10.1016/j.ebiom.2015.08.018

Devereux, G., Steele, S., Griffiths, K., Devlin, E., Fraser-Pitt, D., Cotton, S., et al. (2016). An open-label investigation of the pharmacokinetics and tolerability of oral cysteamine in adults with cystic fibrosis. *Clin. Drug Investig.* 36, 605–612. doi: 10.1007/s40261-016-0405-z

Donaldson, S. H., Solomon, G. M., Zeitlin, P. L., Flume, P. A., Casey, A., McCoy, K., et al. (2017). Pharmacokinetics and safety of cavosonstat (N91115) in healthy and cystic fibrosis adults homozygous for F508DEL-CFTR. *J. Cyst. Fibros* 16, 371–379. doi: 10.1016/j.jcf.2017.01.009

Emoto, C., Fukuda, T., Cox, S, Christians, U., and Vinks, A. A. (2013). Development of a physiologically-based pharmacokinetic model for sirolimus: predicting bioavailability based on intestinal CYP3A content. *CPT Pharmacomet. Syst. Pharmacol.* 2:e59. doi: 10.1038/psp.2013.33

Esposito, S., Tosco, A., Villella, V. R., Raia, V., Kroemer, G., and Maiuri, L. (2016). Manipulating proteostasis to repair the F508del-CFTR defect in cystic fibrosis. *Mol. Cell Pediatr.* 3:13. doi: 10.1186/s40348-016-0040-z

Falkenberg, K. J., and Johnstone, R. W. (2014). Histone deacetylases and their inhibitors in cancer, neurological diseases and immune disorders. *Nat. Rev. Drug Discov.* 13, 673–691. doi: 10.1038/nrd4360

Felice, C., Lewis, A., Armuzzi, A., Lindsay, J. O., and Silver, A. (2015). Review article: selective histone deacetylase isoforms as potential therapeutic targets in inflammatory bowel diseases. *Aliment Pharmacol. Ther.* 41, 26–38. doi: 10.1111/apt.13008

Feng, G., Jiang, Z. Y., Sun, B., Fu, J., and Li, T. Z. (2016). Fisetin alleviates lipopolysaccharide-induced acute lung injury via TLR4-mediated NF-κB signaling pathway in rats. *Inflammation* 39, 148–57. doi: 10.1007/s10753-015-0233-y

Ferrari, E., Monzani, R., Villella, V. R., Esposito, S., Saluzzo, F., Rossin, F., et al. (2017). Cysteamine re-establishes the clearance of *Pseudomonas aeruginosa* by macrophages bearing the cystic fibrosis-relevant F508del-CFTR mutation. *Cell Death Dis.* 8:e2544. doi: 10.1038/cddis.2016.476

Fraser-Pitt, D., and O'Neil, D. (2015). Cystic fibrosis – A multiorgan protein misfolding disease. *Future Sci. OA* 1:FSO57. doi: 10.4155/fso.15.57

Fraser-Pitt, D. J., Mercer, D. K., Smith, D., Kowalczuk, A., Robertson, J., Lovie, E., et al. (2018). Cysteamine, an endogenous aminothiol, and cystamine, the disulfide product of oxidation, increase *Pseudomonas aeruginosa* sensitivity to reactive oxygen and nitrogen species and potentiate therapeutic antibiotics against bacterial infection. *Infect. Immun.* 86:e00947-17. doi: 10.1128/IAI.00947-17

Frost, L., Suryadevara, P., Cannell, S. J., Groundwater, P. W., Hambleton, P. A., Anderson, R. J., et al. (2016). Synthesis of diacylated γ-glutamyl-cysteamine prodrugs, and in vitro evaluation of their cytotoxicity and intracellular delivery of cysteamine. *Eur. J. Med. Chem.* 109, 206–215. doi: 10.1016/j.ejmech.2015.12.027

Gao, N., Zhang, T., Ji, J., Xu, K F., and Tian, X. (2018). The efficacy and adverse events of mTOR inhibitors in lymphangioleiomyomatosis: systematic review and meta-analysis. *Orphanet J. Rare Dis.* 13:134. doi: 10.1186/s13023-018-0874-7

Garaci, E. (2018). From thymus to cystic fibrosis: the amazing life of thymosin alpha 1. *Expert Opin. Biol. Ther.* 18(Suppl1), 9–11. doi: 10.1080/14712598.2018.1484447

Goh, F. Y., Upton, N., Guan, S., Cheng, C., Shanmugam, M. K., Sethi, G., et al. (2012). Fisetin, a bioactive flavonol, attenuates allergic airway inflammation through negative regulation of NF-kappaB. *Eur. J. Pharmacol.* 679, 109–116. doi: 10.1016/j.ejphar.2012.01.002

Gomes-Alves, P., Couto, F., Pesquita, C., Coelho, A. V., and Penque, D. (2010). Rescue of F508del-CFTR by RXR motif inactivation triggers proteome modulation associated with the unfolded protein response. *Biochim. Biophys. Acta* 1804, 856–865. doi: 10.1016/j.bbapap.2009.12.013

Govindaraju, V. K., Bodas, M., and Vij, N. (2017). Cigarette smoke induced autophagy-impairment regulates AMD pathogenesis mechanisms in ARPE-19 cells. *PLoS One* 12:e0182420. doi: 10.1371/journal.pone.0182420

Grassme, H., Henry, B., Ziobro, R., Becker, K. A., Riethmuller, J., Gardner, A., et al. (2017). beta1-integrin accumulates in cystic fibrosis luminal airway epithelial membranes and decreases sphingosine. *Promot. Bact. Infections Cell Host Microbe* 21, 707.e8–718.e8. doi: 10.1016/j.chom.2017.05.001

Guri, Y., Nordmann, T. M., and Roszik, J. (2018). mTOR at the transmitting and receiving ends in tumor immunity. *Front. Immunol.* 9:578. doi: 10.3389/fimmu.2018.00578

Haeri, A., Osouli, M., Bayat, F., Alavi, S., and Dadashzadeh, S. (2017). Nanomedicine approaches for sirolimus delivery: a review of pharmaceutical properties and preclinical studies. *Artif Cells Nanomed. Biotechnol.* doi: 10.1080/21691401.2017.1408123 [Epub ahead of print].

Han, D. Y., Di, X. J., Fu, Y. L., and Mu, T. W. (2015). Combining valosin-containing protein (VCP) inhibition and suberanilohydroxamic acid (SAHA) treatment additively enhances the folding, trafficking, and function of epilepsy-associated γ-aminobutyric acid, type A (GABAA) receptors. *J. Biol. Chem.* 290, 325–337. doi: 10.1074/jbc.M114.580324

Hartl, F. U. (2017). Protein misfolding diseases. *Annu. Rev. Biochem.* 86, 21–26. doi: 10.1146/annurev-biochem-061516-044518

Heras-Sandoval, D., Pérez-Rojas, J. M., Hernández-Damián, J., and Pedraza-Chaverri, J. (2014). The role of PI3K/AKT/mTOR pathway in the modulation of autophagy and the clearance of protein aggregates in neurodegeneration. *Cell Signal.* 26, 2694–2701. doi: 10.1016/j.cellsig.2014.08.019

Hidvegi, T., Stolz, D. B., Alcorn, J. F., Yousem, S. A., Wang, J., Leme, A. S., et al. (2015). Enhancing autophagy with drugs or lung-directed gene therapy reverses the pathological effects of respiratory epithelial cell proteinopathy. *J. Biol. Chem.* 290, 29742–29757. doi: 10.1074/jbc.M115.691253

Holroyd, A. K., and Michie, A. M. (2018). The role of mTOR-mediated signaling in the regulation of cellular migration. *Immunol. Lett.* 196, 74–79. doi: 10.1016/j.imlet.2018.01.015

Houssaini, A., Breau, M., Kebe, K., Abid, S., Marcos, E., Lipskaia, L., et al. (2018). mTOR pathway activation drives lung cell senescence and emphysema. *JCI Insight* 3:93203. doi: 10.1172/jci.insight.93203

Hudock, K. M., and Clancy, J. P. (2017). An update on new and emerging therapies for cystic fibrosis. *Expert Opin Emerg. Drugs* 22, 331–346. doi: 10.1080/14728214.2017.1418324

Hull, E. E., Montgomery, M. R., and Leyva, K. J. (2016). HDAC inhibitors as epigenetic regulators of the immune system: impacts on cancer therapy and inflammatory diseases. *Biomed. Res. Int.* 2016:8797206. doi: 10.1155/2016/8797206

Hutt, D. M., Herman, D., Rodrigues, A. P., Noel, S., Pilewski, J. M., Matteson, J., et al. (2010). Reduced histone deacetylase 7 activity restores function to misfolded CFTR in cystic fibrosis. *Nat. Chem. Biol.* 6, 25–33. doi: 10.1038/nchembio.275

Hutt, D. M., Mishra, S. K., Roth, D. M., Larsen, M. B., Angles, F., Frizzell, R. A., et al. (2018). Silencing of the Hsp70-specific nucleotide-exchange factor BAG3 corrects the F508del-CFTR variant by restoring autophagy. *J. Biol. Chem.* 293, 13682–13695. doi: 10.1074/jbc.RA118.002607

Hutt, D. M., Olsen, C. A., Vickers, C. J., Herman, D., Chalfant, M., Montero, A., et al. (2011). Potential agents for treating cystic fibrosis: cyclic tetrapeptides that restore trafficking and activity of DeltaF508-CFTR. *ACS Med. Chem. Lett.* 2, 703–707. doi: 10.1021/ml200136e

Jung, S., L. Gámez-Díaz, Proietti, M., and Grimbacher, B. (2018). "Immune TOR-opathies," a novel disease entity in clinical immunology. *Front. Immunol.* 9:966. doi: 10.3389/fimmu.2018.00966

Junkins, R. D., McCormick, C., and Lin, T. J. (2014). The emerging potential of autophagy-based therapies in the treatment of cystic fibrosis lung infections. *Autophagy* 10, 538–547. doi: 10.4161/auto.27750

Kadari, A., Gudem, S., Kulhari, H., Bhandi, M. M., Borkar, R. M., Kolapalli, V. R., et al. (2017). Enhanced oral bioavailability and anticancer efficacy of fisetin by encapsulating as inclusion complex with HPβCD in polymeric nanoparticles. *Drug Deliv.* 24, 224–232. doi: 10.1080/10717544.2016.1245366

Kelly, W. K., O'Connor, O. A., Krug, L. M., Chiao, J. H., Heaney, M., Curley, T., et al. (2005). Phase I study of an oral histone deacetylase inhibitor, suberoylanilide hydroxamic acid, in patients with advanced cancer. *J. Clin. Oncol.* 23, 3923–3931. doi: 10.1200/JCO.2005.14.167

Khan, M., Sakakima, H., Dhammu, T. S., Shunmugavel, A., Im, Y. B., Gilg, A. G., et al. (2011). S-nitrosoglutathione reduces oxidative injury and promotes mechanisms of neurorepair following traumatic brain injury in rats. *J. Neuroinflamm.* 8:78. doi: 10.1186/1742-2094-8-78

Khan, N., Syed, D. N., Ahmad, N., and Mukhtar, H. (2013). Fisetin: a dietary antioxidant for health promotion. *Antioxid. Redox Signal.* 19, 151–162. doi: 10.1089/ars.2012.4901

Kim, M. S., Kim, J. S., Park, H. J., Cho, W. K., Cha, K. H., Hwang, S. J., et al. (2011). Enhanced bioavailability of sirolimus via preparation of solid dispersion nanoparticles using a supercritical antisolvent process. *Int. J. Nanomed.* 6, 2997–3009. doi: 10.2147/IJN.S26546

Kim, Y. C., and Guan, K. L. (2015). mTOR: a pharmacologic target for autophagy regulation. *J. Clin. Invest.* 125, 25–32. doi: 10.1172/JCI73939

Klaips, C. L., Jayaraj, G. G., and Hartl, F. U. (2018). Pathways of cellular proteostasis in aging and disease. *J. Cell. Biol.* 217, 51–63. doi: 10.1083/jcb.201709072

Korovila, I., Hugo, M., Castro, J. P., Weber, D., Höhn, A., Grune, T., et al. (2017). Proteostasis, oxidative stress and aging. *Redox Biol.* 13, 550–567. doi: 10.1016/j.redox.2017.07.008

Lamming, D. W. (2016). Inhibition of the mechanistic target of rapamycin (mtor)-rapamycin and beyond. *Cold Spring Harb. Perspect. Med.* 6:a025924. doi: 10.1101/cshperspect.a025924

Lawrence, J., and Nho, R. (2018). The role of the mammalian target of rapamycin (mTOR) in pulmonary fibrosis. *Int. J. Mol. Sci.* 19:E778. doi: 10.3390/ijms19030778

Li, J., Kim, S. G., and Blenis, J. (2014). Rapamycin: one drug, many effects. *Cell Metab.* 19, 373–379. doi: 10.1016/j.cmet.2014.01.001

Liu, N., and Zhuang, S. (2015). Treatment of chronic kidney diseases with histone deacetylase inhibitors. *Front. Physiol.* 6:121. doi: 10.3389/fphys.2015.00121

Lopes-Pacheco, M. (2016). CFTR modulators: shedding light on precision medicine for cystic fibrosis. *Front. Pharmacol.* 7:275. doi: 10.3389/fphar.2016.00275

Luciani, A., Villella, V. R., Esposito, S., Brunetti-Pierri, N., Medina, D., Settembre, C., et al. (2010). Defective CFTR induces aggresome formation and lung inflammation in cystic fibrosis through ROS-mediated autophagy inhibition. *Nat. Cell Biol.* 12, 863–875. doi: 10.1038/ncb2090

Luciani, A., Villella, V. R., Esposito, S., Brunetti-Pierri, N., Medina, D. L., Settembre, C., et al. (2011). Cystic fibrosis: a disorder with defective autophagy. *Autophagy* 7, 104–106. doi: 10.4161/auto.7.1.13987

Lukacs, G. L., Chang, X. B., Bear, C., Kartner, N., Mohamed, A., Riordan, J. R., et al. (1993). The delta F508 mutation decreases the stability of cystic fibrosis transmembrane conductance regulator in the plasma membrane. Determination of functional half-lives on transfected cells. *J. Biol. Chem.* 268, 21592–21598.

Lukacs, G. L., and Verkman, A. S. (2012) CFTR: folding, misfolding and correcting the DeltaF508 conformational defect. *Trends Mol. Med.* 18, 81–91. doi: 10.1016/j.molmed.2011.10.003

Maiuri, L., Raia, V., and Kroemer, G. (2017). Strategies for the etiological therapy of cystic fibrosis. *Cell Death Differ.* 24, 1825–1844. doi: 10.1038/cdd.2017.126

Mall, M. A. (2016). Unplugging mucus in cystic fibrosis and chronic obstructive pulmonary disease. *Ann. Am. Thorac. Soc.* 13(Suppl. 2), S177–S185. doi: 10.1513/AnnalsATS.201509-641KV

Marozkina, N. V., Yemen, S., Borowitz, M., Liu, L., Plapp, M., Sun, F., et al. (2010). Hsp 70/Hsp 90 organizing protein as a nitrosylation target in cystic fibrosis therapy. *Proc. Natl. Acad. Sci. U.S.A.* 107, 11393–11398. doi: 10.1073/pnas.0909128107

Matthes, E., Hanrahan, J. W., and Cantin, A. M. (2018). F508del-CFTR is not corrected by thymosin α1. *Nat. Med.* 24, 890–891. doi: 10.1038/s41591-018-0079-6

Mayer, M. (2016). Lumacaftor-ivacaftor (Orkambi) for cystic fibrosis: behind the 'breakthrough'. *Evid. Based. Med.* 21, 83–86. doi: 10.1136/ebmed-2015-110325

Mehta, P., Pawar, A., Mahadik, K., and Bothiraja, C. (2018). Emerging novel drug delivery strategies for bioactive flavonol fisetin in biomedicine. *Biomed. Pharmacother.* 106, 1282–1291. doi: 10.1016/j.biopha.2018.07.079

Mohamed, E. A., Zhao, Y., Meshali, M. M., Remsberg, C. M., Borg, T. M., Foda, A. M., et al. (2012). Vorinostat with sustained exposure and high solubility in poly(ethylene glycol)-b-poly(DL-lactic acid) micelle nanocarriers:

characterization and effects on pharmacokinetics in rat serum and urine. *J. Pharm. Sci.* 101, 3787–3798. doi: 10.1002/jps.23265

Montagna, C., Rizza, S., Maiani, E., Piredda, L., Filomeni, G., and Cecconi, F., et al. (2016). To eat, or NOt to eat: S-nitrosylation signaling in autophagy. *FEBS J.* 283, 3857–3869. doi: 10.1111/febs.13736

O'Connor, O. A., Heaney, M. L., Schwartz, L., Richardson, S., Willim, R., MacGregor-Cortelli, B., et al. (2006). Clinical experience with intravenous and oral formulations of the novel histone deacetylase inhibitor suberoylanilide hydroxamic acid in patients with advanced hematologic malignancies. *J. Clin. Oncol.* 24, 166–173. doi: 10.1200/JCO.2005.01.9679

Odunuga, O. O., Longshaw, V. M., and Blatch, G. L. (2004). Hop: more than an Hsp70/Hsp90 adaptor protein. *Bioessays* 26, 1058–1068. doi: 10.1002/bies.20107

Oh, B. R., Suh, D. H., Bae, D., Ha, N., Choi, Y. I., Yoo, H. J., et al. (2017). Therapeutic effect of a novel histone deacetylase 6 inhibitor, CKD-L, on collagen-induced arthritis in vivo and regulatory T cells in rheumatoid arthritis in vitro. *Arthritis Res. Ther.* 19:154. doi: 10.1186/s13075-017-1357-2

Pal, H. C., Pearlman, R. L., and Afaq, F. (2016). Fisetin and its role in chronic diseases. *Adv. Exp. Med. Biol.* 928, 213–244. doi: 10.1007/978-3-319-41334-1_10

Paquette, M., El-Houjeiri, L., and Pause, A. (2018). mTOR pathways in cancer and autophagy. *Cancers (Basel)* 10:E18. doi: 10.3390/cancers10010018

Paranjape, S. M., and Mogayzel, P. J. (2018). Cystic fibrosis in the era of precision medicine. *Paediatr. Respir. Rev.* 25, 64–72. doi: 10.1016/j.prrv.2017.03.001

Pehote, G., Bodas, M., Brucia, K., and Vij, N. (2017). Cigarette smoke exposure inhibits bacterial killing via TFEB-mediated autophagy impairment and resulting phagocytosis defect. *Mediat. Inflamm.* 2017:3028082. doi: 10.1155/2017/3028082

Pesce, E., Sondo, E., Ferrerra, L., Tomati, V., Caci, E., Scudieri, P., et al. (2018). Emerging therapeutic approaches for cystic fibrosis. *Front. Pharmacol.* 13:1464. doi: 10.3389/fphar.2018.01464

Que, L. G., Yang, Z., Stamler, J. S., Lugogo, N. L., and Kraft, M. (2009). S-nitrosoglutathione reductase: an important regulator in human asthma. *Am. J. Respir. Crit Care Med.* 180, 226–231. doi: 10.1164/rccm.200901-0158OC

Rabal, O., Sánchez-Arias, J. A., Cuadrado-Tejedor, M., de Miguel, I., Pérez-González, M., García-Barroso, C., et al. (2016). Design, synthesis, and biological evaluation of first-in-class dual acting histone deacetylases (HDACs) and phosphodiesterase 5 (PDE5) inhibitors for the treatment of Alzheimer's disease. *J. Med. Chem.* 59, 8967–9004. doi: 10.1021/acs.jmedchem.6b00908

Rabanal-Ruiz, Y., Otten, E. G., and Korolchuk, V. I. (2017). mTORC1 as the main gateway to autophagy. *Essays Biochem.* 61, 565–584. doi: 10.1042/EBC20170027

Rafeeq, M. M., and Murad, H. A. S. (2017). Cystic fibrosis: current therapeutic targets and future approaches. *J. Transl. Med.* 15:84. doi: 10.1186/s12967-017-1193-9

Ragelle, H., Crauste-Manciet, S., Seguin, J., Brossard, D., Scherman, D., Arnaud, P., et al. (2012). Nanoemulsion formulation of fisetin improves bioavailability and antitumour activity in mice. *Int. J. Pharm.* 427, 452–459. doi: 10.1016/j.ijpharm.2012.02.025

Rauhala, P., Lin, A. M., and Chiueh, C. C. (1998). Neuroprotection by S-nitrosoglutathione of brain dopamine neurons from oxidative stress. *FASEB J.* 12, 165–173. doi: 10.1096/fasebj.12.2.165

Reilly, R., Mroz, M. S., Dempsey, E., Wynne, K., Keely, S. J., McKone, E. F., et al. (2017). Targeting the PI3K/Akt/mTOR signalling pathway in cystic fibrosis. *Sci. Rep.* 7:7642. doi: 10.1038/s41598-017-06588-z

Romani, L., Oikonomou, V., Moretti, S., Iannitti, R. G., D'Adamo, M. C., Villella, V. R., et al. (2017). Thymosin α1 represents a potential potent single-molecule-based therapy for cystic fibrosis. *Nat. Med.* 23, 590–600. doi: 10.1038/nm.4305

Rubin, B. K (2018). Unmet needs in cystic fibrosis. *Expert Opin. Biol. Ther.* 18(Supl), 49–52. doi: 10.1080/14712598.2018.1484101

Sala, M. A., and Jain, M. (2018). Tezacaftor for the treatment of cystic fibrosis. *Expert Rev. Respir Med.* 12, 725–732. doi: 10.1080/17476348.2018.1507741

Saxton, R. A., and Sabatini, D. M. (2017). mTOR signaling in growth. *Metabol. Dis. Cell* 168, 960–976. doi: 10.1016/j.cell.2017.02.004

Seguin, J., Brullé, L., Boyer, R., Lu, Y. M., Ramos Romano, M., Touil, Y. S., et al. (2013). Liposomal encapsulation of the natural flavonoid fisetin improves bioavailability and antitumor efficacy. *Int. J. Pharm.* 444, 146–154. doi: 10.1016/j.ijpharm.2013.01.050

Shi, J., Li, H., Yuan, C., Luo, M., Wei, J., and Liu, X. (2018). Cigarette smoke-induced acquired dysfunction of cystic fibrosis transmembrane conductance regulator in the pathogenesis of chronic obstructive pulmonary disease. *Oxid. Med. Cell Longev.* 2018:6567578. doi: 10.1155/2018/6567578

Shrestha, C. L., Assani, K. D., Rinehardt, H., Albastroiu, F., Zhang, S., Shell, R., et al. (2017). Cysteamine-mediated clearance of antibiotic-resistant pathogens in human cystic fibrosis macrophages. *PLoS One* 12:e0186169. doi: 10.1371/journal.pone.0186169

Sondo, E., Tomati, V., Caci, E., Esposito, A. I., Pfeffer, U., Pedemonte, N., et al. (2011). Rescue of the mutant CFTR chloride channel by pharmacological correctors and low temperature analyzed by gene expression profiling. *Am. J. Physiol. Cell Physiol.* 301, C872–C885. doi: 10.1152/ajpcell.00507.2010

Stincardini, C., Renga, G., Villella, V., Pariano, M., Oikonomou, V., Borghi, M., et al. (2018). Cellular proteostasis: a new twist in the action of thymosin α1. *Expert Opin. Biol. Ther.* 18, 43–48. doi: 10.1080/14712598.2018.1484103

Stoltz, D. A., Meyerholz, D. K., and Welsh, M. J. (2015). Origins of cystic fibrosis lung disease. *N. Engl. J. Med.* 372, 351–362. doi: 10.1056/NEJMra1300109

Sun, X., Wasley, J. W., Qiu, J., Blonder, J. P., Stout, A. M., Green, L. S., et al. (2011). Discovery of s-nitrosoglutathione reductase inhibitors: potential agents for the treatment of asthma and other inflammatory diseases. *ACS Med. Chem. Lett.* 2, 402–406. doi: 10.1021/ml200045s

Svedin, E., Utorova, R., Hühn, M. H., Larsson, P. G., Stone, V. M., Garimella, M., et al. (2017). A link between a common mutation in CFTR and impaired innate and adaptive viral defense. *J. Infect. Dis.* 216, 1308–1317. doi: 10.1093/infdis/jix474

Tazi, M. F., and Amer, A. (2015). OhioLINK Electronic Theses and Dissertations Center, Ohio State University. Integrated Biomedical Science Graduate Program and Ohio State University: Improving autophagy in cystic fibrosis : the effects of epigenetic regulation.

Tazi, M. F., Dakhlallah, D. A., Caution, K., Gerber, M. M., Chang, S. W., Khalil, H., et al. (2016). Elevated mirc1/Mir17-92 cluster expression negatively regulates autophagy and CFTR (cystic fibrosis transmembrane conductance regulator) function in CF macrophages. *Autophagy* 12, 2026–2037. doi: 10.1080/15548627.2016.1217370

Teichgraber, V., Ulrich, M., Endlich, N., Riethmuller, J., Wilker, B., De Oliveira-Munding, C. C., et al. (2008). Ceramide accumulation mediates inflammation, cell death and infection susceptibility in cystic fibrosis. *Nat. Med.* 14, 382–391. doi: 10.1038/nm1748

Tomati, V., Caci, E., Ferrera, L., Pesce, E., Sondo, E., Cholon, D. M., et al. (2018). Thymosin α-1 does not correct F508del-CFTR in cystic fibrosis airway epithelia. *JCI Insight* 3:e98699. doi: 10.1172/jci.insight.98699

Tosco, A., De Gregorio, F., Esposito, S.,. De Stefano, D, Sana, I., Ferrari, E., et al. (2016). A novel treatment of cystic fibrosis acting on-target: cysteamine plus epigallocatechin gallate for the autophagy-dependent rescue of class II-mutated CFTR. *Cell Death Differ.* 23, 1380–1393. doi: 10.1038/cdd.2016.22

Tran, I., Ji, C., Ni, I., Min, T., Tang, D., and Vij, N. (2015). Role of cigarette smoke-induced aggresome formation in chronic obstructive pulmonary disease-emphysema pathogenesis. *Am J. Respir Cell. Mol. Biol.* 53, 159–173. doi: 10.1165/rcmb.2014-0107OC

Tran, T. H., Ramasamy, T., Truong, D. H., Shin, B. S., Choi, H. G., Yong, C. S., et al. (2014). Development of vorinostat-loaded solid lipid nanoparticles to enhance pharmacokinetics and efficacy against multidrug-resistant cancer cells. *Pharm. Res.* 31, 1978–1988. doi: 10.1007/s11095-014-1300-z

Valle, C. W., and Vij, N. (2012). Can correcting the ΔF508-CFTR proteostasis-defect rescue CF lung disease? *Curr. Mol. Med.* 12, 860–871. doi: 10.2174/156652412801318773

Van Goor, F., Hadida, S., Grootenhuis, P. D., Burton, B., Stack, J. H., Straley, K. S., et al. (2011). Correction of the F508del-CFTR protein processing defect in vitro by the investigational drug VX-809. *Proc. Natl. Acad. Sci. U.S.A.* 108, 18843–18848. doi: 10.1073/pnas.1105787108

van Rijt, S. H., Bein, T., and Meiners, S. (2014). Medical nanoparticles for next generation drug delivery to the lungs. *Eur. Respir. J.* 44, 765–774. doi: 10.1183/09031936.00212813

Veys, K. R., Besouw, M. T., Pinxten, A. M., Dyck, M. V., Casteels, I., and Levtchenko, E. N. (2016). Cystinosis: a new perspective. *Acta Clin. Belg.* 71, 131–137. doi: 10.1179/2295333714Y.0000000113

Vij, N. (2017). Nano-based rescue of dysfunctional autophagy in chronic obstructive lung diseases. *Expert Opin. Drug Deliv.* 14, 483–489. doi: 10.1080/17425247.2016.1223040

Vij, N. (2011). Nano-based theranostics for chronic obstructive lung diseases: challenges and therapeutic potential. *Expert Opin. Drug Deliv.* 8, 1105–1109. doi: 10.1517/17425247.2011.597381

Vij, N., Chandramani-Shivalingappa, P., Van Westphal, C., Hole, R., and Bodas, M. (2018). Cigarette smoke-induced autophagy impairment accelerates lung aging, COPD-emphysema exacerbations and pathogenesis. *Am. J. Physiol. Cell Physiol.* 314, C73–C87. doi: 10.1152/ajpcell.00110.2016

Vij, N., Mazur, S., and Zeitlin, P. L. (2009). CFTR is a negative regulator of NFkappaB mediated innate immune response. *PLoS One* 4:e4664. doi: 10.1371/journal.pone.0004664

Vij, N., Min, T., Marasigan, R., Belcher, C. N., Mazur, S., Ding, H., et al. (2010). Development of PEGylated PLGA nanoparticle for controlled and sustained drug delivery in cystic fibrosis. *J. Nanobiotechnol.* 8:22. doi: 10.1186/1477-3155-8-22

Villella, V. R., Esposito, S., Bruscia, E. M., Maiuri, M. C., Raia, V., Kroemer, G., et al. (2013a). Targeting the intracellular environment in cystic fibrosis: restoring autophagy as a novel strategy to circumvent the CFTR defect. *Front. Pharmacol.* 4:1. doi: 10.3389/fphar.2013.00001

Villella, V. R., Esposito, S., Maiuri, M. C., Raia, V., Kroemer, G., and Maiuri, L. (2013b). Towards a rational combination therapy of cystic fibrosis: how cystamine restores the stability of mutant CFTR *Autophagy* 9, 1431–1434. doi: 10.4161/auto.25517

Vu, C. B., Bridges, R. J., Pena-Rasgado, C., Lacerda, A. E., Bordwell, C., Sewell, A., et al. (2017). Fatty acid cysteamine conjugates as novel and potent autophagy activators that enhance the correction of misfolded f508del-cystic fibrosis transmembrane conductance regulator (CFTR). *J. Med. Chem.* 60, 458–473. doi: 10.1021/acs.jmedchem.6b01539

Wainwright, C. E., Elborn, J. S., and Ramsey, B. W. (2015). Lumacaftor-ivacaftor in patients with cystic fibrosis homozygous for Phe508del CFTR. *N. Engl. J. Med.* 373, 1783–1784. doi: 10.1056/NEJMc1510466

Wang, Y., Liu, J., Zhou, J. S., Huang, H. Q., Li, Z. Y., Xu, X. C., et al. (2018). MTOR suppresses cigarette smoke-induced epithelial cell death and airway inflammation in chronic obstructive pulmonary disease. *J. Immunol.* 200, 2571–2580. doi: 10.4049/jimmunol.1701681

Welsh, M. J., Denning, G. M., Ostedgaard, L. S., and Anderson, M. P. (1993). Dysfunction of CFTR bearing the delta F508 mutation. *J. Cell Sci. Suppl.* 17, 235–239. doi: 10.1242/jcs.1993.Supplement_17.33

West, A. C., and Johnstone, R. W. (2014). New and emerging HDAC inhibitors for cancer treatment. *J. Clin. Invest.* 124, 30–39. doi: 10.1172/JCI69738

West, N. E., and Flume, P. A. (2018). Unmet needs in cystic fibrosis: the next steps in improving outcomes. *Expert Rev. Respir. Med.* 12, 585–593. doi: 10.1080/17476348.2018.1483723

Xu, Y., Xu, S., Liu, P., Koroleva, M., Zhang, S., Si, S., et al. (2017). Suberanilohydroxamic acid as a pharmacological kruppel-like factor 2 activator that represses vascular inflammation and atherosclerosis. *J. Am. Heart Assoc.* 6:e007134. doi: 10.1161/JAHA.117.007134

Yang, Y. P., Hu, L. F., Zheng, H. F., Mao, C. J., Hu, W. D., Xiong, K. P., et al. (2013). Application and interpretation of current autophagy inhibitors and activators. *Acta Pharmacol. Sin.* 34, 625–635. doi: 10.1038/aps.2013.5

Yu, J. S., and Cui, W. (2016). Proliferation, survival and metabolism: the role of PI3K/AKT/mTOR signalling in pluripotency and cell fate determination. *Development* 143, 3050–3060. doi: 10.1242/dev.137075

Zaman, K., Bennett, D., Fraser-Butler, M., Greenberg, Z., Getsy, P., Sattar, A., et al. (2014). S-Nitrosothiols increases cystic fibrosis transmembrane regulator expression and maturation in the cell surface. *Biochem. Biophys. Res. Commun.* 443, 1257–1262. doi: 10.1016/j.bbrc.2013.12.130

Zaman, K., Carraro, S., Doherty, J., Henderson, E. M., Lendermon, E., Liu, L., et al. (2006). S-nitrosylating agents: a novel class of compounds that increase cystic fibrosis transmembrane conductance regulator expression and maturation in epithelial cells. *Mol. Pharmacol.* 70, 1435–1442. doi: 10.1124/mol.106.023242

Zaman, K., Sawczak, V., Zaidi, A., Butler, M., Bennett, D., Getsy, P., et al. (2016). Augmentation of CFTR maturation by S-nitrosoglutathione reductase. *Am. J. Physiol. Lung Cell Mol. Physiol.* 310, L263–L270. doi: 10.1152/ajplung.00269.2014

Zhang, S., Stoll, G., Pedro, J., M. B. S., Sica, V., Sauvat, A., Obrist, F., et al. (2018). Evaluation of autophagy inducers in epithelial cells carrying the ΔF508 mutation of the cystic fibrosis transmembrane conductance regulator CFTR. *Cell Death Dis.* 9:191. doi: 10.1038/s41419-017-0235-9

10

TMEM16A in Cystic Fibrosis: Activating or Inhibiting?

Karl Kunzelmann[1], Jiraporn Ousingsawat[1], Inês Cabrita[1], Tereza Doušová[2], Andrea Bähr[3,4], Melanie Janda[3], Rainer Schreiber[1] and Roberta Benedetto[1]*

[1] Institut für Physiologie, Universität Regensburg, Regensburg, Germany, [2] Department of Pediatrics, Second Faculty of Medicine, University Hospital Motol, Charles University in Prague, Prague, Czechia, [3] Institute of Molecular Animal Breeding and Biotechnology, Ludwig-Maximilians-Universität München, Munich, Germany, [4] Innere Medizin I, Klinikum Rechts der Isar der TU München, München, Germany

***Correspondence:**
Karl Kunzelmann
karl.kunzelmann@ur.de

The inflammatory airway disease cystic fibrosis (CF) is characterized by airway obstruction due to mucus hypersecretion, airway plugging, and bronchoconstriction. The cystic fibrosis transmembrane conductance regulator (CFTR) chloride channel is dysfunctional in CF, leading to defects in epithelial transport. Although CF pathogenesis is still disputed, activation of alternative Cl^- channels is assumed to improve lung function in CF. Two suitable non-CFTR Cl^- channels are present in the airway epithelium, the Ca^{2+} activated channel TMEM16A and SLC26A9. Activation of these channels is thought to be feasible to improve hydration of the airway mucus and to increase mucociliary clearance. Interestingly, both channels are upregulated during inflammatory lung disease. They are assumed to support fluid secretion, necessary to hydrate excess mucus and to maintain mucus clearance. During inflammation, however, TMEM16A is upregulated particularly in mucus producing cells, with only little expression in ciliated cells. Recently it was shown that knockout of TMEM16A in ciliated cells strongly compromises Cl^- conductance and attenuated mucus secretion, but does not lead to a CF-like lung disease and airway plugging. Along this line, activation of TMEM16A by denufosol, a stable purinergic ligand, failed to demonstrate any benefit to CF patients in earlier studies. It rather induced adverse effects such as cough. A number of studies suggest that TMEM16A is essential for mucus secretion and possibly also for mucus production. Evidence is now provided for a crucial role of TMEM16A in fusion of mucus-filled granules with the apical plasma membrane and cellular exocytosis. This is probably due to local Ca^{2+} signals facilitated by TMEM16A. Taken together, TMEM16A supports fluid secretion by ciliated airway epithelial cells, but also maintains excessive mucus secretion during inflammatory airway disease. Because TMEM16A also supports airway smooth muscle contraction, inhibition rather than activation of TMEM16A might be the appropriate treatment for CF lung disease, asthma and COPD. As a number of FDA-approved and well-tolerated drugs have been shown to inhibit TMEM16A, evaluation in clinical trials appears timely.

Keywords: TMEM16A, anoctamin 1, mucus secretion, cystic fibrosis, asthma, COPD, Ca^{2+} signaling

INTRODUCTION

The inflammatory airway disease cystic fibrosis (CF) is characterized by airway obstruction due to mucus hypersecretion, mucus plugging, and bronchoconstriction. The cystic fibrosis transmembrane conductance regulator (CFTR) chloride channel is dysfunctional in CF, leading to a loss of fluid secretion and probably impaired bicarbonate transport, along with Na^+ hyperabsorption (Boucher, 2007; Stoltz et al., 2015). Dehydration of the airway surface (periciliary) fluid layer (ASL) covering the airway epithelium is thought to be the crucial factor leading to abnormal rheological properties of the mucus and occlusion of smaller airways (Boucher, 2007). Independent of the underlying precise molecular defect, tremendous effort was put into identification of small molecules, and natural compounds that would correct the basic defect by restoring CFTR function (Amaral and Kunzelmann, 2007; Verkman and Galietta, 2009). This, however, turned out to be a long and stony path that has finally provided effective drugs that correct and potentiate mutant CFTR. Moreover, the search is on to identify compounds that inhibit salt hyperabsorption in CF, and to find molecules that activate alternative Cl^- secretory pathways. What has not been in the minds of CF researchers is to look for inhibitors of certain types of Cl^- channels as a treatment for inflammatory airway disease (Li et al., 2017).

STILL UNRESOLVED: THE PATHOGENESIS OF CF

Lack of appropriate Cl^- secretion due to defective CFTR was long regarded as the essential, if not only cause for CF lung disease. However, a pathogenic concept proposing Na^+ hyperabsorption relative to attenuated Cl^- secretion, leading to airway dehydration and mucus plugging, has also been put forward in a number of studies (Boucher et al., 1986; Grubb et al., 1994; Mall et al., 1998a, 2004). We detected enhanced Na^+ conductances in nasal *ex vivo* tissue and freshly isolated intestinal cells from CF patients (Mall et al., 1998a, 2000). Along this line, reduced ASL would lead to thickened airway mucus, airway plugging and impaired mucociliary clearance with subsequent chronic bacterial infections. Yet, this concept has been questioned by Welsh and collaborators as well as other investigators, who did not find evidence for Na^+ hyperabsorption. In contrast, reduced airway Na^+ absorption in CF was claimed, leading to salt accumulation in the ASL, which under normal conditions might be even hypotonic when compared with the interstitial fluid. Thus, hypertonic ASL was blamed to inactivate ß-defensins, thereby causing a predisposition toward bacterial infections (Zabner et al., 1998; Chen et al., 2010; Itani et al., 2011). In contrast, the Boucher team and others found neither evidence for a hypotonic ASL under normal conditions, nor any salt concentration (hypertonic ASL) in CF airways (Matsui et al., 1998). Given the fact that the airway epithelium is relatively leaky and has a large hydraulic conductivity, it appears somewhat unlikely that it maintains a large transepithelial osmotic gradient.

A similar controversy arose around the pH value of the ASL. It had been shown that CFTR is permeable for bicarbonate (HCO_3^-), or contributes to HCO_3^- transport as a Cl^- recycling pathway in a number of epithelial organs [reviewed in (Kunzelmann et al., 2017)]. To what extend HCO_3^- is conducted by CFTR or rather operates indirectly as a Cl^- recycling channel that drives HCO_3^- secretion by Cl^-/HCO_3^- exchangers, is still a matter of debate. At any rate, Smith and Welsh were among the first to show defective cAMP-induced bicarbonate secretion in airways of CF patients (Smith and Welsh, 1992), while others showed that CFTR is permeable for HCO_3^- (Poulsen et al., 1994; Tang et al., 2009). It should be noted that patch clamp and other types of experiments with isotonic concentrations of HCO_3^- are not trivial and may be compromised by pH fluctuations (Kunzelmann et al., 1991). Attenuated fluid/HCO_3^- secretion in CF airways was shown to have adverse effects on the biophysical properties of airway mucus (Trout et al., 1998). Quinton and others provided further evidence that bicarbonate transport is essential for proper mucus release and viscosity (Choi et al., 2001; Quinton, 2001). In fact, HCO_3^- transport is impaired in a number of different epithelial tissues derived from CF patients (Kunzelmann et al., 2017). Importantly, human lung pathology was brilliantly reproduced in a CF pig model. Using this CF pig model, reduced airway surface liquid pH, impaired bacterial killing, and mucus abnormalities were demonstrated (Pedersen et al., 1999; Stoltz et al., 2010; Pezzulo et al., 2012; Hoegger et al., 2014). Interestingly, Hoegger et al. demonstrated abnormal mucociliary transport in CF in submerged epithelia, which somewhat questions the role of surface dehydration in CF (Hoegger et al., 2014). In sharp contrast to these results, Schultz and coworkers found no evidence for acidic airway surface liquid pH in lungs of CF children, using a novel optical pH probe and a specialized bronchoscope (Schultz et al., 2017).

Stick and Schulz claimed that only a small fraction of infants diagnosed early with CF through the Australian AREST CF early surveillance program, present lower airway infection (Stick and Schultz, 2018). This may support the "inflammation first" concept, proposing that inflammation in CF lungs is present early in life and clearly before airway infection (Khan et al., 1995; Doring and Worlitzsch, 2000). Thus, CF epithelia appear to be in an inflammatory, pro-proliferative, and constantly remodeling state, even without any bacterial infection (Hajj et al., 2007; Rottner et al., 2007, 2009; Martins et al., 2011). CF epithelial cells were also shown to have a compromised anti-oxidant defense by superoxide dismutase (Rottner et al., 2011). Notably, some CFTR knockout mouse models do show signs of lung/airway inflammation even in the absence of mucus obstruction (Tirkos et al., 2006; Wilke et al., 2011). Moreover, airways of newborn CF pigs demonstrate developmental defects, such as cartilage abnormalities, muscle bundles, and smaller airways, which may support progression into a CF lung disease (Chen et al., 2010; Stoltz et al., 2010; Klymiuk et al., 2012). Considerable insight into epithelial ion transport and its defect in CF, was also obtained in studies with wt and transgenic mice, although mouse airways show differences in structure, distribution of submucosal glands and contribution of CFTR to Cl^- transport. While identical ion channels and transporters are expressed in human and mouse airway, intestinal epithelium, and other epithelial organs, the course of lung disease is mild in CF mice and airway plugging is not observed (Wilke et al., 2011). Nevertheless, because of the available broad range of tools in mouse genetics, valuable insights into organ physiology and pathological changes in CF have been gained in the different mouse CF models.

IS ABNORMAL ION TRANSPORT RELEVANT IN CF OR ONLY AN EPIPHENOMENON?

Others argue that airway inflammation is second to the transport defect and to bacterial colonization (Ribeiro et al., 2005). At any rate, the most impressive clinical symptom in CF lung disease is accumulation of large amounts of airway mucus. Yet, are low pH, Na^+ hyperabsorption, or lack of Cl^- secretion are truly the cause for mucus plugging and obstruction of airways? If we compare the changes in absorptive and secretory ion transport present in ßENaC-overexpressing mice (Mall et al., 2004), with the changes in ion transport in kcne3 knockout mice (Preston et al., 2010), or mice lacking TMEM16A in ciliated epithelial cells (Benedetto et al., 2017), the contribution of ion transport appears less clear. In the three mouse models we find a shift toward enhanced net absorptive transport: (i) pronounced increase in Na^+ absorption with unchanged Cl^- secretion (Mall et al., 2004), (ii) milder increase in Na^+ absorption but strongly reduced Cl^- secretion (Preston et al., 2010), (iii) partial reduction in Na^+ absorption but pronounced inhibition of Cl^- secretion (Benedetto et al., 2017) (**Table 1**). Only the ßENaC mice develop a CF like lung phenotype, which may suggest that indeed Na^+ absorption by ENaC is rate limiting and determines the direction of net flux of ions and water through an otherwise relatively leaky airway epithelium (Cotton et al., 1983; Donaldson and Boucher, 2007). This may explains why loss of Cl^- secretion in the airways of adult *kcne3* and *tmem16A* knockout mice does not lead to a CF like lung phenotype.

As discussed below, basal airway mucus secretion is attenuated in mice lacking TMEM16A in ciliated epithelial cells. This leads to mucus accumulation in secretory epithelial cells (Benedetto et al., 2019) (**Figure 1**). The mechanism of crosstalk between the two cell types is currently unclear. However, it is likely that ciliated cells secrete a factor that is required to release mucus from club cells. This factor could be ATP, which is found in the airway surface liquid, and which is assumed to control basal mucus secretion. Evidence has been presented that TMEM16A supports vesicular/granular exocytosis and subsequent insertion of transmembrane proteins into the plasma membrane. Moreover, it was also shown to control paracrine release of inflammatory mediators (Benedetto et al., 2016, 2017, 2019; Cabrita et al., 2017). We would favor a pathogenic mechanism that initiates the disease by intrinsic inflammation caused by dyslocalization/dysfunction of CFTR, and in the absence of bacterial infection. Intrinsic inflammation is followed by upregulation of TMEM16A, particularly in mucus producing cells, with consecutive mucus hyperproduction/hypersecretion. Accordingly, inflammation and mucus hyperproduction/hypersecretion should be pharmacologically targeted. Along this line it appears noteworthy that treatment with the anti-inflammatory drug ibuprofen was able to rescue trafficking mutant F508del-CFTR (Carlile et al., 2015).

CORRECTING AND POTENTIATING CFTR

Pharmacological restoration of defective CFTR chloride transport has been the primary goal over the past decade and has led to considerable success in correcting the gating mutant G551D-CFTR by the potentiator compound VX-770 (ivacaftor, kalydeco) (Van Goor et al., 2009; Accurso et al., 2010). G551D accounts for only a small fraction (about 5%) of all CF cases (De Boeck et al., 2014). Thus, US-based Vertex developed the small molecule CFTR-corrector VX-809 (lumacaftor), a compound that is able to rescue a fraction of the class two mutant F508del-CFTR *in vitro* (Van Goor et al., 2011; Pranke et al., 2017). Large phase 3 studies demonstrated a moderate improvement in the percentage of predicted FEV1 between 2.6 and 4.0% (Wainwright et al., 2015). Studies with next generation compounds, e.g., VX-661 (Tezacaftor), reported improvement in FEV1 in the range of 7% (Rowe et al., 2017; Taylor-Cousar et al., 2017; Donaldson et al., 2018). Recent clinical trials reported great therapeutic success with triple combinations of the corrector VX661 with VX-445 or VX-659, together with the potentiator VX-770. The combinations increased the percentage of predicted FEV1 by more than 10% (Davies et al., 2018; Keating et al., 2018). Despite such great success in correcting mutant CFTR, critical voices were raised regarding a combinatorial drug treatment. For example, adverse effects of VX-770 were reported on VX-809-corrected F508del-CFTR in the combinatorial preparation Orkambi. Moreover, long-term effects of these drugs on CFTR expression could be negative (Cholon et al., 2014; Veit et al., 2014; Chin et al., 2018). Finally, the costs for treatment by these drugs are often prohibitive (Ferkol and Quinton, 2015). Thus, there is a need for alternative drug treatments.

A number of other strategies to correct biosynthesis of misfolded CFTR are currently under investigation Recent screening efforts identified the translation initiation factor 3a (eIF3a) as a potentially druggable central hub for the biogenesis of CFTR (Hutt et al., 2018). FDA-approved histone deacetylase (HDAC) inhibitors such as panobinostat (LBH-589) and romidepsin (FK-228) can help to correct misfolded CFTR, particularly in combination with other correctors such as VX809 (Angles et al., 2018). Promising results were also obtained with combinations of pharmacological chaperones with different sites of action, such as VX-809, RDR1, and MCG1516A (Carlile et al., 2018). All these recent results are rather encouraging, however, as not every CFTR mutation is accessible to such a CFTR-based therapy, activation of other airway epithelial Cl^- channels was proposed to compensate for defective CFTR (De Boeck and Amaral, 2016).

TABLE 1 | Ion transport assessed by the measurement of short circuit currents in different adult mouse models [wild type (wt) littermates vs. transgenic (trans) mice].

Mouse model	Amiloride-sensitive I_{SC} ($\mu A/cm^2$)			cAMP-activated I_{SC}			Ca^{2+}-activated I_{SC}			Phenotype
	wt	trans	%↓↑	wt	trans	%↓↑	wt	trans	%↓↑	
ßENaC overexpressing mouse (Mall et al., 2004)	22	59	↑168	25	27	↑11	79	84	↑6	CF-like lung disease
Kcne3-knockout mouse (Preston et al., 2010)	48	84	↑ 75	83	17	↓80	294	50	↓83	No lung phenotype
FOXJ1-Cre-TMEM16Aflox/flox mice (Benedetto et al., 2017)	104	49	↓ 47	99	58	↓42	176	74	↓58	No lung phenotype

Shown are approximate I_{SC} values. %↓↑, percent decrease or increase in unidirectional ion transport.

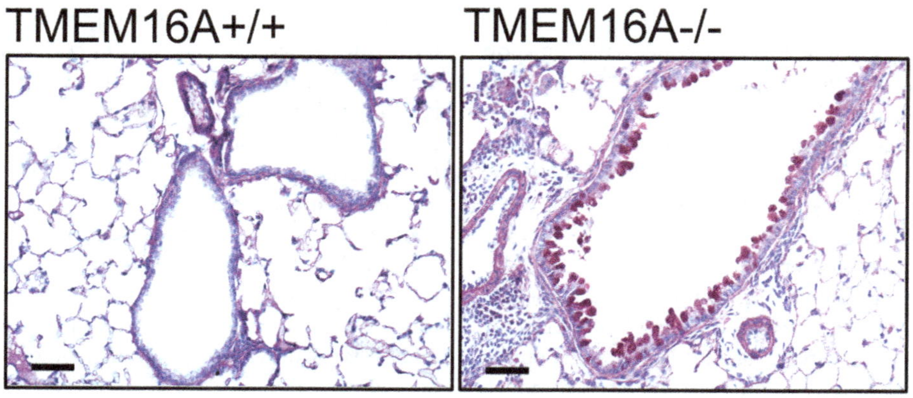

FIGURE 1 | Accumulation of mucus in airways of TMEM16A$^{-/-}$ mice. Mucus staining (PAS) in bronchi of wild type littermates (TMEM16Aflox/flox; TMEM16A$^{+/+}$) and mice with an airway epithelial-specific knockout of TMEM16A (FOXJ1-Cre-TMEM16Aflox/flox; TMEM16A$^{-/-}$). Strong accumulation of mucus in airway epithelial cells is observed in TMEM16A$^{-/-}$ mice. Bars indicate 20 µm (Benedetto et al., 2019).

AIRWAY CHLORIDE CHANNELS: SLC26A9

Apart from CFTR, there are two other major Cl^- channels present in human and mouse airways, namely SLC26A9 and TMEM16A. How much both Cl^- channels quantitatively contribute to production of the ASL and support mucociliary clearance is currently not known (**Figure 2**). SLC26 proteins typically operate as anion exchangers, but for SLC26A9 it was shown to function as a Cl^- channel (Mount and Romero, 2004; Ousingsawat et al., 2011b; Bertrand et al., 2017). In contrast to CFTR, SLC26A9 is spontaneously active, once inserted into the apical membrane of airway epithelial cells. However, it is also regulated by Cl^- feedback/WNK kinases and surprisingly is controlled by the Cl^- channel CFTR (Dorwart et al., 2007; Bertrand et al., 2009). SLC26A9 is likely to provide the basal Cl^- conductance that is found in airways in the absence of any secretagogue (Bertrand et al., 2017). Absence of basal Cl^- secretion in airways of CF patients carrying the type II mutation F508del-CFTR (De Boeck and Amaral, 2016), is probably due to the lack of expression of SLC26A9 in the apical membrane (**Figure 2B**) (El Khouri and Toure, 2014; Bertrand et al., 2017). SLC26A9 and CFTR form a complex with the help of PDZ scaffold proteins such as NHERF1 (**Figure 3**). When coexpressed with wtCFTR, SLC26A9 is co-trafficked together with CFTR from the ER to the plasma membrane. However, if coexpressed with F508del-CFTR, SLC26A9 will remain intracellularly and will be degraded (Bertrand et al., 2017). As shown recently, also CFTR and TMEM16A do interact via PDZ-domain proteins, and TMEM16A has an impact on plasma membrane expression of CFTR (Benedetto et al., 2017).

Furthermore, SLC26A9 may be regulated by the R domain of CFTR through STAS domain interaction (Chang et al., 2009). Indeed, SLC26A9 has been demonstrated to be a genetic modifier in CF (Sun et al., 2012; Miller et al., 2015), and the CFTR corrector VX-809 partially rescued SLC26A9, probably by facilitating trafficking of F508del-CFTR to the plasma membrane (Strug et al., 2016). Similar to TMEM16A, SLC26A9 is upregulated during airway inflammation and exposure of the airway cells to IL-13 (Anagnostopoulou et al., 2012). It will be interesting to learn more about the regulation of SLC26A9 expression, and whether SLC26A9 is upregulated in CF airways in ciliated or in mucus secreting cells. Taken together, SLC26A9 could potentially serve as an alternative Cl^- channel in CF, but compromised biosynthesis of CFTR carrying type two mutations need to be corrected. Identifying small molecules that would interfere with the formation of the F508del-CFTR/SLC26A9 complex could be an interesting therapeutic option in CF.

AIRWAY CHLORIDE CHANNELS: TMEM16A

TMEM16A is a Ca^{2+} activated Cl^- channel (CaCC) that belongs to a larger family of 10 paralogous proteins (TMEM16A-K), also

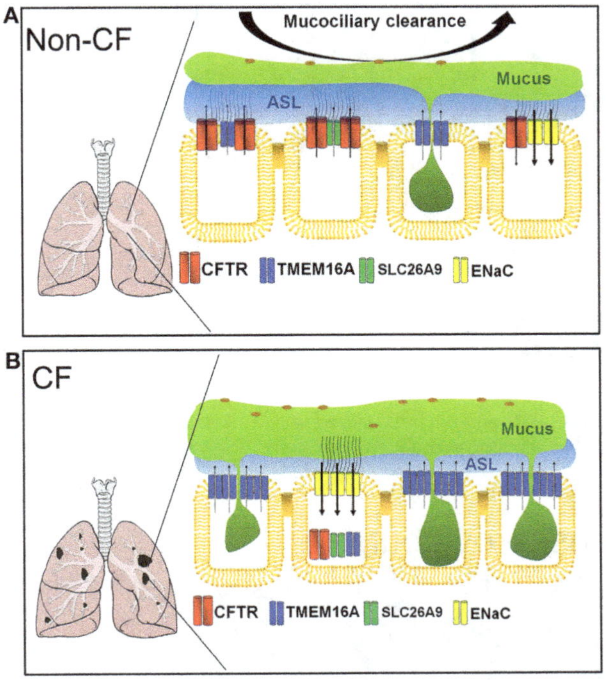

FIGURE 2 | Ion channels contributing to fluid/mucus balance in non-CF and CF airways. **(A)** In non-CF airways, CFTR is expressed in ciliated epithelial cells and ionocytes (not shown). Ca^{2+} activated Cl^- channels are sparsely expressed in both ciliated and secretory club and goblet cells. SLC26A9, TMEM16A and CFTR located in ciliated epithelial cells and probably in ionocytes are in charge of fluid secretion, while TMEM16A expressed in secretory club/goblet cells support mucus secretion. Epithelial Na^+ channels reabsorb Na^+ thereby causing fluid absorption. **(B)** In inflamed CF airways, CFTR is dysfunctional and often dislocated intracellularly together with SLC26A9 and TMEM16A in ciliated epithelial cells. TMEM16A is upregulated in secretory cells strongly contributing to mucus secretion. Na^+ absorption by ENaC is augmented. Inflammation and transport abnormalities lead to excessive mucus production/secretion, airway plugging, and reduced water secretion, strongly reducing mucociliary clearance.

called anoctamins (ANO1-ANO10) (Kunzelmann et al., 2011; Pedemonte and Galietta, 2014). The majority of these double-barreled channels are operating as phospholipid scramblases, i.e., they transport phospholipids from one site of the bilayer membrane to the other, once activated by a strong increase in intracellular Ca^{2+} (Suzuki et al., 2010). TMEM16A and B are solely CaCCs, whose structure and gating has been largely uncovered in cryo-EM studies (Paulino et al., 2017a,b). TMEM16A is typically localized in the apical plasma membrane of epithelial cells. However, it is also found to be expressed basolateral and in intracellular compartments (Schreiber et al., 2010, 2014). TMEM16F is a phospholipid scramblase that also conducts Cl^- and other ions (Yang et al., 2012; Grubb et al., 2013; Shimizu et al., 2013; Kunzelmann et al., 2014; Ousingsawat et al., 2015; Scudieri et al., 2015; Drumm et al., 2017; Schreiber et al., 2018). Although endogenous TMEM16 proteins are mostly localized intracellularly, overexpression of these proteins together with purinergic receptors allows partial trafficking to the plasma membrane (Tian et al., 2012a). TMEM16A is clearly the epithelial airway CaCC (Benedetto et al., 2017), but a number of other TMEM16 paralogues are also coexpressed in mouse airways and in human large and small bronchi, bronchiole and alveoli, such as TMEM16C, F, J (Kunzelmann et al., 2012). Particularly TMEM16F may participate as well in epithelial Cl^- transport.

UPREGULATION OF TMEM16A DURING INFLAMMATORY LUNG DISEASE: GOOD OR BAD?

TMEM16A is strongly upregulated during inflammation, a fact that was utilized to identify the molecular nature of CaCC (Galietta et al., 2002; Caputo et al., 2008). TMEM16A is strongly upregulated in CF and asthma, which parallels goblet cell metaplasia and mucus hypersecretion (Huang et al., 2012; Kondo et al., 2017), and is also upregulated by bacterial components (Caci et al., 2015). Upregulation of TMEM16A is predominant in mucus producing cells and to a much lesser degree in ciliated epithelial cells (Huang et al., 2012; Scudieri et al., 2012). Expression of TMEM16A is almost undetectable by immunocytochemistry in normal adult human and mouse airways; although CaCC is clearly present (Huang et al., 2009, 2012; Benedetto et al., 2017). While this may be explained by the limited sensitivity of the available antibodies, it also raises questions as to what degree other members of the TMEM16 family might participate in CaCC. As mentioned above, TMEM16C, F, and J are also expressed in mouse airway epithelium (Kunzelmann et al., 2012). On the other hand, knockout of TMEM16A completely abolished CaCC activated by purinergic stimulation (Benedetto et al., 2017). We will discuss below that TMEM16A has a strong impact on intracellular Ca^{2+} signals triggered by stimulation of G-protein coupled receptors (GPCRs), which then activate phospholipase C, increase inositol trisphosphate and intracellular Ca^{2+} (Kunzelmann et al., 2016)

As mentioned above, expression of TMEM16A in normal adult airways is hardly detectable by immunohistochemistry (Ousingsawat et al., 2009; Benedetto et al., 2017) (**Figure 4**). However, induction of airway inflammation in an ovalbumin asthma model induced a pronounced upregulation of TMEM16A in mucus producing club/goblet cells, but induced little expression in ciliated epithelial cells (Benedetto et al., 2019) (**Figure 4**). Ciliated epithelial cells, and particularly the recently identified ionocytes express CFTR and are in charge of fluid secretion (Montoro et al., 2018; Plasschaert et al., 2018). Expression of TMEM16A is low in ciliated cells when compared to mucus producing club and goblet cells. The contribution of TMEM16A to overall fluid secretion by the airway epithelium might therefore be limited, while it plays a central role for basal mucus secretion (Benedetto et al., 2019). This will be further outlined below.

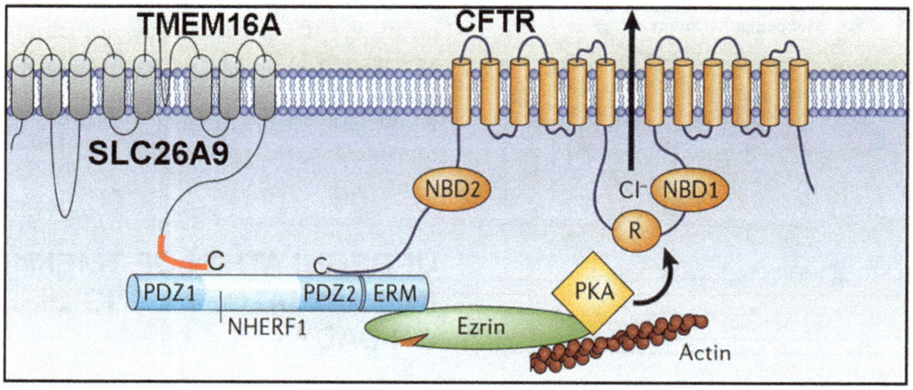

FIGURE 3 | Molecular and functional relationship of CFTR, SLC26A9 and TMEM16A. Both SLC26A9 and TMEM16A interact with CFTR via their C-terminal PDZ (PSD-95/Discs-large/ZO1) -binding domains with the help of the PDZ-protein NHERF1 (Na^+/H^+ exchanger regulatory factor 1).

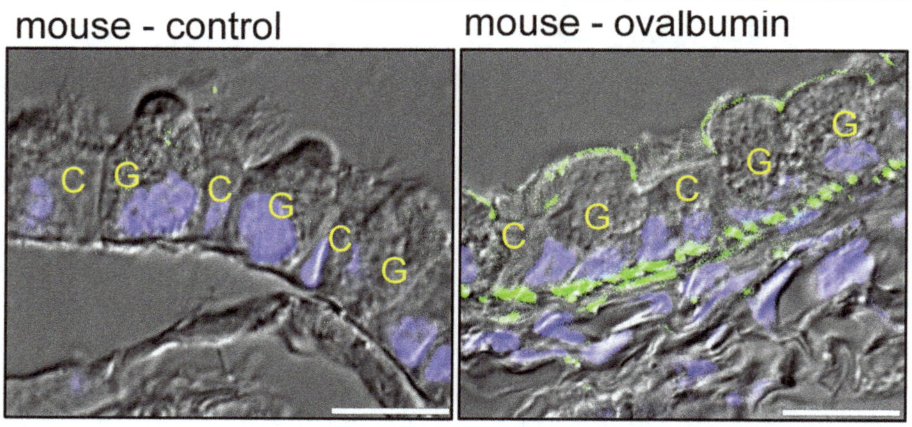

FIGURE 4 | Predominant expression of TMEM16A in mucus producing cells. Distal airways of a control mouse and an ovalbumin-sensitized (asthmatic) mouse. Expression of TMEM16A (green fluorescence) is hardly detectable in control airways, but is clearly detectable in mucus producing club/goblet cells (G) of asthmatic mice with inflamed airways. Little expression of TMEM16A is found in ciliated epithelial cells (C). Blue, DAPI staining of nuclei. Bars indicate 20 μm (Benedetto et al., 2019).

F508DEL-CFTR ATTENUATES EXPRESSION OF TMEM16A IN THE APICAL MEMBRANE

A functional coupling between TMEM16A and CFTR has been described in a number of previous publications (Kunzelmann et al., 1997; Wei et al., 1999; Ousingsawat et al., 2011a). Subsequent studies reported attenuated expression of TMEM16A in the apical membrane of airway epithelial cells by coexpressed F508del-CFTR (Ruffin et al., 2013; Benedetto et al., 2017). We demonstrated that TMEM16A and CFTR directly interact through PSD-95/Dlg/ZO-1 (PDZ) domain proteins, similar to SLC26A9 (**Figure 3**). The functional interaction between TMEM16A and CFTR is also demonstrated by a crosstalk of intracellular Ca^{2+} and cAMP-dependent signaling. This compartmentalized crosstalk is facilitated by exchange protein directly activated by cAMP (EPAC1) and Ca^{2+} -sensitive adenylate cyclase type 1 (ADCY1). Assembly of such a local signalosome was shown to depend on the number of phospholipase C coupled GPCRs (Lerias et al., 2018).

These studies suggest a significant overlap of cAMP- and Ca^{2+} activated Cl^- currents. Along this line, our early studies also showed that epithelial cAMP-dependent and Ca^{2+}-activated Cl^- currents cannot be easily separated based on apparently specific ion channel inhibitors (Kunzelmann et al., 1992; Benedetto et al., 2017; Lerias et al., 2018). Moreover, in both airway and intestinal epithelium, most of the Ca^{2+} activated Cl^- secretion is in fact through CFTR and not through TMEM16A Cl^- channels (Mall et al., 1998b; Namkung et al., 2010a; Billet and Hanrahan, 2013; Benedetto et al., 2017). The actual purinergic (ATP-activated) Cl^- secretion via TMEM16A is very transient, as TMEM16A deactivates quickly within 1–5 min after activation by ATP when examined in *Xenopus* oocytes (Faria et al., 2009), HEK293 cells (Tian et al., 2012b), mouse trachea (Kunzelmann et al., 2002), and human airways (Mall et al.,

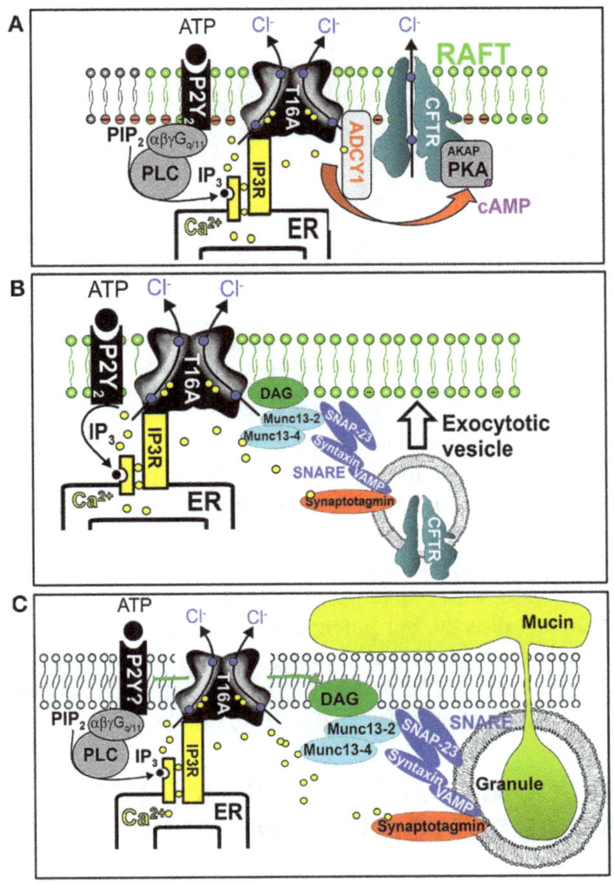

FIGURE 5 | Impact of TMEM16A on intracellular Ca^{2+}, exocytosis, and mucus secretion. **(A)** TMEM16A is colocalized with purinergic P2Y receptors and CFTR within the apical membrane. Stimulation of purinergic receptors leads to endoplasmic reticulum (ER) Ca^{2+} store release through IP3 receptors (IP3R). Ca^{2+} not only activates TMEM16A (T16A) but also stimulates adenylate cyclase type 1 (ADCY1) to produce cAMP and to activate CFTR via protein kinase A (PKA). TMEM16A binds to IP3 receptors and tethers the ER to the apical membrane, thereby facilitating effective compartmentalized Ca^{2+} signaling. **(B)** Effective apical Ca^{2+} signaling by TMEM16A leads to activation of the exocytic SNARE machinery insertion and improved expression of CFTR in the apical plasma membrane. **(C)** Effective apical Ca^{2+} signaling by TMEM16A leads to fusion of mucus containing granules, exocytosis, and release of mucus.

2003). Analysis of freshly isolated human nasal epithelial cells demonstrates ATP-induced steady-state secretion only in non-CF cells, but not in CF nasal cells. Thus, the direct contribution of TMEM16A to the epithelial secretory Cl^- transport is small. However, the non-transient steady component of purinergic Cl^- secretion that is produced by CFTR is essential for fluid secretion (Mall et al., 2003; Benedetto et al., 2017). The traffic mutant F508del is by far the most common mutation in CF that also compromises biosynthesis of TMEM16A. Therefore, the pro-secretory function of TMEM16A in CF is probably limited, and inhibition of TMEM16A may not much reduce Cl^- secretion in CF (Ruffin et al., 2013; Benedetto et al., 2017).

UPREGULATION OF TMEM16A IN AIRWAY SMOOTH MUSCLES

Upon induction of asthma, we also observed an upregulation of TMEM16A in mouse airway smooth muscle (ASM) cells (Benedetto et al., 2017; Miner et al., 2019) (**Figure 4**). This has already been described in a number of previous studies (Huang et al., 2009, 2012; Gallos et al., 2013; Danielsson et al., 2015). Inhibitors of TMEM16A were shown to induce hyperpolarization of ASM and airway relaxation (Yim et al., 2013; Danielsson et al., 2017; Miner et al., 2019). Airway inflammation is well-known to induce hyperresponsiveness of ASM (Brightling et al., 2002; Galli et al., 2008). Inflammatory mediators binding to GPCRs activate TMEM16A channels; depolarize the membrane voltage and cause airway contraction, a process that is upregulated in asthma (Wang et al., 2018). Expression of TMEM16A is not only upregulated in allergic asthma, but also in airway epithelial cells and probably ASM of CF patients (Caci et al., 2015). Moreover, the signaling cascade comprising GPCR - TMEM16A - intracellular Ca^{2+} is further augmented by inflammatory mediators and cholinergic stimuli.

TMEM16A CONTROLS Ca^{2+} SIGNALS, MEMBRANE EXOCYTOSIS AND MUCUS SECRETION

As pointed out above, membrane expression and activity of CFTR strongly relies on TMEM16A (Benedetto et al., 2017; Lerias et al., 2018). We showed that augmentation of apical Ca^{2+} signals in the presence of TMEM16A activates adenylate cyclase type 1, enhances local cAMP levels and boosts CFTR activity (**Figure 5A**). The enhanced plasma membrane expression of CFTR in the presence of TMEM16A may be caused by enhanced Ca^{2+} levels in the apical submembranous compartment, which triggers the exocytic machinery and membrane insertion of CFTR in ciliated epithelial cells and possibly ionocytes (Benedetto et al., 2017) (**Figure 5B**). A similar exocytic mechanism may apply to the process of mucus secretion by club and goblet cells. We found that ATP-induced mucus secretion by secretory cells is strongly compromised in the absence of TMEM16A. Without TMEM16A, intracellular Ca^{2+} concentrations in the apical pole of club and goblet cells are attenuated. These Ca^{2+} ions are required for basal and acute ATP-activated mucus release (Benedetto et al., 2019) (**Figure 5C**). ATP-dependent mucus secretion is characterized by Ca^{2+} dependent single granule docking to the apical membrane which requires Munc13 proteins and the SNARE (soluble N-ethylmaleimide–sensitive factor attachment protein receptor) machinery (Fahy and Dickey, 2010). Taken together, in healthy non-CF airways TMEM16A may support CFTR-driven fluid secretion in ciliated cells and possibly ionocytes, and supports basal mucus release by club and goblet cells. In inflammatory CF airway disease, the function of TMEM16A may be marginal in ciliated cells and ionocytes, but may be pronounced in secretory cells due to strong upregulation of expression.

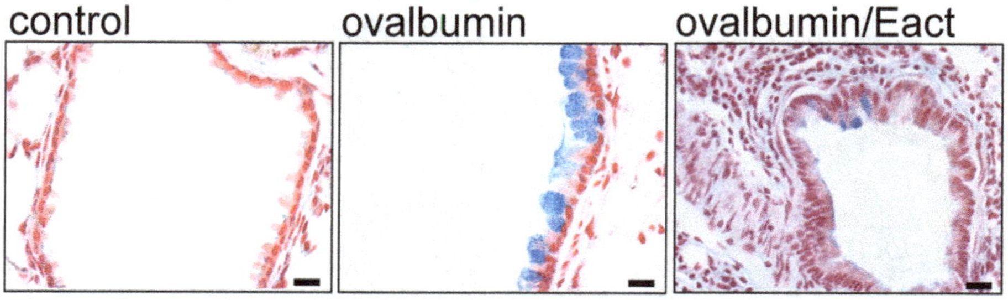

FIGURE 6 | Activation of TMEM16A leads to mucus release and airway contraction. Control mouse airways show very little mucus (alcian blue). In contrast, airways from ovalbumin-sensitized mice show pronounced mucus accumulation. Acute exposure of an ovalbumin-sensitized mouse to the known activator of TMEM16A, Eact (4.8 μg, tracheal instillation), induced a rapid mucus release and airway contraction (Benedetto et al., 2019). Bars indicate 20 μm.

According to this, pharmacological activation of TMEM16A in CF and asthma patients could have adverse effects on lung function due to its prosecretory effect on mucus release. Correspondingly, we found in OVA-sensitized asthmatic mice that activation of TMEM16A by the compound Eact (Namkung et al., 2011b) induced massive mucus release and a considerable expiratory stridor, suggesting airway contraction. Airway narrowing was confirmed by analysis of the airway cross section (Benedetto et al., 2019) (**Figure 6**). It may be argued that Eact raises intracellular Ca^{2+} and therefore induces adverse effects independent of TMEM16A. However, increase in intracellular Ca^{2+} by Eact is expected. As outlined below, activation of TMEM16A is known to increase intracellular Ca^{2+} (Cabrita et al., 2017). Activation of TMEM16A by Eact depolarizes the membrane voltage, which leads to an increase in intracellular Ca^{2+}. Notably, increase in intracellular Ca^{2+} by Eact was inhibited by 1 μM of the TMEM16A blocker niclosamide (Benedetto et al., 2019).

INHIBITORS AND ACTIVATORS OF TMEM16A

Meanwhile a larger number of inhibitors of TMEM16A has been identified, but there is only one published group of N-aroylaminothiazole "activators" (Eact) (Namkung et al., 2011b), apart from some herbal compounds like Ginsenoside Rb1 and Resveratrol, which apparently activate TMEM16A in a Ca^{2+} independent manner (Chai et al., 2017; Guo et al., 2017) (**Table 2**). Enterprise therapeutics (Sussex, UK; http://www.enterprisetherapeutics.com/) is currently working on potentiators of TMEM16A, but details on potentiating molecules are not yet available. Silurian pharmaceuticals (Oakland, US; http://www.silurianpharma.com/index.php) reported brevenal to activate Ca^{2+} activated Cl^- channels, possibly in a Ca^{2+} independent fashion. Denufusol was developed by Inspire pharmaceuticals (later taken over by Merck). Denufosol is a deoxycytidine-uridine dinucleotide with enhanced metabolic stability, to activate purinergic P2Y2 receptors which stimulate TMEM16A (Yerxa et al., 2002) and inhibit ENaC (Kunzelmann et al., 2002) (c.f. below). An interesting group of lipids was identified originally to uncouple GPCR-mediated Ca^{2+} increase from inactivation/desensitization of Ca^{2+} activated Cl^- channels. These D-myo-inositol 3,4,5,6-tetrakisphosphate [Ins(3,4,5,6)P4] (Vajanaphanich et al., 1994) were synthetically modified to result in the membrane permeable analog INO4995, which was shown to inhibit ENaC (Moody et al., 2005) and to activate TMEM16A (Tian et al., 2012b). INO4995 did not increase intracellular Ca^{2+}. It activated overexpressed TMEM16A directly, but potentiated ATP-dependent activation of TMEM16A expressed endogenously. Preliminary data suggested enhanced membrane localization of TMEM16A induced by INO4995 (Tian et al., 2012b) (**Table 3**).

BIOLOGICAL EFFECTS OF INHIBITORS AND ACTIVATORS OF TMEM16A

TMEM16A is broadly expressed in many epithelial and non-epithelial tissues. It is therefore expected that inhibition or activation of TMEM16A through systemic drug application might have a number of side effects. Apart from inhibiting mucus production and mucus secretion, TMEM16A-inhibitors will induce bronchorelaxation by blocking TMEM16A in airway smooth muscle (Huang et al., 2012; Gallos et al., 2013; Zhang et al., 2013; Danielsson et al., 2015; Wang et al., 2018; Miner et al., 2019). Another desired lung-specific effect of TMEM16A-inhibitors is the inhibition of release of inflammatory mediators (Knight, 2004; Danielsson et al., 2017; Benedetto et al., 2019).

Some inhibitors of TMEM16A have additional beneficial effects, such as protection from reactive oxygen species (idebenone, Villalba et al., 2010), and general inhibition of inflammation (Knight, 2004; Schreiber et al., 2018). Many studies demonstrate inhibition of proliferation and anti-cancer effects by blocking TMEM16A (Wanitchakool et al., 2014; Wang et al., 2017). General anti-hypertensive effects are likely (Namkung et al., 2010b; Heinze et al., 2014), as well as inhibition of nociception, itching, and heat perception (Cho et al., 2012; Lee et al., 2014; Pusch and Zifarelli, 2014; Deba and Bessac, 2015). Inhibition of saliva production and dry mouth may occur mediation with TMEM16A-inhibitors (Ousingsawat et al., 2009; Catalan et al., 2015). Inhibition of TMEM16A may also attenuate intestinal contraction and abdominal peristalsis (Sanders et al., 2012; Singh et al., 2014), and therefore could have antidiarrheal effects (Tradtrantip et al., 2010; Namkung et al., 2011b; Jiang et al., 2016). Finally, inhibition of renal TMEM16A could

TABLE 2 | Inhibitors of TMEM16A.

Inhibitor	IC50 (μM)	Structural formula	References
10bm	0.03	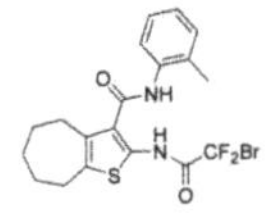	Truong et al., 2017
Monna	0.08	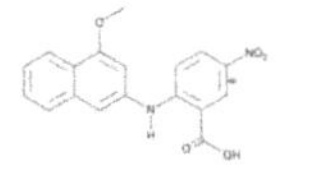	Oh et al., 2013
Niclosamide	0.7	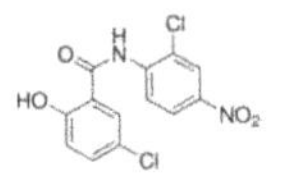	Miner et al., 2019
Ani9	0.1	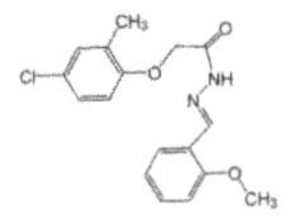	Seo et al., 2016
Tannic acid	0.323	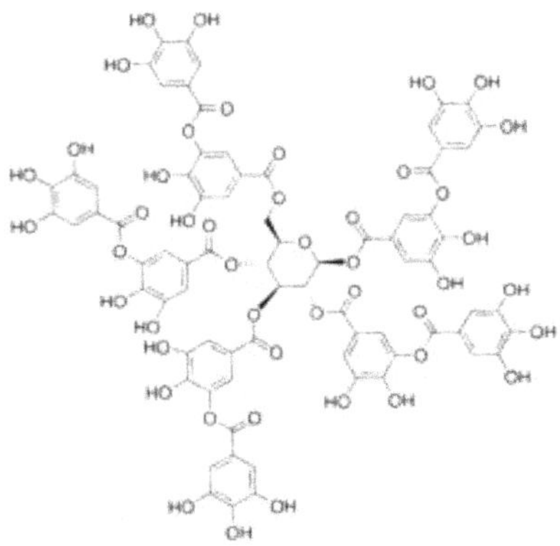	Namkung et al., 2010b
T16A-A01	1.1	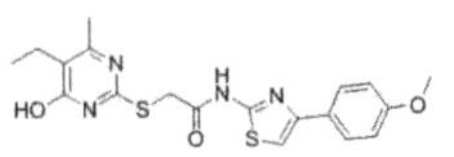	Namkung et al., 2011a; Fedigan et al., 2017
Dichlorophen	5.49	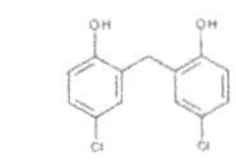	Huang et al., 2012
Idebenone	5.52	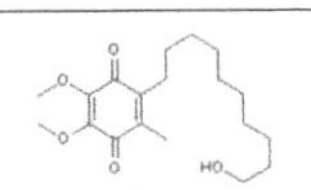	Seo et al., 2015
Shikonin	6.5	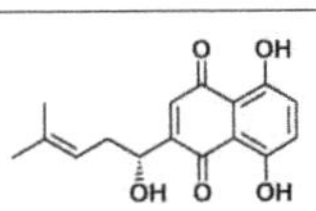	Jiang et al., 2016
Benzbromarone	9.97	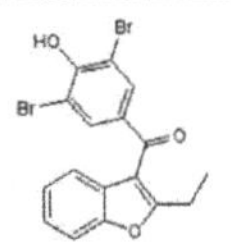	Huang et al., 2012
CaCC-A01	10	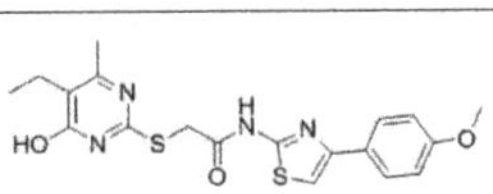	de La Fuente et al., 2007; Gianotti et al., 2016; Fedigan et al., 2017

(Continued)

TABLE 2 | Continued

Inhibitor	IC50 (μM)	Structural formula	References
9-Phenanthrol	12	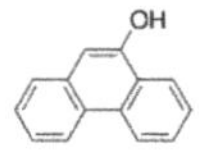	Burris et al., 2015)
Niflumic Acid	12	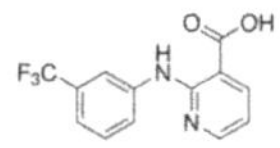	Hogg et al., 1994
Flufenamic acid	28	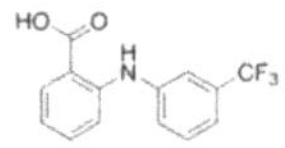	White and Aylwin, 1990
Talniflumate	–	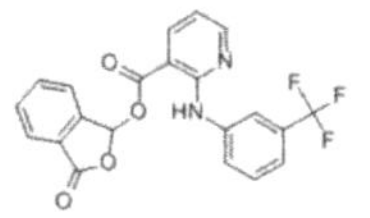	Walker et al., 2006
A9C	58	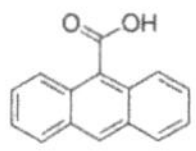	Baron et al., 1991
Dehydroandrographolide	20–30	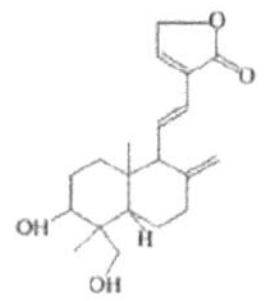	Sui et al., 2015
DIDS	10–100	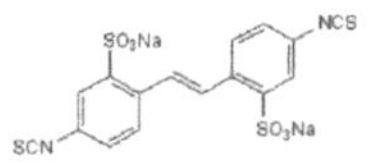	Kubitz et al., 1992
NPPB	15–150	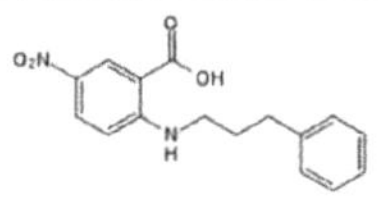	Kubitz et al., 1992; Yang et al., 2008
Rice bran extract			Sharm et al., 2017
Matrine	28 μM	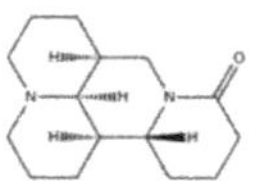	Guo et al., 2018
(Ani9 derivative) 5f	22 nM	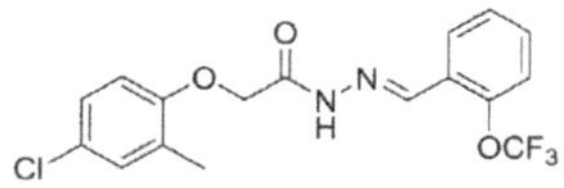	Seo et al., 2018

potentially lead to proteinuria and acidosis (Faria et al., 2014; Schenk et al., 2018). For activators of TMEM16A, opposite effects are possible, which is why local application via aerosol may be recommended for the treatment of CF lung disease. Nevertheless, oral application of a TMEM16A-blocker was shown to increase survival of CFTR-knockout mice (Walker et al., 2006).

ACTIVATING OR INHIBITING TMEM16A?

Under physiological conditions, airway mucus represents an innate defense mechanism against pathogens. It traps inhaled pathogens and particles and is part of the mucociliary clearance (Knowles and Boucher, 2002). However, mucus becomes a serious problem when hypersecreted in inflammatory lung diseases, such as asthma, COPD, and CF (Dunican et al., 2018). Despite many pathological findings and pathogenic mechanisms proposed for CF lung disease (c.f. above), the single most prominent finding is the excessive overproduction of highly viscous mucus with adhesive and cohesive properties in CF patients (Button et al., 2018). It causes airway obstruction and a reduced mucociliary clearance, and it thereby drives chronic inflammatory lung disease (Fahy and Dickey, 2010). Thus, inhibition of mucus production/secretion is likely to be the most

TABLE 3 | Activators of TMEM16A.

Activator	IC50 (μM)	Structural formula	References
Brevenal	–	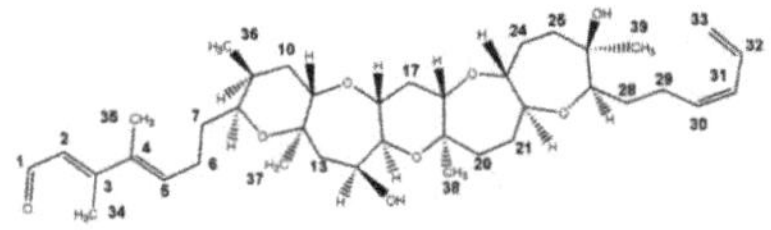	http://www.silurianpharma.com/index.php
Eact	3	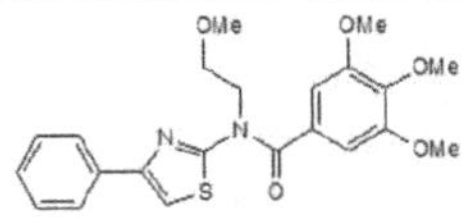	Namkung et al., 2011b
INO-4995	5	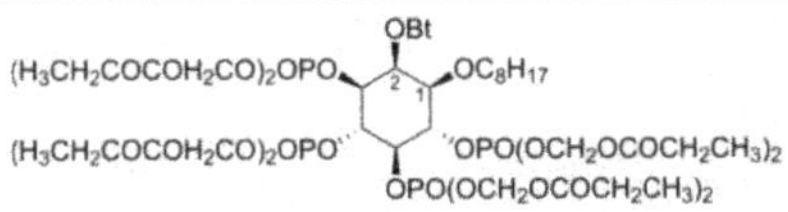	Tian et al., 2012b
Denufosol	10	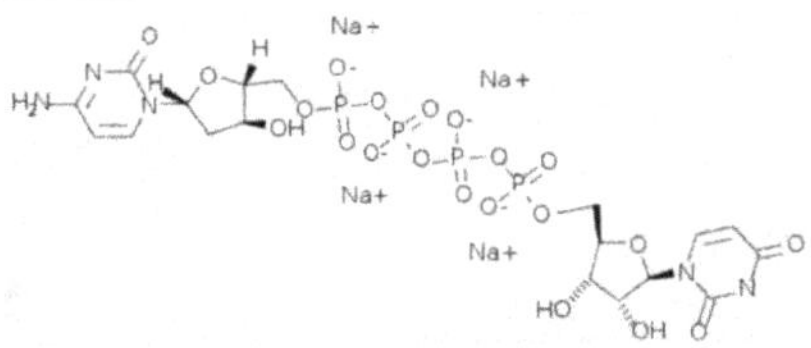	Yerxa et al., 2002
Cinnamaldehyde	10	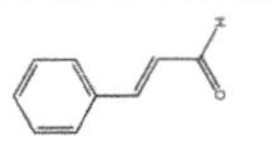	Huang et al., 2018
Ginsenoside Rb1	38.4	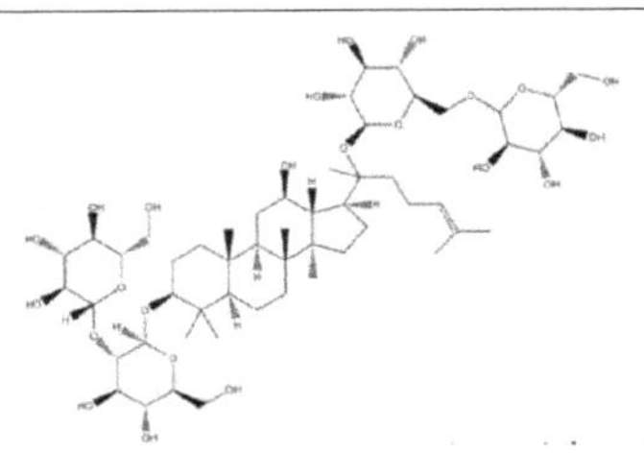	Guo et al., 2017
Resveratrol	47.9	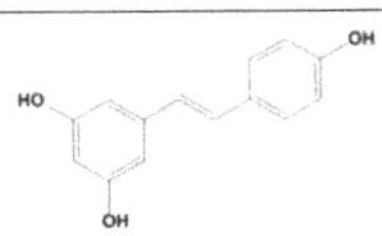	Chai et al., 2017
A9C	100–1000	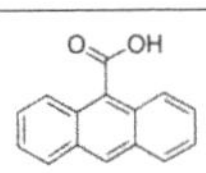	Ta et al., 2016

effective treatment of CF lung disease, normalizing the imbalance between excessive mucus secretion and reduced ASL (**Figure 7**). Our recent data show that TMEM16A and other TMEM16 proteins are essential for mucus production and basal secretion of mucus in airways and intestine (Benedetto et al., 2019). These findings open up a new avenue for the therapy of inflammatory airway diseases, and particularly for the treatment of airway mucus plugging and CF lung disease.

In contrast, activation of TMEM16A in CF to facilitate fluid secretion may be rather ineffective due to the reasons outlined above (**Figure 7A**). An earlier clinical trial was performed using stabilized dinucleotides (Denufosol) to induce purinergic Ca^{2+} dependent Cl^- secretion and to restore ASL with the goal of improving lung function in CF. However, the clinical trial failed to demonstrate any benefit of denufosol (Ratjen et al., 2012; Moss, 2013). As an adverse effect, the aerosol induced cough in 52% of all patients. It may be speculated that denufosol may have induced additional mucus secretion and even additional airway obstruction. Being strongly upregulated in inflammatory airway disease in secretory cells and in ASM, activation of TMEM16A could induce adverse effects by augmenting mucus secretion and bronchoconstriction (**Figure 7B**).

Inhibition of TMEM16A in CF may appear counterintuitive in the first place (assuming a potential inhibition of fluid secretion), however, the available data suggest otherwise. As outlined above, in CF TMEM16A membrane expression is

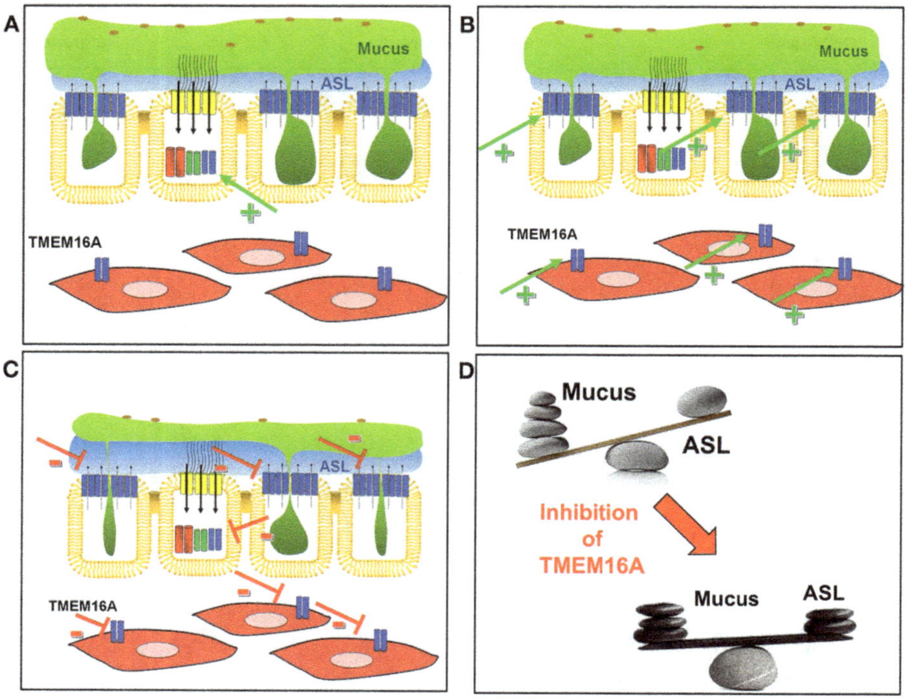

FIGURE 7 | Activation of inhibition of TMEM16A in airways of CF patients. **(A)** Activators of TMEM16A (green arrow, +) will find only few TMEM16A channels in the apical membrane of ciliated epithelial cells, which could enhance fluid secretion by ciliated epithelial cells. **(B)** In contrast, activators of TMEM16A will prominently activate TMEM16A strongly upregulated in mucus producing cells and airway smooth muscle cells during airway inflammation. This leads to hypersecretion of mucus along with airway contraction. **(C)** Inhibitors of TMEM16A will have an only limited (adverse) effect on TMEM16A channels expressed (fluid secreting) ciliated epithelial cells. In contrast, inhibition of TMEM16 channels in mucus producing cells and airway smooth muscle cells will inhibit mucus production/secretion and induce bronchodilation. **(D)** Inhibition of TMEM16 channels are likely to restore the balance between mucus and fluid in CF airways.

compromised (Ruffin et al., 2013; Benedetto et al., 2017), Cl^- secretion through CFTR is missing (Namkung et al., 2010a; Billet and Hanrahan, 2013; Benedetto et al., 2017; Lerias et al., 2018), and most TMEM16A is expressed in mucus secreting cells (Benedetto et al., 2019). Therefore, inhibition of TMEM16A may not substantially lower fluid secretion. In contrast, interfering with mucus and cytokine secretion by blocking upregulated TMEM16A is likely to improve mucociliary clearance and to improve lung function (**Figure 7C**). Along this line, talniflumate, the anti-inflammatory pro-drug of the common TMEM16A-inhibitor NFA that was originally developed by Argentinian Laboratorios Bago, increased survival of CF mice remarkably (Walker et al., 2006). Talniflumate had been further developed by the former company Genaera, as a mucoregulator for cystic fibrosis, chronic obstructive pulmonary disease, and asthma. Sadly, phase II trials have never been finished due to the shutdown of the company (Knight, 2004). In a large number of studies, mucus production, and secretion, as well as airway constriction were inhibited by niflumic acid and other inhibitors of TMEM16A (Kondo et al., 2012; Yim et al., 2013; Lin et al., 2015; Danielsson et al., 2017; Miner et al., 2019). The inhibitors niflumic acid, CaCCinhAO1, T16Ainh-A01, 17 benzbromarone, or niclosamide have been examined *in vivo* as well as *in vitro* in the low micromolecular range. Despite voltage dependence of TMEM16A-inhibition by NFA and other inhibitors, *in vivo* application to airway epithelial cells maintaining their intrinsic hyperpolarized membrane voltage demonstrated remarkable biological effects. Similar has been observed when TMEM16A inhibitors were applied to tracheal ring preparations *ex vivo*. Presumably TMEM16A is partially active in the airways, as low levels of ATP in the airway surface liquid maintain a basal activity of TMEM16A.

Because TMEM16A currents are blocked by niflumic acid, the published reports suggest that TMEM16A is in charge of both production and secretion of mucus. Niflumic acid, however, is a rather non-specific drug that inhibits a number of ion channels and blocks intracellular Ca^{2+} signals (Cabrita et al., 2017). Suppression of Ca^{2+} signals by niflumic acid is probably due to inhibition of TMEM16A. Other TMEM16A inhibitors such as CaCCinhAO1, T16Ainh-A01, benzbromarone, or niclosamide also inhibit intracellular Ca^{2+} and mucus release (de La Fuente et al., 2007; Kondo et al., 2017; Miner et al., 2019). It is important to note that other TMEM16 paralogues are also blocked by inhibitors of TMEM16A (Sirianant et al., 2015; Wanitchakool et al., 2016). Because several TMEM16 paralogues are expressed in airway epithelial cells, the possible contribution of other TMEM16 proteins to Ca^{2+} signaling and mucus production/secretion is currently unknown. Using different TMEM16 knockout mice and TMEM16 knockout cell lines, we found that most TMEM16 paralogues affect intracellular

Ca^{2+} signals (Kunzelmann et al., 2016; Cabrita et al., 2017). It is currently assumed that at least two TMEM16 members, TMEM16A and TMEM16F control mucus production and mucus secretion (Benedetto et al., 2019).

CONCLUSION

Despite significant progress in the development of CFTR–specific treatments for CF lung disease, it appears reasonable to search for alternative drug targets in CF. Potentiators and correctors of mutant CFTR show benefit in patients carrying the common F508del mutation. Improvement of lung function by the recent combinatorial drugs can be as high as 13%. Insight into mode of action of these compounds is still limited, and the costs for treatment may exclude some patients from therapy (Ferkol and Quinton, 2015). Moreover, a fraction of patients with particular CFTR mutations [type 1,5,6,7 mutations (De Boeck and Amaral, 2016)] will not respond to such a treatment.

Restoration of the mucus/liquid balance has been the driving force behind the search for novel openers of secretory Cl^- channels (SLC26A9 and TMEM16A) and basolateral pro-secretory K^+ channels, as well as for inhibitors of reabsorptive Na^+ channels. The counterintuitive idea of using inhibitors of TMEM16 channels is based on their role for mucus production and mucus secretion, which were uncovered only recently. Overwhelming mucus production and mucus plugging is the central problem in CF lung disease. Therefore, potent and well-tolerated TMEM16-inhibitors, which have FDA-approval for other diseases, should be further examined in preclinical and clinical studies to be use in CF lung disease and other inflammatory airway diseases.

AUTHOR CONTRIBUTIONS

KK wrote manuscript, analyzed data, and designed experiments. RS, JO, and IC analyzed data, designed experiments, and performed experiments. TD, AB, and MJ wrote manuscript. RB wrote manuscript, analyzed data, designed experiments, and performed experiments.

ACKNOWLEDGMENTS

Supported by Cystic Fibrosis Trust, SRC 013, INOVCF, DFG KU756/14-1, DFG KU756/14-1, and Gilead Stiftung 2018: Inhibition of TMEM16A to reduce mucus plugging in CF.

REFERENCES

Accurso, F. J., Rowe, S. M., Clancy, J. P., Boyle, M. P., Dunitz, J. M., Durie, P. R., et al. (2010). Effect of VX-770 in persons with cystic fibrosis and the G551D-CFTR mutation. *N. Engl. J. Med.* 363, 1991–2003. doi: 10.1056/NEJMoa0909825

Amaral, M. D., and Kunzelmann, K. (2007). Molecular targeting of CFTR as a therapeutic approach to cystic fibrosis. *Trends Pharmacol. Sci.* 28, 334–341. doi: 10.1016/j.tips.2007.05.004

Anagnostopoulou, P., Riederer, B., Duerr, J., Michel, S., Binia, A., Agrawal, R., et al. (2012). SLC26A9-mediated chloride secretion prevents mucus obstruction in airway inflammation. *J. Clin. Invest.* 122, 3629–3634. doi: 10.1172/JCI60429

Angles, F., Hutt, D., and Balch, W. E. (2018). HDAC inhibitors rescue multiple disease-causing CFTR variants. *bioRxiv.* doi: 10.1101/399451

Baron, A., Pacaud, P., Loirand, G., Mironneau, C., and Mironneau, J. (1991). Pharmacological block of Ca^{2+}-activated Cl^- current in rat vascular smooth muscle cells in short-term primary culture. *Pflugers Arch.* 419, 553–558. doi: 10.1007/BF00370294

Benedetto, R., Cabrita, I., Schreiber, R., and Kunzelmann, K. (2019). TMEM16A is indispensable for basal mucus secretion in airways and intestine. *FASEB J.* doi: 10.1096/fj.201801333RRR. [Epub ahead of print].

Benedetto, R., Ousingsawat, J., Wanitchakool, P., Zhang, Y., Holtzman, M. J., Amaral, M., et al. (2017). Epithelial chloride transport by CFTR requires TMEM16A. *Sci. Rep.* 7:12397. doi: 10.1038/s41598-017-10910-0

Benedetto, R., Sirianant, L., Pankonien, I., Wanitchakool, P., Ousingsawat, J., Cabrita, I., et al. (2016). Relationship between TMEM16A/anoctamin 1 and LRRC8A. *Pflugers Arch.* 468, 1751–1763. doi: 10.1007/s00424-016-1862-1

Bertrand, C. A., Mitra, S., Mishra, S. K., Wang, X., Zhao, Y., Pilewski, J. M., et al. (2017). The CFTR trafficking mutation F508del inhibits the constitutive activity of SLC26A9. *Am. J. Physiol. Lung Cell. Mol. Physiol.* 312, L912–L925. doi: 10.1152/ajplung.00178.2016

Bertrand, C. A., Zhang, R., Pilewski, J. M., and Frizzell, R. A. (2009). SLC26A9 is a constitutively active, CFTR-regulated anion conductance in human bronchial epithelia. *J. Gen. Physiol.* 133, 421–438. doi: 10.1085/jgp.200810097

Billet, A., and Hanrahan, J. W. (2013). The secret life of CFTR as a calcium-activated chloride channel. *J. Physiol.* 591, 5273–5278. doi: 10.1113/jphysiol.2013.261909

Boucher, R. C. (2007). Airway surface dehydration in cystic fibrosis: pathogenesis and therapy. *Annu. Rev. Med.* 58, 157–170. doi: 10.1146/annurev.med.58.071905.105316

Boucher, R. C., Stutts, M. J., Knowles, M. R., Cantley, L., and Gatzy, J. T. (1986). Na^+ transport in cystic fibrosis respiratory epithelia: abnormal basal rate and response to adenylate cyclase. *J. Clin. Invest.* 78, 1245–1252. doi: 10.1172/JCI112708

Brightling, C. E., Bradding, P., Symon, F. A., Holgate, S. T., Wardlaw, A. J., and Pavord, I. D. (2002). Mast-cell infiltration of airway smooth muscle in asthma. *N. Engl. J. Med.* 346, 1699–1705. doi: 10.1056/NEJMoa012705

Burris, S. K., Wang, Q., Bulley, S., Neeb, Z. P., and Jaggar, J. H. (2015). 9-phenanthrol inhibits recombinant and arterial myocyte TMEM16A channels. *Br. J. Pharmacol.* 172, 2459–2468. doi: 10.1111/bph.13077

Button, B., Goodell, H. P., Atieh, E., Chen, Y. C., Williams, R., Shenoy, S., et al. (2018). Roles of mucus adhesion and cohesion in cough clearance. *Proc. Natl. Acad. Sci. U.S.A.* 115, 12501–12506. doi: 10.1073/pnas.1811787115

Cabrita, I., Benedetto, R., Fonseca, A., Wanitchakool, P., Sirianant, L., Skryabin, B. V., et al. (2017). Differential effects of anoctamins on intracellular calcium signals. *FASEB J.* 31, 2123–2134. doi: 10.1096/fj.201600797RR

Caci, E., Scudieri, P., Di Carlo, E., Morelli, P., Bruno, S., De, F., et al. (2015). Upregulation of TMEM16A protein in bronchial epithelial cells by bacterial pyocyanin. *PLoS ONE* 10:e0131775. doi: 10.1371/journal.pone.0131775

Caputo, A., Caci, E., Ferrera, L., Pedemonte, N., Barsanti, C., Sondo, E., et al. (2008). TMEM16A, a membrane protein associated with calcium-dependent chloride channel activity. *Science* 322, 590–594. doi: 10.1126/science.1163518

Carlile, G. W., Robert, R., Goepp, J., Matthes, E., Liao, J., Kus, B., et al. (2015). Ibuprofen rescues mutant cystic fibrosis transmembrane conductance regulator trafficking. *J. Cyst. Fibros.* 14, 16–25. doi: 10.1016/j.jcf.2014.06.001

Carlile, G. W., Yang, Q., Matthes, E., Liao, J., Radinovic, S., Miyamoto, C., et al. (2018). A novel triple combination of pharmacological chaperones improves F508del-CFTR correction. *Sci. Rep.* 8:11404. doi: 10.1038/s41598-018-29276-y

Catalan, M. A., Kondo, Y., Pena-Munzenmayer, G., Jaramillo, Y., Liu, F., Choi, S., et al. (2015). A fluid secretion pathway unmasked by acinar-specific Tmem16A gene ablation in the adult mouse salivary gland. *Proc. Natl. Acad. Sci U.S.A.* 112, 2263–2268. doi: 10.1073/pnas.1415739112

Chai, R., Chen, Y., Yuan, H., Wang, X., Guo, S., Qi, J., et al. (2017). Identification of resveratrol, an herbal compound, as an activator of the calcium-activated chloride channel, TMEM16A. *J. Membr. Biol.* 250, 483–492. doi: 10.1007/s00232-017-9975-9

Chang, M. H., Plata, C., Sindic, A., Ranatunga, W. K., Chen, A. P., Zandi-Nejad, K., et al. (2009). Slc26a9 is inhibited by the R-region of CFTR via the STAS domain. *J. Biol. Chem.* 284, 28306–28318. doi: 10.1074/jbc.M109.001669

Chen, J. H., Stoltz, D. A., Karp, P. H., Ernst, S. E., Pezzulo, A. A., Moninger, T. O., et al. (2010). Loss of anion transport without increased sodium absorption characterizes newborn porcine cystic fibrosis airway epithelia. *Cell* 143, 911–923. doi: 10.1016/j.cell.2010.11.029

Chin, S., Hung, M., Won, A., Wu, Y. S., Ahmadi, S., Yang, D., et al. (2018). Lipophilicity of the cystic fibrosis drug, ivacaftor (VX-770), and its destabilizing effect on the major CF-causing mutation: F508del. *Mol. Pharmacol.* 94, 917–925. doi: 10.1124/mol.118.112177

Cho, H., Yang, Y. D., Lee, J., Lee, B., Kim, T., Jang, Y., et al. (2012). The calcium-activated chloride channel anoctamin 1 acts as a heat sensor in nociceptive neurons. *Nat. Neurosci.* 15, 1015–1021. doi: 10.1038/nn.3111

Choi, J. Y., Muallem, D., Kiselyov, K., Lee, M. G., Thomas, P. J., and Muallem, S. (2001). Aberrant CFTR-dependent HCO3- transport in mutations associated with cystic fibrosis. *Nature* 410, 94–97. doi: 10.1038/35065099

Cholon, D. M., Quinney, N. L., Fulcher, M. L., Esther, C. R. Jr., Das, J., Dokholyan, N. V., et al. (2014). Potentiator ivacaftor abrogates pharmacological correction of DeltaF508 CFTR in cystic fibrosis. *Sci. Transl. Med.* 6:246ra296. doi: 10.1126/scitranslmed.3008680

Cotton, C. U., Lawson, E. E., Boucher, R. C., and Gatzy, J. T. (1983). Bioelectric properties and ion transport of airways excised from adult and fetal sheep. *J. Appl. Physiol. Respir. Environ. Exerc. Physiol.* 55, 1542–1549. doi: 10.1152/jappl.1983.55.5.1542

Danielsson, J., Mikami, M., and Emala, C. W. (2017). Antagonism of the Tmem16a calcium-activated chloride channel attenuates allergic lung inflammation. *Am. J. Respir. Crit. Care Med.* 195:A5290.

Danielsson, J., Perez-Zoghbi, J., Bernstein, K., Barajas, M. B., Zhang, Y., Kumar, S., et al. (2015). Antagonists of the TMEM16A calcium-activated chloride channel modulate airway smooth muscle tone and intracellular calcium. *Anesthesiology* 123, 569–581. doi: 10.1097/ALN.0000000000000769

Davies, J. C., Moskowitz, S. M., Brown, C., Horsley, A., Mall, M. A., Mckone, E. F., et al. (2018). VX-659-tezacaftor-ivacaftor in patients with cystic fibrosis and one or two Phe508del alleles. *N. Engl. J. Med.* 379, 1599–1611. doi: 10.1056/NEJMoa1807119

De Boeck, K., and Amaral, M. D. (2016). Progress in therapies for cystic fibrosis. *Lancet Respir. Med.* 4, 662–674. doi: 10.1016/S2213-2600(16)00023-0

De Boeck, K., Zolin, A., Cuppens, H., Olesen, H. V., and Viviani, L. (2014). The relative frequency of CFTR mutation classes in European patients with cystic fibrosis. *J. Cyst. Fibros.* 13, 403–409. doi: 10.1016/j.jcf.2013.12.003

de La Fuente, R., Namkung, W., Mills, A., and Verkman, A. S. (2007). Small molecule screen identifies inhibitors of a human intestinal calcium activated chloride channel. *Mol. Pharmacol.* 73, 758–768. doi: 10.1124/mol.107.043208

Deba, F., and Bessac, B. F. (2015). Anoctamin-1 Cl channels in nociception: activation by an N-aroylaminothiazole and capsaicin and inhibition by T16A[inh]-A01. *Mol. Pain* 11:55. doi: 10.1186/s12990-015-0061-y

Donaldson, S. H., and Boucher, R. C. (2007). Sodium channels and cystic fibrosis. *Chest* 132, 1631–1636. doi: 10.1378/chest.07-0288

Donaldson, S. H., Pilewski, J. M., Griese, M., Cooke, J., Viswanathan, L., Tullis, E., et al. (2018). Tezacaftor/Ivacaftor in subjects with cystic fibrosis and F508del/F508del-CFTR or F508del/G551D-CFTR. *Am. J. Respir. Crit. Care Med.* 197, 214–224. doi: 10.1164/rccm.201704-0717OC

Doring, G., and Worlitzsch, D. (2000). Inflammation in cystic fibrosis and its management. *Paediatr. Respir. Rev.* 1, 101–106. doi: 10.1053/prrv.2000.0030

Dorwart, M. R., Shcheynikov, N., Wang, Y., Stippec, S., and Muallem, S. (2007). SLC26A9 is a Cl(-) channel regulated by the WNK kinases. *J. Physiol.* 584, 333–345. doi: 10.1113/jphysiol.2007.135855

Drumm, B. T., Hennig, G. W., Battersby, M. J., Cunningham, E. K., Sung, T. S., Ward, S. M., et al. (2017). Clustering of Ca^{2+}) transients in interstitial cells of cajal defines slow wave duration. *J. Gen. Physiol.* 149, 703–725. doi: 10.1085/jgp.201711771

Dunican, E. M., Elicker, B. M., Gierada, D. S., Nagle, S. K., Schiebler, M. L., Newell, J. D., et al. (2018). Mucus plugs in patients with asthma linked to eosinophilia and airflow obstruction. *J. Clin. Invest.* 128, 997–1009. doi: 10.1172/JCI 95693

El Khouri, E., and Toure, A. (2014). Functional interaction of the cystic fibrosis transmembrane conductance regulator with members of the SLC26 family of anion transporters (SLC26A8 and SLC26A9): physiological and pathophysiological relevance. *Int. J. Biochem. Cell Biol.* 52, 58–67. doi: 10.1016/j.biocel.2014.02.001

Fahy, J. V., and Dickey, B. F. (2010). Airway mucus function and dysfunction. *N. Engl. J. Med.* 363, 2233–2247. doi: 10.1056/NEJMra0910061

Faria, D., Schlatter, E., Witzgall, R., Grahammer, F., Bandulik, S., Schweda, F., et al. (2014). The calcium activated chloride channel Anoctamin 1 contributes to the regulation of renal function. *Kindey Int.* 85, 1369–1381. doi: 10.1038/ki.2013.535

Faria, D., Schreiber, R., and Kunzelmann, K. (2009). CFTR is activated through stimulation of purinergic P2Y2 receptors. *Pflügers Arch.* 457, 1373–1380. doi: 10.1007/s00424-008-0606-2

Fedigan, S., Bradley, E., Webb, T., Large, R. J., Hollywood, M. A., Thornbury, K. D., et al. (2017). Effects of new-generation TMEM16A inhibitors on calcium-activated chloride currents in rabbit urethral interstitial cells of cajal. *Pflugers Arch.* 469, 1443–1455. doi: 10.1007/s00424-017-2028-5

Ferkol, T., and Quinton, P. (2015). Precision medicine: at what price? *Am. J. Respir. Crit. Care Med.* 192, 658–659. doi: 10.1164/rccm.201507-1428ED

Galietta, L. J., Pagesy, P., Folli, C., Caci, E., Romio, L., Costes, B., et al. (2002). IL-4 is a potent modulator of ion transport in the human bronchial epithelium *in vitro*. *J. Immunol.* 168, 839–845. doi: 10.4049/jimmunol.168.2.839

Galli, S. J., Tsai, M., and Piliponsky, A. M. (2008). The development of allergic inflammation. *Nature* 454, 445–454. doi: 10.1038/nature07204

Gallos, G., Remy, K. E., Danielsson, J., Funayama, H., Fu, X. W., Chang, H. Y., et al. (2013). Functional expression of the TMEM16 family of calcium activated chloride channels in airway smooth muscle. *Am. J. Physiol. Lung Cell. Mol. Physiol.* 305, L625–L634. doi: 10.1152/ajplung.00068.2013

Gianotti, A., Ferrera, L., Philp, A. R., Caci, E., Zegarra-Moran, O., Galietta, L. J., et al. (2016). Pharmacological analysis of epithelial chloride secretion mechanisms in adult murine airways. *Eur. J. Pharmacol.* 787, 100–108. doi: 10.1016/j.ejphar.2016.04.007

Grubb, B. R., Vick, R. N., and Boucher, R. C. (1994). Hyperabsorption of Na^+ and raised Ca^{2+} mediated Cl^- secretion in nasal epithelia of CF mice. *Am. J. Physiol.* 266, C1478–C1483. doi: 10.1152/ajpcell.1994.266.5.C1478

Grubb, S., Poulsen, K. A., Juul, C. A., Kyed, T., Klausen, T. K., Larsen, E. H., et al. (2013). TMEM16F (Anoctamin 6), an anion channel of delayed Ca^{2+} activation. *J. Gen. Physiol.* 141, 585–600. doi: 10.1085/jgp.201210861

Guo, S., Chen, Y., Pang, C., Wang, X., Qi, J., Mo, L., et al. (2017). Ginsenoside Rb1, a novel activator of the TMEM16A chloride channel, augments the contraction of guinea pig ileum. *Pflugers Arch.* 469, 681–692. doi: 10.1007/s00424-017-1934-x

Guo, S., Chen, Y., Pang, C., Wang, X., Shi, S., Zhang, H., et al. (2018). Matrine is a novel inhibitor of the TMEM16A chloride channel with antilung adenocarcinoma effects. *J. Cell Physiol.* doi: 10.1002/jcp.27529. [Epub ahead of print].

Hajj, R., Lesimple, P., Nawrocki-Raby, B., Birembaut, P., Puchelle, E., and Coraux, C. (2007). Human airway surface epithelial regeneration is delayed and abnormal in cystic fibrosis. *J. Pathol.* 211, 340–350. doi: 10.1002/path.2118

Heinze, C., Seniuk, A., Sokolov, M. V., Huebner, A. K., Klementowicz, A. E., Szijarto, I. A., et al. (2014). Disruption of vascular Ca^{2+}-activated chloride currents lowers blood pressure. *J. Clin. Invest.* 124, 675–686. doi: 10.1172/JCI70025

Hoegger, M. J., Fischer, A. J., Mcmenimen, J. D., Ostedgaard, L. S., Tucker, A. J., Awadalla, M. A., et al. (2014). Impaired mucus detachment disrupts mucociliary transport in a piglet model of cystic fibrosis. *Science* 345, 818–822. doi: 10.1126/science.1255825

Hogg, R. C., Wang, Q., and Large, W. A. (1994). Action of niflumic acid on evoked and spontaneous calcium-activated chloride and potassium currents in smooth muscle cells from rabbit portal vein. *Br. J. Pharmacol.* 112, 977–984. doi: 10.1111/j.1476-5381.1994.tb13177.x

Huang, F., Rock, J. R., Harfe, B. D., Cheng, T., Huang, X., Jan, Y. N., et al. (2009). Studies on expression and function of the TMEM16A calcium-activated chloride channel. *Proc. Natl. Acad. Sci. U.S.A.* 106, 21413–21418. doi: 10.1073/pnas.0911935106

Huang, F., Zhang, H., Wu, M., Yang, H., Kudo, M., Peters, C. J., et al. (2012). Calcium-activated chloride channel TMEM16A modulates mucin secretion and airway smooth muscle contraction. *Proc. Natl. Acad. Sci. U.S.A.* 109, 16354–16359. doi: 10.1073/pnas.12145 96109

Huang, Y., Guo, S., Ren, S., Chen, Y., Zhan, Y., and An, H. (2018). The natural compound cinnamaldehyde is a novel activator of calcium-activated chloride channel. *J. Membr. Biol.* 251, 747–756. doi: 10.1007/s00232-018-0052-9

Hutt, D. M., Loguercio, S., Roth, D. M., Su, A. I., and Balch, W. E. (2018). Correcting the F508del-CFTR variant by modulating eukaryotic translation initiation factor 3-mediated translation initiation. *J. Biol. Chem.* 293, 13477–13495. doi: 10.1074/jbc.RA118.003192

Itani, O. A., Chen, J. H., Karp, P. H., Ernst, S., Keshavjee, S., Parekh, K., et al. (2011). Human cystic fibrosis airway epithelia have reduced Cl^- conductance but not increased Na^+ conductance. *Proc. Natl. Acad. Sci. U.S.A.* 108, 10260–10265. doi: 10.1073/pnas.1106695108

Jiang, Y., Yu, B., Yang, H., and Ma, T. (2016). Shikonin inhibits intestinal calcium-activated chloride channels and prevents rotaviral diarrhea. *Front. Pharmacol.* 7:270. doi: 10.3389/fphar.2016.00270

Keating, D., Marigowda, G., Burr, L., Daines, C., Mall, M. A., Mckone, E. F., et al. (2018). VX-445-Tezacaftor-Ivacaftor in patients with cystic fibrosis and one or two Phe508del alleles. *N. Engl. J. Med.* 379, 1612–1620. doi: 10.1056/NEJMoa1807120

Khan, T. Z., Wagener, J. S., Bost, T., Martinez, J., Accurso, F. J., and Riches, D. W. (1995). Early pulmonary inflammation in infants with cystic fibrosis. *Am. J. Respir. Crit. Care Med.* 151, 1075–1082.

Klymiuk, N., Mundhenk, L., Kraehe, K., Wuensch, A., Plog, S., Emrich, D., et al. (2012). Sequential targeting of CFTR by BAC vectors generates a novel pig model of cystic fibrosis. *J. Mol. Med.* 90, 597–608. doi: 10.1007/s00109-011-0839-y

Knight, D. (2004). Talniflumate (Genaera). *Curr. Opin. Investig. Drugs* 5, 557–562.

Knowles, M. R., and Boucher, R. C. (2002). Mucus clearance as a primary innate defense mechanism for mammalian airways. *J. Clin. Invest.* 109, 571–577. doi: 10.1172/JCI0215217

Kondo, M., Nakata, J., Arai, N., Izumo, T., Tagaya, E., Takeyama, K., et al. (2012). Niflumic acid inhibits goblet cell degranulation in a guinea pig asthma model. *Allergol. Int.* 61, 133–142. doi: 10.2332/allergolint.11-OA-0307

Kondo, M., Tsuji, M., Hara, K., Arimura, K., Yagi, O., Tagaya, E., et al. (2017). Chloride ion transport and overexpression of TMEM16A in a guinea pig asthma model. *Clin. Exp. Allergy* 47, 795–804. doi: 10.1111/cea.12887

Kubitz, R., Warth, R., Kunzelmann, K., Grolik, M., and Greger, R. (1992). Small conductance Cl^- channels induced by cAMP, Ca^{2+}, and hypotonicity in HT_{29} cells: ion selectivity, additivity and stilbene sensitivity. *Pflügers Arch.* 421, 447–454. doi: 10.1007/BF00370255

Kunzelmann, K., Cabrita, I., Wanitchakool, P., Ousingsawat, J., Sirianant, L., Benedetto, R., et al. (2016). Modulating Ca^{2+}signals: a common theme for TMEM16, Ist2, and TMC. *Pflügers Arch.* 468, 475–490. doi: 10.1007/s00424-015-1767-4

Kunzelmann, K., Gerlach, L., Fröbe, U., and Greger, R. (1991). Bicarbonate permeability of epithelial chloride channels. *Pflügers Arch.* 417, 616–621. doi: 10.1007/BF00372960

Kunzelmann, K., Kubitz, R., Grolik, M., Warth, R., and Greger, R. (1992). Small conductance Cl^- channels in HT_{29} cells: activation by Ca^{2+}, hypotonic cell swelling and 8-Br-cGMP. *Pflügers Arch.* 421, 238–246. doi: 10.1007/BF00374833

Kunzelmann, K., Mall, M., Briel, M., Hipper, A., Nitschke, R., Ricken, S., et al. (1997). The cystic fibrosis transmembrane conductance regulator attenuates the endogenous Ca^{2+} activated Cl^- conductance in *Xenopus* ooyctes. *Pflügers Arch.* 434, 178–181. doi: 10.1007/s004240050498

Kunzelmann, K., Nilius, B., Owsianik, G., Schreiber, R., Ousingsawat, J., Sirianant, L., et al. (2014). Molecular functions of anoctamin 6 (TMEM16F): a chloride channel, cation channel or phospholipid scramblase? *Pflügers Arch.* 466, 407–414. doi: 10.1007/s00424-013-1305-1

Kunzelmann, K., Schreiber, R., and Cook, D. I. (2002). Mechanisms for inhibition of amiloride-sensitive Na^+ absorption by extracellular nuceotides in mouse trachea. *Pflügers Arch.* 444, 220–226. doi: 10.1007/s00424-002-0796-y

Kunzelmann, K., Schreiber, R., and Hadorn, H. B. (2017). Bicarbonate in cystic fibrosis. *J. Cyst. Fibros.* 16, 653–662. doi: 10.1016/j.jcf.2017.06.005

Kunzelmann, K., Tian, Y., Martins, J. R., Faria, D., Kongsuphol, P., Ousingsawat, J., et al. (2011). Anoctamins. *Pflugers Arch.* 462, 195–208. doi: 10.1007/s00424-011-0975-9

Kunzelmann, K., Tian, Y., Martins, J. R., Faria, D., Kongsuphol, P., Ousingsawat, J., et al. (2012). Cells in focus: airway epithelial cells-Functional links between CFTR and anoctamin dependent Cl(-) secretion. *Int. J. Biochem. Cell Biol.* 44, 1897–1900. doi: 10.1016/j.biocel 2012.06.011

Lee, B., Cho, H., Jung, J., Yang, Y. D., Yang, D. J., and Oh, U. (2014). Anoctamin 1 contributes to inflammatory and nerve-injury induced hypersensitivity. *Mol. Pain* 10:5. doi: 10.1186/1744-8069-10-5

Lerias, J., Pinto, M., Benedetto, R., Schreiber, R., Amaral, M., Aureli, M., et al. (2018). Compartmentalized crosstalk of CFTR and TMEM16A (ANO1) through EPAC1 and ADCY1. *Cell. Signal.* 44, 10–19. doi: 10.1016/j.cellsig.2018.01.008

Li, H., Salomon, J. J., Sheppard, D. N., Mall, M. A., and Galietta, L. J. (2017). Bypassing CFTR dysfunction in cystic fibrosis with alternative pathways for anion transport. *Curr. Opin. Pharmacol.* 34, 91–97. doi: 10.1016/j.coph.2017.10.002

Lin, J., Jiang, Y., Li, L., Liu, Y., Tang, H., and Jiang, D. (2015). TMEM16A mediates the hypersecretion of mucus induced by Interleukin-13. *Exp. Cell Res.* 334, 260–269. doi: 10.1016/j.yexcr.2015.02.026

Mall, M., Bleich, M., Greger, R., Schreiber, R., and Kunzelmann, K. (1998a). The amiloride inhibitable Na^+ conductance is reduced by CFTR in normal but not in CF airways. *J. Clin. Invest.* 102, 15–21. doi: 10.1172/JCI2729

Mall, M., Bleich, M., Greger, R., Schürlein, M., Kühr, J., Seydewitz, H. H., et al. (1998b). Cholinergic ion secretion in human colon requires co-activation by cAMP. *Am. J. Physiol.* 275, G1274–G1281.

Mall, M., Gonska, T., Thomas, J., Schreiber, R., Seydewitz, H. H., Kuehr, J., et al. (2003). Modulation of Ca^{2+} activated Cl^- secretion by basolateral K^+ channels in human normal and cystic fibrosis airway epithelia. *Pediatr. Res.* 53, 608–618. doi: 10.1203/01.PDR.0000057204.51420.DC

Mall, M., Grubb, B. R., Harkema, J. R., O'neal, W. K., and Boucher, R. C. (2004). Increased airway epithelial Na^+ absorption produces cystic fibrosis-like lung disease in mice. *Nat. Med.* 10, 487–493. doi: 10.1038/nm1028

Mall, M., Wissner, A., Kühr, J., Gonska, T., Brandis, M., and Kunzelmann, K. (2000). Inhibition of amiloride sensitive epithelial Na^+ absorption by extracellular nucleotides in human normal and CF airways. *Am. J. Respir. Cell Mol. Biol.* 23, 755–761. doi: 10.1165/ajrcmb.23.6.4207

Martins, J. R., Kongsuphol, P., Sammels, E., Daimène, S., Aldehni, F., Clarke, L., et al. (2011). F508del-CFTR increases intracellular Ca^{2+} signaling that causes enhanced calcium-dependent Cl^- conductance in cystic fibrosis. *Biochim. Biophys. Acta* 1812, 1385–1392. doi: 10.1016/j.bbadis.2011.08.008

Matsui, H., Grubb, B. R., Tarran, R., Randell, S. H., Gatzy, J. T., Davis, C. W., et al. (1998). Evidence for periciliary liquid layer depletion, not abnormal ion composition, in the pathogenesis of cystic fibrosis airways disease. *Cell* 95, 1005–1015. doi: 10.1016/S0092-8674(00)81724-9

Miller, M. R., Soave, D., Li, W., Gong, J., Pace, R. G., Boelle, P. Y., et al. (2015). Variants in solute carrier SLC26A9 modify prenatal exocrine pancreatic damage in cystic fibrosis. *J. Pediatr.* 166, 1152–1157.e1156. doi: 10.1016/j.jpeds.2015.01.044

Miner, K., Mohn, D., Elliot, R., Powers, D., Chen, J., Liu, B., et al. (2019). The anthelminthic niclosamide and related compounds represent potent Tmem16a antagonists that fully relax mouse and human airway rings. *Front. Pharmacol.* (in press).

Montoro, D. T., Haber, A. L., Biton, M., Vinarsky, V., Lin, B., Birket, S. E., et al. (2018). A revised airway epithelial hierarchy includes CFTR-expressing ionocytes. *Nature* 560, 319–324. doi: 10.1038/s41586-018-0393-7

Moody, M., Pennington, C., Schultz, C., Caldwell, R., Dinkel, C., Rossi, M. W., et al. (2005). Inositol polyphosphate derivative inhibits Na^+ transport and improves fluid dynamics in cystic fibrosis airway epithelia. *Am. J. Physiol. Cell Physiol.* 289, C512–C520. doi: 10.1152/ajpcell.00591.2004

Moss, R. B. (2013). Pitfalls of drug development: lessons learned from trials of denufosol in cystic fibrosis. *J. Pediatr.* 162, 676–680. doi: 10.1016/j.jpeds.2012.11.034

Mount, D. B., and Romero, M. F. (2004). The SLC26 gene family of multifunctional anion exchangers. *Pflugers Arch.* 447, 710–721. doi: 10.1007/s00424-003-1090-3

Namkung, W., Finkbeiner, W. E., and Verkman, A. S. (2010a). CFTR-Adenylyl cyclase I association is responsible for UTP activation of CFTR in well-differentiated primary human bronchial cell cultures. *Mol. Biol. Cell* 21, 2639–2648. doi: 10.1091/mbc e09-12-1004

Namkung, W., Phuan, P. W., and Verkman, A. S. (2011a). TMEM16A inhibitors reveal TMEM16A as a minor component of CaCC conductance in airway and intestinal epithelial cells. *J. Biol. Chem.* 286, 2365–2374. doi: 10.1074/jbc.M110.175109

Namkung, W., Thiagarajah, J. R., Phuan, P. W., and Verkman, A. S. (2010b). Inhibition of Ca^{2+}-activated Cl^{-} channels by gallotannins as a possible molecular basis for health benefits of red wine and green tea. *FASEB J.* 24, 4178–4186. doi: 10.1096/fj.10-160648

Namkung, W., Yao, Z., Finkbeiner, W. E., and Verkman, A. S. (2011b). Small-molecule activators of TMEM16A, a calcium-activated chloride channel, stimulate epithelial chloride secretion and intestinal contraction. *FASEB J.* 25, 4048–4062. doi: 10.1096/fj.11-191627

Oh, S. J., Hwang, S. J., Jung, J., Yu, K., Kim, J., Choi, J. Y., et al. (2013). MONNA, a potent and selective blocker for TMEM16A/Anoctamin-1. *Mol. Pharmacol.* 84, 726–735. doi: 10.1124/mol.113.087502

Ousingsawat, J., Kongsuphol, P., Schreiber, R., and Kunzelmann, K. (2011a). CFTR and TMEM16A are separate but functionally related Cl channels. *Cell. Physiol. Biochem.* 28, 715–724. doi: 10.1159/000335765

Ousingsawat, J., Martins, J. R., Schreiber, R., Rock, J. R., Harfe, B. D., and Kunzelmann, K. (2009). Loss of TMEM16A causes a defect in epithelial Ca^{2+} dependent chloride transport. *J. Biol. Chem.* 284, 28698–28703. doi: 10.1074/jbc.M109.012120

Ousingsawat, J., Schreiber, R., and Kunzelmann, K. (2011b). Differential contribution of SLC26A9 to Cl(-) conductance in polarized and non-polarized epithelial cells. *J. Cell. Physiol.* 227, 2323–2329. doi: 10.1002/jcp.22967

Ousingsawat, J., Wanitchakool, P., Kmit, A., Romao, A. M., Jantarajit, W., Schreiber, S., et al. (2015). Anoctamin 6 mediates effects essential for innate immunity downstream of P2X7-receptors in macrophages. *Nat. Commun.* 6:6245. doi: 10.1038/ncomms7245

Paulino, C., Kalienkova, V., Lam, A. K. M., Neldner, Y., and Dutzler, R. (2017a). Activation mechanism of the calcium-activated chloride channel TMEM16A revealed by cryo-EM. *Nature* 552, 421–425. doi: 10.1038/nature24652

Paulino, C., Neldner, Y., Lam, A. K., Kalienkova, V., Brunner, J. D., Schenck, S., et al. (2017b). Structural basis for anion conduction in the calcium-activated chloride channel TMEM16A. *Elife* 6:e26232. doi: 10.7554/eLife.26232

Pedemonte, N., and Galietta, L. J. (2014). Structure and function of TMEM16 proteins (anoctamins). *Physiol. Rev.* 94, 419–459. doi: 10.1152/physrev.00039.2011

Pedersen, K. A., Schroder, R. L., Skaaning-Jensen, B., Strobaek, D., Olesen, S. P., and Christophersen, P. (1999). Activation of the human intermediate-conductance Ca^{2+})-activated K^{+} channel by 1-ethyl-2-benzimidazolinone is strongly Ca^{2+}-dependent. *Biochim. Biophys. Acta* 1420, 231–240. doi: 10.1016/S0005-2736(99)00110-8

Pezzulo, A. A., Tang, X. X., Hoegger, M. J., Alaiwa, M. H., Ramachandran, S., Moninger, T. O., et al. (2012). Reduced airway surface pH impairs bacterial killing in the porcine cystic fibrosis lung. *Nature* 487, 109–113. doi: 10.1038/nature11130

Plasschaert, L. W., Zilionis, R., Choo-Wing, R., Savova, V., Knehr, J., Roma, G., et al. (2018). A single-cell atlas of the airway epithelium reveals the CFTR-rich pulmonary ionocyte. *Nature* 560, 377–381. doi: 10.1038/s41586-018-0394-6

Poulsen, J. H., Fischer, H., Illek, B., and Machen, T. E. (1994). Bicarbonate conductance and pH regulatory capability of cystic fibrosis transmembrane conductance regulator. *Proc. Natl. Acad. Sci. U.S.A* 91, 5340–5344. doi: 10.1073/pnas.91.12.5340

Pranke, I. M., Hatton, A., Simonin, J., Jais, J. P., Le Pimpec-Barthes, F., Carsin, A., et al. (2017). Correction of CFTR function in nasal epithelial cells from cystic fibrosis patients predicts improvement of respiratory function by CFTR modulators. *Sci. Rep.* 7:7375. doi: 10.1038/s41598-017-07504-1

Preston, P., Wartosch, L., Gunzel, D., Fromm, M., Kongsuphol, P., Ousingsawat, J., et al. (2010). Disruption of the K^{+} channel beta-subunit KCNE3 reveals an important role in intestinal and tracheal Cl^{-} transport. *J. Biol. Chem.* 285, 7165–7175. doi: 10.1074/jbc.M109.047829

Pusch, M., and Zifarelli, G. (2014). Thermal sensitivity of CLC and TMEM16 chloride channels and transporters. *Curr. Top. Membr.* 74, 213–231. doi: 10.1016/B978-0-12-800181-3.00008-7

Quinton, P. M. (2001). The neglected ion: HCO_3^{-}. *Nat. Med.* 7, 292–293. doi: 10.1038/85429

Ratjen, F., Durham, T., Navratil, T., Schaberg, A., Accurso, F. J., Wainwright, C., et al. (2012). Long term effects of denufosol tetrasodium in patients with cystic fibrosis. *J. Cyst. Fibros.* 11, 539–549. doi: 10.1016/j.jcf.2012.05.003

Ribeiro, C. M., Paradiso, A. M., Schwab, U., Perez-Vilar, J., Jones, L., O'neal, W., et al. (2005). Chronic airway infection/Inflammation Induces a Ca^{2+}i-dependent hyperinflammatory response in human cystic fibrosis airway epithelia. *J. Biol. Chem.* 280, 17798–17806. doi: 10.1074/jbc.M410618200

Rottner, M., Freyssinet, J. M., and Martinez, M. C. (2009). Mechanisms of the noxious inflammatory cycle in cystic fibrosis. *Respir. Res.* 10:23. doi: 10.1186/1465-9921-10-23

Rottner, M., Kunzelmann, C., Mergey, M., Freyssinet, J. M., and Martinez, M. C. (2007). Exaggerated apoptosis and NF-kappaB activation in pancreatic and tracheal cystic fibrosis cells. *FASEB J.* 21, 2939–2948. doi: 10.1096/fj.06-7614com

Rottner, M., Tual-Chalot, S., Mostefai, H. A., Andriantsitohaina, R., Freyssinet, J. M., and Martinez, M. C. (2011). Increased oxidative stress induces apoptosis in human cystic fibrosis cells. *PLoS ONE* 6:e24880. doi: 10.1371/journal.pone.0024880

Rowe, S. M., Daines, C., Ringshausen, F. C., Kerem, E., Wilson, J., Tullis, E., et al. (2017). Tezacaftor-Ivacaftor in residual-function heterozygotes with cystic fibrosis. *N. Engl. J. Med.* 377, 2024–2035. doi: 10.1056/NEJMoa1709847

Ruffin, M., Voland, M., Marie, S., Bonora, M., Blanchard, E., Blouquit-Laye, S., et al. (2013). Anoctamin 1 dysregulation alters bronchial epithelial repair in cystic fibrosis. *Biochim. Biophys. Acta* 1832, 2340–2351. doi: 10.1016/j.bbadis.2013.09.012

Sanders, K. M., Zhu, M. H., Britton, F., Koh, S. D., and Ward, S. M. (2012). Anoctamins and gastrointestinal smooth muscle excitability. *Exp. Physiol.* 97, 200–206. doi: 10.1113/expphysiol.2011.058248

Schenk, L. K., Buchholz, B., Henke, S. F., Michgehl, U., Daniel, C., Amann, K., et al. (2018). Nephron-specific knockout of TMEM16A leads to reduced number of glomeruli and albuminuria. *Am. J. Physiol. Renal Physiol.* doi: 10.1152/ajprenal.00638.2017. [Epub ahead of print].

Schreiber, R., Faria, D., Skryabin, B. V., Rock, J. R., and Kunzelmann, K. (2014). Anoctamins support calcium-dependent chloride secretion by facilitating calcium signaling in adult mouse intestine. *Pflügers Arch.* 467, 1203–1213. doi: 10.1007/s00424-014-1559-2

Schreiber, R., Ousingsawat, J., Wanitchakool, P., Sirianant, L., Benedetto, R., Reiss, K., et al. (2018). Regulation of TMEM16A/ANO1 and TMEM16F/ANO6 ion currents and phospholipid scrambling by Ca^{2+} and plasma membrane lipid. *J. Physiol.* 596, 217–229. doi: 10.1113/JP275175

Schreiber, R., Uliyakina, I., Kongsuphol, P., Warth, R., Mirza, M., Martins, J. R., et al. (2010). Expression and function of epithelial anoctamins. *J. Biol. Chem.* 285, 7838–7845. doi: 10.1074/jbc.M109.065367

Schultz, A., Puvvadi, R., Borisov, S. M., Shaw, N. C., Klimant, I., Berry, L. J., et al. (2017). Airway surface liquid pH is not acidic in children with cystic fibrosis. *Nat. Commun.* 8:1409. doi: 10.1038/s41467-017-00532-5

Scudieri, P., Caci, E., Bruno, S., Ferrera, L., Schiavon, M., Sondo, E., et al. (2012). Association of TMEM16A chloride channel overexpression with airway goblet cells metaplasia. *J. Physiol.* 590, 6141–6155. doi: 10.1113/jphysiol.2012.240838

Scudieri, P., Caci, E., Venturini, A., Sondo, E., Pianigiani, G., Marchetti, C., et al. (2015). Ion channel and lipid scramblase activity associated with expression of tmem16F/ANO6 isoforms. *J. Physiol.* 593, 3829–3848. doi: 10.1113/JP270691

Seo, Y., Kim, J., Chang, J., Kim, S. S., Namkung, W., and Kim, I. (2018). Synthesis and biological evaluation of novel Ani9 derivatives as potent and selective ANO1 inhibitors. *Eur. J. Med. Chem.* 160, 245–255. doi: 10.1016/j.ejmech.2018.10.002

Seo, Y., Lee, H. K., Park, J., Jeon, D. K., Jo, S., Jo, M., et al. (2016). Ani9, a novel potent small-molecule ANO1 inhibitor with negligible effect on ANO2. *PLoS ONE* 11:e0155771. doi: 10.1371/journal.pone.0155771

Seo, Y., Park, J., Kim, M., Lee, H. K., Kim, J. H., Jeong, J. H., et al. (2015). Inhibition of ANO1/TMEM16A chloride channel by idebenone and its cytotoxicity to cancer cell lines. *PLoS ONE* 10:e0133656. doi: 10.1371/journal.pone.0133656

Sharm, K., Sung, J., Kim, H. J., Oak, M. H., and Yi, E. (2017). Rice bran extract inhibits TMEM16A-Involved activity in the neonatal rat cochlea. *J. Nanosci. Nanotechnol.* 17, 2390–2393. doi: 10.1166/jnn.2017.13333

Shimizu, T., Iehara, T., Sato, K., Fujii, T., Sakai, H., and Okada, Y. (2013). TMEM16F is a component of a Ca^{2+}-activated Cl^{-} channel but not a volume-sensitive outwardly rectifying Cl^{-} channel. *Am. J. Physiol. Cell Physiol.* 304, C748–C759. doi: 10.1152/ajpcell.00228.2012

Singh, R. D., Gibbons, S. J., Saravanaperumal, S. A., Du, P., Hennig, G. W., Eisenman, S. T., et al. (2014). Ano1, a Ca^{2+}-activated Cl^{-}

channel coordinates contractility in mouse intestine by ca^{2+} transient coordination between interstitial cells of cajal. *J. Physiol.* 592, 4051–4068. doi: 10.1113/jphysiol.2014.277152

Sirianant, L., Ousingsawat, J., Wanitchakool, P., Schreiber, R., and Kunzelmann, K. (2015). Cellular volume regulation by anoctamin 6:Ca^{2+}, phospholipase A2,osmosensing. *Pflügers Arch.* 468, 335–349. doi: 10.1007/s00424-015-1739-8

Smith, J. J., and Welsh, M. J. (1992). cAMP stimulates bicarbonate secretion across normal, but not cystic fibrosis airway epithelia. *J. Clin. Invest.* 89, 1148–1153. doi: 10.1172/JCI115696

Stick, S. M., and Schultz, A. (2018). CrossTalk opposing view: mucosal acidification does not drive early progressive lung disease in cystic fibrosis. *J. Physiol.* 596, 3439–3441. doi: 10.1113/JP275426

Stoltz, D. A., Meyerholz, D. K., Pezzulo, A. A., Ramachandran, S., Rogan, M. P., Davis, G. J., et al. (2010). Cystic fibrosis pigs develop lung disease and exhibit defective bacterial eradication at birth. *Sci. Transl. Med.* 2:29ra31. doi: 10.1126/scitranslmed.3000928

Stoltz, D. A., Meyerholz, D. K., and Welsh, M. J. (2015). Origins of cystic fibrosis lung disease. *N. Engl. J. Med.* 372, 351–362. doi: 10.1056/NEJMra1300109

Strug, L. J., Gonska, T., He, G., Keenan, K., Ip, W., Boelle, P. Y., et al. (2016). Cystic fibrosis gene modifier SLC26A9 modulates airway response to CFTR-directed therapeutics. *Hum. Mol. Genet.* 25, 4590–4600. doi: 10.1093/hmg/ddw290

Sui, Y., Wu, F., Lv, J., Li, H., Li, X., Du, Z., et al. (2015). Identification of the novel TMEM16A Inhibitor dehydroandrographolide and its anticancer activity on SW620 cells. *PLoS ONE* 10:e0144715. doi: 10.1371/journal.pone.0144715

Sun, L., Rommens, J. M., Corvol, H., Li, W., Li, X., Chiang, T. A., et al. (2012). Multiple apical plasma membrane constituents are associated with susceptibility to meconium ileus in individuals with cystic fibrosis. *Nat. Genet.* 44, 562–569. doi: 10.1038/ng.2221

Suzuki, J., Umeda, M., Sims, P. J., and Nagata, S. (2010). Calcium-dependent phospholipid scrambling by TMEM16F. *Nature* 468, 834–838. doi: 10.1038/nature09583

Ta, C. M., Adomaviciene, A., Rorsman, N. J., Garnett, H., and Tammaro, P. (2016). Mechanism of allosteric activation of TMEM16A/ANO1 channels by a commonly used chloride channel blocker. *Br. J. Pharmacol.* 173, 511–528. doi: 10.1111/bph.13381

Tang, L., Fatehi, M., and Linsdell, P. (2009). Mechanism of direct bicarbonate transport by the CFTR anion channel. *J. Cyst. Fibros.* 8, 115–121. doi: 10.1016/j.jcf.2008.10.004

Taylor-Cousar, J. L., Munck, A., Mckone, E. F., Van Der Ent, C. K., Moeller, A., Simard, C., et al. (2017). Tezacaftor-Ivacaftor in patients with cystic fibrosis homozygous for Phe508del. *N. Engl. J. Med.* 377, 2013–2023. doi: 10.1056/NEJMoa1709846

Tian, Y., Schreiber, R., and Kunzelmann, K. (2012a). Anoctamins are a family of Ca^{2+} activated Cl^{-} channels. *J. Cell Sci.* 125, 4991–4998. doi: 10.1242/jcs.109553

Tian, Y., Schreiber, R., Wanitchakool, P., Kongsuphol, P., Sousa, M., Uliyakina, I., et al. (2012b). Control of TMEM16A by INO-4995 and other inositolphosphates. *Br. J. Pharmacol.* 168, 253–265. doi: 10.1111/j.1476-5381.2012.02193.x

Tirkos, S., Newbigging, S., Nguyen, V., Keet, M., Ackerley, C., Kent, G., et al. (2006). Expression of S100A8 correlates with inflammatory lung disease in congenic mice deficient of the cystic fibrosis transmembrane conductance regulator. *Respir. Res.* 7:51. doi: 10.1186/1465-9921-7-51

Tradtrantip, L., Namkung, W., and Verkman, A. S. (2010). Crofelemer, an antisecretory antidiarrheal proanthocyanidin oligomer extracted from *Croton lechleri*, targets two distinct intestinal chloride channels. *Mol. Pharmacol.* 77, 69–78. doi: 10.1124/mol.109.061051

Trout, L., King, M., Feng, W., Inglis, S. K., and Ballard, S. T. (1998). Inhibition of airway liquid secretion and its effect on the physical properties of airway mucus. *Am. J. Physiol.* 274, L258–L263. doi: 10.1152/ajplung.1998.274.2.L258

Truong, E. C., Phuan, P. W., Reggi, A. L., Ferrera, L., Galietta, L. J. V., Levy, S. E., et al. (2017). Substituted 2-acylaminocycloalkylthiophene-3-carboxylic acid arylamides as inhibitors of the calcium-activated chloride channel transmembrane protein 16A (TMEM16A). *J. Med. Chem.* 60, 4626–4635. doi: 10.1021/acs.jmedchem.7b00020

Vajanaphanich, M., Schultz, C., Rudolf, M. T., Wasserman, M., Enyedi, P., Craxton, A., et al. (1994). Long-term uncoupling of chloride secretion from intracellular calcium levels by Ins(3,4,5,6)P_4. *Nature* 371, 711–714. doi: 10.1038/371711a0

Van Goor, F., Hadida, S., Grootenhuis, P. D., Burton, B., Cao, D., Neuberger, T., et al. (2009). Rescue of CF airway epithelial cell function *in vitro* by a CFTR potentiator, VX-770. *Proc. Natl. Acad. Sci. U.S.A.* 106, 18825–18830. doi: 10.1073/pnas.0904709106

Van Goor, F., Hadida, S., Grootenhuis, P. D., Burton, B., Stack, J. H., Straley, K. S., et al. (2011). Correction of the F508del-CFTR protein processing defect *in vitro* by the investigational drug VX-809. *Proc. Natl. Acad. Sci. U.S.A.* 108, 18843–18848. doi: 10.1073/pnas.1105787108

Veit, G., Avramescu, R. G., Perdomo, D., Phuan, P. W., Bagdany, M., Apaja, P. M., et al. (2014). Some gating potentiators, including VX-770, diminish DeltaF508-CFTR functional expression. *Sci. Transl. Med.* 6:246ra297. doi: 10.1126/scitranslmed.3008889

Verkman, A. S., and Galietta, L. J. (2009). Chloride channels as drug targets. *Nat. Rev. Drug Discov.* 8, 153–171. doi: 10.1038/nrd2780

Villalba, J. M., Parrado, C., Santos-Gonzalez, M., and Alcain, F. J. (2010). Therapeutic use of coenzyme Q10 and coenzyme Q10-related compounds and formulations. *Expert Opin. Investig. Drugs* 19, 535–554. doi: 10.1517/13543781003727495

Wainwright, C. E., Elborn, J. S., Ramsey, B. W., Marigowda, G., Huang, X., Cipolli, M., et al. (2015). Lumacaftor-Ivacaftor in patients with cystic fibrosis homozygous for Phe508del CFTR. *N. Engl. J. Med.* 373, 220–231. doi: 10.1056/NEJMoa1409547

Walker, N. M., Simpson, J. E., Levitt, R. C., Boyle, K. T., and Clarke, L. L. (2006). Talniflumate increases survival in a cystic fibrosis mouse model of distal intestinal obstructive syndrome. *J. Pharmacol. Exp. Ther.* 317, 275–283. doi: 10.1124/jpet.105.094847

Wang, H., Zou, L., Ma, K., Yu, J., Wu, H., Wei, M., et al. (2017). Cell-specific mechanisms of TMEM16A Ca^{2+}-activated chloride channel in cancer. *Mol. Cancer* 16:152. doi: 10.1186/s12943-017-0720-x

Wang, P., Zhao, W., Sun, J., Tao, T., Chen, X., Zheng, Y. Y., et al. (2018). Inflammatory mediators mediate airway smooth muscle contraction through a GPCR-TMEM16A-VDCC axis and contribute to bronchial hyperresponsiveness in asthma. *J. Allergy Clin. Immunol.* 141, 1259–1268. doi: 10.1016/j.jaci.2017.05.053

Wanitchakool, P., Ousingsawat, J., Sirianant, L., Macaulay, N., Schreiber, R., and Kunzelmann, K. (2016). Cl^{-} channels in apoptosis. *Eur. Biophys. J.* 45, 599–610. doi: 10.1007/s00249-016-1140-3

Wanitchakool, P., Wolf, L., Koehl, G., Sirianant, L., Gaumann, A., Schreiber, R., et al. (2014). Role of anoctamins in cancer and apoptosis. *Philos. Trans. R. Soc. Lond. B Biol. Sci.* 369:20130096. doi: 10.1098/rstb.2013.0096

Wei, L., Vankeerberghen, A., Cuppens, H., Eggermont, J., Cassiman, J. J., Droogmans, G., et al. (1999). Interaction between calcium-activated chloride channels and the cystic fibrosis transmembrane conductance regulator. *Pflugers Arch.* 438, 635–641. doi: 10.1007/s004249900108

White, M. M., and Aylwin, M. (1990). Niflumic and flufenamic acids are potent reversible blockers of Ca^{2+}-activated Cl^{-} channels in *Xenopus* oocytes. *Mol. Pharmacol.* 37, 720–724.

Wilke, M., Buijs-Offerman, R. M., Aarbiou, J., Colledge, W. H., Sheppard, D. N., Touqui, L., et al. (2011). Mouse models of cystic fibrosis: phenotypic analysis and research applications. *J. Cyst. Fibros.* 10 (Suppl. 2), S152–171. doi: 10.1016/S1569-1993(11)60020-9

Yang, H., Kim, A., David, T., Palmer, D., Jin, T., Tien, J., et al. (2012). TMEM16F forms a Ca^{2+}-activated cation channel required for lipid scrambling in platelets during blood coagulation. *Cell* 151, 111–122. doi: 10.1016/j.cell.2012.07.036

Yang, Y. D., Cho, H., Koo, J. Y., Tak, M. H., Cho, Y., Shim, W. S., et al. (2008). TMEM16A confers receptor-activated calcium-dependent chloride conductance. *Nature* 455, 1210–1215. doi: 10.1038/nature07313

Yerxa, B. R., Sabater, J. R., Davis, C. W., Stutts, M. J., Lang-Furr, M., Picher, M., et al. (2002). Pharmacology of INS37217 [P(1)-(uridine 5')-P(4)- (2'-deoxycytidine 5')tetraphosphate, tetrasodium salt], a next-generation P2Y(2) receptor agonist for the treatment of cystic fibrosis. *J Pharmacol. Exp. Ther.* 302, 871–880. doi: 10.1124/jpet.102.035485

Yim, P. D., Gallos, G., Perez-Zoghbi, J. F., Trice, J., Zhang, Y., Siviski, M., et al. (2013). Chloride channel blockers promote relaxation of TEA-induced contraction in airway smooth muscle. *J. Smooth Muscle Res.* 49, 112–124. doi: 10.1540/jsmr.49.112

Zabner, J., Smith, J. J., Karp, P. H., Widdicombe, J. H., and Welsh, M. J. (1998). Loss of CFTR chloride channels alters salt absorption by cystic fibrosis airway epithelia *in vitro*. *Mol. Cell* 2, 397–403. doi: 10.1016/S1097-2765(00)80284-1

Zhang, C. H., Li, Y., Zhao, W., Lifshitz, L. M., Li, H., Harfe, B. D., et al. (2013). The transmembrane protein 16A Ca^{2+}-activated Cl^{-} channel in airway smooth muscle contributes to airway hyperresponsiveness. *Am. J. Respir. Crit. Care Med.* 187, 374–381. doi: 10.1164/rccm.201207-1303OC

11

Anion-Transport Mechanism of a Triazole-Bearing Derivative of Prodigiosine: A Candidate for Cystic Fibrosis Therapy

*Claudia Cossu[1], Michele Fiore[1], Debora Baroni[1], Valeria Capurro[2], Emanuela Caci[2], Maria Garcia-Valverde[3], Roberto Quesada[3] and Oscar Moran[1]**

[1] *Istituto di Biofisica, Consiglio Nazionale Delle Ricerche, Genova, Italy,* [2] *U.O.C. Genetica Medica, Istituto Giannina Gaslini, Genova, Italy,* [3] *Departamento de Química, Facultad de Ciencias, Universidad de Burgos, Burgos, Spain*

***Correspondence:**
Oscar Moran
oscar.moran@cnr.it

Cystic fibrosis (CF) is a genetic lethal disease, originated from the defective function of the CFTR protein, a chloride and bicarbonate permeable transmembrane channel. CF mutations affect CFTR protein through a variety of molecular mechanisms which result in different functional defects. Current therapeutic approaches are targeted to specific groups of patients that share a common functional defect. We seek to develop an innovative therapeutic approach for the treatment of CF using anionophores, small molecules that facilitate the transmembrane transport of anions. We have characterized the anion transport mechanism of a synthetic molecule based on the structure of prodigiosine, a red pigment produced by bacteria. Anionophore-driven chloride efflux from large unilamellar vesicles is consistent with activity of an uniporter carrier that facilitates the transport of anions through lipid membranes down the electrochemical gradient. There are no evidences of transport coupling with protons. The selectivity sequence of the prodigiosin inspired EH160 ionophore is formate > acetate > nitrate > chloride > bicarbonate. Sulfate, phosphate, aspartate, isothionate, and gluconate are not significantly transported by these anionophores. Protonation at acidic pH is important for the transport capacity of the anionophore. This prodigiosin derived ionophore induces anion transport in living cells. Its low toxicity and capacity to transport chloride and bicarbonate, when applied at low concentration, constitute a promising starting point for the development of drug candidates for CF therapy.

Keywords: cystic fibrosis, ionophore, ion transport, phospholipid vesicles, prodigiosin derivatives

INTRODUCTION

Cystic fibrosis (CF), the most common autosomal recessive lethal genetic disease in the Caucasian population (Strausbaugh and Davis, 2007), is caused by mutations on the gene coding for CFTR (cystic fibrosis transmembrane conductance regulator), an anion selective channel that transports chloride and bicarbonate in the apical membrane of epithelium. CFTR regulates salt and water transport across a variety of epithelium, and malfunction of this protein leads to defective mucus and airway surface liquid (ASL) properties, resulting in poor mucus clearance and bacterial infections on the airways (Berger et al., 1991; Saint-Criq and Gray, 2017). More than 1,500 mutations in CFTR, classified in six classes according to the effect of the mutation, lead to anion transport defects in epithelium by various mechanisms (failure to synthesize the protein, processing flaws, gating or conductance defects, reduced expression). In cell models, several small molecules, called correctors, increase CFTR defective expression at the cell membrane, and small molecules called potentiators to enhance the function of the CFTR channel (Zegarra-Moran and Galietta, 2017). While the potentiator ivacaftor (Kalydeco™) is successfully used for treatment in patients with gating mutations (Ramsey et al., 2011; De Boeck and Davies, 2017), the corrector lumacaftor, alone or in the combination with ivacaftor (Orkambi™) resulted on a limited clinical outcome (Clancy et al., 2012; Wainwright et al., 2015).

The discovery of small molecules capable to transport anions across lipid bilayers, named anionophores, has offered the opportunity of designing new substances to be used for pharmacological purposes (Davis et al., 2010; Valkenier et al., 2014; Hernando et al., 2018). The most striking among the potential applications of anionophores is the proposal to use these substances to substitute the defective anion transport in cystic fibrosis (CF). The idea of using anionophores to replace the defective CFTR protein has the advantage to become a general therapy for CF, that would be independent of the specific mutation. Different chemical structures have been described to transport anions across lipid bilayers, including prodigiosin and obatoclax derivatives (Seganish and Davis, 2005; Díaz de Greñu et al., 2011; García-Valverde et al., 2012; Gale et al., 2013), marine alkaloids such as tambjamines (Iglesias Hernández et al., 2012; Saggiomo et al., 2012; Hernando et al., 2014; Soto-Cerrato et al., 2015), steroid-based "cholapods" (Koulov et al., 2003; McNally et al., 2008; Valkenier et al., 2014), and calix[4]pyrrole derivatives (Gale et al., 2017), anion channel-forming peptides (Wallace et al., 2000; Broughman et al., 2004; Pajewski et al., 2006) and Calix[4]arene amides (Sidorov et al., 2002).

We have previously identified several triazole derivatives of prodigiosin with a significant anion transport capacity and relatively low toxicity (Hernando et al., 2018). There, we show that these compounds can transport chloride and bicarbonate across lipid bilayers, and the transport activity increases at acidic pH. Also evidences of anionophore-driven halides transport in cells is provided. Hence, to follow the search of "druggable" anionophores adequate for CF therapy, we have undertaken the analysis of the transmembrane anion transport mechanism of these molecules. Thus, for the functional characterization of this anionophore family, we chose of the most active substance of that series, EH160 (named **1b** in reference Hernando et al., 2018). Here, we have extended the data previously reported (Hernando et al., 2018), analysing the selectivity of the anionophore, demonstrating that the carrier has a good selectivity for physiologically relevant anions, such as chloride and bicarbonate. An important finding was that pH influence on the ionization state determines the anionophore activity, without any proton transport. We showed that this prodigiosin-inspired anionophore act as electro-neutral anion exchanger. To reinforce the concept that anionophores can induce chloride transport in mammalian cells, we repeated chloride efflux and iodide influx experiments in cells, similar to those reported elsewhere (Hernando et al., 2018).

MATERIALS AND METHODS

Synthesis of the Anionophore EH160

EH160 was synthesized as previously described (Hernando et al., 2018). In brief, it was prepared by acid-catalyzed condensation of 3-methoxy-5-(1-butyl-1H-1,2,3-triazol-4-yl)-1H-pyrrole-2-carbaldehyde and 2-methyl-3-pentyl-1H-pyrrole. The precursor aldehyde was prepared by standard click chemistry reaction between 1-azidobutane and the corresponding 5-ethynylpyrrole carbaldehyde. The compound is inspired by the structure of natural products prodiginines, replacing one of the pyrrole groups by a 1,2,3-triazole moiety. EH160 was fully characterized by mass spectroscopy and NMR (Hernando et al., 2018). Except when indicated, all chemicals were purchased from Sigma-Aldrich.

Large Unilamellar Vesicles

Asolectin large unilamellar vesicles (LUV) were made from phospholipids films (Baroni et al., 2014; Nicastro et al., 2016; Hernando et al., 2018). Soybean phospholipids (20 mg/ml) were dissolved in chloroform and lipid films were obtained by evaporation of the solvent under a gentle nitrogen flux; in order to remove all chloroform, films were further dried overnight in vacuum. The phospholipids were hydrated in chloride buffer (in mM: NaCl 450, 20 mM HEPES; pH 7.5, unless other composition was indicated), and vigorously vortex mixed and, to ensure equilibration, sonicated in 5 cycles of 1.5 min each, with 1 min rest, in ice. Liposomes were centrifuged at 2,000 g for 5–10 min to remove any titanium particles released by the sonicator tip. Large unilamellar vesicles (LUV) were then obtained by extrusion through polycarbonate filters mounted in a mini-extruder (Lipofast, Avestin, Mannheim, Germany). Samples were subjected to 19 passes through a single 100 nm mesh filter (MacDonald et al., 1991). External solution was exchanged twice on a Sephadex G25 column previously equilibrated with the external chloride-free solution: $NaNO_3$ 450 mM, 20 mM HEPES; pH 7.5 (unless other composition was indicated).

Chloride Efflux Measurements in LUV

To measure the efflux of chloride from LUV, chloride concentration was measured with an ion-sensitive electrode (Vernier, Beaverton, Oregon, USA) in a constantly stirred 3.5 ml LUV suspension. Data were acquired using a LabQuest mini interface (Vernier). Ionophores were dissolved in DMSO to a concentration of 10 mM. After an initial equilibration, chloride efflux was induced by a small volume (<1%) of ionophore. Control experiments where similar amounts of DMSO (without anionophores) were added demonstrated that these concentrations of DMSO do not induce any chloride efflux (see below). The measurement was concluded with the addition of the detergent polyoxyethylene 10 tridecyl ether (C13E10) to break off the bilayers and measure the maximum chloride encapsulated in the LUV. The time course of the chloride concentration, *Cl*, in the experiment can be described by a single exponential function:

$$Cl^-(t) = Cl_0^- + \Delta Cl^- \left(1 - \exp\left[-tk\right]\right) \qquad (1)$$

where Cl_0^- is the initial chloride concentration, ΔCl^- is the maximum change of the chloride concentration (after addition of detergent), and k is the rate constant of the process. The chloride efflux, J_{cl}, is defined as the time derivative of $Cl^-(t)$. Thus, deriving from equation (1), for $t = 0$, i.e., after the chloride gradient was changed, we obtain the initial chloride efflux-rate, J_0:

$$J_0 = \Delta Cl^- k \qquad (2)$$

To compare different data sets, the chloride concentration was normalized to the maximum concentration change, ΔCl^-. Data are expressed as means ± s.e.m. Experiments were done at 25 ± 1°C. Every experimental condition was repeated at least three times.

Cell Preparation and Viability

The Human embryonic kidney (HEK) cell lines were grown in standard conditions, in Ham's F10 medium supplemented with 2 mM L-glutamine and 10% fetal bovine serum (FBS). Cell toxicity was evaluated by the trypan blue exclusion staining method (Louis and Siegel, 2011). Toxicity data is expressed as the half maximum toxic dose (TD_{50}).

Chloride Efflux in Cells

Cells at 80% confluence were detached from the bottom of the flask by soft scrapping, washed in chloride-free solution, and used immediately. For chloride efflux measurement, ~2×10^6 cells were suspended in 4 ml of buffer containing (in mM): 136 $NaNO_3$, 3 KNO_3, 2 $Ca(NO_3)_2$, 20 HEPES, 11 Glucose, pH 7.4. Ionophores were dissolved in DMSO to a concentration of 10 mM. Chloride concentration in the extracellular solution was continuously measured with a chloride-sensitive electrode. After an initial equilibration, chloride efflux was induced by a small volume (<1%) of ionophore. The measurement was concluded with the addition of the sodium dodecyl sulfate (SDS) to break off the membranes and measure the total chloride content in the cells. Experiments were done at 25 ± 1°C.

Iodine Influx in Cells

The activity of anionophores was determined in Fisher Rat Thyroid (FRT) cells expressing the halide-sensitive YFP protein as previously described (Caci et al., 2008). The assay is based in the fact that the fluorescence of the YFP protein is quenched to a greater extend by I^- than by Cl^- (Galietta et al., 2001). FRT cells stably transfected with a halide-sensitive yellow fluorescent protein (YFP-H148Q/I152L) were plated on 96-well micro-plates at a density of 40,000 cells/well in Coon's modified medium supplemented with 10% serum, 2 mM L-glutamine, 1 mg/ml penicillin, 100 μg/ml streptomycin, and 0.5 mg/ml hygromycin as selection agent for the YFP. Cells were maintained at 37°C in a 5% CO_2 /95% air atmosphere. Functional experiments were done 48 h after cell seeding. Cells were washed twice, with an external solution containing (in mM): NaCl 137, KCl 2.7, Na_2HPO_4 8.1, KH_2PO_4 1.5, $CaCl_2$ 1 and $MgCl_2$ 0.5 (pH 7.3). The solution injected during the assay is similar but contained NaI 137 mM instead of NaCl (pH 7.3). To explore the effect of lowering the extracellular pH, the NaI solution was buffered at pH 6.9 with HEPES, or at pH 6.6 and 6.2 using MES. For the iodide influx assay, after washing, cells were incubated in 60 μl of the 137 mM NaCl-external solution, supplemented with the anionophore or with DMSO as control. A fluorescence baseline was recorded for 2 s after injection of 165 μl of NaI-external solution, so that the final concentration of NaI in the well is 100 mM. The iodide influx was observed as quenching of the YFP fluorescence.

RESULTS

Application of micromolar concentrations of anionophores to a LUV suspension induces a chloride efflux. In **Figure 1A** we show the time course of chloride efflux measured upon the application of 4 μM of prodigiosine and the triazole derivative EH160. The natural product, prodigiosine, is a more effective transporter, with a J_0 of 110.2 ± 1.2 μM/s. Instead, the triazole derivative EH160 induces a slower chloride efflux of 51.8 ± 0.5 μM/s. Application of DMSO does not induce a significant chloride efflux (J_0 of 0.2 ± 2.8 μM/s), confirming that the anion efflux was elicited by the anionophore and not by the solvent. Similar experiments were done using LUV formed with chemically defined phospholipids (palmitoyl-oleyl-phosphatidylcholine,

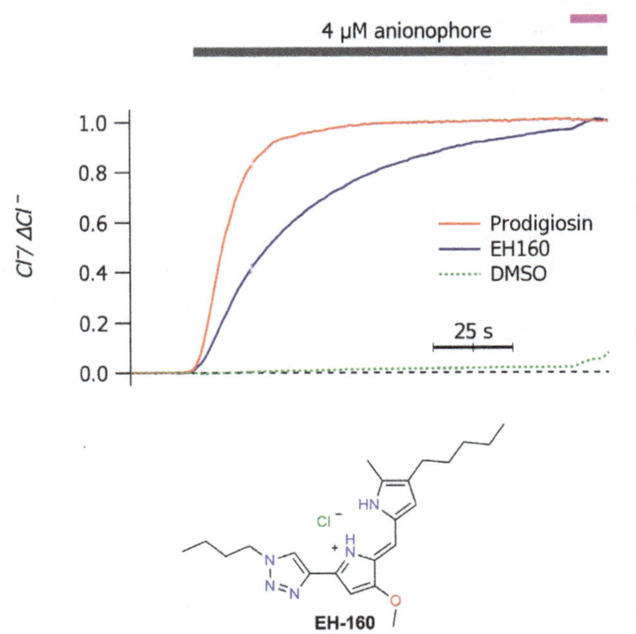

FIGURE 1 | Time course of the external concentration of chloride in a LUV suspension upon application of 4 μM of prodigiosin and EH160, as indicated by the upper bar. The magenta bar indicates the addition of detergent. A control trace was obtained after the application of DMSO. Data was normalized by the maximum chloride change, ΔCl^-. The chemical structure of EH160 is shown at the bottom.

POPC; palmitoyl-oleyl-phosphatidylethanolamine, POPE) and cholesterol (chol). Anionophore-driven chloride efflux measured in LUV composed by POPC:chol (19:1) (48.9 ± 0.4 μM/s), POPC:POPE (9:1) (52.3 ± 0.2 μM/s) and POPC:POPE:chol (8.1:0.9:1) (47.1 ± 0.9 μM/s), was very similar to that measured in asolectin LUV, indicating that the lipid composition is not critical for the anionophore transport (data not shown). Similarly, substitution of sodium by potassium in the internal or in the external solutions does not affect the measured chloride efflux, confirming that EH160 is an anion selective carrier.

The chloride efflux rate depends on the concentration of anionophore (see **Figure 2A**). To evaluate the concentration to induce half of the maximum rate, EC_{50}, was estimated plotting the initial efflux rate, J_0, against the anionophore concentration, [EH160] (**Figure 2B**). Data was fitted with the Equation (3):

$$J_0 = \frac{J_{max}}{1 + \frac{EC_{50}}{[EH160]}} \tag{3}$$

where $Jmax$ is the maximum chloride efflux initial rate. The time course of the traces obtained at EH160 concentration higher than 10 μM was often quite variable. We interpreted these data as a destabilization of the LUV bilayers. Thus, to remove these possible outliers, we fitted iteratively the data, removing data points that lie beyond the 95% confidence prediction interval at each iteration, until no outliers remain. After this procedure, the doses-response fit yielded a maximum initial chloride efflux of 87.3 ± 6.4 μM/s, and an EC_{50} of 5.64 ± 1.28 μM.

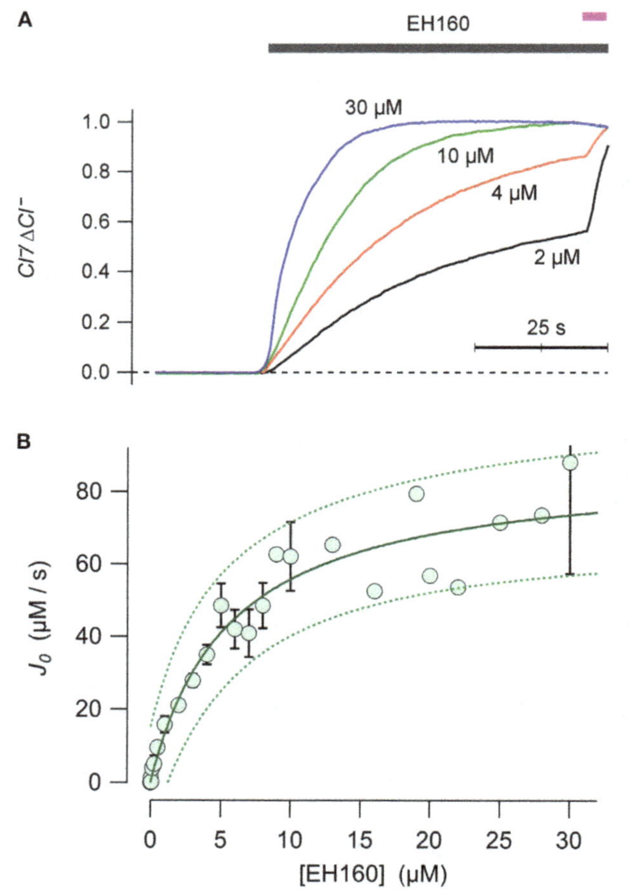

FIGURE 2 | (A) Time course of external concentration of chloride elicited by various concentrations of EH160, as shown near each trace. Application of the anionophore is indicated by the upper horizontal bar, and the addition of detergent is indicated by the magenta bar. Data was normalized by the maximum anion change, ΔCl^-. **(B)** The initial chloride efflux rate, J_0 is plotted against the anionophore concentration. When the measurement was repeated more than once, data represent the average and the bar is the standard error of the mean. The continuous line is the best fit of data with equation 3, yielding the concentration for the half of the maximum effect, $EC_{50} = 5.6$ μM, and a maximum chloride initial efflux rate of 87.3 μmoles/s. Broken lines represent the prediction interval for 95% confidence.

Selectivity of the Anionophore

To evaluate the selectivity of the anionophores, we measured the chloride efflux from LUV with an internal concentration of 450 mM chloride, and the external solution containing an isomolar concentration of different anions. Measurements were done in the presence of 10 mM HEPES to adjust the pH at 7.5 in both compartments. As no differences in the chloride efflux were observed substituting sodium by potassium, neither, in the internal solution nor in the external solutions, the cationic ion was used indifferently in this series of experiments. The time course of the chloride efflux measured with different external anions is shown in **Figure 3A**.

As a first approach, we could hypothesize that the anionophore interchanges the anions from both sides of the bilayer, and the chloride efflux is proportional to the efficiency of the counter-anion influx. Thus, the estimation of the initial rate of the chloride efflux should represent the permeability of the external anion. From these data (**Figure 3B**), we can assert that the anionophore EH160 has a consistent transport rate for small organic anions, as acetate and formate, and in less extend for inorganic anions, as nitrate and bicarbonate. Conversely, transport of bigger, more hydrophilic anions, as aspartate, gluconate, phosphate, sulfate, and isethionate, is more than ten-fold reduced.

However, in this experimental design it is not possible to use external chloride to compare the relative permeability of this anion with other anions. To overcome this limitation we designed a series of experiments in which a fraction of the internal chloride was substituted by nitrate or bicarbonate. Thus, the second anion will compete with chloride for binding the anionophore, and therefore, the chloride efflux will be modified accordingly. The initial chloride efflux rates, measured for different combinations of chloride/nitrate and chloride/bicarbonate at the internal side are shown in **Figures 3C,D**, respectively. The reduction of the chloride efflux, as the concentration of the second anion increases, occurs because the carrier binds bicarbonate or nitrate instead of chloride, resembling a competitive inhibition of an enzyme. Hence, the continuous lines in **Figures 3C,D** represent the best fits of data with:

$$\frac{J_0\left(Cl^-, anion\right)}{J_0\left(Cl^-, 0\right)} = \frac{Cl^-}{K_{Cl}\left(1 + \frac{anion}{K_{anion}}\right) + Cl^-} \tag{4}$$

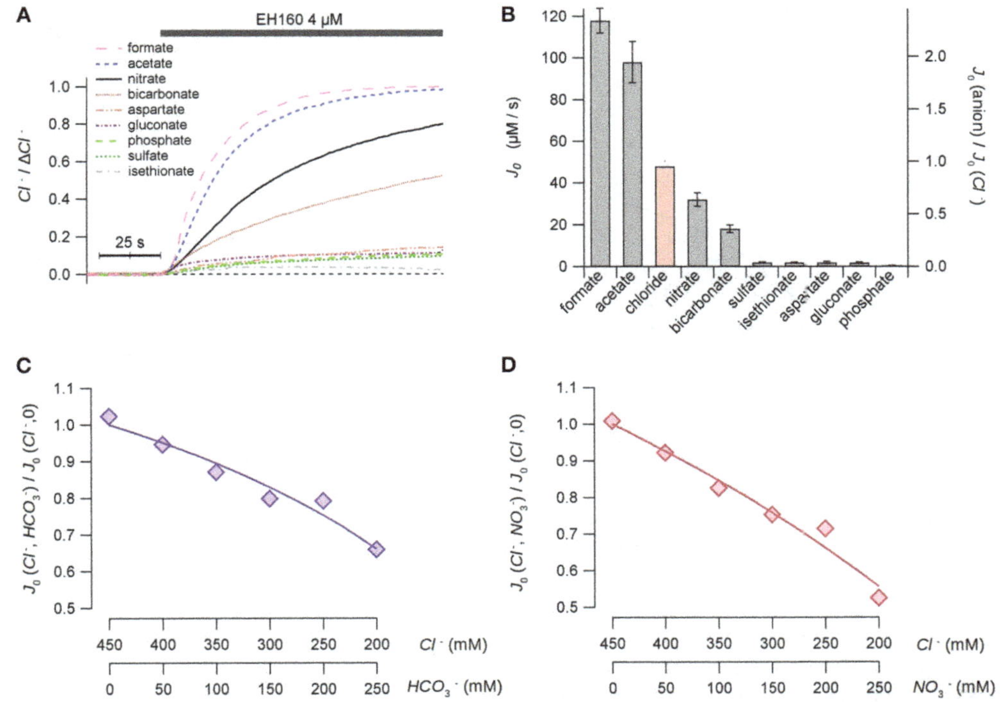

FIGURE 3 | Permeability of the anionophore EH160 to different anions. **(A)** Time course of the external concentration of chloride measured in LUV with 450 mM internal chloride and variable external iso-osmotic anions, as indicated in the figure. The application of the anionophore is indicated in the upper bar. Data was normalized by the maximum anion change, ΔCl^{-}. **(B)** The initial chloride efflux, J_0, measured for different external anions. The red bar is the estimated chloride efflux in the presence of external chloride, calculated from the apparent dissociation constants of the anionophore for chloride bicarbonate and nitrate estimates in the competition experiments. Data represent the average (± s.e.m.) of, at least, three different measurements. Panels **(C,D)** show the results of the bicarbonate/chloride and nitrate/chloride competition experiments, respectively. The concentrations of anions are shown in the bottom axes of the figures. The continuous lines represent the best fit of data with Equation (4).

where K_{cl} and K_{anion} are the apparent dissociation constants of chloride and the second anion (nitrate or bicarbonate), respectively. The average chloride apparent dissociation constant is $K_{cl} = 3.17 \pm 0.48$ mM, and the apparent dissociation constants for nitrate and bicarbonate are $K_{NO_3} = 4.79 \pm 0.67$ mM and $K_{HCO_3} = 8.18 \pm 0.71$ mM. The higher affinity of chloride (lower apparent dissociation constant) clearly reflects a higher permeability of this ion. Thus, we can assume that the ratio of the apparent dissociation constants $K_{NO_3}/K_{HCO_3} = 0.59$ is proportional to the bicarbonate:nitrate permeability ratio. This concept is confirmed by the ratio of the initial efflux rates of 0.57, measured with bicarbonate and nitrate in the external solution (**Figure 3A**). These data allow to estimate the hypothetical chloride initial efflux rate when the external solution is chloride, yielding a value of 48 μM/s. Scaling data to the theoretical chloride initial efflux rate it is possible to estimate the relative permeability of all assayed ions with respect of chloride, as shown in the right axis in **Figure 3B**.

It is intriguing to notice that when nominally impermeable anions, such as sulfate and gluconate, are in the external solution, a tiny chloride efflux induced by anionophores is still measurable, although it is very small (chloride efflux of 1.96 and 1.75 μM/s for sulfate and gluconate, respectively). As previously reported (Hernando et al., 2018), in these cases, after the initial chloride efflux, the system seems to stop transport chloride, and no further changes in the external chloride concentration are measured by the ion sensitive electrode (see **Figure 4**). The trace in **Figure 4** show the time course of the external chloride concentration upon the addition of 8 μM EH160 in a suspension of LUV with the internal solution containing 450 mM chloride and the external solution of 450 μM gluconate. The initial chloride efflux is 3.4 μM/s, and the flux is arrested when the external chloride concentration is 0.11 × ΔCl. The successive addition of a permeable anion to the external solution, to a final concentration of 225 mM of nitrate, induces again a chloride efflux. The restarted efflux, $J_0 = 6.2$ μM/s, is larger than the efflux obtained with only gluconate in the external solution, even after the 11% reduction of the chloride gradient and the dilution of the anionophore. In the presence of external impermeable anions, the initial chloride efflux occurs until the net charge displacement, occurring when the chloride ions move outside from the LUV, is balanced by the potential difference because of the asymmetrical distribution of permeable ions.

Thus, to avoid the charge accumulation and be independent of the potential difference, we "shunted" the LUV bilayer with cationic carriers. The addition of valinomycin (0.5 ng/ml), a

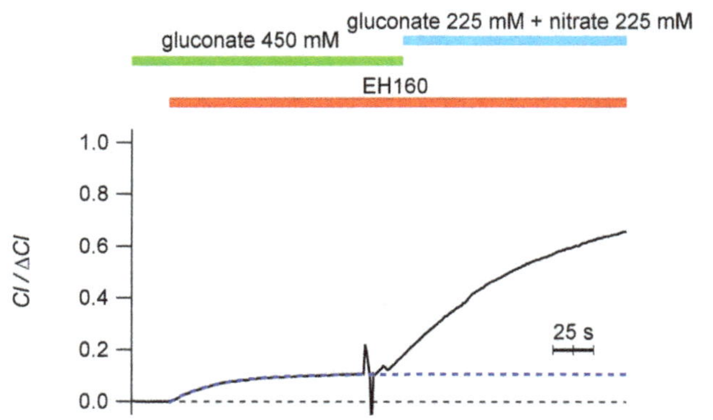

FIGURE 4 | Time course of the external concentration of chloride induced by the anionophore EH160 with different external anions, as indicated in the figure. When gluconate is in the external solution, chloride efflux is small, and is arrested without reaching the equilibria of concentrations (internal *Cl* = 49.5 mM; external *Cl* = 0.099 mM). Further addition of nitrate, a permeable anion, restores the normal anionophore-induced chloride efflux. Data was normalized by the maximum anion change, ΔCl^-.

specific potassium transporter, does not induce any chloride transport in the vesicles (**Figure 5A**), and does not modify the typical chloride efflux induced by the anionophore when the external ion is permeable. Differently, in the presence of an impermeable anion, as sulfate, addition of valinomycin restore the chloride efflux (**Figure 5B**). The same result, reactivation of the chloride efflux halted by an impermeable anion, gluconate outside, is obtained by the addition of 25 μg/ml of carbonyl cyanide-4-phenylhydrazone (FCCP), a proton ionophore (**Figure 5C**). The application of valinomycin before the addition of EH160 serves to condition the system to produce a chloride efflux in the presence of an external impermeable anion, as aspartate (**Figure 5A**, green trace).

Interestingly, in the presence of external impermeable anions, the time course of anionophore-driven chloride efflux favored by valinomycin is not exponential, but linear, as shown by the regression lines represented in blue in **Figure 5**; there, the correlation coefficient for a linear regression is $r > 0.999$, confirming the linearity of the traces. The exponential shape of the chloride efflux is due to the depletion of the anion from the LUV, that reduce the chloride gradient, and according to the Fick law, will reduce the anion flux. Conversely, the linear time course of the chloride efflux reflects a constant chloride gradient during the experiment.

This paradox may occur because, in the presence of the cation ionophore, the efflux of chloride driven by EH160 is accompanied with the facilitated efflux of potassium ions by valinomycin [or protons by cyanide-4-(trifluoromethoxy)phenylhydrazone, FCCP], thus maintaining the electro-neutrality of the process and resulting in a net solute loss from the LUV, with the consequent osmotic water withdrawal. The consequence is the maintenance of the concentration of the solutes, leaving essentially unaltered the ionic gradients.

To examine whether the anionophore-driven transport is affected by the electric field, we measured the chloride efflux at different electric potential differences. To impose a membrane potential difference, we prepared LUV with different combinations of sodium chloride and potassium chloride inside, and sodium nitrate and potassium nitrate outside. The anion

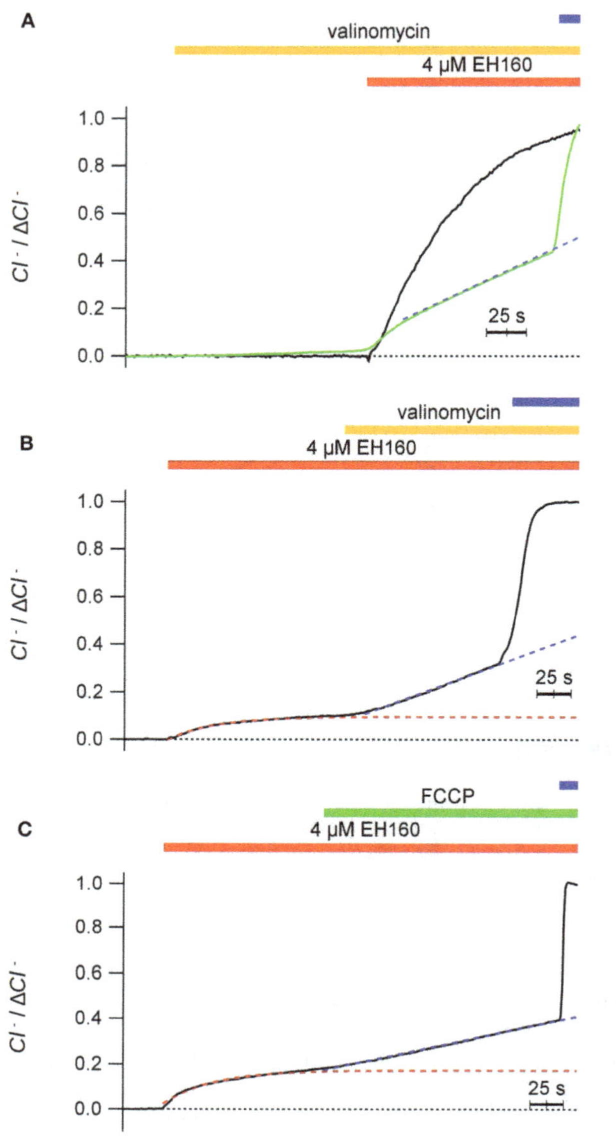

FIGURE 5 | Time course of the external concentration of chloride, revealing the anion efflux induced by the anionophore EH160 recorded in LUV shunted with a second ionophore. In all cases LUV had 450 mM internal potassium chloride and the application of 4 μM of EH160 is indicated by the horizontal (red) bar over the traces. Application of 0.5 ng/ml of valinomycin or 0.25 μg/ml of FCCP is indicated by the middle horizontal bar. The upper horizontal bar indicate the addition of detergent. Data was normalized by the maximum anion change, ΔCl^-. In panel **(A)**, the anionophore was added after the application of valinomicyn in preparations with the external solution containing 450 mM potassium nitrate (black trace) and 450 mM potassium aspartate (green trace); the external solution in panel **(B)** was 300 mM of potassium sulfate, and in panel **(C)** was 450 mM potassium gluconate. The blue broken lines are the lineal fitting of the traces after application of the cation ionophores. The red broken lines in panels **(B,C)** are the exponential fitting of the traces before the application of the cation ionophores.

gradient was always the same (450 mM chloride inside, and 450 mM nitrate outside). Because valinomycin is permeable to potassium, but does not transport sodium, the bilayer potential difference, according to the Nernst equation, depends on the potassium concentration at both sides. The initial chloride efflux, J_0, measured at potential differences between 50 to −150 mV (reference at the external side) resulted virtually independent from the voltage (**Figure 6**), indicating the EH160 activity is not voltage dependent.

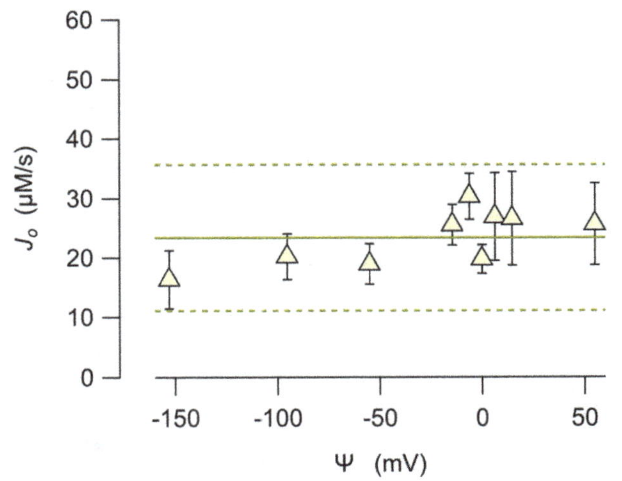

FIGURE 6 | EH160-driven chloride initial efflux, J_0, measured from LUV with 450 mM chloride in the internal solution, and 450 mM nitrate in the external solution. Different potassium concentrations at either side of the bilayer resulted in a potential difference, Ψ, by the presence of valinomycin (0.5 ng/ml). Symbols correspond to the mean values of, at least, three experiments, and the bars are the standard error of the mean. The continuous line is the average of all data, and the broken lines are the prediction limits with 95% confidence.

pH Dependence of EH160 Anionophore Activity

We have previously reported that the transport efficacy of EH160 in LUV strongly depends on pH (Hernando et al., 2018). In LUV with the same values of pH in the internal and external buffers, the rate of the chloride efflux carried by EH160 is faster at acidic pH than at alkaline (**Figure 7A**). This pH dependency of the anionophore activity is similar when the internal pH in the LUV is kept constant at 7.0, and the external pH is varied from 5.0 to 9.0 (**Figure 7B**). Conversely, when the external pH is kept fix at 7.0, variations of the internal pH in LUV from 5.0 to 9.0 does not determine any significant variation of the anionophore induced chloride efflux (**Figure 7C**).

An interesting feature of these observations is that the chloride efflux seems to be independent of the proton gradient. If the anionophore co-transports anions and protons, in absence of an active transport mechanism, it is expected that the gradient of both ligands should determine the transport rate. On the contrary, the chloride efflux in absence of a pH gradient (**Figure 7A**) varies in the same manner as observed in the experiments where a pH gradient was imposed varying the external pH (**Figure 7B**). Moreover, imposing a pH gradient varying the internal LUV pH, but maintaining the external pH constant does not modify the chloride efflux (**Figure 7C**). We conclude that the anionophore chloride transport is independent of the pH gradient, but depends only on the external pH. These data is consistent with the influence of pH in the ionization state at which the anionophore is incorporated into the membrane, but does not affect the ionic transport itself. To test this hypothesis, we compared the pH dependency of the initial chloride efflux, J_0, with the titration curve of the EH160. The titration curve was constructed plotting the ratio of absorbance measured at 502 and 474 nm of 20 μM EH160 against the pH of solvent buffer (**Figure 7D**, blue circles). These data were fitted with the Henderson–Hasselbach equation, yielding a pK_A of 6.47 ± 0.05. This titration curve can be superimposed with the plot of J_0 vs. the external pH (**Figure 7D**, pink squares), confirming that the pH dependence of the anionophore-driven chloride efflux corresponds to the ionization state of EH160. Noteworthy, in mammalian cells the maximum quenching rate of the YFP fluorescence measured at different extracellular pH can be easily superimposed to the EH160 titration curve (**Figure 7D**, green diamonds), further confirming the similarity of the behavior of EH160 in plasma membranes and in model bilayers. Remarkably, the pK_A values estimated for the measurement of chloride efflux in LUV, 6.66 ± 0.07, and influx of iodide in cells, 6.54 ± 0.19, are not significantly different from the pK_A yielded from the EH160 titration.

To further reinforce the idea that anion transport is not coupled with proton (or hydroxide) transport, we measured the EH160 induced chloride efflux in LUV with different pH gradients, to observe the effect of the collapse of the gradient with the proton carrier FCCP. In these experiments, 0.25 μg/ml of FCCP were added to the external solution before the application of the anionophore (**Figure 7E**). The collapse of the pH gradient, induced putative proton transport induced by the FCCP, does not produce any significant chloride efflux; then, application of the anionophore induced a measurable chloride efflux corresponding to the external pH. Similarly, a chloride efflux, correspondent to the external pH, is observed upon application of EH160, but further application of FCCP does not modify the chloride efflux time course (**Figure 7F**). Application of FCCP will plausibly equilibrate the pH to values near to the external pH, thus dissipating the pH gradient. Similar results were obtained in experiments where the pH gradient was dissipated with nigericin, that is another proton transporter (data not shown). Thus, the lack of effect of this action on the chloride efflux rules out the coupling of anion transport and proton transport for EH160, confirming the independence between the anion transport and the proton gradient present.

Anionophore-Driven Transport in Mammalian Cells

Since the ultimate objective of the characterization and further optimization of the anionophores is to open the possibility to

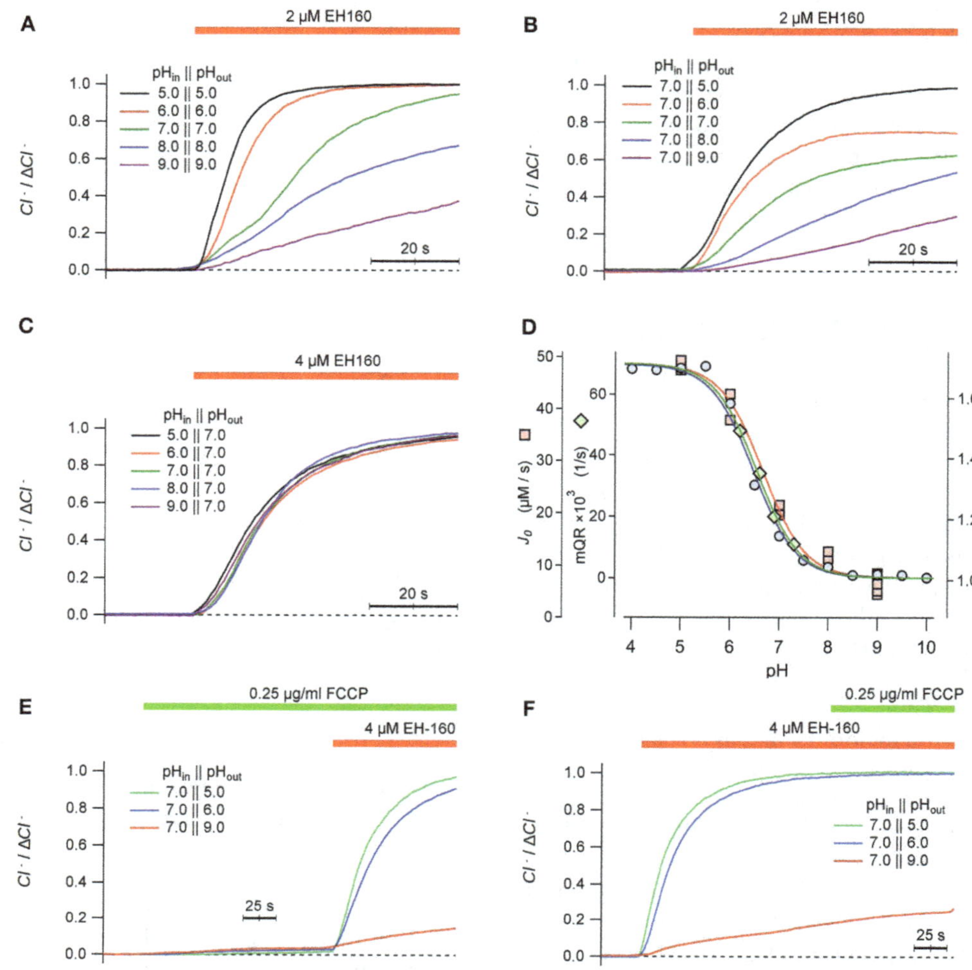

FIGURE 7 | Time course of the external concentration of chloride induced by the anionophore EH-160 was measured in LUV with 450 mM internal chloride and 450 mM external ions, in symmetric pH buffer **(A)** and asymmetrical pH buffer, varying either the external pH **(B)** and the internal pH **(C)**, as indicated in the figure. The application of the anionophore is indicated by the horizontal bar. **(D)** The initial influx rate measured in LUV, J_0, at different external pH is represented by squares; the maximum YFP-quenching rate, mQR, representing the iodide influx in FRT cells measured at different extracellular pH values, is pictured by diamonds. The ionic state of EH160, expressed as the ratios of absorbances at 502 and 474 nm (circles) is also plotted against the pH. The three continuous lines are the corresponding best fits of data with the Henderson-Hasselbach equation, normalized by the maximum and the minimum asymptotes. The time course of the external concentration of chloride measured in LUV treated with the proton ionophore FCCP prior the application of EH-160 **(E)**, or applying the proton ionophore FCCP after the induction of chloride efflux by the anionophore **(F)**, as shown by the horizontal bars.

use them in cells as therapeutic agents, we report the proof of concept that this class of carriers is able to transport anions in mammalian cells. Therefore, we have repeated the measurements of anionophore-driven iodine influx and chloride efflux in mammalian cells. The toxicity of EH-160 ($TD_{50} = 7.1 \pm 1.1\,\mu M$) is reduced respect to that of prodigiosin ($TD_{50} = 2.9 \pm 2.4\,\mu M$). **Figure 8A** shows the time course of the iodide quenching of the YFP fluorescence, representing the influx of the halide into the FRT cells. The iodide influx is clearly dependent of the concentration of EH160. Similarly, a chloride efflux was observed in HEK cells upon the application of the anionophore at different concentrations (**Figure 8C**). Quantification of the chloride efflux under these conditions was difficult because the removal of chloride from the external solution modifies the membrane potential and activates endogenous mechanism to maintain the cell homoeostasis that partially hidden the signal of anionophore-driven transport. It is, however, clear that EH160 induces halide transport in living mammalian cells.

Interestingly, the transport capacity of the anionophore also depends on the extracellular pH. Using both methods to display the anion transport in cells, the fluorescent probe to measure the iodide influx (**Figure 8B**), and the use of ISE to evaluate the chloride efflux (**Figure 8D**), we observed that the efficacy of transport increases as the extracellular pH is more acidic, similarly as observed for the measurements in LUV. We conclude that the transport properties of the triazole derivative of prodigiosine in mammalian cells are similar to those observed in LUV.

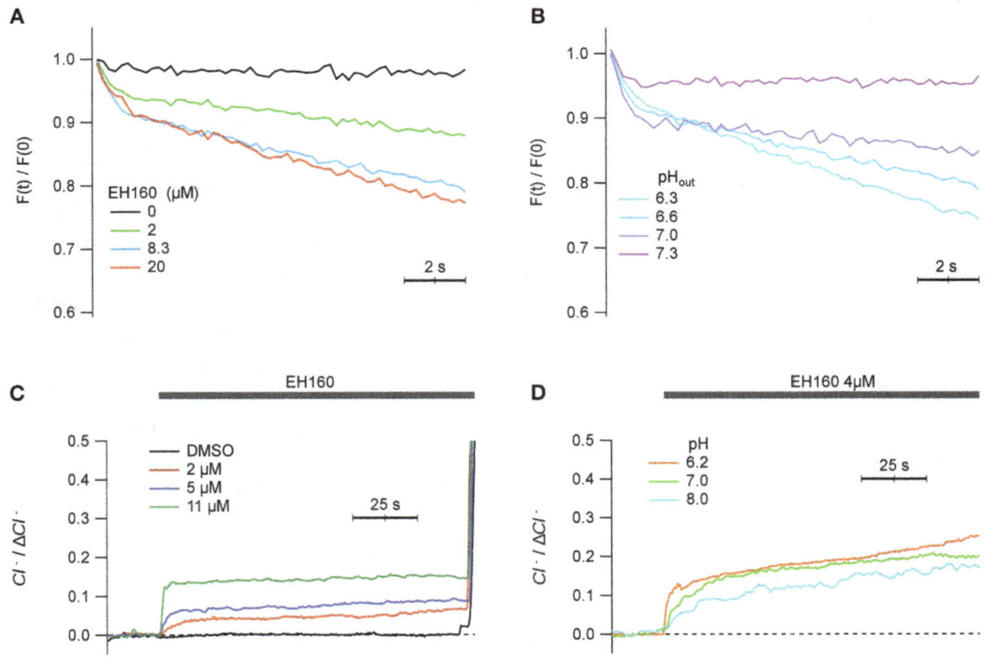

FIGURE 8 | Anionophore-driven transport in mammalian cells. **(A,B)** show the time course of the iodide-sensitive YFP fluorescence, normalized by the initial fluorescence [F(t)/F(0)], measured in FRT cells after the addition of 100 mM iodide in the external solution. The decrease of the fluorescence, due to the quenching of YFP fluorescence by iodide, represents the influx of the halide. Each trace is the average of three measurements. **(A)** Traces obtained with the treatment of cells with different concentrations of EH160, at pH 6.6. **(B)** Different efficacy of 8.2 μM EH160 at different extracellular pH. **(C,D)** represents the time course of the external concentration of chloride on HEK cells perfused with different EH160 concentrations **(C)** and at different pH **(D)**. Data was normalized by the maximum anion change, ΔCl^{-}.

DISCUSSION

We have examined the properties of a prodigiosin-inspired anionophore to characterize its anion transport properties. A detectable chloride efflux was measured in LUV for the 1,2,3-triazole heterocycle assayed, EH160 at micromolar concentrations (**Figure 1A**). At equimolar concentrations, the natural product prodigiosin showed a considerable higher potency than EH160. Notably, the application of the anionophore solvent, DMSO, does not induce any chloride efflux in LUV (**Figure 1A**), confirming that the results reflect the anion transport driven by the anionophore. The dose-response curves for anionophores shown in **Figure 2** further confirm that the examined molecules are responsible for the observed chloride efflux. These data indicated that EH160 in LUV exerts the half of its maximum activity at 5.6 μM (**Figure 2B**). This value is two orders of magnitude higher than that we reported before (Hernando et al., 2018). This discrepancy is due to the different method employed to calculate this EC_{50} value. In our previous work the dose response curves were empirically constructed plotting the amount of chloride transported after a time interval (300 s). This is an arbitrary time interval and this measurement is useful to compare the potency of series of compounds. Here we have obtained this EC_{50} value fitting the initial chloride flux calculated according to Equations (1, 2). This is thus an absolute measurement of the potency of the compound in the assayed conditions. The main advantage of the triazole derivatives is that they exhibit a reduced toxicity while retaining a remarkably high transport activity. Prodigiosine is a highly toxic compound ($TD_{50} = 2.9$ μM), as reported in numerous studies (Manderville, 2001). Although it is likely that cytotoxicity account for some of the intriguing pharmacological properties of this compound it jeopardizes its potential application as CFTR replacement therapy. The TD_{50} of EH160 is 7.1 μM, that is, indeed, no very different of the EC_{50} of 5.4 μM. Although the difference is small, it should be possible to optimize the anionophores to obtain less toxic substances. In any case, to apply these transporters for therapeutic uses, one have to consider also the efficacy of the anionophores. The efficacy (maximum quenching rate) of the iodide influx driven by the anionophore EH160 is similar to the CFTR activated by applying 20 μM forskolin and 10 μM genistein in FRT cells (Hernando et al., 2018). Since the CFTR activity of the CFTR transfected in the FRT cells is more than 13-fold greater that expected in human bronchial cells (Taddei et al., 2004; Moran et al., 2005; Kreindler et al., 2009; Melani et al., 2010; Gianotti et al., 2013, 2016).Thus, to induce an anion transport equivalent to that expected in bronchial cells, it would be necessary to apply <0.5 μM of EH160, significantly increasing the width of the therapeutic window.

Experiments were done with a very simple system, unilamellar vesicles, to avoid the contribution of other anion transport mechanisms present in cells. Another advantage to use such artificial system is the possibility to create large anion gradients, up to 450 mM, that improves the resolution of the measurements. Noteworthy, the phospholipid composition seems not to modify significantly the transport capacity of the anionophores. We cannot exclude, however, that mayor modifications in surface charge or membrane viscosity could induce differences on chloride efflux. We have also assayed the two most biological relevant cations, sodium and potassium, and could not find any difference on chloride efflux. Thus, we concluded that these cations very unlikely contribute to anionophore-driven chloride transport.

To better explain the EH160-driven transport we propose the model presented in **Figure 9**, where the carrier incorporated in the bilayer has three states, the free carrier, $\mathbf{TH^+}$, the carrier bound to chloride, **THCl**, and the carrier bound to a second anion, **THA**, for example nitrate, bicarbonate or gluconate. The binding to the carrier occurs in the aqueous solution-bilayer interface with the first order equilibrium constants $\mathbf{K_{Cl}}$ and $\mathbf{K_A}$ for chloride and the second ion, respectively. The internal solution (**in**) has a high concentration of chloride and there is no second anion; on the other hand, the concentration of the second anion is high in the external solution (**out**), meanwhile chloride is virtually absent. Thus, when the anionophore is on the internal face of the bilayer, the binding of chloride and the release of the second anion are favored, while the unbinding of chloride and the binding of the second anion takes place on the outer face of the bilayer. In this manner, as the anionophore diffuses across the bilayer, a chloride efflux, as a result of the exchange with the second anion, is established.

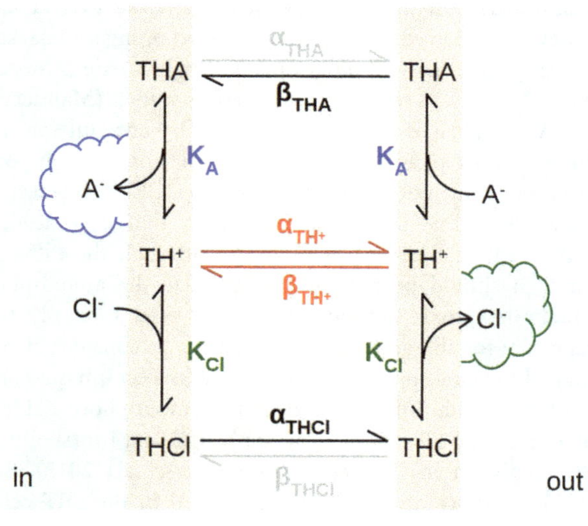

FIGURE 9 | Scheme of the mechanism of transport of anions across a bilayer driven by the anionophore EH160. $\mathbf{TH^+}$, **TCl**, and **TA** are anion-free, chloride-bound, and any other anion-bound forms of the EH160 transporter, respectively. These three carrier forms are located in the aqueous solution-bilayer interface, where they can reversibly bind anions, with a binding equilibrium constant, $\mathbf{K_{Cl}}$ and $\mathbf{K_A}$, for chloride and the second anion, respectively. Each anionophore form can diffuse across the hydrophobic region of the bilayer with a rate constant α and β. The high chloride concentration at the internal side **(in)**, and the high concentration of a second permeable anion (nitrate or bicarbonate) at the outer side **(out)**, will produce a chloride efflux.

These three anionophore forms diffuse across the hydrocarbon chains with rates of α and β. If we assume that the bilayer is symmetric and homogeneous, for a given carrier state, rate constants α and β are equivalent. However, the diffusion of the carrier will be determined by the binding state of the anionophore significantly. The diffusion rates for the free carrier, $\mathbf{TH^+}$, are probably lower than for the chloride bound form, **THCl**, or the **THA** form where $\mathbf{A^-}$ is a permeable anion as bicarbonate or nitrate. It is possible to speculate that the energy barrier to cross the hydrophobic region of the membrane is higher for the $\mathbf{TH^+}$ form, bearing a the positive net charge (see **Figure 1**), than the complexes **THCl** and **THA**. Complexed anions form a tightly bound ion par with the carrier which is overall neutral, and undergoes the diffusion across the hydrophobic environment easily. Thus, the permeability of different anions will depend on both, the binding equilibrium constant, and the diffusion rate of the anion-EH160 complex.

Comparing with permeable ions (chloride, nitrate, bicarbonate), the impermeable anions, such as sulfate, phosphate or gluconate, are characterized by a more stable interaction with water, with a more negative hydration enthalpy and Gibbs energy (Marcus, 1987, 1991). The structural study and theoretical analysis of synthetic prodigiosines have shown that anions bind the molecule in a groove formed by the three N–H groups (Díaz de Greñu et al., 2011; García-Valverde et al., 2012; Hernando et al., 2018). A similar binding of anions was also described for analogs of the marine alkaloids tambjamines (Iglesias Hernández et al., 2012; Hernando et al., 2014). Accordingly, the difficulty to remove the hydration water from these impermeable anions, and their larger molecular volumes (Marcus, 1993) will contribute to reduce the affinity of these anions for the carrier, and therefore the form **THA** is virtually absent, abolishing the flux of these anions across the bilayer. However, as long as electroneutrality conditions are maintained, shunting the bilayer with a cation carrier, the chloride flux is appropriately restored (**Figure 5**). Albeit, the chloride efflux occurring in absence of counter-anion influx (see **Figure 5**), when the **THA** state is not present, demonstrates that the free, unbounded anionophore $\mathbf{TH^+}$, is able to diffuse across the bilayer. At this point we could delineate the transport mechanism of EH160 as a molecular carrier embedded in the lipid bilayer. It should bind an anion at the bilayer interface at one side, cross the bilayer, and release the anion at the other side; the same mechanism occurs when the second ion is transported in the opposite direction, closing the transport cycle.

Interestingly, in the presence of external impermeable anions, the time course of anionophore-driven chloride efflux favored by valinomycin is not exponential, as described by equation 1, but becomes linear (**Figures 5B,C**). The exponential shape of the chloride efflux curve is due to the depletion of the anion from the LUV, that reduces the chloride gradient. According to the Fick law, this results in the reduction of the anion flux (observed as the derivative of the time course). Hypothetically the linear time course of the chloride efflux is due to a shrinking volume of LUV, as the efflux of a chloride ion should be accompanied with the efflux of a potassium ion mediated by valinomycin (or protons through FCCP), to maintain the electroneutrality. The result should be a net solute lost, with the consequent water osmotic withdrawal. These movements, within the measuring time interval, would result in the maintenance of the concentration of the solutes, and the consequent maintenance of the ionic gradients.

In the model depicted in **Figure 9** the movement of anions facilitated by the EH160 carrier has been illustrated. According to this scheme, EH160 is a reversible uniporter, and the direction of the flux is driven by the chemical gradient. Conversely, due to the fact that the measurements of the effect of prodigiosine and its derivatives in cells have shown that they induce cellular death accompanied with modifications of intracellular pH levels (Ohkuma et al., 1998; Castillo-Avila et al., 2005; Seganish and Davis, 2005; Díaz de Greñu et al., 2011; Gale et al., 2013; Cheung et al., 2018), it has been suggested that this class of anionophores are H^{+}/Cl^{-}-symporters. However, we have seen that the pH influence of the EH160-transport activity is independent of the H^{+} gradient (**Figures 7, 8**), but just on the ionization state of the carrier (**Figure 7D**). Indeed, there is no modification of the chloride efflux when the proton gradient is dissipated using proton carriers like FCCP (**Figures 7E,F**) or nigericin (data not shown). This is consistent with the conformational analysis showing that the anion binding is favored by the protonated form of a model prodigiosine (García-Valverde et al., 2012). Therefore, amount of an active protonated carrier in the bilayer will be determined by the pH in the external solution, which has a several orders of magnitude larger volume, and will dominate the equilibria in the three-compartment system formed by the internal space, the external space and the bilayer.

To estimate the chloride exchange rate in LUV we have to take into account the concentration of the anionophore in the bilayer membrane based on the concentration of EH160 in the aqueous solution. The average radius of the LUV, 47 nm, and the bilayer thickness of 3.75 nm, were obtained by small angle x-ray scattering (Baroni et al., 2014). It follows that the bilayer volume per vesicle is 3.39×10^{-16} cm^3. From the final external chloride concentration, $\Delta Cl \approx 0.9$ mM, and the total volume of the assay, 3.5 cm^3 we can estimate the total number of vesicles 1.61×10^{13}, and the total bilayer volume in the sample, 1.55×10^{-3} cm^3. To estimate the concentration of the anionophore in the bilayer, we used the water/*n*-octanol partition coefficient as calculated by the computational chemistry suite Marvin Sketch (https://www.chemaxon.com). It allows to calculate the partition coefficient of ionized and non-ionized species from the molecular structure (Viswanadhan et al., 1989), taking into account the ionization at a given pH, and the effect of the counter ion concentration. Thus, the *n*-octanol/buffer partition coefficient for EH160 in 450 mM NaCl (or KCl) at pH 7.5 is $P_{octanol/buffer} = 68.1$ (logP = 1.83). Hence, for an anionophore concentration of 1 μM, we expect a bilayer anionophore concentration of 6.62×10^{-8} moles cm^3, that corresponds to 6.18×10^{13} molecules of EH160 in the bilayers. The initial chloride efflux expected for 1 μM EH160 is 1.31×10^{-5} M/s, that corresponds to a transport rate of 7.45×10^{-22} moles of chloride/s per anionophore molecule, that represents 449 chloride ions/s per anionophore molecule. It is important to highlight that the efflux, and consequently the transport rate, depends on the chloride gradient, that for LUV experiments is ~450 mM. In contrast, in mammalian cells, we could assume that the chloride gradient is ~120 mM (≥30 mM intracellular and 150 mM extracellular), therefore, the transport rate should be scaled accordingly, resulting in 120 chloride ions/s per anionophore molecule. These values are similar to the exchange rates reported for other natural ion carriers in membranes, like the bacterial sugar transporters 2×10^2 (Waygood and Steeves, 1980), or the sodium calcium exchangers 5×10^3 (Baazov et al., 1999), but significantly lower than those characteristic of ion channel transport (6×10^6-12×10^7; Hille, 2001). A detailed calculation of the chloride turnover is presented as **Supplementary Material**.

We assayed the anionophores in a cellular model to assess whether anionophores could transport halides across the plasma membrane. By using an iodide-sensitive YFP to monitor the intracellular iodide concentration, we could demonstrate that, as described for other small organic molecules such as calix[4]pyrroles (Ko et al., 2014), tambjamines (Soto-Cerrato et al., 2015), ortho-phenylene bis-ureas (Dias et al., 2018), and bis-(p-nitrophenyl)ureidodecalins (Li et al., 2016), EH160 is able to transport this ion through the cell membrane (**Figures 8A,B**). The advantage of the iodide influx measurements is that the ion gradient driving the flux is well-controlled in the experiment. On the other hand, measurements of the chloride efflux revealed difficult because cells regulate the intracellular chloride concentration maintaining it low: in epithelium chloride concentration is ≤30 mM; in an experiment, when the extracellular chloride is removed, the effective gradient is 15-fold smaller that used in LUV experiments, and the efflux must be proportionally smaller. On the other hand, the cell homoeostasis implies a series of mechanisms that transport different ions, including several chloride and bicarbonate transporters, that may conceal a proper estimation of the anionophore- driven chloride efflux. Nevertheless, we could demonstrate that anionophores do induce chloride efflux in mammalian cells, with general characteristics similar to those observed in LUV bilayers (**Figures 8C,D**). Chloride efflux was observed when substituting the extracellular chloride by nitrate.

Here we have complemented the data previously reported (Hernando et al., 2018), designing a series of experiments useful to understand the transport mechanism of triazol derivatives of prodigiosine. These experiments demonstrate that these anionophores could be used to promote chloride and bicarbonate transport in cells, i.e., are good candidates to replace the defective or missing CFTR in an attempt to design a new cystic fibrosis therapy, as proposed for other anion transporters (Shen et al., 2012; Valkenier et al., 2014; Li et al., 2016, 2017; Liu et al., 2016; Dias et al., 2018). The analysis of anionophore-induced anion transport in cells needs, in any case, to be extended, studying the anionophore-induced ion transport in epithelial models, where the polarization of cells plays a fundamental role on the directionality of ion transport, to find the best suited compounds to become candidates for cystic fibrosis therapy. Preliminary experiments on other prodigiosine and tambjamine derivatives have shown that the properties of the anionophore EH160 could be extended to other analogous compounds, opening the possibility to design molecules optimized for clinical development. This proof of concept represents an encouraging promise for future developments toward a mutant-independent cystic fibrosis therapy.

AUTHOR CONTRIBUTIONS

OM and RQ planned the study. OM, RQ, and EC designed the experiments and analyzed data. RQ and MG-V synthesized the anionophores. CC performed the experiment on vesicles under the supervision of OM. VC, DB, and MF performed the experiments on cells under the supervision of OM and EC. OM and RQ wrote the manuscript.

FUNDING

This work has received funding from the European Union's Horizon 2020 research and innovation programme under grant agreement No 667079 and Consejería de Educación de la Junta de Castilla y León (Project BU092U16).

REFERENCES

Baazov, D., Wang, X., and Khananshvili, D. (1999). Time-resolved monitoring of electrogenic Na^{+}-Ca^{2+} exchange in the isolated cardiac sarcolemma vesicles by using a rapid-response fluorescent probe. *Biochemistry* 38, 1435–1445. doi: 10.1021/bi981429u

Baroni, D., Zegarra-Moran, O., Svensson, A., and Moran, O. (2014). Direct interaction of a CFTR potentiator and a CFTR corrector with phospholipid bilayers. *Eur. Biophys. J.* 43, 341–346. doi: 10.1007/s00249-014-0 956-y

Berger, H. A., Anderson, M. P., Gregory, R. J., Thompson, S., Howard, P. W., Maurer, R. A., et al. (1991). Identification and regulation of the cystic fibrosis transmembrane conductance regulator-generated chloride channel. *J. Clin. Invest.* 88, 1422–1431. doi: 10.1172/JCI115450

Broughman, J. R., Brandt, R. M., Hastings, C., Iwamoto, T., Tomich, J. M., and Schultz, B. D. (2004). Channel-forming peptide modulates transepithelial electrical conductance and solute permeability. *Am. J. Physiol. Cell Physiol.* 286, C1312–C1323. doi: 10.1152/ajpcell.00426.2002

Caci, E., Caputo, A., Hinzpeter, A., Arous, N., Fanen, P., Sonawane, N., et al. (2008). Evidence for direct CFTR inhibition by CFTR(inh)-172 based on Arg347 mutagenesis. *Biochem. J.* 413, 135–142. doi: 10.1042/BJ20080029

Castillo-Avila, W., Abal, M., Robine, S., and Pérez-Tomás, R. (2005). Non-apoptotic concentrations of prodigiosin (H+/Cl- symporter) inhibit the acidification of lysosomes and induce cell cycle blockage in colon cancer cells. *Life Sci.* 78, 121–127. doi: 10.1016/j.lfs.2005.04.059

Cheung, S., Wu, D., Daly, H. C., Busschaert, N., Morgunova, M., Simpson, J. C., et al. (2018). Real-time recording of the cellular effects of the anion transporter prodigiosin. *Chem* 4, 879–895. doi: 10.1016/j.chempr.2018.02.009

Clancy, J. P., Rowe, S. M., Accurso, F. J., Aitken, M. L., Amin, R. S., Ashlock, M. A., et al. (2012). Results of a phase IIa study of VX-809, an investigational CFTR corrector compound, in subjects with cystic fibrosis homozygous for the F508del-CFTR mutation. *Thorax* 67, 12–18. doi: 10.1136/thoraxjnl-2011-200393

Davis, J. T., Okunola, O., and Quesada, R. (2010). Recent advances in the transmembrane transport of anions. *Chem. Soc. Rev.* 39, 3843–3862. doi: 10.1039/b926164h

De Boeck, K., and Davies, J. C. (2017). Where are we with transformational therapies for patients with cystic fibrosis? *Curr. Opin. Pharmacol.* 34, 70–75. doi: 10.1016/j.coph.2017.09.005

Dias, C. M., Li, H., Valkenier, H., Karagiannidis, L. E., Gale, P. A., Sheppard, D. N., et al. (2018). Anion transport by ortho-phenylene bis-ureas across cell and vesicle membranes. *Organ. Biomol. Chem.* 16, 1083–1087. doi: 10.1039/c7ob02787g

Díaz de Greñu, B., Iglesias Hernández, P., Espona, M., Quiñonero, D., Light, M. E., Torroba, T., et al. (2011). Synthetic prodiginine obatoclax (GX15-070) and related analogues: anion binding, transmembrane transport, and cytotoxicity properties. *Chemistry* 17, 14074–14083. doi: 10.1002/chem.201101547

Gale, P. A., Davis, J. T., and Quesada, R. (2017). Anion transport and supramolecular medicinal chemistry. *Chem. Soc. Rev.* 46, 2497–2519. doi: 10.1039/c7cs00159b

Gale, P. A., Pérez-Tomás, R., and Quesada, R. (2013). Anion transporters and biological systems. *Acc. Chem. Res.* 46, 2801–2813. doi: 10.1021/ar400019p

Galietta, L. J., Haggie, P. M., and Verkman, A. S. (2001). Green fluorescent protein-based halide indicators with improved chloride and iodide affinities. *FEBS Lett.* 499, 220–224. doi: 10.1016/S0014-5793(01)02561-3

García-Valverde, M., Alfonso, I., Quiñonero, D., and Quesada, R. (2012). Conformational analysis of a model synthetic prodiginine. *J. Organ. Chem.* 77, 6538–6544. doi: 10.1021/jo301008c

Gianotti, A., Capurro, V., Scudieri, P., Galietta, L. J., Moran, O., and Zegarra-Moran, O. (2016). Pharmacological rescue of mutant CFTR protein improves the viscoelastic properties of CF mucus. *J. Cyst. Fibros. Off. J. Eur. Cyst. Fibros. Soc.* 15, 295–301. doi: 10.1016/j.jcf.2015.11.003

Gianotti, A., Melani, R., Caci, E., Sondo, E., Ravazzolo, R., Galietta, L. J., et al. (2013). Epithelial sodium channel silencing as a strategy to correct the airway surface fluid deficit in cystic fibrosis. *Am. J. Respir. Cell Mol. Biol.* 49, 445–452. doi: 10.1165/rcmb.2012-0408OC

Hernando, E., Capurro, V., Cossu, C., Fiore, M., García-Valverde, M., Soto-Cerrato, V., et al. (2018). Small molecule anionophores promote transmembrane anion permeation matching CFTR activity. *Sci. Rep.* 8:2608. doi: 10.1038/s41598-018-20708-3

Hernando, E., Soto-Cerrato, V., Cortés-Arroyo, S., Pérez-Tomás, R., and Quesada, R. (2014). Transmembrane anion transport and cytotoxicity of synthetic tambjamine analogs. *Organ. Biomol. Chem.* 12, 1771–1778. doi: 10.1039/c3ob42341g

Hille, B. (2001). *Ionic Channels of Excitable Membranes*. Sunderland, MA: Sinauer.

Iglesias Hernández, P., Moreno, D., Javier, A. A., Torroba, T., Pérez-Tomás, R., and Quesada, R. (2012). Tambjamine alkaloids and related synthetic analogs: efficient transmembrane anion transporters. *Chem. Commun. Camb. Engl.* 48, 1556–1558. doi: 10.1039/c1cc11300c

Ko, S. K., Kim, S. K., Share, A., Lynch, V. M., Park, J., Namkung, W., et al. (2014). Synthetic ion transporters can induce apoptosis by facilitating chloride anion transport into cells. *Nat. Chem.* 6, 885–892. doi: 10.1038/nchem.2021

Koulov, A. V., Lambert, T. N., Shukla, R., Jain, M., Boon, J. M., Smith, B. D., et al. (2003). Chloride transport across vesicle and cell membranes by steroid-based receptors. *Angew. Chem. Int. Ed. Engl.* 42, 4931–4933. doi: 10.1002/anie.200351957

Kreindler, J. L., Bertrand, C. A., Lee, R. J., Karasic, T., Aujla, S., Pilewski, J. M., et al. (2009). Interleukin-17A induces bicarbonate secretion in normal human bronchial epithelial cells. *Am. J. Physiol. Lung Cell. Mol. Physiol.* 296, L257–266. doi: 10.1152/ajplung.00344.2007

Li, H., Salomon, J. J., Sheppard, D. N., Mall, M. A., and Galietta, L. J. (2017). Bypassing CFTR dysfunction in cystic fibrosis with alternative pathways for anion transport. *Curr. Opin. Pharmacol.* 34, 91–97. doi: 10.1016/j.coph.2017.10.002

Li, H., Valkenier, H., Judd, L. W., Brotherhood, P. R., Hussain, S., Cooper, J. A., et al. (2016). Efficient, non-toxic anion transport by synthetic carriers in cells and epithelia. *Nat. Chem.* 8, 24–32. doi: 10.1038/nchem.2384

Liu, P. Y., Li, S. T., Shen, F. F., Ko, W. H., Yao, X. Q., and Yang, D. (2016). A small synthetic molecule functions as a chloride-bicarbonate dual-transporter and induces chloride secretion in cells. *Chem. Commun. Camb. Engl.* 52, 7380–7383. doi: 10.1039/c6cc01964a

Louis, K. S., and Siegel, A. C. (2011). Cell viability analysis using trypan blue: manual and automated methods. *Methods Mol. Biol. Clifton NJ* 740, 7–12. doi: 10.1007/978-1-61779-108-6_2

MacDonald, R. C., MacDonald, R. I., Menco, B. P., Takeshita, K., Subbarao, N. K., and Hu, L. R. (1991). Small-volume extrusion apparatus for preparation of large, unilamellar vesicles. *Biochim. Biophys. Acta* 1061, 297–303.

Manderville, R. A. (2001). Synthesis, proton-affinity and anti-cancer properties of the prodigiosin-group natural products. *Curr. Med. Chem. Anticancer Agents* 1, 195–218. doi: 10.2174/1568011013354688

Marcus, Y. (1987). The thermodynamics of solvation of ions. Part 2.—The enthalpy of hydration at 298.15 K. *J. Chem. Soc. Faraday Trans. 1 Phys. Chem. Condens. Phases* 83, 339–349. doi: 10.1039/F19878300339

Marcus, Y. (1991). Thermodynamics of solvation of ions. Part 5.—Gibbs free energy of hydration at 298.15 K. *J. Chem. Soc. Faraday Trans.* 87, 2995–2999. doi: 10.1039/FT9918702995

Marcus, Y. (1993). Thermodynamics of solvation of ions. Part 6.—The standard partial molar volumes of aqueous ions at 298.15 K. *J. Chem. Soc. Faraday Trans.* 89, 713–718. doi: 10.1039/FT9938900713

McNally, B. A., Koulov, A. V., Lambert, T. N., Smith, B. D., Joos, J. B., Sisson, A. L., et al. (2008). Structure-activity relationships in cholapod anion carriers: enhanced transmembrane chloride transport through substituent tuning. *Chemistry* 14, 9599–9606. doi: 10.1002/chem.200801163

Melani, R., Tomatis, V., Galietta, L. J., and Zegarra-Moran, O. (2010). Modulation of cystic fibrosis transmembrane conductance regulator (CFTR) activity and genistein binding by cytosolic pH. *J. Biol. Chem.* 285, 41591–41596. doi: 10.1074/jbc.M110.166850

Moran, O., Galietta, L. J., and Zegarra-Moran, O. (2005). Binding site of activators of the cystic fibrosis transmembrane conductance regulator in the nucleotide binding domains. *Cell Mol. Life Sci.* 62, 446–460. doi: 10.1007/s00018-004-4422-3

Nicastro, M. C., Spigolon, D., Librizzi, F., Moran, O., Ortore, M. G., Bulone, D., et al. (2016). Amyloid β-peptide insertion in liposomes containing GM1-cholesterol domains. *Biophys. Chem.* 208, 9–16. doi: 10.1016/j.bpc.2015.07.010

Ohkuma, S., Sato, T., Okamoto, M., Matsuya, H., Arai, K., Kataoka, T., et al. (1998). Prodigiosins uncouple lysosomal vacuolar-type ATPase through promotion of H+/Cl- symport. *Biochem. J.* 334(Pt 3), 731–741.

Pajewski, R., Garcia-Medina, R., Brody, S. L., Leevy, W. M., Schlesinger, P. H., and Gokel, G. W. (2006). A synthetic, chloride-selective channel that alters chloride transport in epithelial cells. *Chem. Commun. Camb. Engl.* 329–331. doi: 10.1039/b513940f

Ramsey, B. W., Davies, J., McElvaney, N. G., Tullis, E., Bell, S. C., Drevínek, P., et al. (2011). A CFTR potentiator in patients with cystic fibrosis and the G551D mutation. *N. Engl. J. Med.* 365, 1663–1672. doi: 10.1056/NEJMoa1105185

Saggiomo, V., Otto, S., Marques, I., Félix, V., Torroba, T., and Quesada, R. (2012). The role of lipophilicity in transmembrane anion transport. *Chem. Commun. Camb. Engl.* 48, 5274–5276. doi: 10.1039/c2cc31825c

Saint-Criq, V., and Gray, M. A. (2017). Role of CFTR in epithelial physiology. *Cell. Mol. Life Sci. CMLS* 74, 93–115. doi: 10.1007/s00018-016-2391-y

Seganish, J. L., and Davis, J. T. (2005). Prodigiosin is a chloride carrier that can function as an anion exchanger. *Chem. Commun. Camb. Engl.* 5781–5783. doi: 10.1039/b511847f

Shen, B., Li, X., Wang, F., Yao, X., and Yang, D. (2012). A synthetic chloride channel restores chloride conductance in human cystic fibrosis epithelial cells. *PLoS ONE* 7:e34694. doi: 10.1371/journal.pone.0034694

Sidorov, V., Kotch, F. W., Abdrakhmanova, G., Mizani, R., Fettinger, J. C., and Davis, J. T. (2002). Ion channel formation from a calix[4]arene amide that binds HCl. *J. Am. Chem. Soc.* 124, 2267–2278. doi: 10.1021/ja012338e

Soto-Cerrato, V., Manuel-Manresa, P., Hernando, E., Calabuig-Fariñas, S., Martínez-Romero, A., Fernández-Dueñas, V., et al. (2015). Facilitated anion transport induces hyperpolarization of the cell membrane that triggers differentiation and cell death in cancer stem cells. *J. Am. Chem. Soc.* 137, 15892–15898. doi: 10.1021/jacs.5b09970

Strausbaugh, S. D., and Davis, P. B. (2007). Cystic fibrosis: a review of epidemiology and pathobiology. *Clin. Chest Med.* 28, 279–288. doi: 10.1016/j.ccm.2007.02.011

Taddei, A., Folli, C., Zegarra-Moran, O., Fanen, P., Verkman, A. S., and Galietta, L. J. (2004). Altered channel gating mechanism for CFTR inhibition by a high-affinity thiazolidinone blocker. *FEBS Lett.* 558, 52–56. doi: 10.1016/s0014-5793(04)00011-0

Valkenier, H., Judd, L. W., Li, H., Hussain, S., Sheppard, D. N., and Davis, A. P. (2014). Preorganized bis-thioureas as powerful anion carriers: chloride transport by single molecules in large unilamellar vesicles. *J. Am. Chem. Soc.* 136, 12507–12512. doi: 10.1021/ja507551z

Viswanadhan, V. N., Ghose, A. K., Revankar, G. R., and Robins, R. K. (1989). Atomic physicochemical parameters for three dimensional structure directed quantitative structure-activity relationships. 4. Additional parameters for hydrophobic and dispersive interactions and their application for an automated superposition of certain naturally occurring nucleoside antibiotics. *J. Chem. Inf. Comput. Sci.* 29, 163–172. doi: 10.1021/ci00063a006

Wainwright, C. E., Elborn, J. S., Ramsey, B. W., Marigowda, G., Huang, X., Cipolli, M., et al. (2015). Lumacaftor-ivacaftor in patients with cystic fibrosis homozygous for Phe508del CFTR. *N. Engl. J. Med.* 373, 220–231. doi: 10.1056/NEJMoa1409547

Wallace, D. P., Tomich, J. M., Eppler, J. W., Iwamoto, T., Grantham, J. J., and Sullivan, L. P. (2000). A synthetic channel-forming peptide induces Cl(-) secretion: modulation by Ca(2+)-dependent K(+) channels. *Biochim. Biophys. Acta* 1464, 69–82. doi: 10.1016/S0005-2736(99)00248-5

Waygood, E. B., and Steeves, T. (1980). Enzyme I of the phosphoenolpyruvate: sugar phosphotransferase system of *Escherichia coli*. Purification to homogeneity and some properties. *Can. J. Biochem.* 58, 40–48.

Zegarra-Moran, O., and Galietta, L. J. (2017). CFTR pharmacology. *Cell. Mol. Life Sci.* 74, 117–128. doi: 10.1007/s00018-016-2392-x

12

In vitro Methods for the Development and Analysis of Human Primary Airway Epithelia

Ambra Gianotti[†], *Livia Delpiano*[†] *and Emanuela Caci**

U.O.C. Genetica Medica, IRCSS Istituto Giannina Gaslini, Genoa, Italy

Correspondence:
Emanuela Caci
emanuela.caci@unige.it

[†] These authors have contributed equally to this work

Cystic fibrosis (CF) is a chronic disease caused by mutations in the CF transmembrane conductance regulator (*CFTR*) gene, which encodes for a channel expressed at the apical surface of epithelial tissues. Defective chloride and bicarbonate secretion, arising from CFTR mutations, cause a multi-organ disease. In the airways, impaired ion transport results in a thick mucus, dehydration of the periciliar region and bacterial infections. Over the last years, basic research has sustained a great effort to identify therapies that are able to correct defective CFTR. For this purpose, *in vitro* cell models have played a key role in the study of mechanisms of the disease and to assess CFTR modulator therapies. Cultures of human primary bronchial epithelia are considered a physiologically relevant disease model due to their ability to maintain most of the morphological and functional characteristics of the airway epithelium *in vivo*. Despite their value, these cells are limited by the availability of human lung tissue and by the complexity of the culture procedure. However, primary human nasal cells can be considered as an alternative model for the study of CF pathophysiology since they are easier to obtain and recapitulate the properties of bronchial cultures. Over the years, several groups have optimized a protocol with key steps to culture and fully amplify differentiated primary airway epithelia. Our approach provides epithelia monolayers grown on porous filters, characterized by high transepithelial electrical resistance and an electrical potential difference. These parameters are required to perform electrophysiological experiments devoted to the study of ion transport mechanisms in airway epithelia. The aim of this study was to describe different methods to expand and differentiate isolated cells into fully polarized monolayers of airway epithelium, in order to provide an optimized protocol to support physiopathology analysis and to evaluate therapeutic strategies.

Keywords: cystic fibrosis, bronchus, airway epithelial cells culture, short-circuit current recording, transepithelial electrical resistance measurement, periciliary mucus properties

INTRODUCTION

Cystic fibrosis (CF) is an autosomal recessive disease caused by mutations in the gene coding for the protein cystic fibrosis transmembrane conductance regulator (CFTR). CFTR is a chloride channel expressed at the apical surface of secretory epithelia where it plays an important role in salt and fluid homeostasis (Saint-Criq and Gray, 2017).

The consequences of mutated CFTR are most important in the airways. The resulting defective chloride secretion, coupled to enhanced sodium absorption, impairs normal mucociliary clearance due to dehydration of the airway surface and consequently causes uncontrolled inflammation and chronic bacterial infections (Castellani and Assael, 2017).

Recently, bicarbonate has emerged as another important anion that contributes to the genesis of CF lung disease due to its role in mucus release (Quinton, 2008; Borowitz, 2015).

Over the last years, basic research has sustained a great effort to define a strategy to identify novel therapies that correct the basic defects responsible for CFTR loss-of-function.

Studies have demonstrated that pharmacological rescue of the CFTR protein, in the presence of small molecules called correctors and potentiators, can repair folding and gating defects (Pedemonte et al., 2005; Okiyoneda et al., 2013; Van Goor et al., 2009, 2011).

The most successful compounds, ivacaftor and lumacaftor developed by Vertex Pharmaceuticals company, have been approved for treatment of CF patients (Wainwright et al., 2015).

Drug discovery is supported by *in vitro* cell models that offer the opportunity to study epithelium physiology, the alterations caused by mutated CFTR, and the efficacy of therapies that aim to correct basic CF defects.

In vitro cell models for airway epithelium studies have been mostly based on primary human bronchial epithelial cells (hereafter termed HBEC), obtained from CF lung resection.

HBEC provide the ideal tool since they exhibit several of the morphological and functional defects of airway epithelia. Despite their value, it is difficult to acquire a large amount of cells and they can only be grown for 4–5 passages before reverting to a poorly differentiated phenotype.

Primary nasal epithelial cells (hereafter termed HNEC) have been recently proposed as an alternative method to HBEC culture.

HNEC are easy to collect by nasal brushing and recapitulate the properties of HBEC cultures (McDougall et al., 2008; Mosler et al., 2008). Furthermore, this model is very useful to predict the clinical treatment efficacy in patients (Pranke et al., 2017).

Several research groups have optimized protocols that allow isolation, expansion, and differentiation of primary HBEC and HNEC (Fulcher et al., 2005; Yaghi et al., 2010; Neuberger et al., 2011; Müller et al., 2013; Stokes et al., 2014).

Primary cells have a very limited proliferative capacity *in vitro* and it is possible to culture for at least five-six passages before noting a slowing down of cell growth. To overcome this problem, culturing of bronchial and nasal epithelial cells under CRC conditions, namely irradiated feeder cells and the RhoA kinase inhibitor Y, enhances cell growth and lifespan while preserving electrophysiological and morphological properties (Gentzsch et al., 2017).

The aim of this article was to present a detailed protocol, optimized in our laboratory, for culture and differentiation of airway epithelia. This method results in large-scale production of isolated HBEC and HNEC and fully differentiated epithelia that exhibit the morphological and functional defects of CF airways. Therefore, these cell models are very useful for improving our knowledge about physiopathology mechanisms involved in CF and to support therapeutics strategies.

Our approach is based on the isolation of airway cells from bronchi or nasal brushings obtained from CF and non-CF subjects. Then, isolated cells are cultured and expanded with a high proliferation rate using a proliferative serum-free medium. This step is followed by epithelial cell differentiation on permeable supports, whose ion transport properties can be evaluated with electrophysiological techniques (Galietta et al., 1998; Scudieri et al., 2012).

For this purpose, we review two powerful methods for ion transport measurements underlining the application, advantages, and limits. These include Ussing chamber and Trans-Epithelial Electrical Resistance (TEER) techniques (Li et al., 2004; Srinivasan et al., 2015).

Moreover, we describe a cell culture protocol to achieve a fully differentiated mucociliary airway epithelium to study the properties of periciliary mucus considering its important involvement in the CF pathology. Indeed, the reduction of fluid secretion in CF alters the composition of the airway surface fluid (ASL) and induces the production of mucus with rheological properties making it inadequate for normal physiology (Gianotti et al., 2016).

Finally, our culture protocol allows morphological and functional characteristics of the airway epithelium to be reproduced *in vivo*, supporting the study of CF physiopathology and therapeutic strategies.

MATERIALS AND EQUIPMENTS

Cell Culture

- Petri dishes, culture flasks, Pasteur pipette, physiological saline solution.
- Snapwell permeable support: 3801 (Corning, Tewksbury, MA, United States).
- HTS Transwell permeable support: 3379 (Corning).
- HBSS (hepes buffered saline solution): hepes (20 mM, Sigma #H4034, Saint Louis, MO, United States), sodium chloride (121.0 mM, Sigma #S9888), potassium chloride (2.7 mM, Sigma #P3911), glucose (9.4 mM, Sigma #G7528), sodium phosphate dibasic (7.2 mM, Sigma #S7907), phenol red (1:1000 of 0.5% stock solution, Sigma #P5530). Adjust pH to 7.4 and bring to volume; sterilize with a filter and store at +4°C.
- Protease solution: protease powder of *Streptomyces griseus* XIV (0.3 g, Sigma #P5147) dissolved in 130 ml HBSS and 30 ml Ham's F12 w/o L-glut. Prepare before using, sterilize with a filter and store at +4°C.
- Ca^{2+}/Mg^{2+} – free phosphate buffered saline (PBS).
- Ca^{2+}/Mg^{2+} – Dulbecco's phosphate buffer saline (D-PBS).
- Trypsin solution: Ca^{2+}/Mg^{2+}-free phosphate buffered saline (PBS) containing 0.05% trypsin and 0.02% EDTA solution.
- Rat tail collagen solution: rat tail collagen (1 mg, Sigma #C7661) dissolved in 1 ml acetic acid 0.1 M.
- SMAD inhibitors cocktail: A 83-01 (1 μM, Sigma #SML0788), DMH1 (1 μM, Sigma #D8946).

- Rock inhibitor: Y-27632 2HCl (5 μM, Sigma #SCM075).
- Proliferative serum-free medium: See **Table 1** and **Supplementary Materials**. Sterilize with a filter and store at +4°C. This medium may be frozen. Protect from light with aluminum foil.
- Cryomedium: prepare a solution of fetal bovine serum (FBS) with 10% DMSO. Prepare before using, store at +4°C for no longer than 1 month.
- Medium with serum to neutralize trypsin: DMEM High glucose w/o L-glut, Ham's F12 w/o L-glut, FBS 10%, penicillin (100 U/ml), streptomycin (100 μg/ml), L-glutamine (2 mM). Sterilize with a filter and store at +4°C.
- Differentiation serum-supplemented medium: See **Table 2** and **Supplementary Materials**. Sterilize with a filter and store at +4°C for no longer than 3 weeks. This medium may not be frozen, freezing seems to destroy the ability to induce differentiation and the appearance of electrical resistance. Protect from light with aluminum foil.

TABLE 1 | Proliferative serum-free medium.

Compound	Final concentration
LHC basal medium (Life Technology #12677-019)	500 ml
RPMI 1640	500 ml
Stock 4	5 ml/L
Stock 11	0.5 ml/L
Calcium stock	40.6 μM
Insulin stock	0.4325 μM
Transferrin stock	61.5 μM
EGF stock	0.403 nM
P/E stock	2.5 ml/L
RA/T3 stock	0.05 ml/L
Trace element solution	5 ml/L
HC stock	0.1 μM
Bovine pituitary extract (BPE) (Gibco #13028-014)	25 mg/L
Penicillin	100 U/ml
Streptomycin	100 μg/ml
L-glutamine	2 mM

TABLE 2 | Differentiation serum-supplemented medium.

Compound	Final concentration
DMEM High glucose w/o L-glut	500 ml
Ham's F12 w/o L-glut	500 ml
Insulin stock	0.4325 μM
Transferrin stock	61.5 μM
P/E stock	2.5 ml/L
RA/T3 stock	0.1 ml/L
HC stock	0.2 μM
Bovine pituitary extract (BPE) (Gibco #13028-014)	25 mg/L
New Zealand Serum	20 ml/L
Penicillin	100 U/ml
Streptomycin	100 μg/ml
L-glutamine	2 mM

- Differentiation serum-free medium: See **Table 3** and **Supplementary Materials**. Sterilize with a filter and store at +4°C for no longer than 3 weeks. This medium cannot be frozen, freezing seems to destroy ability to induce differentiation and the appearance of electrical resistance. Protect from light with aluminum foil.

Electrophysiological Equipment

- Epithelial voltohmmeter: EVOM2 [World precision Instrument (WPI), Sarasota, FL, United States].
- Voltage-clamp (DVD-1000 voltage/current clamp, WPI Instruments).
- PowerLab 4/25 (AD Instruments, Colorado Springs, CO, United States).
- Ag/AgCl electrodes: EK1 (WPI Instruments).
- Agar salt bridges (1 M potassium chloride in 2% agar).
- Ussing chambers (Vertical Diffusion Chamber, Warner Instruments, Hamden, CT, United States).
- Latex tubes for perfusion.
- Ringer's Solution for Ussing chamber: sodium chloride (126 mM, Sigma #S9888), potassium dihydrogen phosphate (0.38 mM, Sigma #NIST200B), potassium phosphate dibasic trihydrate (2.13 mM, Sigma #P9666), magnesium sulfate heptahydrate (1 mM, Sigma #M9397), calcium chloride dihydrate (1 mM, Sigma #C8106), glucose (10 mM, Sigma #G7528), sodium bicarbonate (24 mM, Sigma #S5761), phenol red (1:1000 of 0.5% stock solution, Sigma #P5530). Sterilize with a filter and store at +4°C.
- Coon's modified Ham's F-12 medium for TEER: hepes (20 mM), FBS 10%, penicillin (100 U/ml), streptomycin (100 μg/ml), L-glutamine (2 mM). Sterilize with a filter and store at +4°C.
- Amiloride hydrochloride (Sigma #A7410), CPT-cAMP (Sigma #C3912), forskolin (Selleckchem #S2449, Munich, Germany), genistein (Sigma # G6649), lumacaftor (VX-809, Selleckchem #S1565), ivacaftor (VX-770, Selleckchem #S1144), CFTR-inh172 (Selleckchem

TABLE 3 | Differentiation serum-free medium.

Compound	Final concentration
DMEM High glucose w/o L-glut	500 ml
Ham's F12 w/o L-glut	500 ml
Insulin stock	0.87 μM
Transferrin stock	123 μM
EGF stock	0.806 nM
Epinephrine stock	2.73 μM
RA stock	0.099 μM
T3 stock	0.01 μM
HC stock	1.4 μM
Bovine pituitary extract (BPE) (Gibco #13028-014)	50 mg/L
BSA stock	22.58 μM
Penicillin	100 U/ml
Streptomycin	100 μg/ml
L-glutamine	2 mM

#S7139), UTP (Sigma #U6625), ATP (Sigma #A9187), PPQ-102 (Sigma #219677).

STEPWISE PROCEDURES

Primary HBEC and HNEC Culture

In this step, we describe a cell culture protocol which can provide, from a relatively little amount of sample, a large number of polarized bronchial and nasal epithelia useful for the study of airway physiopathology and predicting *in vivo* drug efficacy.

This method is based on two distinct phases:

1. Expansion of HBEC and HNEC using a proliferative serum-free medium. This culture medium allows the expansion of airway epithelial cells with a high proliferation rate and a low density growth for at least five passages before cell proliferation slows down. Cumulative population doubling level at fifth passage is approximately 33.
2. Differentiation of epithelia on permeable supports using a "air liquid interface" (ALI) condition:
   - serum-supplemented medium condition: cells differentiate into fully polarized monolayers of airway epithelium in order to perform electrophysiological experiments.
   - serum-free medium condition: cells form a fully differentiated mucociliary airway epithelium useful for the study of periciliary fluid properties of airways (Hajj et al., 2007).

Isolation and Expansion of Primary HBEC Derived From CF and Non-CF Donors Following Lung Transplantation

1. Dissect and wash the mainstem human bronchus, derived from CF and non-CF individuals undergoing lung transplant, with physiological saline solution. Transfer the sample into a saline solution at +4°C in the laboratory and process within 4 h.
2. To clean the bronchus of the mucus, wash the sample twice in a 50 ml conical tube containing physiological saline solution.
3. Place the bronchus overnight at +4°C in protease XIV solution in order to separate the epithelial cell layer from the underlying connective tissue.
4. Remove the bronchus gently from the protease XIV solution and place it in a 100-mm Petri-dish containing physiological saline solution. Collect epithelial cells by vigorously flushing the bronchial lumen with physiological saline solution (**Figure 1**).
5. Pellet the detached epithelial cells by centrifugation at 900 rpm for 10 min.
6. Resuspend the cells in 3 ml of trypsin solution, gently pipette five times using a 1-ml pipette tip and incubate at 37°C for 5 min.
7. Neutralize trypsin solution by adding an equal volume of medium with serum.

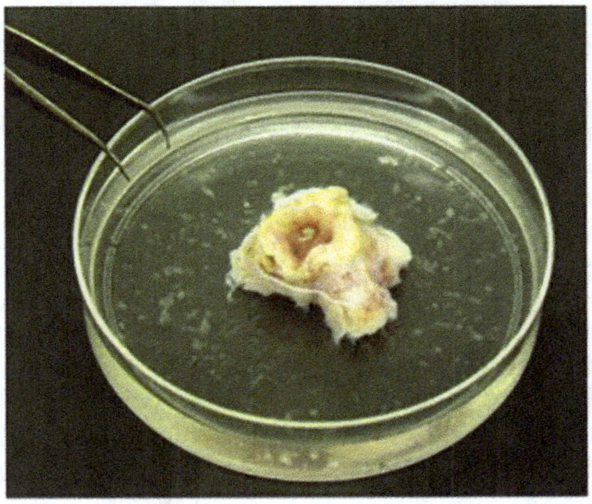

FIGURE 1 | Detached epithelial cells isolated from bronchus. Bronchus is placed in a 100-mm Petri-dish and epithelial cells are collected by flushing the bronchial lumen vigorously with physiological saline solution.

8. Add proliferative medium to bring the final volume to 35 ml.
9. Count the cells to determine the cell yield and then centrifuge at 900 rpm for 10 min.
10. Coat a T150 flask with 100 $\mu l/cm^2$ of rat tail collagen solution and place in an incubator at 37°C (5% CO_2) for at least 15 min or up to 6 h. Before use, carefully aspirate the collagen solution with a Pasteur pipette.
11. Resuspend the pellet in proliferative medium in order to seed approximately 8000 cells/cm^2 in the collagen-coated flask and incubate at 37°C (5% CO_2).
12. To expand the cell culture, replace the proliferative medium every 24 h until the cell density reaches 70% confluence.
13. When the bronchus was derived from a CF patient, treat the medium with antibiotics for the first 6 days to eradicate bacterial contamination. The mixture of antibiotics is designed based on the results of the antibiogram of the bacteria isolated from the patient's most recent expectorate. If the antibiogram is not available use the following cocktail: colistimethate sodium, piperacillin/tazobactam. Use a specific antibiotic cocktail at a 10X concentration for the first 48 h, then reduce every two days by 1:2 to minimize cell toxicity (**Table 4**).
    To overcome fungal contamination, treat the medium with 2.5 $\mu g/ml$ of amphotericin B for at least the first 7 days of culture.
14. When the cell density reaches 70% confluence, harvest HBEC for further expansion or freeze aliquots for future use.
15. To detach HBEC, remove the proliferative media and add 15 ml of warm $Ca^{2+}Mg^{2+}$-free phosphate buffer solution (PBS) and place at 37°C (5% CO_2) for 6 min.
16. Remove PBS and add 2.4 ml of trypsin solution and incubate at 37°C (5% CO_2) until detachment.

TABLE 4 | Antibiotic and antifungal dose concentrations suggested for CF cell culture treatment.

Antibiotic	Dose 10x	Antibiotics type	Indications
Tobramycin	8 μg/mL	Aminoglycoside	Gram-negative Bacteria
Amikacin	25 μg/mL	Aminoglycoside	Gram-negative Bacteria
Gentamicin	40 μg/mL	Aminoglycoside	Gram-negative Bacteria
Piperacillin-Tazobactam	50 μg/mL	Beta-lactamase inhibitors	Gram-positive Bacteria
Ticarcillin	250 μg/mL	Beta-lactamase inhibitors	Gram-positive Bacteria
Imipenem	2000 μg/mL	Beta-lactamase inhibitors	Gram-positive Bacteria
Meropenem	250 μg/mL	Beta-lactamase inhibitors	Gram-positive Bacteria
Ceftazidime	250 μg/mL	Beta-lactamase inhibitors	Gram-positive Bacteria
Oxazolidinone (Linezolid)	2 mg/mL	Inhibitor on the ribosomal 50S	Gram-positive Bacteria
Teicoplanin	60 μg/mL	Semisynthetic glycopeptide	Gram-positive Bacteria
Vancomycin	50 μg/mL	Glycopeptide	Gram-positive Bacteria
Ciprofloxacin	25 μg/mL	Fluoroquinolone	Gram-positive and negative Bacteria
Levofloxacin	100 μg/mL	Fluoroquinolone	Gram-positive and negative Bacteria
Trimethoprim + Sulfamethoxazole	25 μg/mL	Sulfonamides	Gram-positive and negative Bacteria
Colistimethate sodium	50 U/mL	Polymyxin	Multi-drug resistant Bacteria
Amphotericin B	25 μg/mL	Macrocyclic polyene	Antifungal

17. Neutralize the trypsin solution by adding an equal volume of medium with serum.
18. Add 20 ml PBS and gently swirl the flask to collect the cells.
19. Transfer the cell suspension to a 50 ml conical tube.
20. Count the cells to determine the cell yield. The expected yield for one T150 flask is ~6 million cells.
21. Centrifuge at 1500 rpm for 5 min.
22. Resuspend the pellet in 10 ml of proliferative medium and split the cell culture between 3 collagen-coated T150 flasks for further expansion.
23. Replace the growth media every 24 h during the cell expansion phase.
24. Freeze cells every cell splitting in order to have a bio-bank for every passage.
25. For this, resuspend cell culture in cryoprotective-medium at a density of 2 million cells/ml. Place 1 ml of this culture into each cryovial and freeze in a cell freezing container at −80°C for at least 24 h before transferring to a liquid nitrogen tank for long-term storage.
26. To thaw frozen HBEC, place the cryovial in a 37°C water bath for 2 min and then transfer the cell culture into a 15 ml conical tube containing proliferative medium. Centrifuge at 1500 rpm for 5 min.
27. Coat 2 T75 flasks with 100 μl/cm^2 of rat tail collagen solution and place in an incubator at 37°C (5% CO_2) for at least 15 min or up to 6 h. Before use, aspire carefully the collagen solution with a Pasteur pipette.
28. Resuspend the pellet in 8 ml proliferative medium and split the culture in 2 collagen-coated T75 flasks already containing 8 ml growth medium/flask. Replace medium every 2 days and maintain culture as described above.

Isolation and Expansion of Primary HNEC Derived from CF and Non-CF Donors Following Nasal Brushing

1. Collect HNEC by nasal brushing of both nostrils. The nasal brushing is performed without local anesthesia after nasal washings with physiological saline solution, in order to remove the mucus (two washes a day in the previous week and a wash immediately before nasal cells collection).
2. Use a soft sterile interdental brush with 2.5–3 mm bristles scraping along the middle portion of the inferior turbinate with anterior-posterior rotational movements in each nostril, under direct vision.
3. Carefully monitor patient for vital and minor signs, comfort and pain.
4. Place brush in a 15 ml conical tube containing 9 ml of $Ca^{2+}Mg^{2+}$-D-PBS, transfer the sample to the laboratory and process within 4 h.
5. Place the sample in a 37°C water bath for 20 min and then centrifuge at 900 rpm for 5 min to detach all cells from brush.
6. Coat 1 T25 flask with 100 μl/cm^2 of rat tail collagen solution and place in incubator at 37°C (5% CO_2) for at least 15 min until 6 h. Before use, carefully aspirate the collagen solution with a Pasteur pipette.
7. Carefully remove the brush and resuspend the cell pellet in 6 ml of proliferative medium and seed it in the coated T25 flask. To improve growth rate and to extend the number of population doublings *in vitro*, the culture medium is supplemented with a SMAD and Rock inhibitors cocktail required for the conditional reprogramming and immortalization of human epithelial cells (Palechor-Ceron et al., 2013; Mou et al., 2016).
8. Maintain cultures as previously described for HBEC.

Generation of Differentiated Nasal and Bronchial Epithelia With Serum-Supplemented Medium

1. Culture and detach HBEC and HNEC on the fourth passage when the cell density reaches 90% confluence.

2. Count the cells to determine the cell yield. The expected yield for T75 and T150 flasks is ~4 and 8 million cells, respectively.
3. Seed 500.000 cells/insert on Snapwell permeable supports in 500 μl proliferative medium. Add 2 ml proliferative medium on the basolateral side.
4. Alternately, seed 200.000 cells/insert on HTS Transwell permeable supports in 300 μl proliferative medium. Add 25 ml proliferative medium in the bottom well.
5. After 24 h, replace the proliferative medium with differentiation serum-supplemented medium. Add 500 μl and 2 ml of medium on the apical and basolateral sides, respectively, on a Snapwell insert.
6. Alternately, add 200 μl to the apical side and 25 ml in the bottom well of the HTS Transwell insert.
7. Replace medium daily on both sides of the permeable supports until the sixth day (liquid-liquid culture).
8. Check differentiation of cells into a tight epithelium by measuring transepithelial electrical resistance and potential difference with an epithelial voltohmmeter EVOM2.
9. Good values measured in Snapwell supports are ~−40 mV and ~−30 mV for CF and non-CF epithelia, respectively, and 1000–1700 Ω for both genotypes.
10. Subsequently, totally remove the apical medium (ALI condition) and replace medium every two days only in the basolateral side. This condition favors a fully differentiated epithelium.
11. Maintain HBEC and HNEC culture for 2–3 weeks.

Generation of Differentiated Nasal and Bronchial Epithelia With Serum-Free Medium

1. Culture and detach HBEC and HNEC on the fourth passage when cell density reaches 65% confluence.
2. Coat the Snapwell support with 200 μl of rat tail collagen solution and place in an incubator at 37°C (5% CO_2) for at least 15 min or up to 6 h. Before use, carefully aspirate the collagen solution with a Pasteur pipette.
3. Count and seed 150.000 cells/insert on Snapwell supports in 500 μl proliferative medium. Add 2 ml proliferative medium to the basolateral side.
4. After 24 h, replace the proliferative medium with fresh medium at both sides of the permeable support.
5. After 24 h, replace the proliferative medium with serum-free differentiation medium only in the basolateral side (ALI condition).
6. Replace medium every 2 days only on the basolateral side of the permeable support until the 15th day.
7. Check differentiation of cells into a tight epithelium by measuring transepithelial electrical resistance and potential difference with an epithelial voltohmmeter EVOM2.
8. Good values are ~−8 for CF and ~−5 for non-CF epithelia, respectively, and 600–800 Ω for both genotypes.
9. Maintain the ALI culture condition epithelia for 4–5 weeks.

HBEC and HNEC Monolayers Application

Well differentiated HBEC and HNEC epithelia are useful to support the following studies:

1. Electrophysiological experiments aimed at the study of ion transport mechanisms in airway epithelia.
2. Analysis of protein expression with immunofluorescence or Western Blot techniques.
3. Gene expression analysis by RT-qPCR, microarray or RNAseq.
4. Investigation of innate defense mechanisms and response to proinflammatory stimuli.

Important Remarks

1. During the initial isolation from bronchus, columnar cells with rapidly beating cilia should be observed indicating good cell viability. Beating cilia cells will disappear in the culture condition over time. The day after plating, isolated cells from bronchus, many red blood cells, and fibroblasts should be present in the culture and disappear after washing the flask with physiological saline solution. Small spots of epithelial cells should be observed.
2. HBEC from CF patients are frequently infected with antibiotic-resistant organisms. Particular care has been given to eradicate bacterial and fungal contamination with appropriate treatments.
3. During cell expansion HBEC and HNEC can be split up to four times to expand the number of cells available for functional studies. Further expansion may frequently lead to worsening of epithelia performance.
4. During expansion, special care must be taken when splitting cells into new flasks that the cell density reaches no more than 70% confluence. A higher density could induce a squamous differentiation (Sacco et al., 1992) that debars desired morphological and functional properties (**Figure 2**).
5. Measure transepithelial electrical resistance and potential difference with a voltohmmeter to check differentiation of polarized epithelia. We have observed that after 6 days of culture, the value of potential difference in CF epithelia is larger than non-CF.

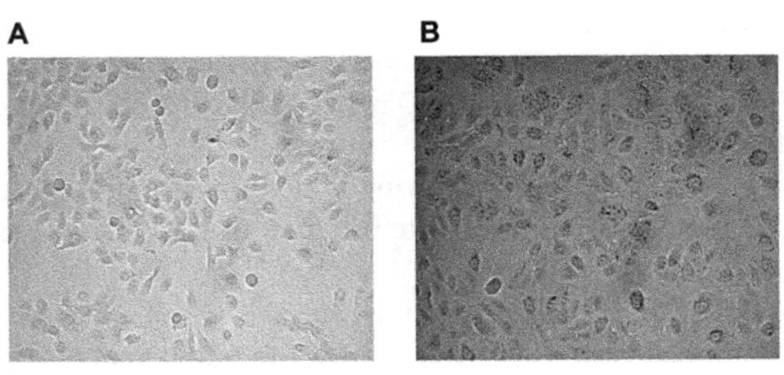

FIGURE 2 | Epithelial cell culture density in the proliferative phase. Epithelial cells with a good morphology and a high proliferation rate **(A)**. Epithelial cells with an increasing number of large squamous cells and decreased cell growth **(B)**.

6. The following remarks contribute to the development of polarized epithelia:
    - Detach cells at the proper growth density.
    - Seed the proper amount of cells on a permeable support.
    - Replace differentiation medium every day.

Recording Transepithelial Ion Transport

The airway epithelium balances Na^+ absorption and Cl^- secretion to carefully regulate the properties of the ASL in order to ensure efficient mucociliary clearance.

Here we present electrophysiological approaches to perform transepithelial ion transport measurements. Moreover, we highlight the applications, the strengths, and limitations of the techniques.

Short-Circuit Current Recordings Using the Ussing Chamber Technique

The Ussing chamber provides a system to measure the transport of ions across epithelial tissues.

Although it can be complicated to perform, it is considered the gold standard for electrophysiological experiments with the aim of studying epithelial transport.

In the most used configuration, the short-circuit current (Isc) technique, the transepithelial potential difference is clamped at zero with a voltage clamp amplifier and the resulting current is recorded.

The Ussing system consists of two hemi-chambers separated by the monolayer of epithelial cells grown on Snapwell supports, a perfusion system, an amplifier, and a data acquisition system.

Both hemichambers are fill with a Ringer's solution, continuously bubbled with a gas mixture containing 5% CO_2 −95% air that maintains the physiological pH. The temperature of the system is kept at 37°C. The voltage-clamp is connected to the apical and basolateral chambers with Ag/AgCl electrodes and agar bridges (two for voltage and two for current). The short-circuit current is recorded with a PowerLab 4/25 analog-to-digital converter connected to a computer.

A typical experiment is conducted as follows:

1. Fresh culture medium is replaced the day before the experiment. The medium may contain drugs or compounds. For example, epithelia from F508del patients may be treated with 1 μM lumacaftor to rescue mutant CFTR protein. As a control, cells are treated with an equal amount of control vehicle (usually DMSO at 0.1%; higher amounts of DMSO may significantly alter epithelial properties).
2. Snapwell support, carrying differentiated bronchial or nasal epithelia, is mounted in a vertical diffusion Ussing chamber.
3. Add 5 ml/hemichamber of warm Ringer's solution and connect each side with the latex tubes that supply the gas mixture for solution bubbling.
4. Insert the current and voltage electrodes into each hemichamber and connect to the voltage-clamp amplifier (follow the instructions of the amplifier manufacturer for correct procedures).
5. Under open-circuit conditions, measure the spontaneous transepithelial electrical potential difference. Then switch the amplifier to voltage-clamp configuration and measure the resulting Isc. Calculate the transepithelial electrical resistance from the values of the transepithelial electrical potential difference and the short-circuit current with Ohm's law. Low resistance values (below 500 Ω) may reflect a "leaky" epithelium that might increase paracellular ion flux.
6. Start recording and allow the transepithelial current to stabilize (10 min) before adding stimuli.
7. Add 10 μM amiloride to apical side to block the ENaC channel. The amplitude of the current drop caused by amiloride is dependent on the expression/function of ENaC. However, it should be kept in mind that experiments are carried out on an intact epithelium. Therefore, transepithelial ion transport is dependent on the coordinated activity of different ion channels and transporters. Changes in amiloride-sensitive current may also occur following modified expression/function of proteins that affect intracellular ion concentrations and membrane potential.
8. Stimulate CFTR channel by adding 5 μM forskolin or 10 μM CPT-cAMP (apical and basolateral sides). Both agents activate CFTR as cAMP agonists therefore they stimulate transepithelial Cl^- and bicarbonate transport. Anion secretion may be also promoted by activation of cAMP-dependent basolateral proteins (e.g., K^+ channels) that generate the required electrochemical driving force.
9. In the case of epithelia from CF patients with CFTR channel gating mutations, add 20 μM forskolin or 100 μM CPT-cAMP in order to maximize CFTR activation, and subsequently add a potentiator compound on apical side (e.g., 50 μM genistein or 1 μM ivacaftor) to further stimulate channel opening.
10. Once the CFTR-dependent current is stabilized, add the CFTR blocker $CFTR_{inh}$-172 (10 μM). The amplitude of the current drop elicited by the inhibitor reflects the extent of CFTR function. However, as discussed for ENaC, other proteins also contribute to CFTR-depedent anion secretion.
11. In the presence of amiloride and $CFTR_{inh}$-172, the activity of other channels can be recorded. For example, stimulation with Ca^{2+} agonists (e.g., apical UTP or ATP) elicits anion secretion through Ca^{2+}- dependent chloride channel (ANO1, a.k.a.TMEM16A).
12. Stop the recording and save the trace.

Ussing Chamber Technique Application

Using *ex vivo* airway epithelia, this technique gives a representation of the functional characteristics and processes involved in the physiological environment.

1. Measurement of physiological ion transport in non-CF epithelia.
2. Study of alterations to ion transport occurring in CF or other pathologies.

3. Evaluation of therapeutic interventions.

Important Remarks

1. Ussing chamber is a valuable technique but its disadvantages include technical expertise, the cost, and space needed for the equipment.
2. It is limited to polarized tissue and it does not allow analysis of a large number of samples, thus this technique has a relatively low throughput.
3. Ussing chamber is not suitable for measuring electroneutral transporters such as the Cl^-/HCO_3^- exchanger (e.g., pendrin protein).
4. Ussing chambers are made of plastic polymers, therefore some compounds used in the experiments (particularly those that work at very low concentrations such as ivacaftor) can penetrate plastic surfaces and be released in subsequent experiments thus altering the results. To overcome this contamination problem, we recommend that the chambers be washed at the end of each experiment in a sodium phosphate tribasic solution (15 g diluted in 1 l of deionized water) for 4 h and then in hydrochloric acid 0.1% solution for 15 min. After that, rinse in deionized water.

   Agar salt bridges represent another source of contamination. We suggest that the bridges be replaced at the end of each experiment.

Electrical Epithelial Properties Measured With the Trans-Epithelial Electrical Resistance (TEER) – Potential Difference (PD) Technique

TEER/PD is a rapid and simple method to quantify ion transport by measuring the electrical resistance and potential difference across the epithelium. TEER/PD is dependent on the expression/activity of channels situated on both apical and basolateral membranes as well as on the properties of tight junctions that control paracellular ion transport.

TEER/PD measurements are performed using the EVOM2 system and placing Ag/AgCl "chopstick" electrodes on both sides of an epithelial monolayer cultured on HTS Transwell permeable supports.

The method is simply based on the separate measurement of TEER and PD values for each epithelium, under resting conditions and following the application of agonists and inhibitors. The equivalent short-circuit current is then calculated from TEER and PD.

Considering the simplicity of the measurement and the data reproducibility compared with the Ussing chamber method, TEER/PD measurements are a good benchmark tool for high-throughput drug discovery screening in CF epithelia.

1. Culture bronchial or nasal epithelial monolayers in HTS Transwell inserts as previously described.
2. Replace the medium the day before the experiment. If needed, treatments can be included (e.g., lumacaftor or other correctors for CF epithelia).
3. Wash the chopstick electrodes with deionized water and equilibrate the electrodes in a Coon's modified solution.
4. Incubate both sides of the epithelia with Coon's modified solution for 1 h at 37°C.
5. Measure TEER and PD under basal conditions.
6. Add 10 μM amiloride solution on the apical side. Blocking ENaC should result in a higher TEER and lower PD due to inhibition of the sodium-dependent current.
7. Wait 10 min at 37°C before recording measurements.
8. Replace the apical and basolateral solution with new solution containing the CFTR activating cocktail (5–20 μM forskolin and, if needed, 50 μM genistein). The apical side should also contain amiloride. Wait 10 min before taking the measurement. It should be noted that genistein is preferred as a low potency CFTR potentiator instead of the high potency ivacaftor. Ivacaftor may stick to electrodes and affect subsequent experiments.
9. The final measurement is performed by adding 30 μM PPQ-102, a CFTR inhibitor, on the apical side. This is done by replacing the apical solution with a new one containing PPQ-102 together with amiloride and a CFTR-activating cocktail at the indicated concentrations. The change in equivalent current elicited by the inhibitor reflects the extent of CFTR function.
10. Wash electrodes with deionized water and 70% ethanol solution.

Important Remarks

1. In the TEER method, CFTR-inh172 does not significantly reduce conductance. We have tested different inhibitors and we have observed that PPQ-102 is the best one for completely blocking CFTR activity (Tradtrantip et al., 2009).

Fluid Absorption Rate Measurements

In CF airways defective ion transport causes a simultaneous reduction of fluid, chloride, and bicarbonate secretion. The altered properties of mucus may be studied in order to understand the pathological mechanisms and to evaluate treatments for recovering hydration of the airways.

Epithelia with serum-free medium reproduces ASL periciliary characteristics with mucus and fluid secretion.

In this section, we present a protocol that allows the measurement of fluid absorption rate.

1. Epithelia begins to secrete mucus and fluids on the apical side after nearly 15 days of culture on Snapwell supports. A fully differentiated epithelia is obtained after 4 weeks of culture.
2. After 15 days of culture, wash the apical surface once a week with D-PBS to remove secreted mucus.
3. Use some of the epithelia of the same cell preparation for short-circuit current recordings to check appropriate ion transport.
4. Apply 130 μl D-PBS on the epithelium surface. We suggest that the apical fluid to recovered between 3 and 48 h after D-PBS incubation.
5. Weigh an empty 1.5 ml collection tube (tare).

6. Carefully collect the fluid remaining after incubation with a pipette and place it in the collection tube (**Figure 3**).
7. Weigh the tube again and estimate the final apical volume collected:
   Vf = (Wf-Wi) × 000/N. Where Wf = tare and collected fluid weight; Wi = tare weight; N = number of pool samples.
8. Calculate fluid transport rate: Jw = (Vi−Vf)/A × t. Where Vi = initial apical volume (130 μl); Vf = final apical volume; A = area of the epithelium (for Snapwell insert: 1.13 cm^2); t = time interval.

Important Remarks

1. During the first days of ALI culture, it is normal to observe some liquid (from the basolateral medium) on the epithelium surface due to the fact that the tight-junctions are not completely formed. This condition will persist in a leaky epithelium.
2. CF secreted mucus is more viscous and difficult to pipette compared to non-CF mucus.

ANTICIPATED RESULTS

To overcome the scarcity of biological material available for primary culture, our group has developed a protocol to extract primary airway epithelial cells from lung resections or nasal brushing and subsequently culture and amplify these cells, maintaining most of the characteristics of the airway epithelium *in vivo*.

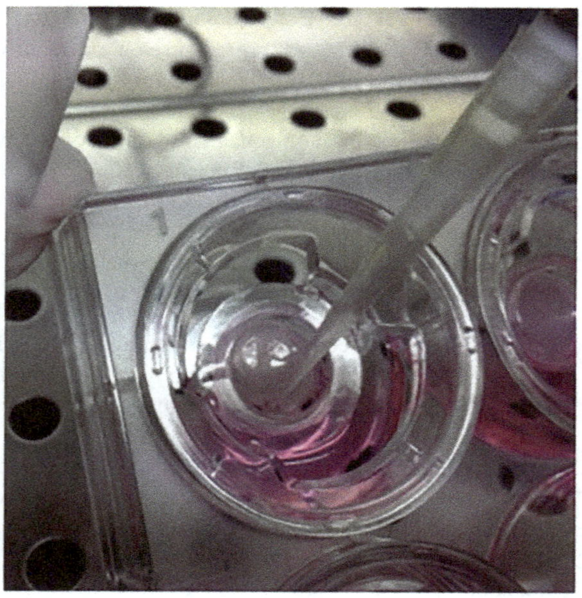

FIGURE 3 | Collection of fluid and mucus secreted from differentiated epithelia. Periciliar fluid collection from surface epithelia after D-PBS incubation.

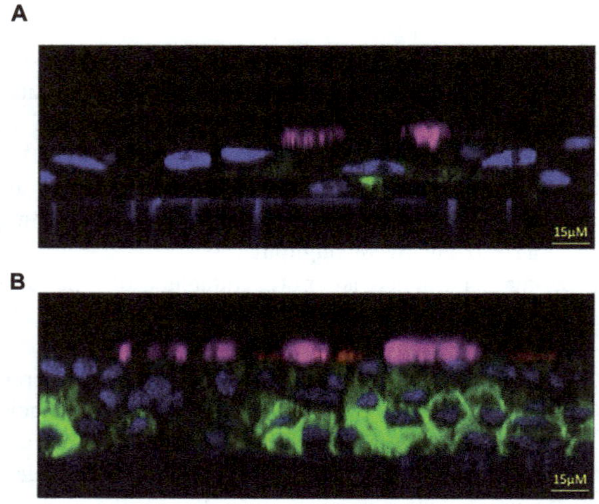

FIGURE 4 | Morphologic properties showing a mature airway epithelium. Representative *xz* immunofluorescence images taken with a confocal microscope (Leica SP8 Laser Scanning Confocal Microscope) to show non-CF bronchial epithelia differentiated with serum-supplemented medium **(A)** or with serum-free medium **(B)**. Cilia are labeled in magenta (anti-tubulin antibody), the goblet cells in red (anti-MUC5AC antibody), the apical membrane in green (anti-TMEM16A antibody) and the nucleus in blue (Hoechst dye). Images kindly provided by Dr. Paolo Scudieri (TIGEM, Pozzuoli, Italy).

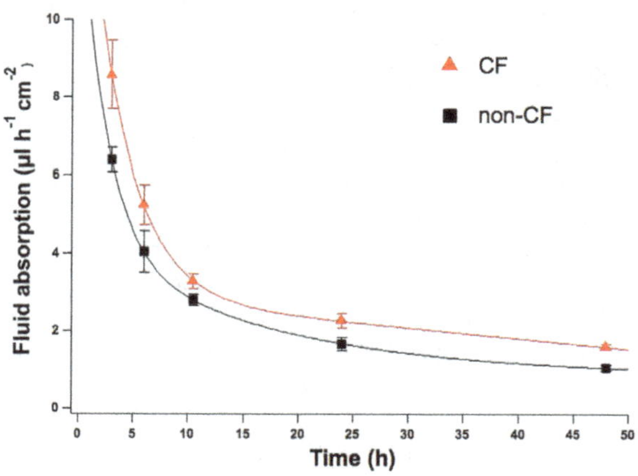

FIGURE 5 | Time course rate of fluid absorption of non-CF and CF epithelia. Net fluid absorption rate measured on non-CF (black squares) and CF (red triangles) epithelia up until 48 h of incubation with D-PBS. Mean values ± SEM are shown, at the timepoints of 24 and 48 h the differences between CF and non-CF epithelia are significant ($p < 0.05$).

The procedure starts by using a proliferative medium that promotes cell growth at a low density and a high proliferation rate in order to obtain a large number of polarized bronchial and nasal epithelia useful for the study of CF physiopathology.

This is followed by a differentiation phase. We have presented two protocols that both require seeding cells on permeable supports and the "ALI" condition, but they differ depending on the final aim of the designed experiments.

The serum-free medium protocol provides a fully differentiated epithelial monolayer that is useful for evaluating morphological and periciliary fluid properties in primary airway epithelia. However, a critical point of this protocol is the prolonged culture time and the cost of medium supplements.

Instead, we suggest that the serum-complemented medium be applied to the protocol for functional electrophysiologic assays, because it still provides a differentiated monolayer with transepithelial ion transport properties similar to *in vivo* conditions, but in a shorter time and with lower costs compared to the serum-free medium protocol. Therefore, this medium is optimal for functional electrophysiologic assays.

To compare the two protocols for evaluating epithelial morphological properties, we have used immunofluorescence combined with confocal microscopy. This technique provides high-resolution imaging of protein localization, expression patterns, and different cell types that characterize the airway of mature epithelium.

Cultured bronchial epithelia are analyzed by immunofluorescence for acetylated tubulin and MUC5AC to identify ciliated and goblet cells, respectively. To distinguish the apical from the basolateral membrane we have used an antibody against the ZO-1 tight junction marker.

The derived staining shows that epithelium differentiated with serum-supplemented medium is pseudo-stratified with a relatively small number of ciliated and goblet cells (**Figure 4A**).

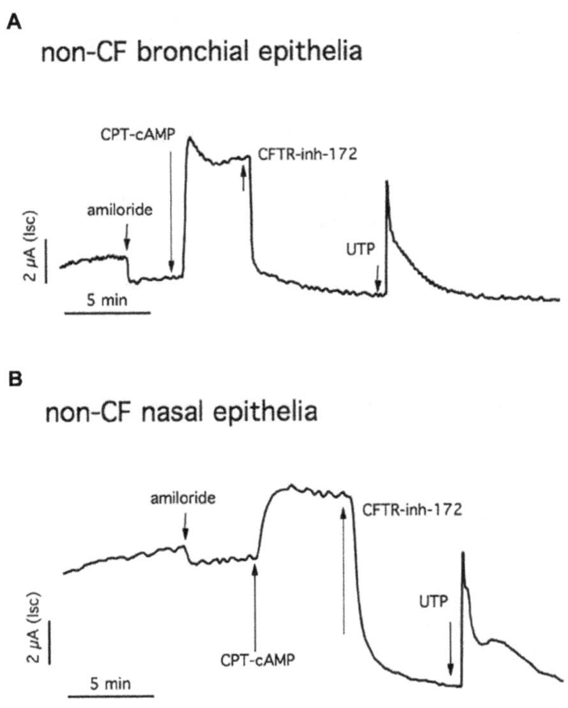

FIGURE 6 | Short circuit currents (Isc) measurements in non-CF epithelia. Representative traces from Ussing chamber recordings of non-CF bronchial **(A)** and nasal epithelia **(B)**. The ENaC channel is blocked with apical amiloride and CFTR activation and inhibition is obtained by adding CPT-cAMP and $CFTR_{inh}$-172, respectively. The Ca^{2+}- dependent chloride channel is stimulated with UTP.

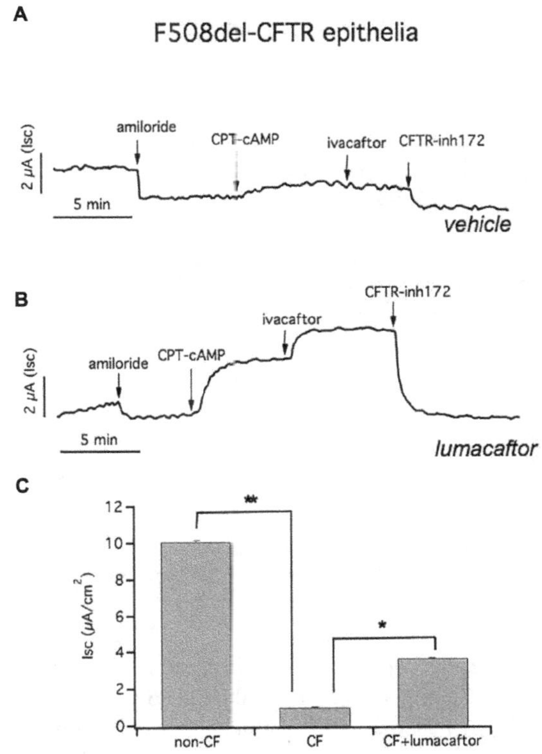

FIGURE 7 | Short circuit currents (Isc) in CF and in lumacaftor-treated CF epithelia. Representative traces from short circuit current (Isc) recordings of homozygous F508del-CFTR epithelia treated with vehicle **(A)** and lumacaftor **(B)**. The ENaC channel is blocked with apical amiloride and CFTR activation and inhibition is obtained by adding CPT-cAMP plus ivacaftor and $CFTR_{inh}$-172, respectively. **(C)** Graph bars summarizing CFTR-mediated currents from Ussing chamber recordings of HBEC derived from 4 non-CF donors (n = 22) and from 4 homozygous F508del-CFTR patients (n = 41). Mean values ± SEM are shown * and ** indicate $p < 0.05$ or $p < 0.001$, respectively.

On the contrary, when using the serum-free medium protocol we obtained a higher pseudo-stratified epithelium characterized by a higher number of ciliated and goblet cells (**Figure 4B**). This result demonstrates that the latter culture condition provides most of the morphological characteristics of the airway epithelium *in vivo*, thus we suggest that it be used to analyse the expression and localization of selected proteins and airway cells.

In the CF lung, the decrease in CFTR-mediated chloride and fluid secretion are believed to cause the dehydration of the airway surface by altering the properties of periciliary mucus. To gather significant information, we have applied the serum-free medium protocol, that reproduces ASL periciliary characteristics with mucus and fluid secretion, to analyse the rate of fluid absorption of non-CF and CF airway mucus recovered from cultured HBEC.

Time course experiments confirmed that the different activities of CFTR in non-CF and F508del-CFTR epithelia resulted in significant differences in the net absorption rate after 24 and 48 h; reflecting the different ASL characteristics.

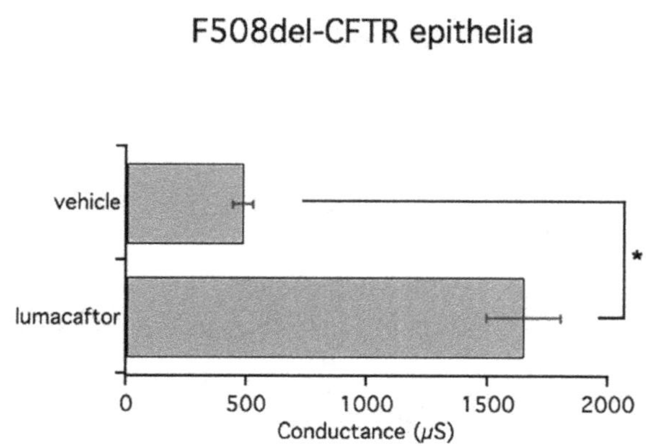

FIGURE 8 | TEER measurements in CF and lumacaftor-treated CF. Graph bars indicate TEER measurements performed on homozygous F508del-CFTR epithelia derived from 4 homozygous F508del-CFTR patients ($n = 12$) treated with vehicle or lumacaftor. The bar graphs show the electrical resistance values measured before and after CFTR inhibition, converted into their reciprocal conductance. Mean values ± SEM are shown, * indicate $p < 0.05$.

While non-CF epithelia absorbed after 24 and 48 h 1.67 ± 0.15 μl/h/cm^2 ($n = 5$) and 1.06 ± 0.06 μl/h/cm^2 ($n = 7$), respectively, in F508del-CFTR epithelia net absorpion rate was 2.25 ± 0.19 μl/h/cm^2 ($n = 5$) and 1.58 ± 0.07 μl/h/cm^2 ($n = 7$) (**Figure 5**).

Moreover, during recovery we observed that the CF fluid is more viscous and difficult to pipette compared to non-CF.

The development and validation of CF-HBEC aims to support drug discovery efforts to correct basic CF defects. For this purpose, electrophysiological approaches allow transepithelial ion transport to be measured in order to assess the efficacy of pre-clinical CFTR modulators in primary human airway cultures.

We have used the Ussing chamber technique to measure short-circuit current as an indication of net ion transport across bronchial and nasal epithelia monolayers maintained in serum-supplemented medium.

Figure 6A shows a representative trace experiment of short-circuit currents of differentiated non-CF bronchial epithelia. The basal current was inhibited by amiloride, indicating the presence of epithelial Na^+ channel (3.1 ± 0.6 μA/cm^2; $n = 25$). To assess the amount of CFTR-dependent Isc, cells are blocked with CFTRinh-172 after maximum CFTR activation using CPT-cAMP. The resulting chloride current is strongly sensitive to CFTRinh-172 (10.08 ± 0.04 μA/cm^2; $n = 31$). Application of UTP generates a very fast calcium-activated chloride current (3.8 ± 1 μA/cm^2; $n = 29$).

Primary human nasal monolayers recapitulate the transepithelial ion transport properties of bronchial cells, confirming the fact that this cell model can predict clinical treatment efficacy in patients (**Figure 6B**).

To further support the conclusion that our culture protocol allows F508del-CFTR-HBEC to reflect the ion transport defects in airway epithelia *in vivo*, we used cells from patients that were homozygous for this mutation; which causes a severe defect in CFTR function. As expected the response to CPT-cAMP and ivacaftor is markedly reduced in negative control cells (1.04 ± 0.023 μA/cm^2; $n = 37$) (**Figure 7A**). However, we have noted that lumacaftor treatment for 24 h induced a significant increase in chloride transport, as indicated by the current blocked by CFTRinh-172 (3.67 ± 0.07 μA/cm^2; $n = 41$) (**Figure 7B**).

Figure 7C summarizes the CFTR-mediated currents from Ussing chamber recordings of HBEC derived from 4 non-CF donors and 4 homozygous F508del-CFTR patients. Transepithelial current measurements showed that there was a significant difference in the CFTR-mediated Isc in cultured F508del-HBE cells compared to non-CF HBE cells, and incubation of CF epithelium with lumacaftor led to a significant improvement in CFTR-dependent chloride secretion.

TEER is a quantitative technique that is useful for predicting the ideal concentration of a drug to be tested, without damaging the epithelium, or to quantify ion transport by measuring the electrical resistance and potential difference across the barrier tissue.

We have performed TEER measurements to evaluate the ability of compounds to correct F508del-CFTR. Bronchial epithelia from patients that were homozygous for the F508del mutation were treated for 24 h with lumacaftor, or vehicle (DMSO), and then assayed. Transepithelial electrical resistance was measured before and after acute stimulation with forskolin and genistein to fully activate CFTR. Subsequently, transepithelial resistance was measured after the addition of the selective CFTR inhibitor, PPQ-102, used to completely block CFTR activity. The delta between the values of electrical resistance before and after CFTR inhibition were then converted into the reciprocal conductance.

In accordance with short-circuit current measurements, treatment with lumacaftor significantly increased transepithelial conductance (1650 ± 153.3 μS/cm^2) compared with the negative control (482 ± 42.2 μS/cm^2). The bar graph shows mean values obtained from four different omozygous F508del-CFTR patients (**Figure 8**).

In conclusion, we have provided evidence that our procedures provide highly differentiated airway epithelial monolayers with morphologic and functional characteristics similar to airway epithelia *in vivo*. These cell models are very useful for improving our knowledge about physiopathology mechanisms involved in CF and to support therapeutics strategies.

ETHICS STATEMENT

The procedure of the bronchus dissection and the informed consent from patients was approved by the Ethical Committee of the Gaslini Institute under the supervision of the Italian Ministry of Health.

AUTHOR CONTRIBUTIONS

AG and LD have performed the procedures and contributed equally to the work. EC has written the manuscript with the help of AG and LD.

ACKNOWLEDGMENTS

This work was supported by grants from the Italian Cystic Fibrosis Foundation (FFC no. CP/2012 with the contribution of "Delegazione FFC di Tradate Gallarate" and "Verbania-V.C.O.") and from European Union's Horizon 2020 research and innovation program under grant agreement no. 667079. We are grateful to Dr. Luis Galietta (TIGEM, Pozzuoli, Italy) for his ongoing support and Amber Philp (Universidad Austral de Chile, Valdivia, Chile) for english editing revision.

REFERENCES

Borowitz, D. (2015). CFTR, bicarbonate, and the pathophysiology of cystic fibrosis. *Pediatr. Pulmonol.* 40, S24–S30. doi: 10.1002/ppul.23247

Castellani, C., and Assael, B. M. (2017). Cystic fibrosis: a clinical view. *Cell. Mol. Life Sci.* 74, 129–140. doi: 10.1007/s00018-016-2393-9

Fulcher, M. L., Gabriel, S., Burns, K. A., Yankaskas, J. R., and Randell, S. H. (2005). Well-differentiated human airway epithelial cell cultures. *Methods Mol. Med.* 2005, 183–206.

Galietta, L. J., Lantero, S., Gazzolo, A., Sacco, O., Romano, L., Rossi, G. A., et al. (1998). An improved method to obtain highly differentiated monolayers of human bronchial epithelial cells. *In Vitro Cell. Dev. Biol. Anim.* 34, 478–481.

Gentzsch, M., Boyles, S. E., Cheluvaraju, C., Chaudhry, I. G., Quinney, N. L., Cho, C., et al. (2017). Pharmacological rescue of conditionally reprogrammed cystic fibrosis bronchial epithelial cells. *Am. J. Respir. Cell Mol. Biol.* 56, 568–574. doi: 10.1165/rcmb.2016-0276MA

Gianotti, A., Capurro, V., Scudieri, P., Galietta, L. J. V., Moran, O., and Zegarra-Moran, O. (2016). Pharmacological rescue of mutant CFTR protein improves the viscoelastic properties of CF mucus. *J. Cyst. Fibros.* 15, 295–301. doi: 10.1016/j.jcf.2015.11.003

Hajj, R., Baranek, T., Le Naour, R., Lesimple, P., Puchelle, E., and Coraux, C. (2007). Basal cells of the human adult airway surface epithelium retain transit-amplifying cell properties. *Stem Cells* 25, 139–148.

Li, H., Sheppard, D. N., and Hug, M. J. (2004). Transepithelial electrical measurements with the Ussing chamber. *J. Cyst. Fibros* 3(Suppl. 2), 123–126. doi: 10.1016/j.jcf.2004.05.026

McDougall, C. M., Blaylock, M. G., Douglas, J. G., Brooker, R. J., Helms, P. J., and Walsh, G. M. (2008). Nasal epithelial cells as surrogates for bronchial epithelial cells in airway inflammation studies. *Am. J. Respir. Cell Mol. Biol.* 39, 560–568. doi: 10.1165/rcmb.2007-0325OC

Mosler, K., Coraux, C., Fragaki, K., Zahm, J., Bajolet, O., Bessaci-Kabouya, K., et al. (2008). Feasibility of nasal epithelial brushing for the study of airway epithelial functions in CF infants. *J. Cyst. Fibros.* 7, 44–53.

Mou, H., Vinarsky, V., Tata, P. R., Brazauskas, K., Choi, S. H., Crooke, A. K., et al. (2016). Dual SMAD signaling inhibition enables long-term expansion of diverse epithelial basal cells. *Cell Stem Cell* 19, 217–231. doi: 10.1016/j.stem.2016.05.012

Müller, L., Brighton, L. E., Carson, J. L., Fischer, W. A. II, and Jaspers, I. (2013). Culturing of human nasal epithelial cells at the air liquid interface. *J. Vis. Exp.* 8:80.

Neuberger, T., Burton, T., Clark, H., and Van Goor, F. (2011). Use of primary cultures of human bronchial epithelial cells isolated from cystic fibrosis patients for the pre-clinical testing of CFTR modulators. *Methods Mol. Biol.* 741, 39–54. doi: 10.1007/978-1-61779-117-8_4

Okiyoneda, T., Veit, G., Dekkers, J. F., Bagdany, M., Soya, N., Xu, H., et al. (2013). Mechanism-based corrector combination restores ΔF508-CFTR folding and function. *Nat. Chem. Biol.* 9, 444–454. doi: 10.1038/nchembio.1253

Palechor-Ceron, N., Suprynowicz, F. A., Upadhyay, G., Dakic, A., Minas, T., Simic, V., et al. (2013). Radiation induces diffusible feeder cell factor(s) that cooperate with ROCK Inhibitor to conditionally reprogram and immortalize epithelial cells. *Am. J. Pathol.* 183, 1862–1870. doi: 10.1016/j.ajpath.2013.08.009

Pedemonte, N., Lukacs, G. L., Du, K., Caci, E., Zegarra-Moran, O., Galietta, L. J. V., et al. (2005). Small-molecule correctors of defective ΔF508-CFTR cellular processing identified by high-throughput screening. *J. Clin. Invest.* 115, 2564–2571.

Pranke, I. M., Hatton, A., Simonin, J., Jais, J. P., Le Pimpec-Barthes, F., Carsin, A., et al. (2017). Correction of CFTR function in nasal epithelial cells from cystic fibrosis patients predicts improvement of respiratory function by CFTR modulators. *Sci. Rep.* 7:7375. doi: 10.1038/s41598-017-07504-1

Quinton, P. M. (2008). Cystic fibrosis: impaired bicarbonate secretion and mucoviscidosis. *Lancet* 372, 415–417. doi: 10.1016/S0140-6736(08)61162-9

Sacco, O., Romberger, D., Rizzino, A., Beckmann, J. D., Rennard, S. I., and Spurzem, J. R. (1992). Spontaneous production of transforming growth factor-beta 2 by primary cultures of bronchial epithelial cells. Effects on cell behavior *in vitro*. *J. Clin. Invest.* 90, 1379–1385.

Saint-Criq, V., and Gray, M. A. (2017). Role of CFTR in epithelial physiology. *Cell. Mol. Life Sci.* 74, 93–115.

Scudieri, P., Caci, E., Bruno, S., Ferrera, L., Schiavon, M., Sondo, E., et al. (2012). Association of TMEM16A chloride channel overexpression with airway goblet cell metaplasia. *J. Physiol.* 590, 6141–6155. doi: 10.1113/jphysiol.2012.240838

Srinivasan, B., Kolli, A. R., Esch, M. B., Abaci, H. E., Shuler, M. L., and Hickman, J. J. (2015). TEER measurement techniques for *in vitro* barrier model systems. *J. Lab. Autom.* 20, 107–126. doi: 10.1177/2211068214561025

Stokes, A. B., Kieninger, E., Schogler, A., Kopf, B. S., Casaulta, C., Geiser, T., et al. (2014). Comparison of three different brushing techniques to isolate and culture primary nasal epithelial cells from human subjects. *Exp. Lung Res.* 40, 327–332. doi: 10.3109/01902148.2014.925987

Tradtrantip, L., Sonawane, N. D., Namkung, W., and Verkman, A. S. (2009). Nanomolar potency pyrimido-pyrrolo-quinoxalinedione CFTR inhibitor reduces cyst size in a polycystic kidney disease model. *J. Med. Chem.* 52, 6447–6455. doi: 10.1021/jm9009873

Van Goor, F., Hadida, S., Grootenhuis, P. D., Burton, B., Cao, D., Neuberger, T., et al. (2009). Rescue of CF airway epithelial cell function *in vitro* by a CFTR potentiator. VX-770. *Proc. Natl. Acad. Sci. U.S.A.* 106, 18825–18830. doi: 10.1073/pnas.0904709106

Van Goor, F., Hadida, S., Grootenhuis, P. D., Burton, B., Stack, J. H., Straley, K. S., et al. (2011). Correction of the F508del-CFTR protein processing defect *in vitro* by the investigational drug VX-809. *Proc. Natl. Acad. Sci. U.S.A.* 108, 18843–18848. doi: 10.1073/pnas.1105787108

Wainwright, C. E., Elborn, J. S., Ramsey, B. W., Marigowda, G., Huang, X., Cipolli, M., et al. (2015). Lumacaftor-Ivacaftor in Patients with Cystic Fibrosis Homozygous for Phe508del CFTR. *N. Engl. J. Med.* 373, 220–231. doi: 10.1056/NEJMoa1409547

Yaghi, A., Zaman, A., and Dolovich, M. (2010). Primary human bronchial epithelial cells grown from explants. *J. Vis. Exp.* 26:37.

13

Peripheral Protein Quality Control as a Novel Drug Target for CFTR Stabilizer

*Ryosuke Fukuda and Tsukasa Okiyoneda**

Department of Biomedical Chemistry, School of Science and Technology, Kwansei Gakuin University, Nishinomiya, Japan

Correspondence:
Tsukasa Okiyoneda
t-okiyoneda@kwansei.ac.jp

Conformationally defective cystic fibrosis transmembrane conductance regulator (CFTR) including rescued ΔF508-CFTR is rapidly eliminated from the plasma membrane (PM) even in the presence of a CFTR corrector and potentiator, limiting the therapeutic effort of the combination therapy. CFTR elimination from the PM is determined by the conformation-dependent ubiquitination as a part of the peripheral quality control (PQC) mechanism. Recently, the molecular machineries responsible for the CFTR PQC mechanism which includes molecular chaperones and ubiquitination enzymes have been revealed. This review summarizes the molecular mechanism of the CFTR PQC and discusses the possibility that the peripheral ubiquitination mechanism becomes a novel drug target to develop the CFTR stabilizer as a novel class of CFTR modulator.

Keywords: peripheral QC, CFTR, stabilizer, ubiquitination, RFFL

INTRODUCTION

Cystic fibrosis (CF) is one of the most lethal autosomal-recessive diseases caused by mutation in CFTR (Lopes-Pacheco, 2016). CFTR mutations are classified as I–VII according to their properties (I-protein synthesis defect, II-maturation defect, III-gating defect, IV-conductance defect, V-reduced quantity, VI-reduced PM stability, VII-no mRNA transcription). The most prevalent CF causing mutation, ΔF508, was classically categorized as class II mutation. However, rescued ΔF508 (rΔF508)-CFTR by corrector (e.g., VX-809/lumacaftor) or low temperature culture shows class III and VI phenotypes (Dalemans et al., 1991; Veit et al., 2016a). Although drug targets of the class II or III mutations are well studied, that of the class VI mutation are not because the mechanism of CFTR PM stability regulation are still veiled by numerous undefined molecules involved in CFTR PQC system. In this review, we summarize accumulated findings regarding the CFTR PQC from the molecular and environmental aspects and also discuss the potential of recently identified PQC machineries including endocytic adaptors and ubiquitination enzymes as targets for CFTR stabilizer which anchors the functional channel at the PM and reduces the degradation (**Figure 1**).

CFTR INSTABILITY AT THE PM

Nascent wild-type (WT) CFTR is *N*-glycosylated at the endoplasmic reticulum (ER) during translation and folded by the aid of chaperones such as calnexin (CNX), HSP70 and HSP90 (Amaral, 2004; Kleizen et al., 2005; Okiyoneda et al., 2008; Rosser et al., 2008; Glozman et al., 2009; Kim and Skach, 2012). Properly folded CFTR is then sorted to the Golgi apparatus and

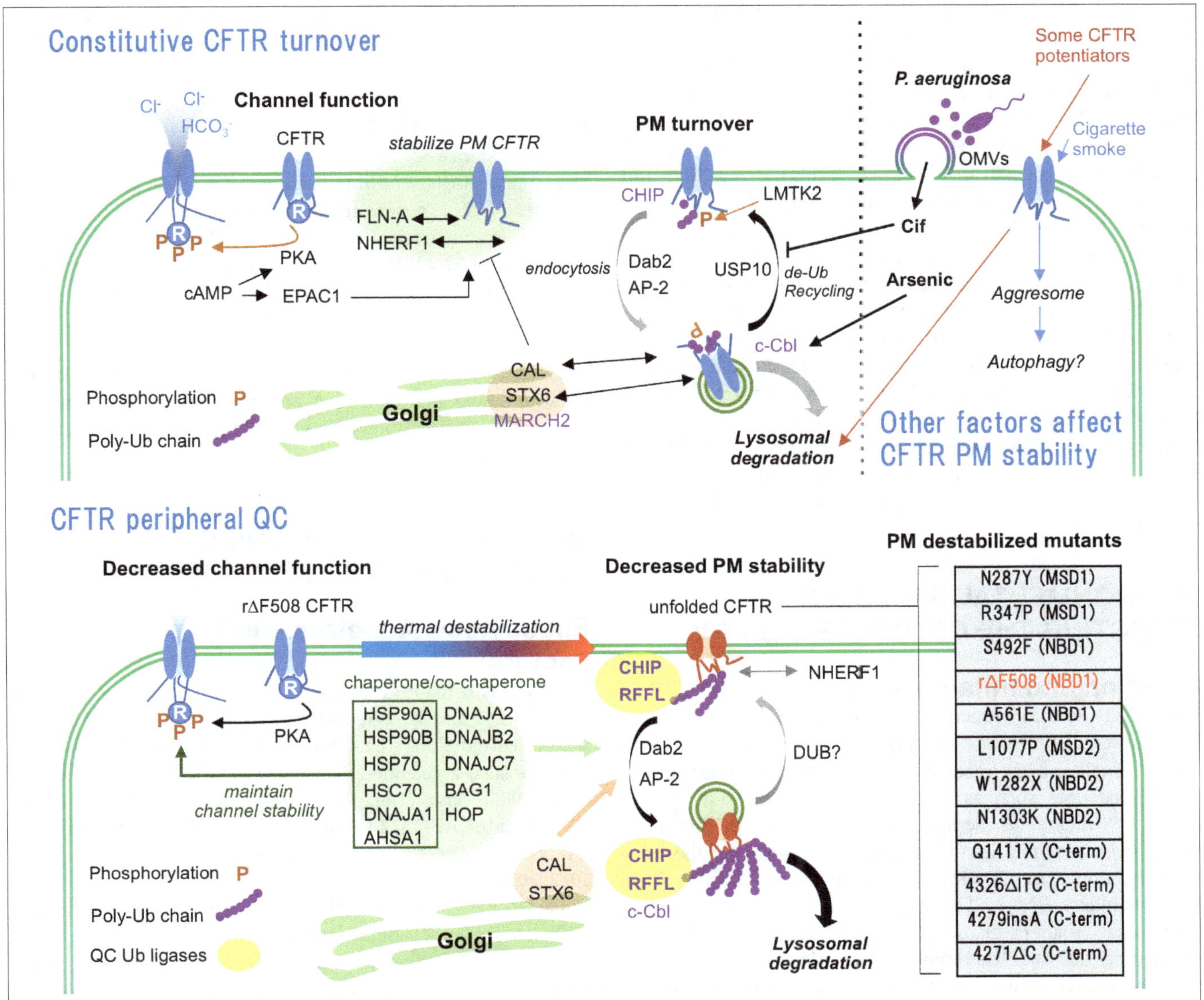

FIGURE 1 | Constitutive turnover and PQC of CFTR. **(Upper)** WT-CFTR is stabilized at the PM by interaction with FLN-A and NHERF1. Internalization of WT-CFTR is regulated by LMTK2-mediated phosphorylation and CHIP-mediated ubiquitination. Predominant endocytosed WT-CFTR is recycled back to the PM by USP10 mediated de-ubiquitination. Golgi localized CAL complex promotes lysosomal sorting of CFTR. CFTR PM stability is deteriorated by infection, CS and CFTR potentiators. **(Lower)** Unfolded rΔF508-CFTR at the PM is ubiquitinated by PQC Ub ligases CHIP and RFFL, and rapidly internalized probably by CME mediated by DAB2 and AP-2. Chaperone/co-chaperone complex also facilitates the unfolded CFTR internalization while it helps the channel functionality at the PM. Internalized unfolded CFTR could be ubiquitinated at endosomes and targeted to lysosomal degradation. CAL also facilitates the lysosomal degradation of internalized CFTR. PM destabilizing CFTR mutations and their locations are listed (Veit et al., 2016a, Cystic Fibrosis Genetic Consortium Database). N287Y mutation increases CFTR endocytosis without affecting maturation (Silvis et al., 2003). R347P, S492F, rΔF508, A561E, L1077P, and N1303K mutations induce severe maturation defect and PM instability (Van Goor et al., 2014). N287Y and L1077P are localized at intracellular loop 2 (ICL2) of MSD1 and ICL4 of MSD2, respectively. Both mutations are predicted to destabilize the MSD1-NBD2 and MSD2-NBD1 interactions that define CFTR conformational stability.

processed to complex glycosylation while misfolded CFTR is retained in the ER and consequently degraded by ER-associated degradation (ERAD). The CFTR ERAD is associated with several ER QC processes such as chaperones binding, ubiquitination and retro-translocation from the ER to cytosol (Younger et al., 2006; Turnbull et al., 2007; Morito et al., 2008; Grove et al., 2011; Nery et al., 2011; El Khouri et al., 2013; Matsumura et al., 2013; Ernst et al., 2016; Gong et al., 2016; McClure et al., 2016; Ramachandran et al., 2016; Hou et al., 2018). Properly folded and matured CFTR is trafficked to the PM to function as an ATP-regulated ion-channel (Chen et al., 2000).

The CFTR is internalized by clathrin-mediated endocytosis (CME) and recycled back to the PM. Conformationally defective CFTR produced by genetic mutations (e.g., ΔF508, T70) and/or environmental stresses (e.g., heat) selectively undergoes ubiquitination at the PM by PQC machineries. The ubiquitinated CFTR is rapidly internalized and delivered to lysosome for degradation (Sharma et al., 2004; Okiyoneda et al., 2010).

Internalized CFTR could be de-ubiquitinated at endosomes by deubiquitinase (DUB) and recycled back to the PM depending on the conformational states. The class VI mutations render the CFTR unstable at the PM. Additionally, the class I, II and some class III CFTR mutants also show PM instability (Lukacs et al., 1993; Haardt et al., 1999; Silvis et al., 2003; Wang et al., 2014; Veit et al., 2016a). *N*-glycosylation, especially the core-glycosylation, determines the CFTR PM stability likely by affecting the CFTR conformational stability (Glozman et al., 2009; Cholon et al., 2010). Protein translation kinetics is also a significant factor that modulates proper co-translational folding. Knock down (KD) of ribosomal protein L12 (RPL12) increases ΔF508-CFTR PM expression and stability (Veit et al., 2016b). RPL12 KD might affect protein translation kinetics associated with co-translational protein folding efficiency (Buhr et al., 2016) and thereby improve CFTR thermodynamic stability which also determines the CFTR PM stability (Okiyoneda et al., 2010; Rabeh et al., 2012). Thus, correcting the CFTR structural defects at the ER could improve the PM stability.

ENVIRONMENTAL STRESSES AFFECTING THE CFTR PM STABILITY

Infection and Inflammation

The CFTR loss of function induces airway surface liquid (ASL) dysregulation which impairs clearance of infected bacteria and/or fungi, and increases the concentration of other soluble signal mediators such as cytokines, chemokines and growth factors. *Pseudomonas aeruginosa* (PA) is one of the most common bacteria found in CF respiratory tissue and responsible for lung injury in CF (Koch, 2002; Bhagirath et al., 2016). PA destabilizes PM CFTR by inhibiting endocytic recycling (Swiatecka-Urban et al., 2006). PA secretes CFTR inhibitory factor (Cif) that stabilizes complex formation of ubiquitin (Ub) specific peptidase 10 (USP10) and GTPase activating protein (SH3 domain) binding protein 1 (G3BP1) and inhibits CFTR-USP10 interaction. Cif inhibits internalized CFTR sorting to recycling pathway by suppressing USP10 dependent CFTR de-ubiquitination at endosome, resulting in the lysosomal degradation of WT-CFTR (Bomberger et al., 2011). PA also activates transforming growth factor β1 (TGF-β1) signaling that is an important modifier of lung disease severity in CF (Harris et al., 2011). TGF-β1 inhibits functional PM expression of WT-CFTR and ΔF508-CFTR by reducing mRNA level (Snodgrass et al., 2013; Sun et al., 2014) although its role in the PQC remains unknown.

Heavy Metals

More than 10 ppb of arsenic induces the WT-CFTR ubiquitination and lysosomal degradation via c-Cbl in CF bronchial epithelial (CFBE) cells (Bomberger et al., 2012). Importantly, the phenotype of arsenic toxicity overlaps with CF patient (Bomberger et al., 2012; Mazumdar et al., 2015). Cadmium (Cd) is a major component of cigarette smoke (CS), and its inhalation is associated with decreased pulmonary function and chronic obstructive pulmonary disease. Cd reduces CFTR PM level, but it remains unknown if it reduces the PM stability (Rennolds et al., 2010).

Cigarette Smoke

Cigarette smoke is a major risk factor of chronic obstructive pulmonary disease and interferes with CFTR functionality. Ten minutes of CS exposure transiently suppresses CFTR function, induces internalization and decreases ASL height in human bronchial epithelial (HBE) cells (Clunes et al., 2012). CS promotes CFTR internalization in BHK cells and results in increased insolubility of CFTR and colocalization with vimentin, a filament protein associated with aggresome Ca^{2+} dependently. This observation suggesting that CS induces PM CFTR destabilization by stimulating internalization and aggregation in addition to suppressing CFTR functionality (Clunes et al., 2012; Rasmussen et al., 2014).

MOLECULAR MACHINERIES DETERMINING THE CFTR PM STABILITY

Endocytosis Adaptors and Tethering Factors

Endocytosis is the critical step of elimination of PM CFTR as a part of PQC and is regulated by several molecules. WT-CFTR is internalized slowly by CME while misfolded rΔF508-CFTR endocytosis is accelerated (Sharma et al., 2004; Swiatecka-Urban et al., 2005; Varga et al., 2008; Okiyoneda et al., 2010). KD of CME adaptor AP-2 μ2 subunit or disabled 2 (DAB2) stabilizes rΔF508-CFTR at the PM by inhibiting endocytosis (Fu et al., 2012, 2015).

CFTR has a postsynaptic density 95, disks large, zonula occludens-1 (PDZ) binding motif at C-terminus and binds with Na^+/H^+ exchanger regulatory factor (NHERF1) PDZ domain. NHERF1 tethers CFTR with Ezrin and works as a scaffold protein that supports CFTR efficient channel activation and apical PM localization (Favia et al., 2010; Arora et al., 2014; Loureiro et al., 2015). NHERF1 also binds to misfolded ΔF508-CFTR and increases the PM stability by inhibiting carboxy terminus of HSP70-interacting protein (CHIP) Ub ligase interaction (Loureiro et al., 2015). An exchange protein directly activated by cAMP1 (EPAC1) selective activating cAMP analog 007-AM promotes WT-CFTR and NHERF1 interaction and increases CFTR PM stability in CFBE cells by suppressing endocytosis (Lobo et al., 2016). EPAC1 activation can rescue ΔF508-CFTR PM expression, and its effect is further improved with VX-809 combination (Lobo et al., 2016).

The CFTR-associated ligand (CAL) negatively regulates ΔF508-CFTR PM abundance through its PDZ domain (Wolde et al., 2007). CAL inhibition enhances the functional stability of ΔF508-CFTR at the apical PM, implying an attractive therapeutic target for CFTR PM stabilizer (Cushing et al., 2010). However, CAL also interacts with syntaxin 6 (STX6) and Golgi-localized E3-ligase membrane associated RING-CH type finger

2 (MARCH2) and regulates WT-CFTR PM expression (Wolde et al., 2007; Cheng and Guggino, 2013).

Filamin-A (FLN-A) is a membrane tethered actin adaptor protein and interacts with CFTR N-terminus region. S13F mutation of CFTR compromises FLN-A binding and consequently destabilizes the PM CFTR (Thelin et al., 2007). FLN-A binds with both WT and rΔF508-CFTR at similar level, however, its contribution to the CFTR PQC remains unclear.

Protein Kinases

The CFTR PM stability is regulated by phosphorylation. CFTR is predominantly phosphorylated at the R domain and also at nucleotide binding domain 1 (NBD1) and C-terminus residues by protein kinase A (PKA), protein kinase C (PKC), casein kinase II (CK2) and AMP-activated protein kinase (AMPK) for the channel function (Chappe et al., 2003; Kongsuphol et al., 2009; Luz et al., 2011). CK2 is predicted to regulate CFTR PM stability by phosphorylation at Thr-1471 where NHERF1 could interact (Venerando et al., 2013). Lemur tyrosine kinase 2 (LMTK2) phosphorylates CFTR at Ser-737 (Wang and Brautigan, 2006) and its KD or mutation at CFTR Ser-737 suppresses the endocytosis and increases CFTR PM density and stability (Luz et al., 2014). However, LMKT2 KD only modestly improves the PM function of rΔF508-CFTR (Luz et al., 2014). Spleen tyrosine kinase (SYK) phosphorylates CFTR at Tyr-512 and decreases CFTR PM levels possibly by triggering endocytosis (Luz et al., 2011; Mendes et al., 2011). Mixed-lineage kinase 3 (MLK3) pathway regulates not only ΔF508-CFTR ERQC, but also the PQC by regulating the CFTR proteostasis (Hegde et al., 2015). Inhibition of MLK3 pathway could regulate ΔF508-CFTR folding/degradation switch by impairing interaction with PQC machinery such as HSP70/HSP90 Organizing Protein (HOP) (Hegde et al., 2015).

Chaperones

Molecular chaperones selectively interact with and stabilize unfolded or partially folded protein to acquire a functionally active conformation. Nascent CFTR interacts with a panel of chaperones and co-chaperones including HSC70, HSP70, HSP90, and CNX at the ER (Yang et al., 1993; Pind et al., 1994; Loo et al., 1998; Meacham et al., 1999; Okiyoneda et al., 2004). Even at the post-ER compartments, conformationally defective CFTR such as unfolded rΔF508-CFTR is recognized by chaperone/co-chaperone complex (Okiyoneda et al., 2010). HSC70/HSP90 complex selectively interacts with unfolded rΔF508-CFTR at the post-Golgi and this interaction is crucial for the unfolding dependent ubiquitination (Okiyoneda et al., 2010). KD of HSC70/HSP90 complex (HSP90, HSC70, HOP, AHA1, DNAJB2, DNAJA1, BAG1) increases the rΔF508-CFTR PM stability in HeLa cells (Okiyoneda et al., 2010). The HSC70/HSP90 complex is also essential for maintaining kinetic and thermodynamic stability of rΔF508-CFTR at the PM by reshaping the CFTR conformation during energetic destabilization (Bagdany et al., 2017). This chaperone activity also maintains rΔF508-CFTR channel function at the PM (Bagdany et al., 2017). Thus, modulating the chaperone activity would be a viable target for attenuating the ubiquitination and for stabilizing the CFTR function at the PM.

Ubiquitination Enzymes

Ubiquitination determines CFTR elimination not only at the ER, but also from the PM. Ubiquitination is mediated by a sequential action of E1, E2, and E3 enzymes and this modification could be removed by DUB. Specifically, E3 Ub ligase has been proposed to determine the substrate specificity. CHIP is the first identified E3 ligase responsible for the CFTR PQC (Okiyoneda et al., 2010). Consistent with the action at the ER (Meacham et al., 2001), CHIP selectively interacts with unfolded ΔF508-CFTR at the post-Golgi through the HSC70/HSP90 chaperones. CHIP KD reduces the ubiquitination of unfolded ΔF508-CFTR, resulting in the decelerated endocytosis and lysosomal delivery in HeLa cells (Okiyoneda et al., 2010). CHIP KD also stabilizes rΔF508-CFTR at the PM of polarized CFBE cells (Fu et al., 2015).

E3 ligase c-Cbl may play a role in the CFTR peripheral QC, but its contribution could be modest since its KD slightly increases rΔF508-CFTR PM stability in CFBE cells (Cihil et al., 2013; Fu et al., 2015). c-Cbl also binds with WT-CFTR and decreases the PM stability without affecting the ubiquitination, suggesting that c-Cbl could regulate constitutive PM turnover of folded CFTR by inducing endocytosis through its C-terminus adaptor function (Ye et al., 2010).

Nedd4-2 is a member of homologous to the E6-AP carboxyl terminus (HECT) E3 which may regulate the CFTR PM expression. Nedd4-2 KD reduces ΔF508-CFTR ubiquitination at the ER, and increases the PM expression and function in CF pancreatic adenocarcinoma cell 1 (CFPAC1) and IB3-1 cells (Caohuy et al., 2009). Nedd4-2 binds both WT- and ΔF508-CFTR while its role in the WT-CFTR ubiquitination remains controversial (Koeppen et al., 2012). However, Nedd4-2 KD does not stabilize the PM rΔF508-CFTR in CFBE cells, implying its marginal contribution to the CFTR PQC (Koeppen et al., 2012; Fu et al., 2015). Nedd4-2 is unlikely a viable CF drug target because its knock out (KO) induces CF-like lung phenotype by excessive function of epithelial Na^+ Channel (ENaC) (Kimura et al., 2011; Rotin and Staub, 2012).

A number of DUBs regulate the CFTR turnover. USP10, a DUB localized at early endosomes, interacts with WT-CFTR and reduces the CFTR poly-ubiquination in CFBE cells. The USP10-mediated deubiquitination enhances the endocytic recycling of WT-CFTR (Bomberger et al., 2009). The role of USP10 in the PM stability of conformationally defective CFTR such as rΔF508-CFTR remains unclear.

Recently, we have discovered RING finger and FYVE like domain containing E3 Ub protein ligase (RFFL) as a novel component of the CFTR PQC machineries by a comprehensive siRNA screen in CFBE cells (Okiyoneda et al., 2018). RFFL selectively recognizes unfolded rΔF508-CFTR through the disordered regions. RFFL promotes K63-linked poly-ubiquitination of the unfolded CFTR in post-Golgi, resulting in accelerated endocytosis and lysosomal degradation. Importantly, RFFL directly interacts with conformationally defective CFTR such as rΔF508-CFTR, but not with folded WT-CFTR at the PM and endosomes. Moreover, the RFFL-mediated ubiquitination is conformation dependent as it selectively ubiquitinates thermally unfolded NBD1. RFFL KD enhances the functional PM expression of rΔF508-CFTR in the presence of VX-809, and this effect is further improved by inhibiting the HSC70-dependent ubiquitination machinery. Thus, RFFL plays an important role in the chaperone-independent CFTR PQC mechanism in HBE cell models.

CFTR MODULATORS AFFECTING THE CFTR PM STABILITY

Pharmacological Chaperones and Chemical Chaperones

Pharmacological chaperones affect the CFTR PM stability by direct stabilization. CFTR corrector VX-809 is the first food and drug administration (FDA) approved CFTR corrector in combination with VX-770/ivacaftor (known as Orkambi). VX-809 selectively improves the processing of misfolded CFTR by stabilizing NBD1-membrane spanning domain (MSD) interface but not other misfolded proteins such as human ether-à-go-go-related gene (hERG) mutants (Van Goor et al., 2011; Okiyoneda et al., 2013; Ren et al., 2013; Farinha et al., 2015). VX-809 repairs not only the CFTR folding defect at the ER but also the CFTR PM instability. VX-809 washout prolongs ΔF508-CFTR functional sustainability (Van Goor et al., 2011), suggesting that improvement of the CFTR folding at the ER could increase the thermal stability and proper co- and/or post-translational modifications that renders CFTR more energetic robust conformations even at the PM. VX-809 also promotes ΔF508-CFTR and NHERF1 interaction, that may increase the PM stability (Arora et al., 2014). C3 (CFcor-325/VRT-325) and C4 (Corr-4a) also extend rΔF508-CFTR PM stability in CFBE cells probably by directing binding (Wang et al., 2007; Varga et al., 2008) although their effect could be not specific to the conformationally defective CFTR (Van Goor et al., 2011). Chemical chaperones such as glycerol also increases the rΔF508-CFTR PM stability probably by non-specifically improving the conformational stability (Okiyoneda et al., 2013).

CFTR Potentiators

The first FDA approved CFTR potentiator VX-770 improves the gating defect of some CFTR mutants. However, chronic VX-770 treatment destabilizes the PM rΔF508-CFTR in CFBE and ΔF508 homozygous CF patient HBE (CF-HBE) cells (Cholon et al., 2014; Veit et al., 2014). Importantly, chronic VX-770 treatment diminishes the VX-809 therapeutic efficacy by stimulating the elimination of PM rΔF508-CFTR (Cholon et al., 2014; Veit et al., 2014). In addition to VX-770, several CFTR potentiators including P1 (VRT-532) and P2 (PG-01) also decrease the rΔF508-CFTR PM stability (Veit et al., 2014). VX-770 and other potentiators could destabilize a variety of CFTR rare mutants referred to as CFTR2 mutants including E92K and L1077P at the PM (Avramescu et al., 2017). Thus, several CFTR potentiators may decrease the thermal stability of metastable mutant CFTR at the PM by inducing conformational change that positively affects for channel gating but negatively affects stability. High-throughput screening has identified several novel CFTR potentiators such as class A analog 4 (A04) and class P analog 12 (P12) that could not destabilize the PM rΔF508-CFTR (Phuan et al., 2015).

Proteostasis Regulating Drugs

Proteostasis regulating drugs that affect array of proteins regulating CFTR folding and QC also affect the CFTR PM stability. Histone deacetylase (HDAC) inhibitor suberoylanilide hydroxamic acid (SAHA) alters expression of a subset of CF-interacting gene products (e.g., chaperones and DAB2) and sustains PM expression of ΔF508-CFTR in CFBE cells (Hutt et al., 2010). Tissue transglutaminase (TGM2) inhibitor cystamine also stabilizes ΔF508-CFTR at the PM of airway epithelial cells by restoring BECN1 interactome which is sequestrated by CFTR dysfunction (Luciani et al., 2012; Villella et al., 2013). MLK3 pathway inhibitor oxozeaenol has been reported to be effective in correcting the ΔF508-CFTR proteostasis defect in the primary HBE cells (Trzcinska-Daneluti et al., 2012). Oxozeaenol could stabilize ΔF508-CFTR at the PM as MLK3 KD reduces mature ΔF508-CFTR elimination by PQC (Hegde et al., 2015).

Cavosonstat and CAL Inhibitor

HSP70/HSP90 Organizing Protein is adaptor protein which coordinates HSP70 and HSP90 function in protein folding and regulates CFTR maturation and PM stability (Odunuga et al., 2004; Okiyoneda et al., 2010). HOP *S*-nitrosylation by *S*-nitrosoglutathione (GSNO) induces HOP degradation and increases ΔF508-CFTR PM expression (Marozkina et al., 2010). Levels of *S*-nitrosothiols such as GSNO are low in CF airway (Grasemann et al., 1999) and *S*-nitrosothiol decreases the internalization rate of rΔF508-CFTR in HBE cells (Grasemann et al., 1999, 2000; Zaman et al., 2014). Cavosonstat (N91115) is an orally bioavailable inhibitor of GSNO reductase and restores GSNO levels (Donaldson et al., 2017). Cavosonstat is the first CFTR stabilizer in phase II trials, but it was not beneficial for improvement of lung function in combination with ivacaftor.

CFTR-associated ligand binds CFTR via a PDZ interaction domain and targets CFTR for lysosomal degradation (Cheng et al., 2004). CAL inhibition increases the PM stability of ΔF508-CFTR (Cushing et al., 2010) and cell penetrating CAL inhibiting peptide is established (Qian et al., 2015). CAL inhibitor has been developed as a cell surface CFTR stabilizer in pre-clinical level while its therapeutic efficacy and conformational selectivity remain unclear.

Ub Ligase Inhibitors

RING finger protein 5 (RNF5/RMA1) is an ER associated E3 Ub ligase that regulates early stage CFTR proteostasis at the ER (Younger et al., 2006). A RNF5 inhibitor Inh-2 identified by homology modeling and virtual ligand screening causes significant rescue of ΔF508-CFTR in immortalized and primary HBE cells from CF patients (Sondo et al., 2018). Intriguingly, Inh-2 modestly increases mature ΔF508-CFTR half-life and this stabilization effect is further improved by VX-809. While the contribution of RNF5 in the CFTR peripheral QC remains unclear, RNF5 inhibitor may be useful to overcome the CFTR instability.

Currently, CHIP and RFFL are the only Ub ligases responsible for the CFTR peripheral QC (Okiyoneda et al., 2010, 2018). Thus, inhibiting their activity could selectively reduce the ubiquitination and elimination of unfolded CFTR from the PM, improving the limited efficacy of CF combination therapy. CHIP binds and regulates a number of substrates via chaperones (Connell et al., 2001). Moreover, inhibiting the CHIP activity induces deleterious effect as the CHIP KO mice result in the abnormal phenotypes including ataxia and pre-mature death[1]. In contrast, RFFL could bind and regulate a limited number of substrates because of its nature of direct binding to the CFTR through the disordered regions (Okiyoneda et al., 2018). More importantly, inhibiting the RFFL activity seems to have no venomousness since the RFFL KO mice exhibit no abnormal phenotype (Ahmed et al., 2009). Therefore, counteracting RFFL activity may provide a preferable therapeutic approach as a CFTR stabilizer that is a class of drugs that extends the PM resident time of CFTR class VI mutants. Although future studies are needed to validate the impact on ΔF508-CFTR in CF-HBE cells, developing agents selectively inhibiting RFFL-mediated CFTR ubiquitination may help improve the efficacy of CF pharmacological therapy.

[1] http://www.informatics.jax.org/marker/phenotypes/MGI:1891731

CONCLUSION AND PERSPECTIVE

Beside the progresses of CF pharmacological therapy, stabilizing the cell surface CFTR remains challenging and is necessary to improve the limited therapeutic efficacy. Recent studies have revealed some of the CFTR PQC mechanism eliminating the functional but conformationally defective CFTR from the PM. Understanding the CFTR PQC mechanism help the development of the CFTR stabilizer, a novel class of CFTR modulator necessary to establish the robust CF pharmacological therapy.

AUTHOR CONTRIBUTIONS

All authors listed have made a substantial, direct and intellectual contribution to the work, and approved it for publication.

FUNDING

This work was supported by JSPS KAKENHI grant numbers JP25893275, 15H05643, and 15H01192.

REFERENCES

Ahmed, A. U., Moulin, M., Coumailleau, F., Wong, W. W., Miasari, M., Carter, H., et al. (2009). CARP2 deficiency does not alter induction of NF-kappaB by TNFalpha. *Curr. Biol.* 19, R15–R17. doi: 10.1016/j.cub.2008.11.040

Amaral, M. D. (2004). CFTR and chaperones: processing and degradation. *J. Mol. Neurosci.* 23, 41–48. doi: 10.1385/JMN:23:1-2:041

Arora, K., Moon, C., Zhang, W., Yarlagadda, S., Penmatsa, H., Ren, A., et al. (2014). Stabilizing rescued surface-localized δf508 CFTR by potentiation of its interaction with Na(+)/H(+) exchanger regulatory factor 1. *Biochemistry* 53, 4169–4179. doi: 10.1021/bi401263h

Avramescu, R. G., Kai, Y., Xu, H., Bidaud-Meynard, A., Schnúr, A., Frenkiel, S., et al. (2017). Mutation-specific downregulation of CFTR2 variants by gating potentiators. *Hum. Mol. Genet.* 26, 4873–4885. doi: 10.1093/hmg/ddx367

Bagdany, M., Veit, G., Fukuda, R., Avramescu, R. G., Okiyoneda, T., Baaklini, I., et al. (2017). Chaperones rescue the energetic landscape of mutant CFTR at single molecule and in cell. *Nat. Commun.* 8:398. doi: 10.1038/s41467-017-00444-4

Bhagirath, A. Y., Li, Y., Somayajula, D., Dadashi, M., Badr, S., and Duan, K. (2016). Cystic fibrosis lung environment and *Pseudomonas aeruginosa* infection. *BMC Pulm. Med.* 16:174. doi: 10.1186/s12890-016-0339-5

Bomberger, J. M., Barnaby, R. L., and Stanton, B. A. (2009). The deubiquitinating enzyme USP10 regulates the post-endocytic sorting of cystic fibrosis transmembrane conductance regulator in airway epithelial cells. *J. Biol. Chem.* 284, 18778–18789. doi: 10.1074/jbc.M109.001685

Bomberger, J. M., Coutermarsh, B. A., Barnaby, R. L., and Stanton, B. A. (2012). Arsenic promotes ubiquitinylation and lysosomal degradation of cystic fibrosis transmembrane conductance regulator (CFTR) chloride channels in human airway epithelial cells. *J. Biol. Chem.* 287, 17130–17139. doi: 10.1074/jbc.M111.338855

Bomberger, J. M., Ye, S., Maceachran, D. P., Koeppen, K., Barnaby, R. L., O'Toole, G. A., et al. (2011). A *Pseudomonas aeruginosa* toxin that hijacks the host ubiquitin proteolytic system. *PLoS Pathog.* 7:e1001325. doi: 10.1371/journal.ppat.1001325

Buhr, F., Jha, S., Thommen, M., Mittelstaet, J., Kutz, F., Schwalbe, H., et al. (2016). Synonymous codons direct cotranslational folding toward different protein conformations. *Mol. Cell.* 61, 341–351. doi: 10.1016/j.molcel.2016.01.008

Caohuy, H., Jozwik, C., and Pollard, H. B. (2009). Rescue of DeltaF508-CFTR by the SGK1/Nedd4-2 signaling pathway. *J. Biol. Chem.* 284, 25241–25253. doi: 10.1074/jbc.M109.035345

Chappe, V., Hinkson, D. A., Zhu, T., Chang, X. B., Riordan, J. R., and Hanrahan, J. W. (2003). Phosphorylation of protein kinase C sites in NBD1 and the R domain control CFTR channel activation by PKA. *J. Physiol.* 548, 39–52. doi: 10.1113/jphysiol.2002.035790

Chen, E. Y., Bartlett, M. C., and Clarke, D. M. (2000). Cystic fibrosis transmembrane conductance regulator has an altered structure when its maturation is inhibited. *Biochemistry* 39, 3797–3803. doi: 10.1021/bi992620m

Cheng, J., and Guggino, W. (2013). Ubiquitination and degradation of CFTR by the E3 ubiquitin ligase MARCH2 through its association with adaptor proteins CAL and STX6. *PLoS One* 8:e68001. doi: 10.1371/journal.pone.0068001

Cheng, J., Wang, H., and Guggino, W. B. (2004). Modulation of mature cystic fibrosis transmembrane regulator protein by the PDZ domain protein CAL. *J. Biol. Chem.* 279, 1892–1898 doi: 10.1074/jbc.M308640200

Cholon, D. M., O'Neal, W. K., Randell, S. H., Riordan, J. R., and Gentzsch, M. (2010). Modulation of endocytic trafficking and apical stability of CFTR in primary human airway epithelial cultures. *Am. J. Physiol. Lung. Cell Mol. Physiol.* 298, L304–L314. doi: 10.1152/ajplung.00016.2009

Cholon, D. M., Quinney, N. L., Fulcher, M. L., Esther, C. R., Das, J., Dokholyan, N. V., et al. (2014). Potentiator ivacaftor abrogates pharmacological correction of ΔF508 CFTR in cystic fibrosis. *Sci. Transl. Med.* 6:246ra96. doi: 10.1126/scitranslmed.3008680

Cihil, K. M., Zimnik, A., and Swiatecka-Urban, A. (2013). c-Cbl reduces stability of rescued ΔF508-CFTR in human airway epithelial cells: implications for cystic fibrosis treatment. *Commun. Integr. Biol.* 6:e23094. doi: 10.4161/cib.23094

Clunes, L. A., Davies, C. M., Coakley, R. D., Aleksandrov, A. A., Henderson, A. G., Zeman, K. L., et al. (2012). Cigarette smoke exposure induces CFTR internalization and insolubility, leading to airway surface liquid dehydration. *FASEB J.* 26, 533–545. doi: 10.1096/fj.11-192377

Connell, P., Ballinger, C. A., Jiang, J., Wu, Y., Thompson, L. J., Höhfeld, J., et al. (2001). The co-chaperone CHIP regulates protein triage decisions mediated by heat-shock proteins. *Nat. Cell Biol.* 3, 93–96. doi: 10.1038/35050618

Cushing, P. R., Vouilleme, L., Pellegrini, M., Boisguerin, P., and Madden, D. R. (2010). A stabilizing influence: CAL PDZ inhibition extends the half-life of ΔF508-CFTR. *Angew. Chem. Int. Ed. Engl.* 49, 9907–9911. doi: 10.1002/anie.201005585

Dalemans, W., Barbry, P., Champigny, G., Jallat, S., Dott, K., Dreyer, D., et al. (1991). Altered chloride ion channel kinetics associated with the delta F508 cystic fibrosis mutation. *Nature* 354, 526–528. doi: 10.1038/354526a0

Donaldson, S. H., Solomon, G. M., Zeitlin, P. L., Flume, P. A., Casey, A., McCoy, K., et al. (2017). Pharmacokinetics and safety of cavosonstat (N91115) in healthy and cystic fibrosis adults homozygous for *F508DEL-CFTR*. *J. Cyst. Fibros* 16, 371–379. doi: 10.1016/j.jcf.2017.01.009

El Khouri, E., Le Pavec, G., Toledano, M. B., and Delaunay-Moisan, A. (2013). RNF185 is a novel E3 ligase of endoplasmic reticulum-associated degradation (ERAD) that targets cystic fibrosis transmembrane conductance regulator (CFTR). *J. Biol. Chem.* 288, 31177–31191. doi: 10.1074/jbc.M113.470500

Ernst, W. L., Shome, K., Wu, C. C., Gong, X., Frizzell, R. A., and Aridor, M. (2016). VAMP-associated Proteins (VAP) as receptors that couple cystic fibrosis transmembrane conductance regulator (CFTR). proteostasis with lipid homeostasis. *J. Biol. Chem.* 291, 5206–5220. doi: 10.1074/jbc.M115.692749

Farinha, C. M., Sousa, M., Canato, S., Schmidt, A., Uliyakina, I., and Amaral, M. D. (2015). Increased efficacy of VX-809 in different cellular systems results from an early stabilization effect of F508del-CFTR. *Pharmacol. Res. Perspect.* 3:e00152. doi: 10.1002/prp2.152

Favia, M., Guerra, L., Fanelli, T., Cardone, R. A., Monterisi, S., Di Sole, F., et al. (2010). Na + /H + exchanger regulatory factor 1 overexpression-dependent increase of cytoskeleton organization is fundamental in the rescue of F508del cystic fibrosis transmembrane conductance regulator in human airway CFBE41o- cells. *Mol. Biol. Cell* 21, 73–86. doi: 10.1091/mbc.E09-03-0185

Fu, L., Rab, A., Tang, L., Bebok, Z., Rowe, S. M., Bartoszewski, R., et al. (2015). ΔF508 CFTR surface stability is regulated by DAB2 and CHIP-mediated ubiquitination in post-endocytic compartments. *PLoS One* 10:e0123131. doi: 10.1371/journal.pone.0123131

Fu, L., Rab, A., Tang, L. P., Rowe, S. M., Bebok, Z., and Collawn, J. F. (2012). Dab2 is a key regulator of endocytosis and post-endocytic trafficking of the cystic fibrosis transmembrane conductance regulator. *Biochem. J.* 441, 633–643. doi: 10.1042/BJ20111566

Glozman, R., Okiyoneda, T., Mulvihill, C. M., Rini, J. M., Barriere, H., and Lukacs, G. L. (2009). N-glycans are direct determinants of CFTR folding and stability in secretory and endocytic membrane traffic. *J. Cell Biol.* 184, 847–862. doi: 10.1083/jcb.200808124

Gong, X., Ahner, A., Roldan, A., Lukacs, G. L., Thibodeau, P. H., and Frizzell, R. A. (2016). Non-native conformers of cystic fibrosis transmembrane conductance regulator NBD1 are recognized by Hsp27 and conjugated to SUMO-2 for degradation. *J. Biol. Chem.* 291, 2004–2017. doi: 10.1074/jbc.M115.685628

Grasemann, H., Gaston, B., Fang, K., Paul, K., and Ratjen, F. (1999). Decreased levels of nitrosothiols in the lower airways of patients with cystic fibrosis and normal pulmonary function. *J. Pediatr.* 135, 770–772. doi: 10.1016/S0022-3476(99)70101-0

Grasemann, H., Knauer, N., Büscher, R., Hübner, K., Drazen, J. M., and Ratjen, F. (2000). Airway nitric oxide levels in cystic fibrosis patients are related to a polymorphism in the neuronal nitric oxide synthase gene. *Am. J. Respir. Crit. Care Med.* 162, 2172–2176. doi: 10.1164/ajrccm.162.6.2003106

Grove, D. E., Fan, C. Y., Ren, H. Y., and Cyr, D. M. (2011). The endoplasmic reticulum-associated Hsp40 DNAJB12 and Hsc70 cooperate to facilitate RMA1 E3-dependent degradation of nascent CFTRDeltaF508. *Mol. Biol. Cell* 22, 301–314. doi: 10.1091/mbc.E10-09-0760

Haardt, M., Benharouga, M., Lechardeur, D., Kartner, N., and Lukacs, G. L. (1999). C-terminal truncations destabilize the cystic fibrosis transmembrane conductance regulator without impairing its biogenesis. A novel class of mutation. *J. Biol. Chem.* 274, 21873–21877. doi: 10.1074/jbc.274.31.21873

Harris, W. T., Muhlebach, M. S., Oster, R. A., Knowles, M. R., Clancy, J. P., and Noah, T. L. (2011). Plasma TGF-β^1 in pediatric cystic fibrosis: potential biomarker of lung disease and response to therapy. *Pediatr. Pulmonol.* 46, 688–695. doi: 10.1002/ppul.21430

Hegde, R. N., Parashuraman, S., Iorio, F., Ciciriello, F., Capuani, F., Carissimo, A., et al. (2015). Unravelling druggable signalling networks that control F508del-CFTR proteostasis. *Elife* 4:e10365. doi: 10.7554/eLife.10365

Hou, X., Wei, H., Rajagopalan, C., Jiang, H., Wu, Q., Zaman, K., et al. (2018). Dissection of the Role of VIMP in endoplasmic reticulum-associated degradation of CFTRΔF508. *Sci. Rep.* 8:4764. doi: 10.1038/s41598-018-23284-8

Hutt, D. M., Herman, D., Rodrigues, A. P., Noel, S., Pilewski, J. M., Matteson, J., et al. (2010). Reduced histone deacetylase 7 activity restores function to misfolded CFTR in cystic fibrosis. *Nat. Chem. Biol.* 6, 25–33. doi: 10.1038/nchembio.275

Kim, S. J., and Skach, W. R. (2012). Mechanisms of CFTR folding at the endoplasmic reticulum. *Front. Pharmacol.* 3:201. doi: 10.3389/fphar.2012.00201

Kimura, T., Kawabe, H., Jiang, C., Zhang, W., Xiang, Y. Y., Lu, C., et al. (2011). Deletion of the ubiquitin ligase Nedd4L in lung epithelia causes cystic fibrosis-like disease. *Proc. Natl. Acad. Sci. U.S.A.* 108, 3216–3221. doi: 10.1073/pnas.1010334108

Kleizen, B., van Vlijmen, T., de Jonge, H. R., and Braakman, I. (2005). Folding of CFTR is predominantly cotranslational. *Mol. Cell.* 20, 277–287. doi: 10.1016/j.molcel.2005.09.007

Koch, C. (2002). Early infection and progression of cystic fibrosis lung disease. *Pediatr. Pulmonol.* 34, 232–236. doi: 10.1002/ppul.10135

Koeppen, K., Chapline, C., Sato, J. D., and Stanton, B. A. (2012). Nedd4-2 does not regulate wt-CFTR in human airway epithelial cells. *Am. J. Physiol. Lung. Cell Mol. Physiol.* 303, L720–L727. doi: 10.1152/ajplung.00409.2011

Kongsuphol, P., Cassidy, D., Hieke, B., Treharne, K. J., Schreiber, R., Mehta, A., et al. (2009). Mechanistic insight into control of CFTR by AMPK. *J. Biol. Chem.* 284, 5645–5653. doi: 10.1074/jbc.M806780200

Lobo, M. J., Amaral, M. D., Zaccolo, M., and Farinha, C. M. (2016). EPAC1 activation by cAMP stabilizes CFTR at the membrane by promoting its interaction with NHERF1. *J. Cell Sci.* 129, 2599–2612. doi: 10.1242/jcs.185629

Loo, M. A., Jensen, T. J., Cui, L., Hou, Y., Chang, X. B., and Riordan, J. R. (1998). Perturbation of Hsp90 interaction with nascent CFTR prevents its maturation and accelerates its degradation by the proteasome. *EMBO J.* 17, 6879–6887. doi: 10.1093/emboj/17.23.6879

Lopes-Pacheco, M. (2016). CFTR modulators: shedding light on precision medicine for cystic fibrosis. *Front. Pharmacol.* 7:275. doi: 10.3389/fphar.2016.00275

Loureiro, C. A., Matos, A. M., Dias-Alves, Â, Pereira, J. F., Uliyakina, I., Barros, P., et al. (2015). A molecular switch in the scaffold NHERF1 enables misfolded CFTR to evade the peripheral quality control checkpoint. *Sci. Signal* 8:ra48. doi: 10.1126/scisignal.aaa1580

Luciani, A., Villella, V. R., Esposito, S., Gavina, M., Russo, I., Silano, M., et al. (2012). Targeting autophagy as a novel strategy for facilitating the therapeutic action of potentiators on ΔF508 cystic fibrosis transmembrane conductance regulator. *Autophagy* 8, 1657–1672. doi: 10.4161/auto.21483

Lukacs, G. L., Chang, X. B., Bear, C., Kartner, N., Mohamed, A., Riordan, J. R., et al. (1993). The delta F508 mutation decreases the stability of cystic fibrosis transmembrane conductance regulator in the plasma membrane. Determination of functional half-lives on transfected cells. *J. Biol. Chem.* 268, 21592–21598.

Luz, S., Cihil, K. M., Brautigan, D. L., Amaral, M. D., Farinha, C. M., and Swiatecka-Urban, A. (2014). LMTK2-mediated phosphorylation regulates CFTR endocytosis in human airway epithelial cells. *J. Biol. Chem.* 289, 15080–15093. doi: 10.1074/jbc.M114.563742

Luz, S., Kongsuphol, P., Mendes, A. I., Romeiras, F., Sousa, M., Schreiber, R., et al. (2011). Contribution of casein kinase 2 and spleen tyrosine kinase to CFTR trafficking and protein kinase A-induced activity. *Mol. Cell. Biol.* 31, 4392–4404. doi: 10.1128/MCB.05517-11

Marozkina, N. V., Yemen, S., Borowitz, M., Liu, L., Plapp, M., Sun, F., et al. (2010). Hsp 70/Hsp 90 organizing protein as a nitrosylation target in cystic fibrosis therapy. *Proc. Natl. Acad. Sci. U.S.A.* 107, 11393–11398. doi: 10.1073/pnas.0909128107

Matsumura, Y., Sakai, J., and Skach, W. R. (2013). Endoplasmic reticulum protein quality control is determined by cooperative interactions between Hsp/c70 protein and the CHIP E3 ligase. *J. Biol. Chem.* 288, 31069–31079. doi: 10.1074/jbc.M113.479345

Mazumdar, M., Christiani, D. C., Biswas, S. K., Ibne-Hasan, O. S., Kapur, K., and Hug, C. (2015). Elevated sweat chloride levels due to arsenic toxicity. *N. Engl. J. Med.* 372, 582–584. doi: 10.1056/NEJMc1413312

McClure, M. L., Barnes, S., Brodsky, J. L., and Sorscher, E. J. (2016). Trafficking and function of the cystic fibrosis transmembrane conductance regulator: a complex network of posttranslational modifications. *Am. J. Physiol. Lung. Cell Mol. Physiol.* 311, L719–L733. doi: 10.1152/ajplung.00431.2015

Meacham, G. C., Lu, Z., King, S., Sorscher, E., Tousson, A., and Cyr, D. M. (1999). The Hdj-2/Hsc70 chaperone pair facilitates early steps in CFTR biogenesis. *EMBO J.* 18, 1492–1505. doi: 10.1093/emboj/18.6.1492

Meacham, G. C., Patterson, C., Zhang, W., Younger, J. M., and Cyr, D. M. (2001). The Hsc70 co-chaperone CHIP targets immature CFTR for proteasomal degradation. *Nat. Cell Biol.* 3, 100–105. doi: 10.1038/35050509

Mendes, A. I., Matos, P., Moniz, S., Luz, S., Amaral, M. D., Farinha, C. M., et al. (2011). Antagonistic regulation of cystic fibrosis transmembrane conductance regulator cell surface expression by protein kinases WNK4 and spleen tyrosine kinase. *Mol. Cell. Biol.* 31, 4076–4086. doi: 10.1128/MCB.05152-11

Morito, D., Hirao, K., Oda, Y., Hosokawa, N., Tokunaga, F., Cyr, D. M., et al. (2008). Gp78 cooperates with RMA1 in endoplasmic reticulum-associated degradation of CFTRDeltaF508. *Mol. Biol. Cell* 19, 1328–1336. doi: 10.1091/mbc.E07-06-0601

Nery, F. C., Armata, I. A., Farley, J. E., Cho, J. A., Yaqub, U., Chen, P., et al. (2011). TorsinA participates in endoplasmic reticulum-associated degradation. *Nat. Commun.* 2:393. doi: 10.1038/ncomms1383

Odunuga, O. O., Longshaw, V. M., and Blatch, G. L. (2004). Hop: more than an Hsp70/Hsp90 adaptor protein. *Bioessays* 26, 1058–1068. doi: 10.1002/bies.20107

Okiyoneda, T., Barrière, H., Bagdány, M., Rabeh, W. M., Du, K., Höhfeld, J., et al. (2010). Peripheral protein quality control removes unfolded CFTR from the plasma membrane. *Science* 329, 805–810. doi: 10.1126/science.1191542

Okiyoneda, T., Harada, K., Takeya, M., Yamahira, K., Wada, I., Shuto, T., et al. (2004). Delta F508 CFTR pool in the endoplasmic reticulum is increased by calnexin overexpression. *Mol. Biol. Cell* 15, 563–574. doi: 10.1091/mbc.e03-06-0379

Okiyoneda, T., Niibori, A., Harada, K., Kohno, T., Michalak, M., Duszyk, M., et al. (2008). Role of calnexin in the ER quality control and productive folding of CFTR; differential effect of calnexin knockout on wild-type and DeltaF508 CFTR. *Biochim. Biophys. Acta* 1783, 1585–1594. doi: 10.1016/j.bbamcr.2008.04.002

Okiyoneda, T., Veit, G., Dekkers, J. F., Bagdany, M., Soya, N., Xu, H., et al. (2013). Mechanism-based corrector combination restores ΔF508-CFTR folding and function. *Nat. Chem. Biol.* 9, 444–454. doi: 10.1038/nchembio.1253

Okiyoneda, T., Veit, G., Sakai, R., Aki, M., Fujihara, T., Higashi, M., et al. (2018). Chaperone-independent peripheral quality control of CFTR by RFFL E3 ligase. *Dev. Cell* 44, 694–708.e7. doi: 10.1016/j.devcel.2018.02.001

Phuan, P. W., Veit, G., Tan, J. A., Finkbeiner, W. E., Lukacs, G. L., and Verkman, A. S. (2015). Potentiators of defective ΔF508-CFTR gating that do not interfere with corrector action. *Mol. Pharmacol.* 88, 791–799. doi: 10.1124/mol.115.099689

Pind, S., Riordan, J. R., and Williams, D. B. (1994). Participation of the endoplasmic reticulum chaperone calnexin (p88, IP90) in the biogenesis of the cystic fibrosis transmembrane conductance regulator. *J. Biol. Chem.* 269, 12784–12788.

Qian, Z., Xu, X., Amacher, J. F., Madden, D. R., Cormet-Boyaka, E., and Pei, D. (2015). Intracellular delivery of peptidyl ligands by reversible cyclization: discovery of a PDZ domain inhibitor that rescues CFTR activity. *Angew. Chem. Int. Ed. Engl.* 54, 5874–5878. doi: 10.1002/anie.201411594

Rabeh, W. M., Bossard, F., Xu, H., Okiyoneda, T., Bagdany, M., Mulvihill, C. M., et al. (2012). Correction of both NBD1 energetics and domain interface is required to restore ΔF508 CFTR folding and function. *Cell* 148, 150–163. doi: 10.1016/j.cell.2011.11.024

Ramachandran, S., Osterhaus, S. R., Parekh, K. R., Jacobi, A. M., Behlke, M. A., and McCray, P. B. (2016). SYVN1, NEDD8, and FBXO2 proteins regulate ΔF508 cystic fibrosis transmembrane conductance regulator (CFTR). Ubiquitin-mediated proteasomal degradation. *J. Biol. Chem.* 291, 25489–25504. doi: 10.1074/jbc.M116.754283

Rasmussen, J. E., Sheridan, J. T., Polk, W., Davies, C. M., and Tarran, R. (2014). Cigarette smoke-induced Ca2 + release leads to cystic fibrosis transmembrane conductance regulator (CFTR) dysfunction. *J. Biol. Chem.* 289, 7671–7681. doi: 10.1074/jbc.M113.545137

Ren, H. Y., Grove, D. E., De La Rosa, O., Houck, S. A., Sopha, P., Van Goor, F., et al. (2013). VX-809 corrects folding defects in cystic fibrosis transmembrane conductance regulator protein through action on membrane-spanning domain 1. *Mol. Biol. Cell* 24, 3016–3024. doi: 10.1091/mbc.E13-05-0240

Rennolds, J., Butler, S., Maloney, K., Boyaka, P. N., Davis, I. C., Knoell, D. L., et al. (2010). Cadmium regulates the expression of the CFTR chloride channel in human airway epithelial cells. *Toxicol. Sci.* 116, 349–358. doi: 10.1093/toxsci/kfq101

Rosser, M. F., Grove, D. E., Chen, L., and Cyr, D. M. (2008). Assembly and misassembly of cystic fibrosis transmembrane conductance regulator: folding defects caused by deletion of F508 occur before and after the calnexin-dependent association of membrane spanning domain (MSD). 1 and MSD2. *Mol. Biol. Cell* 19, 4570–4579. doi: 10.1091/mbc.E08-04-0357

Rotin, D., and Staub, O. (2012). Nedd4-2 and the regulation of epithelial sodium transport. *Front. Physiol.* 3:212. doi: 10.3389/fphys.2012.00212

Sharma, M., Pampinella, F., Nemes, C., Benharouga, M., So, J., Du, K., et al. (2004). Misfolding diverts CFTR from recycling to degradation: quality control at early endosomes. *J. Cell Biol.* 164, 923–933. doi: 10.1083/jcb.200312018

Silvis, M. R., Picciano, J. A., Bertrand, C., Weixel, K., Bridges, R. J., and Bradbury, N. A. (2003). A mutation in the cystic fibrosis transmembrane conductance regulator generates a novel internalization sequence and enhances endocytic rates. *J. Biol. Chem.* 278, 11554–11560. doi: 10.1074/jbc.M212843200

Snodgrass, S. M., Cihil, K. M., Cornuet, P. K., Myerburg, M. M., and Swiatecka-Urban, A. (2013). Tgf-β1 inhibits Cftr biogenesis and prevents functional rescue of ΔF508-Cftr in primary differentiated human bronchial epithelial cells. *PLoS One* 8:e63167. doi: 10.1371/journal.pone.0063167

Sondo, E., Falchi, F., Caci, E., Ferrera, L., Giacomini, E., Pesce, E., et al. (2018). Pharmacological inhibition of the ubiquitin ligase RNF5 rescues F508del-CFTR in cystic fibrosis airway epithelia. *Cell Chem. Biol.* 25, 891–905.e8. doi: 10.1016/j.chembiol.2018.04.010

Sun, H., Harris, W. T., Kortyka, S., Kotha, K., Ostmann, A. J., Rezayat, A., et al. (2014). Tgf-beta downregulation of distinct chloride channels in cystic fibrosis-affected epithelia. *PLoS One* 9:e106842. doi: 10.1371/journal.pone.0106842

Swiatecka-Urban, A., Brown, A., Moreau-Marquis, S., Renuka, J., Coutermarsh, B., Barnaby, R., et al. (2005). The short apical membrane half-life of rescued {Delta}F508-cystic fibrosis transmembrane conductance regulator (CFTR).results from accelerated endocytosis of {Delta}F508-CFTR in polarized human airway epithelial cells. *J. Biol. Chem.* 280, 36762–36772. doi: 10.1074/jbc.M508944200

Swiatecka-Urban, A., Moreau-Marquis, S., Maceachran, D. P., Connolly, J. P., Stanton, C. R., Su, J. R., et al. (2006). *Pseudomonas aeruginosa* inhibits endocytic recycling of CFTR in polarized human airway epithelial cells. *Am. J. Physiol. Cell Physiol.* 290, C862–C872. doi: 10.1152/ajpcell.00108.2005

Thelin, W. R., Chen, Y., Gentzsch, M., Kreda, S. M., Sallee, J. L., Scarlett, C. O., et al. (2007). Direct interaction with filamins modulates the stability and plasma membrane expression of CFTR. *J. Clin. Invest.* 117, 364–374. doi: 10.1172/JCI30376

Trzcinska-Daneluti, A. M., Nguyen, L., Jiang, C., Fladd, C., Uehling, D., Prakesch, M., et al. (2012). Use of kinase inhibitors to correct ΔF508-CFTR function. *Mol. Cell. Proteomics* 11, 745–757. doi: 10.1074/mcp.M111.016626

Turnbull, E. L., Rosser, M. F., and Cyr, D. M. (2007). The role of the UPS in cystic fibrosis. *BMC Biochem.* 8(Suppl. 1):S11. doi: 10.1186/1471-2091-8-S1-S11

Van Goor, F., Hadida, S., Grootenhuis, P. D., Burton, B., Stack, J. H., Straley, K. S., et al. (2011). Correction of the F508del-CFTR protein processing defect in vitro by the investigational drug VX-809. *Proc. Natl. Acad. Sci. U.S.A.* 108, 18843–18848. doi: 10.1073/pnas.1105787108

Van Goor, F., Yu, H., Burton, B., and Hoffman, B. J. (2014). Effect of ivacaftor on CFTR forms with missense mutations associated with defects in protein processing or function. *J. Cyst. Fibros* 13, 29–36. doi: 10.1016/j.jcf.2013.06.008

Varga, K., Goldstein, R. F., Jurkuvenaite, A., Chen, L., Matalon, S., Sorscher, E. J., et al. (2008). Enhanced cell-surface stability of rescued DeltaF508 cystic fibrosis transmembrane conductance regulator (CFTR) by pharmacological chaperones. *Biochem. J.* 410, 555–564. doi: 10.1042/BJ20071420

Veit, G., Avramescu, R. G., Chiang, A. N., Houck, S. A., Cai, Z., Peters, K. W., et al. (2016a). From CFTR biology toward combinatorial pharmacotherapy: expanded classification of cystic fibrosis mutations. *Mol. Biol. Cell* 27, 424–433. doi: 10.1091/mbc.E14-04-0935

Veit, G., Avramescu, R. G., Perdomo, D., Phuan, P. W., Bagdany, M., Apaja, P. M., et al. (2014). Some gating potentiators, including VX-770, diminish ΔF508-CFTR functional expression. *Sci. Transl. Med.* 6:246ra97. doi: 10.1126/scitranslmed.3008889

Veit, G., Oliver, K., Apaja, P. M., Perdomo, D., Bidaud-Meynard, A., Lin, S. T., et al. (2016b). Ribosomal stalk protein silencing partially corrects the ΔF508-CFTR functional expression defect. *PLoS Biol.* 14:e1002462. doi: 10.1371/journal.pbio.1002462

Venerando, A., Franchin, C., Cant, N., Cozza, G., Pagano, M. A., Tosoni, K., et al. (2013). Detection of phospho-sites generated by protein kinase CK2 in CFTR: mechanistic aspects of Thr1471 phosphorylation. *PLoS One* 8:e74232. doi: 10.1371/journal.pone.0074232

Villella, V. R., Esposito, S., Bruscia, E. M., Maiuri, M. C., Raia, V., Kroemer, G., et al. (2013). Targeting the intracellular environment in cystic fibrosis: restoring autophagy as a novel strategy to circumvent the CFTR defect. *Front. Pharmacol.* 4:1. doi: 10.3389/fphar.2013.00001

Wang, H., and Brautigan, D. L. (2006). Peptide microarray analysis of substrate specificity of the transmembrane Ser/Thr kinase KPI-2 reveals reactivity with cystic fibrosis transmembrane conductance regulator and phosphorylase. *Mol. Cell. Proteomics* 5, 2124–2130. doi: 10.1074/mcp.M600188-MCP200

Wang, Y., Liu, J., Loizidou, A., Bugeja, L. A., Warner, R., Hawley, B. R., et al. (2014). CFTR potentiators partially restore channel function to A561E-CFTR, a cystic fibrosis mutant with a similar mechanism of dysfunction as F508del-CFTR. *Br. J. Pharmacol.* 171, 4490–4503. doi: 10.1111/bph.12791

Wang, Y., Loo, T. W., Bartlett, M. C., and Clarke, D. M. (2007). Correctors promote maturation of cystic fibrosis transmembrane conductance regulator (CFTR)-processing mutants by binding to the protein. *J. Biol. Chem.* 282, 33247–33251. doi: 10.1074/jbc.C700175200

Wolde, M., Fellows, A., Cheng, J., Kivenson, A., Coutermarsh, B., Talebian, L., et al. (2007). Targeting CAL as a negative regulator of DeltaF508-CFTR cell-surface expression: an RNA interference and structure-based mutagenetic approach. *J. Biol. Chem.* 282, 8099–8109. doi: 10.1074/jbc.M611049200

Yang, Y., Janich, S., Cohn, J. A., and Wilson, J. M. (1993). The common variant of cystic fibrosis transmembrane conductance regulator is recognized by hsp70 and degraded in a pre-Golgi nonlysosomal compartment. *Proc. Natl. Acad. Sci. U.S.A.* 90, 9480–9484. doi: 10.1073/pnas.90.20.9480

Ye, S., Cihil, K., Stolz, D. B., Pilewski, J. M., Stanton, B. A., and Swiatecka-Urban, A. (2010). c-Cbl facilitates endocytosis and lysosomal degradation of cystic fibrosis transmembrane conductance regulator in human airway epithelial cells. *J. Biol. Chem.* 285, 27008–27018. doi: 10.1074/jbc.M110.139881

Younger, J. M., Chen, L., Ren, H. Y., Rosser, M. F., Turnbull, E. L., Fan, C. Y., et al. (2006). Sequential quality-control checkpoints triage misfolded cystic fibrosis transmembrane conductance regulator. *Cell* 126, 571–582. doi: 10.1016/j.cell.2006.06.041

Zaman, K., Bennett, D., Fraser-Butler, M., Greenberg, Z., Getsy, P., Sattar, A., et al. (2014). S-Nitrosothiols increases cystic fibrosis transmembrane regulator expression and maturation in the cell surface. *Biochem. Biophys. Res. Commun.* 443, 1257–1262. doi: 10.1016/j.bbrc.2013.12.130

14

Challenges Facing Airway Epithelial Cell-Based Therapy for Cystic Fibrosis

*Andrew Berical[1,2], Rhianna E. Lee[3], Scott H. Randell[3,4] and Finn Hawkins[1,2]**

[1] Center for Regenerative Medicine, Boston Medical Center and Boston University, Boston, MA, United States, [2] The Pulmonary Center, Boston University School of Medicine, Boston, MA, United States, [3] Cystic Fibrosis Research Center, Marsico Lung Institute, University of North Carolina at Chapel Hill, Chapel Hill, NC, United States, [4] Department of Cell Biology and Physiology, University of North Carolina at Chapel Hill, Chapel Hill, NC, United States

***Correspondence:**
Finn Hawkins
hawk@bu.edu

Mutations in the cystic fibrosis transmembrane conductance regulator (*CFTR*) gene cause the life-limiting hereditary disease, cystic fibrosis (CF). Decreased or absent functional CFTR protein in airway epithelial cells leads to abnormally viscous mucus and impaired mucociliary transport, resulting in bacterial infections and inflammation causing progressive lung damage. There are more than 2000 known variants in the *CFTR* gene. A subset of CF individuals with specific *CFTR* mutations qualify for pharmacotherapies of variable efficacy. These drugs, termed CFTR modulators, address key defects in protein folding, trafficking, abundance, and function at the apical cell membrane resulting from specific *CFTR* mutations. However, some *CFTR* mutations result in little or no CFTR mRNA or protein expression for which a pharmaceutical strategy is more challenging and remote. One approach to rescue CFTR function in the airway epithelium is to replace cells that carry a mutant *CFTR* sequence with cells that express a normal copy of the gene. Cell-based therapy theoretically has the potential to serve as a one-time cure for CF lung disease regardless of the causative *CFTR* mutation. In this review, we explore major challenges and recent progress toward this ambitious goal. The ideal therapeutic cell would: (1) be autologous to avoid the complications of rejection and immune-suppression; (2) be safely modified to express functional CFTR; (3) be expandable *ex vivo* to generate sufficient cell quantities to restore CFTR function; and (4) have the capacity to engraft, proliferate and persist long-term in recipient airways without complications. Herein, we explore human bronchial epithelial cells (HBECs) and induced pluripotent stem cells (iPSCs) as candidate cell therapies for CF and explore the challenges facing their delivery to the human airway.

Keywords: cystic fibrosis, cell-based therapy, induced pluripotent stem cells, human bronchial epithelial cells, engraftment

INTRODUCTION

Cystic fibrosis (CF) is an autosomal recessive, multisystem, genetic disease caused by mutations in the cystic fibrosis transmembrane conductance regulator (*CFTR*) gene resulting in deficient and/or defective CFTR protein (Cutting, 2014; Ratjen et al., 2015). CFTR is an anion channel present across a number of epithelia including the lungs, intestine, sinuses, pancreas, biliary tree, and vas deferens. The consequences of CFTR dysfunction are pronounced in the lungs where ineffective chloride and bicarbonate ion transport results in an abnormally viscous and acidic apical surface layer (ASL). This abnormal environment is colonized by bacteria in early life and a cycle of infection and inflammation results in bronchiectasis and end-stage lung disease (Ratjen et al., 2015). Disease severity is determined to a large extent by the causative *CFTR* mutation(s). Over 2,000 variants in *CFTR* have been described, of which approximately 300 have been determined to be pathogenic (cftr2.org). These variants or combinations of variants have differing effects on the amount and function of CFTR protein. Some variants are associated with milder disease or particular organ involvement while others may be associated with very severe disease. For classification purposes, these mutations are grouped into six classes (I-VI) based on their effect on CFTR including: no protein synthesis (class I), protein misfolding (class II), dysfunctional channel gating (class III), reduced conductance (class IV), insufficient CFTR protein due to abnormal RNA splicing (class V), or increased protein turnover (class VI).

Mucus clearance techniques, antibiotics, and lung transplantation significantly improve the life expectancy of CF individuals. The recent discovery of CFTR modulators has ushered in a new era of precision medicine for CF patients with mutations that result in some residual druggable CFTR protein. For example, the major defect in patients with the class III mutation G551D is diminished channel activity at the apical surface. Ivacaftor is an FDA approved CFTR potentiator that increases CFTR activity and results in clinical improvement in patients with at least one copy of the G551D mutation (Ramsey et al., 2011). F508del is the most common CFTR mutation affecting approximately 90% of CF patients (Cutting, 2014). This mutation results in defective folding and trafficking of the CFTR protein. Corrector molecules such as lumacaftor and tezacaftor in conjunction with ivacaftor result in increased CFTR activity and some clinical improvement though not as robust as the response of gating and residual function mutations to ivacaftor therapy (Rowe et al., 2017; Taylor-Cousar et al., 2018). Recent progress with "triple combination" regimens including two correctors plus the potentiator ivacaftor indicates increased efficacy for those harboring the class II F508del mutation (Davies et al., 2018; Keating et al., 2018). Class I mutations are non-sense, frameshift or splice variants that result in premature termination of the CFTR transcript and no CFTR protein. These patients currently have no targeted therapies available and there are many barriers to a pharmacological approach to treatment.

The challenge is clear, how do we identify and develop effective therapies for all CF individuals? In theory, replacing the mutant *CFTR* sequence with the normal sequence could restore CFTR function regardless of mutation. Generally, this might be achieved by one of three approaches: (1) *in vivo* delivery of normal *CFTR* sequence, e.g., via viral vectors, (2) *in vivo* editing of the mutant *CFTR* sequence or, (3) delivery of cells carrying the normal *CFTR* sequence to replace cells carrying the mutant sequence. In this review, we focus on the approach of cell-based therapy for CF lung disease. Although there are compelling examples of effective cell-based therapies, such as hematopoietic stem cell transplantation, there are many challenges facing such an approach for lung disease. What cell type is best suited to restore CFTR function to the airways? How might cells be effectively but safely delivered to a CF patient's lungs? Here we will review the most promising cellular candidates to treat CF, human bronchial epithelial cells (HBECs) and induced pluripotent stem cells (iPSCs). Finally, we will discuss the major hurdles facing the field of CF cell-based therapeutics, including delivery and engraftment of cells into a diseased host.

OVERVIEW OF AIRWAY EPITHELIAL BIOLOGY IN CF

Airway epithelial cells, including club, goblet, multi-ciliated, basal and neuroendocrine cells occupy a vital environmental interface. Their normal physiological function is essential to maintain respiratory tract health, and the cells are intimately involved in the pathogenesis of multiple respiratory tract maladies, including the common diseases asthma and chronic obstructive pulmonary disease (Randell et al., 2009). In CF, a dehydrated and acidic ASL impairs critical innate defense mechanisms including mucociliary clearance (Randell et al., 2006; Button et al., 2012; Stoltz et al., 2015). There is current debate on the airway cell types that express *CFTR*, but it is detected in the submucosal glands (Jiang and Engelhardt, 1998) of the airway and in certain surface epithelial cells including multi-ciliated cells (low expression) and in the recently described pulmonary ionocyte (high expression) (Jiang and Engelhardt, 1998; Montoro et al., 2018; Plasschaert et al., 2018). There is debate whether cell autonomous loss of CFTR is hyper-inflammatory *per se*, but the combination of mucus stasis and chronic infection clearly results in highly inflamed CF airways (Roesch et al., 2018). Complex interactions during infection stemming from the epithelial defect ultimately cascade into pathologic changes including extensive mucus obstruction, ectasis of bronchi and bronchioles, and consequent loss of pulmonary function (**Figure 1**). It is likely that significant structural damage to the airways and surrounding parenchyma becomes irreversible, and a goal for airway epithelial cell therapy is to intervene early, likely in childhood.

HUMAN BRONCHIAL AND BRONCHIOLAR EPITHELIAL CELLS (HBECS)

Epithelial cell proliferation in the lung is relatively quiescent at steady state, but this organ retains the ability to regenerate rapidly after injury (Hegab et al., 2012). Much has been learned in recent years about lung stem cells and their roles in repair and regeneration, with particular emphasis on the alveolar parenchyma (Hogan et al., 2014; Kotton and Morrisey, 2014). Cell-based therapy for CF will logically be focused on the conducting airway epithelium, the primary site for mucus stasis, infection, and inflammation. The airways harbor distinct cell populations along the proximal to distal axis that exhibit self-renewal and differentiation capacity. Here, we propose that HBECs may serve as candidates for autologous cell therapy of CF. We review the stem cell properties of HBECs with

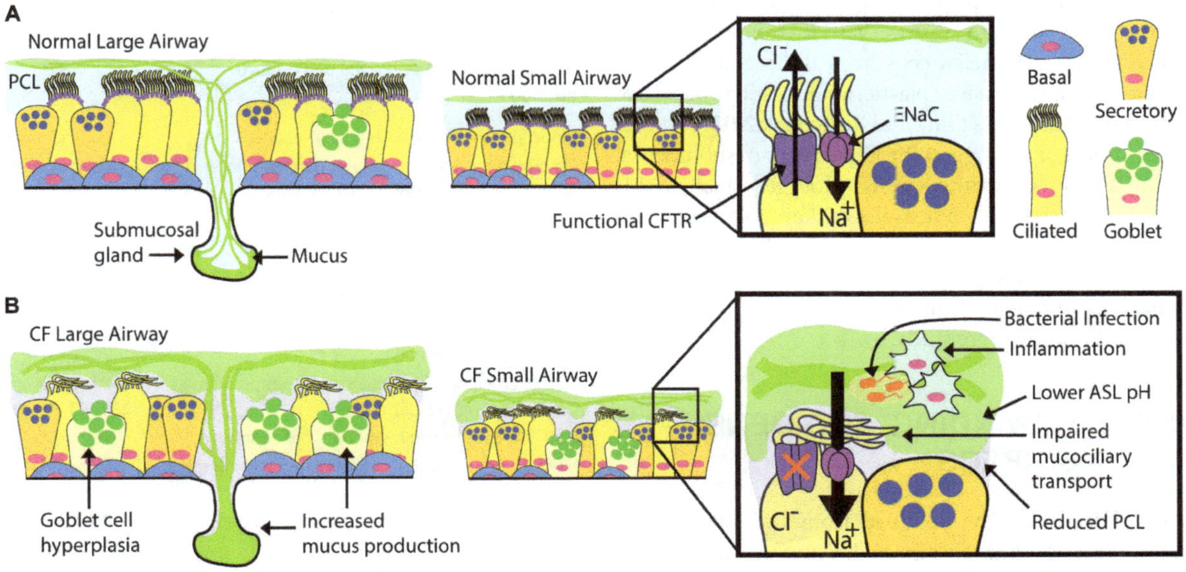

FIGURE 1 | Normal vs. CF Airway. Schematic drawings of normal and CF airways, illustrating selected components of epithelial apical ion transport. **(A)** Secreted mucins are produced by submucosal glands in the large airways and surface goblet cells, forming the overlying, mucin-rich component of the airway surface layer (ASL). This layer is normally transported by effective beating of cilia in the periciliary layer (PCL). ASL hydration is largely controlled by the balance of chloride secretion through CFTR and sodium reabsorption by the epithelial sodium channel (ENaC). **(B)** Mucin overproduction from hypertrophic submucosal glands and hyperplastic surface goblet cells characterize the CF large airways. Non-functional or absent CFTR leads to diminished chloride transport and increased sodium transport through ENaC. Airway dehydration reduces the PCL, impairing mucociliary transport. Accumulation of thick, sticky mucus increases overall ASL thickness and promotes a low pH environment favoring chronic bacterial infection and inflammation. The CF ASL environment is a likely barrier for cell therapy.

a focus on the unique advantages and challenges posed for therapeutic translation.

STEM CELLS IN THE CONDUCTING AIRWAYS

The human conducting airways are composed of a pseudo-stratified epithelium extending from the trachea to the proximal end of small bronchioles. The predominant evidence is that basal cells are the stem cells in this region (Rock et al., 2009). Basal cells are relatively undifferentiated and express a number of classic markers including *TP63* and *KRT5*. The regenerative capacity of basal cells has been extensively demonstrated through *in vitro* clonal growth assays, tracheal graft regeneration, and *in vivo* lineage tracing studies (Gray et al., 1991; Liu et al., 1994; Hong et al., 2004; Rock et al., 2009). Basal cells have the capacity to differentiate into the major cell types of the conducting airways including club (previously Clara) cells (Schoch et al., 2004; Rock et al., 2009), pulmonary neuroendocrine cells (Montoro et al., 2018), the recently described pulmonary ionocyte (Montoro et al., 2018; Plasschaert et al., 2018), and serous and mucus cells in the glands (Hegab et al., 2012, 2014). It is thought that ciliated and goblet cells are generated through a club cell intermediate (Tata et al., 2013; Widdicombe and Wine, 2015), but recent single cell mRNA sequencing studies also suggests direct differentiation of basal cells into ciliated cells (Plasschaert et al., 2018). Basal cell differentiation into pulmonary ionocytes and ciliated cells (either directly or indirectly) is of particular interest for CF cell therapy as these cell types express CFTR and are primarily responsible for epithelial ion transport (Rock et al., 2009; Montoro et al., 2018). The ability of lung basal cells to self-renew and replace luminal CFTR-expressing cell types is vital for cell therapy to be long-lasting.

The basal cell population is likely heterogeneous, containing subpopulations with different proliferation and differentiation capacities. At steady state, basal cell subsets express early differentiation markers for club or ciliated cells including the intracellular domain of Notch2 (N2ICD) or the proto-oncogene transcription factor MYB (C-Myb), respectively, suggesting subpopulations already primed for differentiation (Pardo-Saganta et al., 2015; Watson et al., 2015). Mechanisms regulating lung cell development, homeostatic maintenance, and repair have been recently reviewed (Lee and Rawlins, 2018). However, there is still debate about which cell lineage model is most applicable to the human pseudostratified airway epithelium. Are there rare populations of stem cells in specific niches that undergo asymmetric divisions, generating committed downstream progenitors, or is the stem cell compartment more widely distributed and stochastically regulated? While cell harvesting, gene correction, expansion, and delivery of intermediate progenitors may be efficacious, it is logical that starting with cells exhibiting extensive growth potential and differentiation capacity would be advantageous. Thus, identifying basal cell subsets and gene signatures corresponding to high clonal growth capacity remains an important goal that will theoretically serve as the basis for efficacious CF cell therapy.

Additional cell types within the airways should be considered as alternative candidates to restore CFTR function to the epithelium. Columnar epithelial cells from the pseudostratified regions demonstrate extensive plasticity in which they can dedifferentiate into basal cells (Tata and Rajagopal, 2017). Studies in the porcine model of CF suggest the importance of submucosal gland dysfunction in CF pathogenesis (Hoegger et al., 2014) and lineage tracing in mice illustrates a key role for gland myoepithelial cells in repair (Lynch et al., 2018; Tata et al., 2018). The ability to access, propagate and correct human gland myoepithelial cells, and their ultimate return to gland tubular and acinar niches will require more study.

OBTAINING, EXPANDING, AND GENE CORRECTING HBECS

Conceptually, HBECs can be obtained from the lungs of CF individuals using one of three minimally invasive techniques, induced sputum sample collection, bronchiolar lavage, and endobronchial brushing or biopsy. These methods yield approximately 2×10^3, 5.5×10^3, and 2×10^6 cells, respectively (Mou et al., 2012; Pollock et al., 2013; Butler et al., 2016). Considering how few cells effectively engraft by current approaches, the paucity of HBEC starting materials poses a considerable challenge to their use in cell therapy. As such, autologous cell-based therapy for CF with somatic epithelial cells will likely require *in vitro* culture for both cell expansion and gene correction. Fortunately, there is a long history of cell culture techniques to expand and subsequently differentiate a predominantly basal cell population from mouse and human large airways (see **Table 1** and Bove and Randell, 2015). Conventional expansion methods can be augmented to increase population doublings using dual SMAD inhibition or Rho kinase inhibition along with irradiated mouse 3T3-J2 fibroblasts co-culture (Suprynowicz et al., 2012; Mou et al., 2016). Key reagents such as irradiated 3T3-J2 feeder cells and irradiated serum developed for keratinocytes have been approved for clinical applications by some regulatory authorities and can be, similarly, employed in modern protocols to expand primary HBECs (Suprynowicz et al., 2012; Gentzsch et al., 2017).

While the larger airways are lined by a tall pseudostratified epithelium the more distal bronchi and bronchioles are lined by a progressively shorter epithelium, in which basal cells eventually extinguish. In the last generations of the small airways, the epithelium becomes simple columnar to cuboidal where stem cells are thought to be contained in the club cell compartment, with an independent lineage existing among pulmonary neuroendocrine cells (Hogan et al., 2014), although pulmonary neuroendocrine cell generation of club and ciliated cells has been observed (Song et al., 2012). This distal region is an important target since small airway obstruction and air trapping is thought to be a defining feature of early CF (Rosenow et al., 2017). Culture methods for human small airway epithelial cells are less well developed than for the large airway, and cells of the smallest bronchioles appear to be more dependent on mesenchymal signals (Lee et al., 2017; Zepp et al., 2017). Specific efforts to better understand human small airway stem cells, their propagation, and eventual engraftment are required.

TABLE 1 | Key studies in the development of culture methods for HBECs and directed differentiation protocols to derive airway epithelial cells from iPSCs.

Human bronchial epithelial cell culture methods	Reference
Clonal growth of human bronchial epithelial cells	Lechner et al., 1981
Detailed description of a media for proliferation of human bronchial epithelial cells on plastic	Lechner and LaVeck, 1985
Differentiation of serially passaged cells at an air-liquid interface (ALI)	Gray et al., 1996
Current detailed methods for ALI cultures using proprietary reagents	Neuberger et al., 2011
Current detailed methods for ALI cultures using non-proprietary reagents	Fulcher and Randell, 2013
Detailed methods for Conditionally Reprogrammed Cells (CRC, with feeder cells)	Gentzsch et al., 2017; Liu et al., 2017
Dual SMAD inhibition method for cell expansion	Mou et al., 2016
Method allowing clonal expansion of CRC primary HBECs	Peters-Hall et al., 2018
CRC method with proprietary media and no feeder cells	Zhang et al., 2018
Derivation of human airway epithelial cells from iPSCs	
TGFβ/BMP inhibition required to generate anterior foregut endoderm from iPSC	Green et al., 2011
Differentiation of human CF iPSCs into airway epithelial cells	Mou et al., 2012
Efficient differentiation of human iPSCs into lung epithelial cells comprised of both proximal and distal epithelial cells	Huang et al., 2013
Generation of multiciliated cells from human iPSCs	Firth et al., 2014
Human iPSC-derived lung organoids composed of epithelium and mesoderm	Dye et al., 2015
Surface marker sort method (Carboxypeptidase M) and culture conditions to generate neuroendocrine and functional multiciliated cells	Konishi et al., 2016
Fluorescent lineage reporters to purify early lung progenitors and generate epithelial-only organoid	Hawkins et al., 2017
Wnt withdrawal after early lung specification required for airway patterning	McCauley et al., 2017
Engraftment of iPSC-derived similar to embryonic lung-tips into immunocompromised mouse lungs	Miller et al., 2018

There have been tremendous advances in genome editing techniques in the last decade, including zinc-finger nucleases, transcription activator-like effector nucleases (TALENs), and the clustered regularly interspaced short palindromic repeats (CRISPR)/Cas9 technique (Zhang et al., 2014). While of utmost importance for correcting a monogenic but complex lung disease such as CF, optimal methods for *CFTR* gene correction of HBECs with minimal off target, potentially carcinogenic risks, followed by cell expansion that maintains long-lived basal stem cells remain to be determined.

INDUCED PLURIPOTENT STEM CELLS (iPSCS)

iPSCs have several features relevant to their suitability as a source for cell-based therapies. Pluripotency refers to the capacity to differentiate into all cell types in the body. iPSCs can now be routinely generated from any human while retaining an individual's unique genetic information, without the need for an invasive procedure. The capacity of these cells to proliferate while retaining pluripotency means sufficient numbers for cell-based therapy might someday be feasible. In the following section we review the essential studies that made the discovery of iPSCs possible, summarize the recent progress in deriving lung epithelial cells from iPSCs (**Table 1**), particularly cell types relevant to CF, and finally highlight the many challenges to be addressed before these cells can be transplanted into CF recipients.

HISTORY OF iPSCS

In 2006, Takahashi and Yamanaka made the remarkable discovery that the overexpression of four key factors in somatic cells could "re-program" cells into iPSCs (Takahashi and Yamanaka, 2006; Takahashi et al., 2007). This breakthrough was made possible by decades of prior work in the field of embryonic stem cells (ESCs) that identified: (1) the transient presence of a population of pluripotent stem cells in the developing embryo, (2) the culture conditions sufficient to capture, *in vitro* expand, and maintain the pluripotency of cells isolated from early embryos, and (3) the gene-regulatory networks that control the ground-state of pluripotency (Solter et al., 1970; Stevens, 1970; Evans and Kaufman, 1981; Smith, 2001). Given the regenerative potential of ESCs there was much initial enthusiasm for their therapeutic promise but also controversy over the ethical and moral considerations regarding the use of fetal tissue. From a scientific perspective the main drawback for using ESCs as a cell-based therapy was that even if the cell type of interest could be generated efficiently and safely, the cells would be allogeneic to the recipient and the issues of rejection and immunosuppression that limit the effectiveness of solid organ transplants would persist. Dr. Jim Gurdon's pioneering nuclear transfer experiments in the 1960s first suggested the feasibility of reprogramming a somatic cell into an autologous pluripotent stem cell (Gurdon, 1962). When a frog egg nucleus was replaced with an intestinal cell nucleus a viable tadpole was produced confirming that the cellular identity could be "reset" to a pluripotent state. Takahashi and Yamanaka set about screening candidate factors that might have the same effect. They identified four factors, *Oct4*, *Sox2*, *Klf4*, and *c-Myc* that were sufficient to reprogram mouse somatic cells (initially skin fibroblasts) into pluripotent stem cells. These "induced" pluripotent stem cells were virtually indistinguishable from ESCs based on their similar transcriptional profiles and capacity to differentiate into all three germ layers when injected subcutaneously in a teratoma assay. Remarkably, iPSCs also contributed to embryogenesis when injected into a blastocyst. One year later, the same four factors were confirmed to reprogram human fibroblasts into iPSCs. Crucial to the emerging field of regenerative medicine, iPSCs have four key characteristics: (1) they are generated from the potential recipient, i.e., autologous, (2) they provide an unlimited supply of pluripotent stem cells without the need for embryonic tissues, (3) they are amenable to gene correction approaches, and (4) they are now routinely derived.

DIRECTED DIFFERENTIATION OF iPSCS INTO LUNG EPITHELIUM

Over the past decade, many groups contributed to major progress toward generating lung epithelial cells from iPSCs (**Table 1**). Directed differentiation refers to the approach of recapitulating, *in vitro*, the key embryonic developmental milestones that lead to the specification of the cell(s) of interest. This is typically achieved through the stepwise addition of signaling factors identified in mouse studies of organogenesis. The field of lung directed differentiation has evolved from generating relatively immature lung epithelial cells to recent reports of increasingly sophisticated protocols that produce relatively mature and functional lung epithelial cells that are currently being applied to lung disease modeling, drug screening and the first forays into *in vivo* transplantation.

In order to understand the directed differentiation process, a brief overview of lung development is first required. The lung develops from the foregut endoderm and is first identified by the expression of *Nkx2-1*, a key transcription factor. *Nkx2-1* is first detected at E9.0 in mice and day 28 in human embryos (Lazzaro et al., 1991; Morrisey and Hogan, 2010). During the first stages of lung organogenesis *Nkx2-1*$^+$ cells form two primary lung buds and the adjacent foregut separates into two tubes, a ventral trachea and dorsal esophagus. During the pseudoglandular stage, the lung buds undergo branching morphogenesis and proximal-distal patterning. This process, controlled by reciprocal signaling between the lung epithelium and surrounding mesenchyme, gives rise to a highly branched airway tree composed of basal, secretory, multi-ciliated and neuroendocrine cells and an alveolar compartment composed of types 1 and 2 pneumocytes. A number of signaling pathways are involved in the epithelial-mesenchymal interactions that control these stages of lung development including SHH, WNTs, FGFs, retinoic acid and BMPs (Hawkins et al., 2016).

To differentiate iPSCs into lung epithelial cells researchers seek to reproduce these key developmental events *in vitro*. The first major developmental stage in the road map of lung development is the formation of definitive endoderm. Mimicking the *in vivo* patterning of the primitive streak, the addition of the Nodal agonist Activin-A to iPSCs or ESCs produces a highly enriched population of endodermal cells that express classic endoderm markers (including *FOXA2* and *SOX17*) (Kubo et al., 2004; D'Amour et al., 2005; Christodoulou et al., 2011). The protocols to generate definitive endoderm are now well established and form the basis of all endodermal differentiation protocols including lung, liver, pancreas and intestine. The next important developmental step is directing definitive endodermal cells (*FOXA2*$^+$) toward an anterior-foregut fate (*FOXA2*$^+$/*SOX2*$^+$), analogous to the anterior-posterior axis patterning in the primitive gut tube. The field of lung directed differentiation is relatively new and not surprisingly the published protocols from different groups vary significantly in terms of the timing and combination of growth factors and inhibitors applied at different stages. For example, differing approaches have achieved *in vitro* foregut patterning. In one method antagonism of BMP and TGFβ pathways after endoderm induction was identified as the most potent condition to maintain *FOXA2* expression, and to induce the anterior endoderm marker *SOX2* while suppressing a hindgut fate that expresses *CDX2* (Green et al., 2011). The inclusion of BMP and/or TGFβ inhibition has been adopted by others (Longmire et al., 2012; Mou et al., 2012; Firth et al., 2014; Dye et al., 2015; Hawkins et al., 2017). Alternative approaches include the combination of FGF2 and SHH signaling (Wong et al., 2012). Lung specification is the next major developmental milestone and is indicated by the expression of *NKX2-1* in foregut endoderm cells. Several groups have concluded that WNT, through recombinant WNT3a or glycogen synthase kinase 3 inhibitors, BMP4, and retinoic acid pathway activation are required for lung specification (Huang et al., 2013; Gotoh et al., 2014; Hawkins et al., 2017). Others have developed quite different approaches that led to specification of a lung program, for example using a combination of BMP and TGFβ inhibition, plus SHH and WNT activation (Dye et al., 2015). Early reports demonstrated lung competence of these cells via upregulation of differentiation markers over time. However, both proximal and distal lung markers were frequently present suggesting that the precise signals patterning lung progenitors toward proximal vs. distal fates and to specific differentiated cell types are incompletely known. Competence of these cells to differentiate into functional airway lineages was demonstrated by transitioning to air-liquid interface conditions used to differentiate primary HBECs, or by injecting the cells into the flank or kidney capsule of immune-deficient mice (Wong et al., 2012; Huang et al., 2013; Firth et al., 2014). More recently, there has been progress in generating lung organoids from iPSC-derived lung epithelium, reminiscent of the 3-D organization of lung tissue (Gotoh et al., 2014; Dye et al., 2015; Chen et al., 2017; Hawkins et al., 2017; Miller et al., 2018). In some cases, these protocols involve the co-development of mesodermal and endodermal compartments. To overcome the heterogeneity of cell types produced in these protocols, fluorescent lineage reporters or surface markers have been employed to prospectively isolate the lung epithelial cells of interest. Surface markers including Carboxypeptidase M or the combination of $CD47^{hi}/CD26^{lo}$ were identified to isolate immature $NKX2\text{-}1^{+}$ lung epithelial cells and to generate lung epithelial organoids depleted of other endodermal and mesodermal cell types (Gotoh et al., 2014; Hawkins et al., 2017). Although less relevant as a cell-based therapy for CF, it is worth highlighting some of the most compelling progress toward generating relatively mature, functional type 2 pneumocytes from iPSCs. Two groups, adopting the approach of targeting fluorescent reporters to the endogenous *SFTPC* locus, developed similar protocols to isolate and propagate long term a population of $SFTPC^{+}$ cells highly reminiscent of alveolar type 2 cells (Jacob et al., 2017; Yamamoto et al., 2017).

DIRECTED DIFFERENTIATION OF iPSCS INTO AIRWAY EPITHELIUM

To cure CF airway disease, a cell-based therapy would ideally replace the CFTR-expressing columnar luminal epithelial cells, including terminally differentiated multi-ciliated cells and perhaps ionocytes, but also the stem/progenitor cells that maintain the luminal cells. A number of groups have demonstrated the feasibility of generating CFTR expressing airway epithelium composed of multi-ciliated cells and cells reminiscent of basal and secretory cells (Wong et al., 2012; Firth et al., 2014; Konishi et al., 2016; McCauley et al., 2017). These airway epithelial cells broadly recapitulate the CFTR dysfunction seen in the primary cells of CF patients when interrogated using established CFTR functional assays including ion transport in Ussing chambers and forskolin-induced spheroid swelling. In an important proof-of-concept study, Crane et al., demonstrated the correction of the F508del mutation in iPSCs using zinc-finger nucleases and restoration of CFTR function in those cells after lung differentiation (Crane et al., 2015). Based on our current knowledge, an ideal iPSC-derived candidate cell for engraftment into CF airways is the airway basal cell. A number of groups have described the presence of a subset of basal-like cells after directed lung differentiation as evidenced by the expression of key basal cell markers (e.g., *TP63*, *KRT5*) (Dye et al., 2015; Konishi et al., 2016; Chen et al., 2017; Hawkins et al., 2017; McCauley et al., 2017). However, the efficient derivation of bonafide basal cells, as evidenced by transcriptional profiling and functional demonstration of differentiation into multi-ciliated and secretory cells comparable to those generated by primary basal cell controls, has not yet been convincingly achieved.

IN VIVO ENGRAFTMENT OF iPSC-DERIVED LUNG EPITHELIAL CELLS

Provided that it is possible to derive a candidate cell type *in vitro*, would that cell engraft and function once transplanted? This is a major question now facing this field and very little is known about the *in vivo* potential of iPSC-derived cells in the lung. Recently, the first report of human iPSC-derived lung epithelial cells engrafting in a murine lung injury model was described (Miller et al., 2018). Miller et al., identified conditions to capture and expand cells with a transcriptional profile similar to the multipotent cells of the developing lung bud tip. The iPSC-derived lung tip cells were delivered intra-tracheally into immunocompromised mice following airway injury with naphthalene. Engrafted cells persisted for up to 6 weeks after transplantation and these cells had adopted a predominantly airway and mostly secretory cell fate with rare multi-ciliated cells. This study is an important first step establishing the feasibility of using animal models to develop engraftment strategies, and suggests that the micro-environment or niche may play an important role in the cell fate decisions of transplanted cells.

CHALLENGES FACING iPSCS AS A CELL-BASED THERAPY

Despite the progress made in the field of iPSC directed differentiation into lung cells, there are major challenges facing the application of cell-based therapy for the treatment of CF. To date, the derivation of a pure population of airway epithelial cells from iPSCs in sufficient numbers to engraft in human airways has not yet been achieved. How will adequate numbers of differentiated cells be generated for patients? How safe are iPSC-derived lung epithelial cells? The same factors and culture conditions that allow for the unimpeded self-renewal and pluripotency also predispose to tumorigenicity; in fact, a survey of the exomes of 117 human iPSC lines identified nine with mutations in the tumor suppressor gene, *TP53,* with evidence that iPSCs with the mutation had a survival advantage (Ben-David and Benvenisty, 2011; Merkle et al., 2017). Other groups have confirmed that gene editing with CRISPR/Cas9 selects against cells with a normal p53 pathway (Haapaniemi et al., 2018; Ihry et al., 2018). Initially iPSCs were generated using viral vectors that randomly integrated into the genome (Takahashi and Yamanaka, 2006). This approach raised obvious concerns about the malignant potential of iPSCs if an important tumor suppressor locus was disrupted. A non-integrating episomal-based method, such as Sendai virus, is a more logical approach to derive clinical-grade iPSCs (Fusaki et al., 2009). The delivery of safe cells will require a robust and reproducible process to generate iPSCs and differentiated cells, compliant with relevant current good manufacturing practice (cGMP) and regulatory agency approval. Confirmation that the resulting cells are free of integrations and somatic mutations will be needed (Baghbaderani et al., 2015). Transplanted cells will require *in vitro* gene-correction to express functional CFTR. With reprogramming and passaging, and additional time needed to gene-edit and expand cells, the probability of somatic mutations will increase. Furthermore, the process of gene-editing brings additional risk of off-target double-stranded breaks with the potential of disrupting other genetic loci (Zhang et al., 2015). As the goal of cell-based therapy is to replace diseased endogenous lung epithelium with engineered cells, it will be essential to generate pure populations of lung epithelial cells that are highly similar to their *in vivo* counterparts. The field is relatively new and most reports have not focused on the non-lung cells that might also be produced during the differentiation process. For example, an iPSC line expressing GFP from the NKX2-1 locus (*NKX2-1*^{GFP}) identified significant variability in the percentage of GFP^{+} cells, and analysis of the GFP^{-} population confirmed expression of liver and intestine markers (Hawkins et al., 2017; Serra et al., 2017). Even after a purification step to sort *NKX2-1*$^{\mathrm{GFP}+}$ cells, McCauley et al. applied single-cell RNA sequencing to airway and alveolar iPSC-derived organoids and identified distinct populations of non-lung endoderm including hepatic-like and gastric-like cells (McCauley et al., 2018). The quest to generate pure populations of well-defined lung epithelial cells will continue and be aided by powerful new techniques such as single-cell RNA sequencing and expanding knowledge of the transcriptional profile and signaling pathways involved in human lung development (Treutlein et al., 2014; Nikolić et al., 2017; Miller et al., 2018). The appropriate number of donor cells required to repopulate a sufficient portion of the diseased airway epithelium is unknown. CFTR levels 15–20% of normal airway expression may be enough to effectively treat CF airway disease (McKone et al., 2003). Building on these aforementioned advances, the ultimate final hurdle to a cell-based therapeutic approach for CF is engraftment.

ENGRAFTMENT

The gold standard for cell-based therapy is hematopoietic cell transplantation. This now commonplace and life-saving procedure relies on delivering hematopoietic progenitor cells after inducing tissue receptivity through marrow-ablative doses of cytotoxic agents and radiation. The term engraftment is used to describe the reconstitution of host bone marrow by donor cells. For CF, successful airway engraftment is thought of in similar terms, recipient airway priming, donor cell survival and regeneration of the airway epithelium (**Figure 2**). The ideal strategy to deliver a cell-based therapy for CF, or any lung disease, has yet to be developed and the prospect of deliberately injuring the lungs of CF recipients to ablate endogenous cells is daunting. An ideal engraftment strategy would involve the minimal airway injury necessary, in particular to the small airways, to promote a microenvironment conducive to long-lived engraftment of cells in numbers sufficient to restore CFTR function. There are many hurdles the scientific community must overcome to achieve human airway engraftment such as determining: (1) the most suitable cell type(s), (2) the methods to safely scale-up cell production, (3) the optimal injury, (4) supportive measures for oxygenation/ventilation and (5) methods to control mucus and infection to allow engraftment of cells. Despite these challenges, there are promising reports of effective cell therapies for other organ systems that support the overall feasibility of this approach. Based on pioneering work from the laboratory of Howard Green, autologous epidermal keratinocytes have been extensively evaluated as treatment for burns (Green et al., 1979; Ter Horst et al., 2018). Recently, transgenic autologous keratinocytes with a correct copy of a gene mutated in the blistering skin disease junctional epidermolysis bullosa were used to replace nearly the entire epidermis of a critically ill child with 60% skin loss, miraculously allowing hospital discharge and return to school (Hirsch et al., 2017). This remarkable achievement not only alleviated patient suffering, but also provided vital insights about epidermal keratinocyte stem cell dynamics, indicating the importance of long-lived stem cells for epidermal restoration. Additional experience comes from corneal limbal epithelial stem cell transplantation in which damage to one eye can be treated with autologous stem cells from the contralateral eye (Rama et al., 2017; Sasamoto et al., 2018). In the lung field, a number of groups have recently reported evidence of lung engraftment in animal models (Rosen et al., 2015; Vaughan et al., 2015;

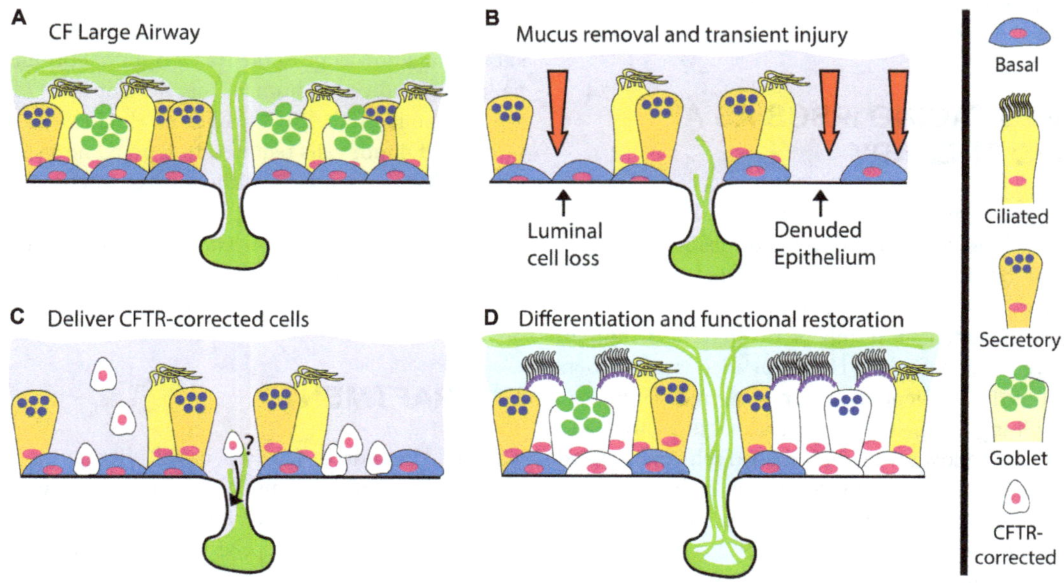

FIGURE 2 | A Cell-Based Therapy Model for CF. **(A)** The pre-treatment CF large airway. **(B–D)** A depiction of cell-based therapy in three steps: **(B)** Mucus removal and transient preconditioning of the airway epithelium, potentially requiring luminal epithelial surface cell loss and partial epithelial denudation; **(C)** Delivery of CFTR-corrected stem and progenitor cells to the surface epithelium and possibly the submucosal glands; **(D)** Differentiation of delivered CFTR-corrected cells into all relevant cell types, restoration of functional CFTR ion-transport and a return to normal airway physiology.

Ghosh et al., 2017; Nichane et al., 2017; Ma et al., 2018; Miller et al., 2018). Here we will briefly review this progress and highlight important next steps.

A number of injury models, including naphthalene, sulfur dioxide, radiation and detergents, have been developed to study the biology of the airway epithelium (Lamb and Reid, 1968; Plopper et al., 1992; Borthwick et al., 2001; Leblond et al., 2009; Rosen et al., 2015). It is unclear to what extent, if any, these models might be used in humans but they have provided a platform to study and develop engraftment strategies. Embryonic lung, both mouse and human, contain stem/progenitor populations with engraftment capacity (Rosen et al., 2015; Nichane et al., 2017). In one approach, intravenous administration of a single cell suspension of whole canalicular stage lung (mouse E15-16 or human week 20–22) into mice pre-conditioned with both naphthalene and total body irradiation, resulted in epithelial, mesenchymal, and endothelial patches of engrafted cells (Rosen et al., 2015). Higher rates of chimerism were detected in mouse-into-mouse compared to human-into-mouse experiments. It is surprising that intravenous delivery of a mixture of embryonic lung cell types resulted in homing of cells to their unique anatomic compartments. Further work is required to understand the safety of this approach including the consequence of cells being delivered to the wrong compartment within the lung or even to other organs. In terms of an approach for CF, the majority of epithelial engrafted cells had an alveolar phenotype although some airway-like cells were detected and some expressed CFTR. Interestingly, the co-administration of mesenchymal and endothelial cells was associated with improved epithelial cell engraftment. The multitude of practical, ethical and political issues surrounding the use of fetal tissue make this an unlikely future option for cell-based therapy. However, iPSCs may provide access to autologous cells at embryonic time points with capacity to engraft (Miller et al., 2018). Adult airway epithelial cells can also engraft in the lung (Vaughan et al., 2015; Ghosh et al., 2017; Nichane et al., 2017). The environment induced by H1N1 influenza infection has garnered much interest for its engraftment potential (Kumar et al., 2011; Vaughan et al., 2015). The viral infection causes widespread damage to the airway and alveolar epithelium and activates rare immature (*TP63*$^+$/*KRT5*$^-$) basal cells in the small airways (Yang et al., 2018). Orthotopic transplantation of a variety of airway epithelial cells into influenza-injured mice led to varying levels of engraftment (Vaughan et al., 2015). Perhaps most relevant to the CF field is a recent report of successful engraftment of primary airway basal cells into naphthalene injured mice (Ghosh et al., 2017). Transplanted mouse or human basal cells reconstituted patches of epithelium in the trachea and small airways with evidence of multi-lineage differentiation into secretory and multi-ciliated cells. Themes common to each of the above experiments include: (1) lung injury is required for engraftment of donor cells, (2) different injury models likely result in unique regenerative niches and (3) successful strategies to date suggest multipotent input donor cells are the most promising candidates for engraftment. Looking forward, a number of approaches might accelerate the field of cell-based therapy for lung disease. Engraftment after hematopoietic cell transplantation is monitored by sampling the peripheral blood. Assessing lung engraftment is far more challenging. Methods to interrogate whether donor cells are functionally integrated into the airway epithelium will be essential. Animal studies to optimize injury models and the efficiency, function and safety of engrafted cells are necessary, but are rate-limiting due to low throughput, particularly in larger animals. Developing non-lethal experimental methods, including targeted airway injury and bioluminescent reporter cell lines to track engrafted cells in real-time without the need for necropsy would increase the efficiency of animal engraftment studies.

Methods to incite a targeted, clinically tolerable airway epithelial injury have been tested in humans albeit not in the context of cell-based therapy. Bronchial thermoplasty, an FDA-approved treatment for refractory severe persistent asthma, delivers brief thermal energy to the airways via flexible bronchoscopy and leads to initial epithelial sloughing and a prolonged decrease in smooth muscle with improvement in asthma severity (Miller et al., 2005). In a small pilot study, airway delivery of a metered liquid nitrogen cryospray via bronchoscopy resulted in airway epithelial damage followed by regeneration (Slebos et al., 2017). An alternative approach, with potential for clinical translation, is targeted airway de-epithelialization achieved by instilling mild detergents intratracheally (Dorrello et al., 2017). Despite the many limitations of these approaches in the context of CF, including the small size and large number of airways needed to treat CF, they provide preliminary support for the feasibility of a human injury platform. The situation is further complicated for targeting CF in more advanced disease where successful cell-based therapy must also overcome a highly inflamed, architecturally distorted organ characterized by thick mucus and superinfection. Similar to the blood product and growth factor support necessary after hematopoietic cell transplant, lung engraftment strategies will likely require lung supportive measures. The advances and more widespread use of extracorporeal membrane oxygenation (ECMO) provides a means of supporting oxygenation during respiratory failure (Squiers et al., 2016). Advances in the technology to maintain human lungs using *ex vivo* lung perfusion (EVLP) may provide insights into supporting the injured and regenerating lung (Makdisi et al., 2017). Future approaches for cell-based therapy incorporating these evolving technologies may be necessary. Alternatively, devising injury-independent strategies to promote lung engraftment of therapeutic cells may be an avenue for future research and development.

CONCLUSION

To date, CF remains the most common life-limiting hereditary lung disease. Decades of work resulted in important strides to understand molecular mechanisms in CF and treatment options for many patients. Despite this progress, a subset of patients lack effective treatment options and cell-based therapies could theoretically cure CF lung disease. The ideal cell type for this purpose would repopulate the airway epithelium with autologous, functional, and CFTR-expressing cells. Progress in our understanding of airway epithelial biology and endogenous stem/progenitor populations has revealed a number of candidate cell types for airway regeneration, in particular basal cells. The recent revolution in gene-editing techniques means genetic correction of the *CFTR* mutation in basal cells will likely be achieved in the near future and would provide a source of autologous airway stem cells with the normal *CFTR* sequence. In the iPSC field, directed differentiation protocols have evolved from initial studies demonstrating the presence of immature lung-like cells to more recent reports of increasingly efficient protocols to derive functional alveolar and airway epithelial cells. We have detailed some of the major challenges that must be overcome both in terms of generating the cells of interest and engrafting those cells in a safe and effective manner. While there is work yet to be done, there is cautious optimism that a curative cell-based therapy for CF will be achieved in the future.

AUTHOR CONTRIBUTIONS

All authors contributed to this manuscript. In collaboration, AB, FH, RL, and SR wrote all sections of this review. RL illustrated the figures. All authors read, edited, and approved of the final version of the manuscript.

FUNDING

The authors received funding support from NIH grants T32HL0007025 (AB) and R01HL139799 (FH), Cystic Fibrosis Foundation grants RANDEL15XX0 (SR), RANDEL17XX0 (SR), and HAWKIN15XX0 (FH), and Emily's Entourage (FH and SR).

REFERENCES

Baghbaderani, B. A., Tian, X., Neo, B. H., Burkall, A., Dimezzo, T., Sierra, G., et al. (2015). cGMP-manufactured human induced pluripotent stem cells are available for pre-clinical and clinical applications. *Stem Cell Rep.* 5, 647–659. doi: 10.1016/j.stemcr.2015.08.015

Ben-David, U., and Benvenisty, N. (2011). The tumorigenicity of human embryonic and induced pluripotent stem cells. *Nat. Rev. Cancer* 11, 268–277. doi: 10.1038/nrc3034

Borthwick, D. W., Shahbazian, M., Krantz, Q. T., Dorin, J. R., and Randell, S. H. (2001). Evidence for stem-cell niches in the tracheal epithelium. *Am. J. Respir. Cell Mol. Biol.* 24, 662–670. doi: 10.1165/ajrcmb.24.6.4217

Bove, P. F., and Randell, S. H. (2015). "Comparative mammalian lung primary surface epithelial cell culture," in *Comparative Biology of the Normal Lung*, (Cambridge, MA: Academic Press), 129–139. doi: 10.1016/B978-0-12-404577-4.00011-4

Butler, C. R., Hynds, R. E., Gowers, K. H. C., Lee, D. D. H., Brown, J. M., Crowley, C., et al. (2016). Rapid expansion of human epithelial stem cells suitable for airway tissue engineering. *Am. J. Respir. Crit. Care Med.* 194, 156–168. doi: 10.1164/rccm.201507-1414OC

Button, B., Cai, L.-H., Ehre, C., Kesimer, M., Hill, D. B., Sheehan, J. K., et al. (2012). A periciliary brush promotes the lung health by separating the mucus layer from airway epithelia. *Science* 337, 937–941. doi: 10.1126/science.1223012

Chen, Y.-W., Huang, S. X., de Carvalho, A. L. R. T., Ho, S.-H., Islam, M. N., Volpi, S., et al. (2017). A three-dimensional model of human lung development and disease from pluripotent stem cells. *Nat. Cell Biol.* 19, 542–549. doi: 10.1038/ncb3510

Christodoulou, C., Longmire, T. A., Shen, S. S., Bourdon, A., Sommer, C. A., Gadue, P., et al. (2011). Mouse ES and iPS cells can form similar definitive endoderm despite differences in imprinted genes. *J. Clin. Investig.* 121, 2313–2325. doi: 10.1172/JCI43853

Crane, A. M., Kramer, P., Bui, J. H., Chung, W. J., Li, X. S., Gonzalez-Garay, M. L., et al. (2015). Targeted correction and restored function of the CFTR gene in cystic fibrosis induced pluripotent stem cells. *Stem Cell Rep.* 4, 569–577. doi: 10.1016/j.stemcr.2015.02.005

Cutting, G. R. (2014). Cystic fibrosis genetics: from molecular understanding to clinical application. *Nat. Rev. Genet.* 16, 45–56. doi: 10.1038/nrg3849

D'Amour, K. A., Agulnick, A. D., Eliazer, S., Kelly, O. G., Kroon, E., and Baetge, E. E. (2005). Efficient differentiation of human embryonic stem cells to definitive endoderm. *Nat. Biotechnol.* 23, 1534–1541. doi: 10.1038/nbt1163

Davies, J. C., Moskowitz, S. M., Brown, C., Horsley, A., Mall, M. A., McKone, E. F., et al. (2018). VX-659-tezacaftor-ivacaftor in patients with cystic fibrosis and one or two phe508del alleles. *N. Engl. J. Med.* 379, 1599–1611. doi: 10.1056/NEJMoa1807119

Dorrello, N. V., Guenthart, B. A., O'Neill, J. D., Kim, J., Cunningham, K., Chen, Y.-W., et al. (2017). Functional vascularized lung grafts for lung bioengineering. *Sci. Adv.* 3:e1700521. doi: 10.1126/sciadv.1700521

Dye, B. R., Hill, D. R., Ferguson, M. A., Tsai, Y.-H., Nagy, M. S., Dyal, R., et al. (2015). *In vitro* generation of human pluripotent stem cell derived lung organoids. *eLife* 4, 1999–1925. doi: 10.7554/eLife.05098

Evans, M. J., and Kaufman, M. H. (1981). Establishment in culture of pluripotential cells from mouse embryos. *Nature* 292, 154–156. doi: 10.1038/292154a0

Firth, A. L., Dargitz, C. T., Qualls, S. J., Menon, T., Wright, R., Singer, O., et al. (2014). Generation of multiciliated cells in functional airway epithelia from human induced pluripotent stem cells. *Proc. Natl. Acad. Sci. U.S.A.* 111, E1723–E1730. doi: 10.1073/pnas.1403470111

Fulcher, M. L., and Randell, S. H. (2013). Human nasal and tracheo-bronchial respiratory epithelial cell culture. *Methods Mol. Biol.* 945, 109–121. doi: 10.1007/978-1-62703-125-7_8

Fusaki, N., Ban, H., Nishiyama, A., Saeki, K., and Hasegawa, M. (2009). Efficient induction of transgene-free human pluripotent stem cells using a vector based on Sendai virus, an RNA virus that does not integrate into the host genome. *Proc. Jpn. Acad. Series B Phys. Biol. Sci.* 85, 348–362. doi: 10.2183/pjab.85.348

Gentzsch, M., Boyles, S. E., Cheluvaraju, C., Chaudhry, I. G., Quinney, N. L., Cho, C., et al. (2017). Pharmacological rescue of conditionally reprogrammed cystic fibrosis bronchial epithelial cells. *Am. J. Respir. Cell Mol. Biol.* 56, 568–574. doi: 10.1165/rcmb.2016-0276MA

Ghosh, M., Ahmad, S., White, C. W., and Reynolds, S. D. (2017). Transplantation of airway epithelial stem/progenitor cells: a future for cell-based therapy. *Am. J. Respir. Cell Mol. Biol.* 56, 1–10. doi: 10.1165/rcmb.2016-0181MA

Gotoh, S., Ito, I., Nagasaki, T., Yamamoto, Y., Konishi, S., Korogi, Y., et al. (2014). Generation of alveolar epithelial spheroids via isolated progenitor cells from human pluripotent stem cells. *Stem Cell Rep.* 3, 394–403. doi: 10.1016/j.stemcr.2014.07.005

Gray, T., Rundhaug, J., and Nettesheim, P. (1991). Critical variables controlling cell proliferation in primary cultures of rat tracheal epithelial cells. *In Vitro* cellular & developmental biology. *J. Tissue Cult. Assoc.* 27A, 805–814. doi: 10.1007/BF02631247

Gray, T. E., Guzman, K., Davis, C. W., Abdullah, L. H., and Nettesheim, P. (1996). Mucociliary differentiation of serially passaged normal human tracheobronchial epithelial cells. *Am. J. Respir. Cell Mol. Biol.* 14, 104–112. doi: 10.1165/ajrcmb.14.1.8534481

Green, H., Kehinde, O., and Thomas, J. (1979). Growth of cultured human epidermal cells into multiple epithelia suitable for grafting. *Proc. Natl. Acad. Sci. U.S.A.* 76, 5665–5668. doi: 10.1073/pnas.76.11.5665

Green, M., Chen, A., Nostro, M.-C., d'Souza, S. L., Schaniel, C., Lemischka, I. R., et al. (2011). Generation of anterior foregut endoderm from human embryonic and induced pluripotent stem cells. *Nat. Biotechnol.* 29, 267–272. doi: 10.1038/nbt.1788

Gurdon, J. B. (1962). The developmental capacity of nuclei taken from intestinal epithelium cells of feeding tadpoles. *J. Embryol. Exp. Morphol.* 10, 622–640.

Haapaniemi, E., Botla, S., Persson, J., Schmierer, B., and Taipale, J. (2018). CRISPR-Cas9 genome editing induces a p53-mediated DNA damage response. *Nat. Med.* 24, 927–930. doi: 10.1038/s41591-018-0049-z

Hawkins, F., Kramer, P., Jacob, A., Driver, I., Thomas, D. C., McCauley, K. B., et al. (2017). Prospective isolation of NKX2-1-expressing human lung progenitors derived from pluripotent stem cells. *J. Clin. Investig.* 127, 2277–2294. doi: 10.1172/JCI89950

Hawkins, F., Rankin, S. A., Kotton, D. N., and Zorn, A. M. (2016). "The genetic programs regulating embryonic lung development and induced pluripotent stem cell differentiation," in *Fetal and Neonatal Lung Development*, eds A. Jobe, J. Whitsett, and S. Abman (Cambridge: Cambridge University Press), 1–21. doi: 10.1017/CBO9781139680349.002

Hegab, A. E., Ha, V. L., Bisht, B., Darmawan, D. O., Ooi, A. T., Zhang, K. X., et al. (2014). Aldehyde dehydrogenase activity enriches for proximal airway basal stem cells and promotes their proliferation. *Stem Cells Dev.* 23, 664–675. doi: 10.1089/scd.2013.0295

Hegab, A. E., Ha, V. L., Darmawan, D. O., Gilbert, J. L., Ooi, A. T., Attiga, Y. S., et al. (2012). Isolation and in vitro characterization of basal and submucosal gland duct stem/progenitor cells from human proximal airways. *Stem Cells Transl. Med.* 1, 719–724. doi: 10.5966/sctm.2012-0056

Hirsch, T., Rothoeft, T., Teig, N., Bauer, J. W., Pellegrini, G., De Rosa, L., et al. (2017). Regeneration of the entire human epidermis using transgenic stem cells. *Nature* 551, 327–332. doi: 10.1038/nature24487

Hoegger, M. J., Fischer, A. J., McMenimen, J. D., Ostedgaard, L. S., Tucker, A. J., Awadalla, M. A., et al. (2014). Impaired mucus detachment disrupts mucociliary transport in a piglet model of cystic fibrosis. *Science* 345, 818–822. doi: 10.1126/science.1255825

Hogan, B. L. M., Barkauskas, C. E., Chapman, H. A., Epstein, J. A., Jain, R., Hsia, C. C. W., et al. (2014). Repair and regeneration of the respiratory system: complexity, plasticity, and mechanisms of lung stem cell function. *Cell Stem Cell* 15, 123–138. doi: 10.1016/j.stem.2014.07.012

Hong, K. U., Reynolds, S. D., Watkins, S., Fuchs, E., and Stripp, B. R. (2004). Basal cells are a multipotent progenitor capable of renewing the bronchial epithelium. *Am. J. Pathol.* 164, 577–588. doi: 10.1016/S0002-9440(10)63147-1

Huang, S. X. L., Islam, M. N., O'Neill, J., Hu, Z., Yang, Y.-G., Chen, Y.-W., et al. (2013). Efficient generation of lung and airway epithelial cells from human pluripotent stem cells. *Nat. Biotechnol.* 32, 84–91. doi: 10.1038/nbt.2754

Ihry, R. J., Worringer, K. A., Salick, M. R., Frias, E., Ho, D., Theriault, K., et al. (2018). p53 inhibits CRISPR-Cas9 engineering in human pluripotent stem cells. *Nat. Med.* 24, 939–946. doi: 10.1038/s41591-018-0050-6

Jacob, A., Morley, M., Hawkins, F., McCauley, K. B., Jean, J. C., Heins, H., et al. (2017). Differentiation of human pluripotent stem cells into functional lung alveolar epithelial cells. *Cell Stem Cell* 21, 472.e10–488.e10. doi: 10.1016/j.stem.2017.08.014

Jiang, Q., and Engelhardt, J. F. (1998). Cellular heterogeneity of CFTR expression and function in the lung: implications for gene therapy of cystic fibrosis. *Eur. J. Hum. Genet.* 6, 12–31. doi: 10.1038/sj.ejhg.5200158

Keating, D., Marigowda, G., Burr, L., Daines, C., Mall, M. A., McKone, E. F., et al. (2018). VX-445-tezacaftor-ivacaftor in patients with cystic fibrosis and one or two Phe508del alleles. *N. Engl. J. Med.* 379, 1612–1620. doi: 10.1056/NEJMoa1807120

Konishi, S., Gotoh, S., Tateishi, K., Yamamoto, Y., Korogi, Y., Nagasaki, T., et al. (2016). Directed induction of functional multi-ciliated cells in proximal airway epithelial spheroids from human pluripotent stem cells. *Stem Cell Rep.* 6, 18–25. doi: 10.1016/j.stemcr.2015.11.010

Kotton, D. N., and Morrisey, E. E. (2014). Lung regeneration: mechanisms, applications and emerging stem cell populations. *Nat. Med.* 20, 822–832. doi: 10.1038/nm.3642

Kubo, A., Shinozaki, K., Shannon, J. M., Kouskoff, V., Kennedy, M., Woo, S., et al. (2004). Development of definitive endoderm from embryonic stem cells in culture. *Development* 131, 1651–1662. doi: 10.1242/dev.01044

Kumar, P. A., Hu, Y., Yamamoto, Y., Hoe, N. B., Wei, T. S., Mu, D., et al. (2011). Distal airway stem cells yield alveoli *in vitro* and during lung regeneration following H1N1 influenza infection. *Cell* 147, 525–538. doi: 10.1016/j.cell.2011.10.001

Lamb, D., and Reid, L. (1968). Mitotic rates, goblet cell increase and histochemical changes in mucus in rat bronchial epithelium during exposure to sulphur dioxide. *J. Pathol. Bacteriol.* 96, 97–111. doi: 10.1002/path.1700960111

Lazzaro, D., Price, M., de Felice, M., and Di Lauro, R. (1991). The transcription factor TTF-1 is expressed at the onset of thyroid and lung morphogenesis and in restricted regions of the foetal brain. *Development* 113, 1093–1104.

Leblond, A.-L., Naud, P., Forest, V., Gourden, C., Sagan, C., Romefort, B., et al. (2009). Developing cell therapy techniques for respiratory disease: intratracheal delivery of genetically engineered stem cells in a murine model of airway injury. *Hum. Gene Ther.* 20, 1329–1343. doi: 10.1089/hum.2009.035

Lechner, J. F., Haugen, A., Autrup, H., McClendon, I. A., Trump, B. F., and Harris, C. C. (1981). Clonal growth of epithelial cells from normal adult human bronchus. *Cancer Res.* 41, 2294–2304.

Lechner, J. F., and LaVeck, M. A. (1985). A serum-free method for culturing normal human bronchial epithelial cells at clonal density. *J. Tiss. Cult. Methods* 9, 43–48. doi: 10.1007/BF01797773

Lee, J.-H., and Rawlins, E. L. (2018). Developmental mechanisms and adult stem cells for therapeutic lung regeneration. *Dev. Biol.* 433, 166–176. doi: 10.1016/j.ydbio.2017.09.016

Lee, J.-H., Tammela, T., Hofree, M., Choi, J., Marjanovic, N. D., Han, S., et al. (2017). Anatomically and functionally distinct lung mesenchymal populations marked by Lgr5 and Lgr6. *Cell* 170, 1149.e–1163.e. doi: 10.1016/j.cell.2017.07.028

Liu, J. Y., Nettesheim, P., and Randell, S. H. (1994). Growth and differentiation of tracheal epithelial progenitor cells. *Am. J. Physiol.* 266(3 Pt 1), L296–L307. doi: 10.1152/ajplung.1994.266.3.L296

Liu, X., Krawczyk, E., Suprynowicz, F. A., Palechor-Ceron, N., Yuan, H., Dakic, A., et al. (2017). Conditional reprogramming and long-term expansion of normal and tumor cells from human biospecimens. *Nat. Protoc.* 12, 439–451. doi: 10.1038/nprot.2016.174

Longmire, T. A., Ikonomou, L., Hawkins, F., Christodoulou, C., Cao, Y., Jean, J. C., et al. (2012). Efficient derivation of purified lung and thyroid progenitors from embryonic stem cells. *Stem Cell* 10, 398–411. doi: 10.1016/j.stem.2012.01.019

Lynch, T. J., Anderson, P. J., Rotti, P. G., Tyler, S. R., Crooke, A. K., Choi, S. H., et al. (2018). Submucosal gland myoepithelial cells are reserve stem cells that can regenerate mouse tracheal epithelium. *Cell Stem Cell* 22, 653.e5–667.e5. doi: 10.1016/j.stem.2018.04.007

Ma, Q., Ma, Y., Dai, X., Ren, T., Fu, Y., Liu, W., et al. (2018). Regeneration of functional alveoli by adult human SOX9+ airway basal cell transplantation. *Protein Cell* 9, 267–282. doi: 10.1007/s13238-018-0506-y

Makdisi, G., Makdisi, T., Jarmi, T., and Caldeira, C. C. (2017). *Ex vivo* lung perfusion review of a revolutionary technology. *Ann. Transl. Med.* 5, 343–343. doi: 10.21037/atm.2017.07.17

McCauley, K. B., Alysandratos, K.-D., Jacob, A., Hawkins, F., Caballero, I. S., Vedaie, M., et al. (2018). Single-cell transcriptomic profiling of pluripotent stem cell-derived SCGB3A2+ airway epithelium. *Stem Cell Rep.* 10, 1579–1595. doi: 10.1016/j.stemcr.2018.03.013

McCauley, K. B., Hawkins, F., Serra, M., Thomas, D. C., Jacob, A., and Kotton, D. N. (2017). Efficient derivation of functional human airway epithelium from pluripotent stem cells via temporal regulation of wnt signaling. *Cell Stem Cell* 20, 844.e6–857.e6. doi: 10.1016/j.stem.2017.03.001

McKone, E. F., Emerson, S. S., Edwards, K. L., and Aitken, M. L. (2003). Effect of genotype on phenotype and mortality in cystic fibrosis: a retrospective cohort study. *Lancet* 361, 1671–1676. doi: 10.1016/S0140-6736(03)13368-5

Merkle, F. T., Ghosh, S., Kamitaki, N., Mitchell, J., Avior, Y., Mello, C., et al. (2017). Human pluripotent stem cells recurrently acquire and expand dominant negative P53 mutations. *Nature* 545, 229–233. doi: 10.1038/nature22312

Miller, A. J., Hill, D. R., Nagy, M. S., Aoki, Y., Dye, B. R., Chin, A. M., et al. (2018). *InVitro* induction and *InVivo* engraftment of lung bud tip progenitor cells derived from human pluripotent stem cells. *Stem Cell Rep.* 10, 101–119. doi: 10.1016/j.stemcr.2017.11.012

Miller, J. D., Cox, G., Vincic, L., Lombard, C. M., Loomas, B. E., and Danek, C. J. (2005). A prospective feasibility study of bronchial thermoplasty in the human airway. *Chest* 127, 1999–2006. doi: 10.1378/chest.127.6.1999

Montoro, D. T., Haber, A. L., Biton, M., Vinarsky, V., Lin, B., Birket, S. E., et al. (2018). A revised airway epithelial hierarchy includes CFTR-expressing ionocytes. *Nature* 560, 319–324. doi: 10.1038/s41586-018-0393-7

Morrisey, E. E., and Hogan, B. L. M. (2010). Preparing for the first breath: genetic and cellular mechanisms in lung development. *Dev. Cell* 18, 8–23. doi: 10.1016/j.devcel.2009.12.010

Mou, H., Vinarsky, V., Tata, P. R., Brazauskas, K., Choi, S. H., Crooke, A. K., et al. (2016). Dual SMAD signaling inhibition enables long-term expansion of diverse epithelial basal cells. *Cell Stem Cell* 19, 217–231. doi: 10.1016/j.stem.2016.05.012

Mou, H., Zhao, R., Sherwood, R., Ahfeldt, T., Lapey, A., Wain, J., et al. (2012). Generation of multipotent lung and airway progenitors from mouse ESCs and patient-specific cystic fibrosis iPSCs. *Cell Stem Cell* 10, 385–397. doi: 10.1016/j.stem.2012.01.018

Neuberger, T., Burton, B., Clark, H., and Van Gf. (2011). Use of primary cultures of human bronchial epithelial cells isolated from cystic fibrosis patients for the pre-clinical testing of CFTR modulators. *Methods Mol. Biol.* 741, 39–54. doi: 10.1007/978-1-61779-117-8_4

Nichane, M., Javed, A., Sivakamasundari, V., Ganesan, M., Ang, L. T., Kraus, P., et al. (2017). Isolation and 3D expansion of multipotent Sox9+ mouse lung progenitors. *Nat. Methods* 14, 1205–1212. doi: 10.1038/nmeth.4498

Nikolić, M. Z., Caritg, O., Jeng, Q., Johnson, J.-A., Sun, D., Howell, K. J., et al. (2017). Human embryonic lung epithelial tips are multipotent progenitors that can be expanded *in vitro* as long-term self-renewing organoids. *eLife* 6:e26575. doi: 10.7554/eLife.26575

Pardo-Saganta, A., Tata, P. R., Law, B. M., Saez, B., Chow, R. D.-W., Prabhu, M., et al. (2015). Parent stem cells can serve as niches for their daughter cells. *Nature* 523, 597–601. doi: 10.1038/nature14553

Peters-Hall, J. R., Coquelin, M. L., Torres, M. J., LaRanger, R., Alabi, B. R., Sho, S., et al. (2018). Long-term culture and cloning of primary human bronchial basal cells that maintain multipotent differentiation capacity and CFTR channel function. *Am. J. Physiol. Lung Cell. Mol. Physiol.* 315, L313–L327. doi: 10.1152/ajplung.00355.2017

Plasschaert, L. W., Žilionis, R., Choo-Wing, R., Savova, V., Knehr, J., Roma, G., et al. (2018). A single-cell atlas of the airway epithelium reveals the CFTR-rich pulmonary ionocyte. *Nature* 3, 545–523. doi: 10.1038/s41586-018-0394-6

Plopper, C. G., Suverkropp, C., Morin, D., Nishio, S., and Buckpitt, A. (1992). Relationship of cytochrome P-450 activity to clara cell cytotoxicity. i. histopathologic comparison of the respiratory tract of mice, rats and hamsters after parenteral administration of naphthalene. *J. Pharmacol. Exp. Ther.* 261, 353–363.

Pollock, K., Albares, L., Wendt, C., and Hubel, A. (2013). Isolation of fibroblasts and epithelial cells in bronchoalveolar lavage (BAL). *Exp. Lung Res.* 39, 146–154. doi: 10.3109/01902148.2013.781720

Rama, P., Ferrari, G., and Pellegrini, G. (2017). Cultivated limbal epithelial transplantation. *Curr. Opin. Ophthalmol.* 28, 387–389. doi: 10.1097/ICU.0000000000000382

Ramsey, B. W., Davies, J., McElvaney, N. G., Tullis, E., Bell, S. C., Dřevínek, P., et al. (2011). A CFTR potentiator in patients with cystic fibrosis and the G551D mutation. *N. Engl. J. Med.* 365, 1663–1672. doi: 10.1056/NEJMoa1105185

Randell, S. H., Boucher, R. C., and University of North Carolina Virtual Lung Group. (2006). Effective mucus clearance is essential for respiratory health. *Am. J. Respir. Cell Mol. Biol.* 35, 20–28. doi: 10.1165/rcmb.2006-0082SF

Randell, S. H., Burns, K., and Boucher, R. C. (2009). *Epithelial Cells.* New York, NY: Elsevier Ltd., 201–210. doi: 10.1016/B978-0-12-374001-4.00016-X

Ratjen, F., Bell, S. C., Rowe, S. M., Goss, C. H., Quittner, A. L., and Bush, A. (2015). Cystic fibrosis. *Nat. Rev. Dis. Primers* 1;15010. doi: 10.1038/nrdp.2015.10

Rock, J. R., Onaitis, M. W., Rawlins, E. L., Lu, Y., Clark, C. P., Xue, Y., et al. (2009). Basal cells as stem cells of the mouse trachea and human airway epithelium. *Proc. Natl. Acad. Sci. U.S.A.* 106, 12771–12775. doi: 10.1073/pnas.0906850106

Roesch, E. A., Nichols, D. P., and Chmiel, J. F. (2018). Inflammation in cystic fibrosis: an update. *Pediatr. Pulmonol.* 23, S30–S50. doi: 10.1002/ppul.24129

Rosen, C., Shezen, E., Aronovich, A., Klionsky, Y. Z., Yaakov, Y., Assayag, M., et al. (2015). Preconditioning allows engraftment of mouse and human embryonic lung cells, enabling lung repair in mice. *Nat. Med.* 21, 869–879. doi: 10.1038/nm.3889

Rosenow, T., Ramsey, K., Turkovic, L., Murray, C. P., Mok, L. C., Hall, G. L., et al. (2017). Air trapping in early cystic fibrosis lung disease-Does CT tell the full story? *Pediatr. Pulmonol.* 52, 1150–1156. doi: 10.1002/ppul.23754

Rowe, S. M., Daines, C., Ringshausen, F. C., Kerem, E., Wilson, J., Tullis, E., et al. (2017). Tezacaftor-ivacaftor in residual-function heterozygotes with cystic fibrosis. *N. Engl. J. Med.* 377, 2024–2035. doi: 10.1056/NEJMoa1709847

Sasamoto, Y., Ksander, B. R., Frank, M. H., and Frank, N. Y. (2018). Repairing the corneal epithelium using limbal stem cells or alternative cell-based therapies. *Expert Opin. Biol. Ther.* 18, 505–513. doi: 10.1080/14712598.2018.1443442

Schoch, K. G., Lori, A., Burns, K. A., Eldred, T., Olsen, J. C., and Randell, S. H. (2004). A subset of mouse tracheal epithelial basal cells generates large colonies *in vitro*. *Am. J. Physiol. Lung Cell. Mol. Physiol.* 286, L631–L642. doi: 10.1152/ajplung.00112.2003

Serra, M., Alysandratos, K.-D., Hawkins, F., McCauley, K. B., Jacob, A., Choi, J., et al. (2017). Pluripotent stem cell differentiation reveals distinct developmental pathways regulating lung- versus thyroid-lineage specification. *Development* 144, 3879–3893. doi: 10.1242/dev.150193

Slebos, D.-J., Breen, D., Coad, J., Klooster, K., Hartman, J., Browning, R., et al. (2017). Safety and histological effect of liquid nitrogen metered spray cryotherapy in the lung. *Am. J. Respir. Crit. Care Med.* 196, 1351–1352. doi: 10.1164/rccm.201611-2220LE

Smith, A. G. (2001). Embryo-derived stem cells: of mice and men. *Ann. Rev. Cell Dev. Biol.* 17, 435–462. doi: 10.1146/annurev.cellbio.17.1.435

Solter, D., Skreb, N., and Damjanov, I. (1970). Extrauterine growth of mouse egg cylinders results in teratoma formation. *Nature* 227, 503–504. doi: 10.1038/227503a0

Song, H., Yao, E., Lin, C., Gacayan, R., Chen, M.-H., and Chuang, P.-T. (2012). Functional characterization of pulmonary neuroendocrine cells in lung development, injury, and tumorigenesis. *Proc. Natl. Acad. Sci. U.S.A.* 109, 17531–17536. doi: 10.1073/pnas.1207238109

Squiers, J. J., Lima, B., and DiMaio, J. M. (2016). Contemporary extracorporeal membrane oxygenation therapy in adults: fundamental principles and systematic review of the evidence. *J. Thorac. Cardiovasc. Surg.* 152, 20–32. doi: 10.1016/j.jtcvs.2016.02.067

Stevens, L. C. (1970). The development of transplantable teratocarcinomas from intratesticular grafts of pre- and post-implantation mouse embryos. *Dev. Biol.* 21, 364–382. doi: 10.1016/0012-1606(70)90130-2

Stoltz, D. A., Meyerholz, D. K., and Welsh, M. J. (2015). Origins of cystic fibrosis lung disease. *N. Engl. J. Med.* 372, 351–362. doi: 10.1056/NEJMra1300109

Suprynowicz, F. A., Upadhyay, G., Krawczyk, E., Kramer, S. C., Hebert, J. D., Liu, X., et al. (2012). Conditionally reprogrammed cells represent a stem-like state of adult epithelial cells. *Proc. Natl. Acad. Sci. U.S.A.* 109, 20035–20040. doi: 10.1073/pnas.1213241109

Takahashi, K., Tanabe, K., Ohnuki, M., Narita, M., Ichisaka, T., Tomoda, K., et al. (2007). Induction of pluripotent stem cells from adult human fibroblasts by defined factors. *Cell* 131, 861–872. doi: 10.1016/j.cell.2007.11.019

Takahashi, K., and Yamanaka, S. (2006). Induction of pluripotent stem cells from mouse embryonic and adult fibroblast cultures by defined factors. *Cell* 126, 663–676. doi: 10.1016/j.cell.2006.07.024

Tata, A., Kobayashi, Y., Chow, R. D., Tran, J., Desai, A., Massri, A. J., et al. (2018). Myoepithelial cells of submucosal glands can function as reserve stem cells to regenerate airways after injury. *Cell Stem Cell* 22, 668.e6–683.e6. doi: 10.1016/j.stem.2018.03.018

Tata, P. R., Mou, H., Pardo-Saganta, A., Zhao, R., Prabhu, M., Law, B. M., et al. (2013). Dedifferentiation of committed epithelial cells into stem cells in vivo. *Nature* 503, 218–223. doi: 10.1038/nature12777

Tata, P. R., and Rajagopal, J. (2017). Plasticity in the lung: making and breaking cell identity. *Development* 144, 755–766. doi: 10.1242/dev.143784

Taylor-Cousar, J. L., Jain, M., Barto, T. L., Haddad, T., Atkinson, J., Tian, S., et al. (2018). Lumacaftor/ivacaftor in patients with cystic fibrosis and advanced lung disease homozygous for F508del-CFTR. *J. Cyst. Fibros.* 17, 228–235. doi: 10.1016/j.jcf.2017.09.012

Ter Horst, B., Chouhan, G., Moiemen, N. S., and Grover, L. M. (2018). Advances in keratinocyte delivery in burn wound care. *Adv. Drug Deliv. Rev.* 123, 18–32. doi: 10.1016/j.addr.2017.06.012

Treutlein, B., Brownfield, D. G., Wu, A. R., Neff, N. F., Mantalas, G. L., Espinoza, F. H., et al. (2014). Reconstructing lineage hierarchies of the distal lung epithelium using single-cell RNA-seq. *Nature* 509, 371–375. doi: 10.1038/nature13173

Vaughan, A. E., Brumwell, A. N., Xi, Y., Gotts, J. E., Brownfield, D. G., Treutlein, B., et al. (2015). Lineage-negative progenitors mobilize to regenerate lung epithelium after major injury. *Nature* 517, 621–625. doi: 10.1038/nature14112

Watson, J. K., Rulands, S., Wilkinson, A. C., Wuidart, A., Ousset, M., Van Keymeulen, A., et al. (2015). Clonal dynamics reveal two distinct populations of basal cells in slow-turnover airway epithelium. *Cell Rep.* 12, 90–101. doi: 10.1016/j.celrep.2015.06.011

Widdicombe, J. H., and Wine, J. J. (2015). Airway gland structure and function. *Physiol. Rev.* 95, 1241–1319. doi: 10.1152/physrev.00039.2014

Wong, A. P., Bear, C. E., Chin, S., Pasceri, P., Thompson, T. O., Huan, L.-J., et al. (2012). Directed differentiation of human pluripotent stem cells into mature airway epithelia expressing functional CFTR protein. *Nat. Biotechnol.* 30, 876–882. doi: 10.1038/nbt.2328

Yamamoto, Y., Gotoh, S., Korogi, Y., Seki, M., Konishi, S., Ikeo, S., et al. (2017). Long-term expansion of alveolar stem cells derived from human iPS cells in organoids. *Nat. Methods* 14, 1097–1106. doi: 10.1038/nmeth.4448

Yang, Y., Riccio, P., Schotsaert, M., Mori, M., Lu, J., Lee, D.-K., et al. (2018). Spatial-temporal lineage restrictions of embryonic p63+ progenitors establish distinct stem cell pools in adult airways. *Dev. Cell* 44, 752.e4–761.e4. doi: 10.1016/j.devcel.2018.03.001

Zepp, J. A., Zacharias, W. J., Frank, D. B., Cavanaugh, C. A., Zhou, S., Morley, M. P., et al. (2017). Distinct mesenchymal lineages and niches promote epithelial self-renewal and myofibrogenesis in the lung. *Cell* 170, 1134.e10–1148.e10. doi: 10.1016/j.cell.2017.07.034

Zhang, C., Lee, H. J., Shrivastava, A., Wang, R., McQuiston, T. J., Challberg, S. S., et al. (2018). Long-term *in vitro* expansion of epithelial stem cells enabled by pharmacological inhibition of PAK1-ROCK-Myosin II and TGF-β signaling. *Cell Rep.* 25, 598–610. doi: 10.1016/j.celrep.2018.09.072

Zhang, F., Wen, Y., and Guo, X. (2014). CRISPR/Cas9 for genome editing: progress, implications and challenges. *Hum. Mol. Genet.* 23, R40–R46. doi: 10.1093/hmg/ddu125

Zhang, X.-H., Tee, L. Y., Wang, X.-G., Huang, Q.-S., and Yang, S.-H. (2015). Off-target effects in CRISPR/Cas9-mediated genome engineering. *Mol. Ther. Nucleic Acids* 4:e264. doi: 10.1038/mtna.2015.37

15

Use of a Primary Epithelial Cell Screening Tool to Investigate Phage Therapy in Cystic Fibrosis

Stephanie Trend[1,2], Barbara J. Chang[3], Mark O'Dea[4], Stephen M. Stick[1,2,5,6], Anthony Kicic[1,2,5,6,7]*, WAERP†, AusREC† and AREST CF†

[1] Telethon Kids Institute, Perth, WA, Australia, [2] Division of Paediatrics, School of Biomedical Sciences, The University of Western Australia, Perth, WA, Australia, [3] The Marshall Centre for Infectious Diseases Research and Training, School of Biomedical Sciences, The University of Western Australia, Perth, WA, Australia, [4] School of Veterinary and Life Sciences, Murdoch University, Perth, WA, Australia, [5] Department of Respiratory Medicine, Perth Children's Hospital, Perth, WA, Australia, [6] Centre for Cell Therapy and Regenerative Medicine, School of Medicine and Pharmacology, The University of Western Australia and Harry Perkins Institute of Medical Research, Perth, WA, Australia, [7] Occupation and the Environment, School of Public Health, Curtin University, Perth, WA, Australia

***Correspondence:**
Anthony Kicic
Anthony.Kicic@telethonkids.org.au

† The members of these groups are listed in the Acknowledgments section.

Antimicrobial-resistant microbes are an increasing threat to human health. In cystic fibrosis (CF), airway infections with *Pseudomonas aeruginosa* remain a key driver of lung damage. With few new antibiotics on the development horizon, alternative therapeutic approaches are needed against antimicrobial-resistant pathogens. Phage therapy, or the use of viruses that infect bacteria, is one proposed novel therapy to treat bacterial infections. However, the airways are complex microenvironments with unique characteristics that may affect the success of novel therapies. Here, three phages of *P. aeruginosa* (E79, F116, and one novel clinically derived isolate, designated P5) were screened for activity against 21 *P. aeruginosa* strains isolated from children with CF. Of these, phage E79 showed broad antibacterial activity (91% of tested strains sensitive) and was selected for further assessment. E79 genomic DNA was extracted, sequenced, and confirmed to contain no bacterial pathogenicity genes. High titre phage preparations were then purified using ion-exchange column chromatography and depleted of bacterial endotoxin. Primary airway epithelial cells derived from children with CF (n = 8, age range 0.2–5.5 years, 5 males) or healthy non-CF controls (n = 8, age range 2.5–4.0 years, 4 males) were then exposed to purified phage for 48 h. Levels of inflammatory IL-1β, IL-6, and IL-8 cytokine production were measured in culture supernatant by immunoassays and the extent of cellular apoptosis was measured using a ssDNA kit. Cytokine and apoptosis levels were compared between E79-stimulated and unstimulated controls, and, encouragingly, purified preparations of E79 did not stimulate any significant inflammatory cytokine responses or induce apoptosis in primary epithelial cells derived from children with or without CF. Collectively, this study demonstrates the feasibility of utilizing pre-clinical *in vitro* culture models to screen therapeutic candidates, and the potential of E79 as a therapeutic phage candidate in CF.

Keywords: cystic fibrosis, phage therapy, preclinical models, airway epithelial cells, *Pseudomonas aeruginosa*, infection

INTRODUCTION

Cystic fibrosis (CF) is the most common autosomal recessive lethal genetic disease of Caucasian populations (Tian et al., 2016). In the lung, loss of CFTR function leads to production of viscous mucus, which is difficult to clear by standard mucociliary action (Koehler et al., 2004). This in turn contributes to the development of chronic infections with opportunistic bacterial pathogens such as *Pseudomonas aeruginosa* (Friman et al., 2013). The severity of lung bronchiectasis, excessive lung inflammation in children, and rate of decline in lung function in infants with CF is directly correlated with airway infections with *P. aeruginosa* (Koehler et al., 2004; Farrell et al., 2009; Pillarisetti et al., 2011).

Current therapies for CF lung infections include intravenous or inhaled antibiotics (National Guideline Alliance, 2017). However, antibiotic-resistant bacterial strains have emerged as major causes of mortality in hospitals worldwide, and in Western Australia, approximately 30% of *P. aeruginosa* isolates from CF patients are carbapenem-resistant (Tai et al., 2015). The World Health Organization has recognized antibiotic resistance as a significant threat to human health requiring urgent action (World Health Organization, 2014). Bacteriophages (phages) are viruses that infect bacteria, and present a novel treatment option in CF, however, little has been investigated regarding their potential in this setting. Concomitant with this need for new antibacterial treatments is the need for relevant *in vitro* models to screen potentially therapeutic phages and facilitate understanding of how these preparations act in the context of the human airway (Trend et al., 2017). Phage therapy holds enormous potential benefit for people with CF, and may complement existing antimicrobial strategies, since phages can replicate at the site of infection inside the target bacterial cells and subvert existing antimicrobial resistance in bacterial pathogens (Alemayehu et al., 2012; Sahota et al., 2015).

While the investigation and development of phage-derived products as therapeutic agents requires employment of *in vitro* antimicrobial assays, the effectiveness of any antimicrobial therapy *in vivo* may not always correspond to expected outcomes, due to a range of human factors not considered in the models (Henry et al., 2013). For example, host immune mediators directly interact with phage particles to inactivate them *in vivo* (Majewska et al., 2015). Furthermore, the patient's innate immune system may induce an inflammatory response upon exposure to the phage, particularly if the phage preparations derived from culture in bacterial hosts are inadequately purified. Relevant *in vitro* models are thus essential in order to elucidate and understand the responses of the airway to this new potential therapy.

To develop phages for clinical trials, researchers should characterize and screen candidates for antimicrobial activity and carriage of bacterial pathogenicity genes. Given the inflammatory nature of many bacterial-derived products, stringent purification steps must be applied to phage preparations after propagation in bacterial hosts (Merabishvili et al., 2009), the success of which can then be confirmed on human cells using relevant exposure models. Previous investigations of this type have utilized immortal cell lines or animal models. Although the ability to screen the suitability of phage preparations using human CF airways cells would lead to more relevant findings, investigations involving primary airway epithelial cells have traditionally been limited due to their restricted expansion potential (Lane et al., 2005). However, our laboratory has recently described the development of an *in vitro* culture expansion methodology of primary airway epithelial cells in a realistic model of the airway (Martinovich et al., 2017). Using primary airway cells derived utilizing this technique, we performed screening analyses of a number of phages. Due to its broad range of activity against CF clinical isolates, phage E79 was purified using ion-exchange chromatography and endotoxin depleted to clinically acceptable levels. We showed that purified E79 does not induce apoptosis or inflammatory cytokine production in primary airway cells derived from children with CF or healthy non-CF individuals exposed to the phage preparations for 48 h. Moreover, the phage was virulent, stable, and genome sequencing did not reveal any known bacterial virulence genes. Collectively, these findings suggest that E79 may be a good candidate for phage therapy.

MATERIALS AND METHODS

Bacteriophage and Bacterial Sources and Culture

E79 and F116 bacteriophages (Slayter et al., 1964) were obtained from the University of Western Australia Department of Microbiology Culture Collection (MCC), and utilized as examples of virulent and temperate phages to compare to novel phage isolates. Novel *P. aeruginosa* phage P5 was isolated from pediatric CF patient sputum. A panel of 21 isolates of *P. aeruginosa* (designated PMH-) were derived from sputum of patients with CF-related infections, supplied by PathWest Laboratory Medicine, Perth, Western Australia. An independent collection of 14 isolates of *P. aeruginosa* isolated from sputa of children with CF were derived from the AREST CF culture collection (designated ARESTCF-). Reference strain PAO1 (Dunn and Holloway, 1971) was obtained from MCC. *P. aeruginosa* strains were routinely propagated in heart infusion agar (HIA) or broth (HIB) aerobically at 37°C.

Antimicrobial Susceptibility of Clinical *P. aeruginosa* Isolates

Sensitivity of 14 clinical isolates (AREST CF collection) of *P. aeruginosa* to gentamicin, ceftazidime, meropenem, amikacin, piperacillin, cefepime, tobramycin, ciprofloxacin, norfloxacin, timentin, piperacillin/tazobactam, and aztreonam was determined by the Royal Children's Hospital Melbourne pathology laboratory using disk diffusion assays. Susceptibility was determined according to Clinical and Laboratory Standards Institute (CLSI) breakpoints (CLSI, 2016).

Isolation of Clinically Derived Phages

Sputa from 20 CF patients were screened for the presence of phages that were able to infect any member of the panel of 21 clinical *P. aeruginosa* isolates (PMH collection). Sputa were mixed, and large materials sedimented by centrifugation at 1,750 × *g* for 20 min at room temperature (RT). Following filter-sterilization of the supernatant using a 0.22 μm pore sterile membrane, an aliquot (10 μL) was pipetted onto a lawn of each bacterial strain as described for phage propagation. Plaques appearing on bacterial lawns, either derived from sputa or from lysogenic phage spontaneously induced from the bacterial genome, were transferred to 150 μL of phage buffer (Tris-HCl 10 mM, $MgCl_2$ 10 mM [pH 8]) (Matsumoto et al., 1986). The suspension was purified as described for phage propagation and tested for phage titre. Phages were plaque-purified twice, prepared at high titre and stored at 4°C.

Phage Imaging and Classification

Electron microscopy was performed on phage suspensions that were purified using a modified methodology (Bruttin and Brussow, 2005). Briefly, following centrifugation at 4,000 × *g* for 15 min at RT the resulting supernatant was separated by centrifugation at 35,000 × *g* for 25 min at RT. The phage-containing pellet was resuspended and applied to carbon-coated formvar grids for 5 min, which were charged prior to phage co-incubation using 1% (w/v) Alcian blue. Grids were negatively stained for 10 min using a 2% sodium silicotungstate solution, dried at RT, then analyzed using Transmission Electron Microscopy (TEM) using a Philips 401 TE microscope. Phage head, tail, and sheath sizes were measured, and data presented as a mean and standard deviation of three particle measurements.

For classification, phage genetic material was treated with the class II restriction endonucleases, either *Bam*HI or *Hind*III, for 2 h at 37°C. A 2 μL sample was then combined with 3 μL of tracking dye containing bromophenol blue (2.5 mg/mL) and sucrose (400 mg/mL) and electrophoresed on a 0.8% (w/v) agarose gel containing ethidium bromide (10 μg/mL) in Tris-Acetate Buffer with Ethylenediaminetetraacetic acid (0.5 M) for 60 min at 90 V. The gel was then photographed using UV illumination to detect if multiple bands were present, indicating digested DNA. The genome size was estimated by comparison to a *Hind*III ladder, while the genome sequencing results provided a more precise genome size.

Phage Propagation and Host Range

Phages were propagated to high titre according to a modified version of the double agar layer method (Adams, 1959). Molten overlay agar containing 1% Bacto agar and HIB, supplemented with calcium and magnesium (0.01 M) was mixed with an aliquot of overnight broth culture of host bacteria and phage at approximately 10^5 PFU/mL. The mixture was overlaid onto a HIA plate, allowed to set at RT and then incubated overnight at 37°C in 5% CO_2. The following day, the overlay agar with semi-confluent phage plaques was scraped off the HIA plate and mixed with 3.5 mL of isotonic saline. All phage preparations were preliminarily purified by mixing followed by centrifugation at 1,750 × *g* at RT. The supernatant was filtered through a 0.22 μm pore-size membrane. Phage titre was then determined using the drop-on plate method. Briefly, 10 μL of 10-fold dilutions of phage preparations were dropped in triplicate onto a HIA plate overlaid with overlay agar containing an overnight culture of PAO1, and the plaques in the bacterial lawn counted after incubation overnight at 37°C in 5% CO_2.

Host range experiments were carried out on 21 clinical *P. aeruginosa* strains. Sensitivity to a phage was determined by a zone of clearing or plaques on a bacterial lawn where 10 μL of high titre phage preparation (10^8–10^{12} PFU/mL) was spotted onto the lawn in triplicate, followed by incubation at 37°C overnight.

Growth Inhibition by E79

The inhibitory capacity of E79 for clinical *P. aeruginosa* isolates (AREST CF collection) was determined using the following method. Briefly, bacteria were grown to approximately 0.5 MacPharland standard (~1 × 10^8 CFU/mL,) determined by spectroscopy and 100 μL of bacterial suspension was then added to wells of a 96-well flat-bottom polypropylene plate. E79 was diluted to 10^9 PFU/mL in sterile isotonic saline, then serially diluted in 10-fold dilutions down to 10^4 PFU/mL. Dilutions of phage or a control of saline only were added in equal volumes at a multiplicity of infection (MOI) of 10:1 and 1:1, and plates incubated at 37°C in 5% CO_2 overnight. Optical density of wells was then measured at 595 nm, and the percentage of growth in treated wells quantified by dividing this value by the absorbance in the control well. A bacterial strain was considered sensitive to phage at that MOI if the optical density in the test well was ≥10% lower than that of the untreated well.

Phage DNA Extraction and Genome Sequencing

High titre E79 was pre-treated with DNase I to reduce contaminating bacterial DNA. A 200 μL aliquot containing ~10^{11} PFU of phage was incubated for 30 min at 37°C with 1 U of DNase I from the Invitrogen PureLink RNA Mini Kit. DNA was subsequently extracted using a QIAamp DNA mini spin column kit (QIAGEN) per manufacturer's instructions and sequenced (LotteryWest Sequencing Facility, University of Western Australia, Perth, WA, Australia). The concentration of DNA was determined using a Qubit fluorometer according to manufacturer's instructions. The sample (10 ng) was sheared using a S2 ultrasonicator (Covaris) and sequencing libraries prepared using a NEBnext Ultra library kit (New England Biosciences). Sequencing was performed on a 318 chip using an Ion Torrent PGM semiconductor sequencer for 820 flows. Data were collected using Torrent Suite 5.0. Reads were imported into CLC Genomics Workbench V 10.1.2, and *de novo* assembled, before the phage genome was annotated using RASTtk (Brettin et al., 2015). The annotated phage genome was then imported into Geneious V10.2.4 for visualization and manual curation.

Purification of High Titre Phage Preparation for Cellular Assays

Filter-sterilized high titre phage preparations were purified using a CIMmultus quaternary amine (QA) advanced composite monolithic column (BIA separations) in combination with a Bio-Rad Econopump. Phage was diluted 1:10 in 20 mM Tris-HCl (pH 7.5) loading buffer, and 10 mL was passed through the column.

TABLE 1 | Clinical details of CF-related characteristics in cell donors with CF at time of cell collection.

Sample	CFTR genotype	CFTR mutation class	Neutrophil elastase (nM)	Bronchiectasis (0–12 score)	Respiratory pathogens
CF1	p.Gly85Glu/Unknown	–/–	100	0	Mixed oral flora
CF2	p.Phe508del/p.Phe508del	II/II	1260	n/a	None
CF3	p.Phe508del/p.Phe508del	II/II	270	n/a	*Moraxella catarrhalis, Haemophilus influenzae,* MRSA, Mixed oral flora
CF4	p.Phe508del/p.Asn1303Lys	II/II	270	n/a	*Aspergillus fumigatus, Stenotrophomonas maltophilia*
CF5	p.Phe508del/p.Thr966ArgfsX2	#N/A	170	n/a	None
CF6	p.Phe508del/Ala455Glu	#N/A	70	n/a	*H. influenzae*
CF7	p.Phe508del/p.Phe508del	II/II	140	n/a	*Streptococcus pneumoniae*
CF8	p.Phe508del/p.Phe508del	II/II	60	n/a	None

CF, cystic fibrosis; CFTR, cystic fibrosis transmembrane conductance regulator; MRSA, methicillin-resistant Staphylococcus aureus.

The column was washed with 20 volumes of loading buffer, and then 20 mM Tris–HCl supplemented with successive increases of saline (250 mM–1.2 M NaCl) in 2 mL volumes, which were collected as separate fractions. The titre of phage in each fraction was tested as previously described and the fraction with the highest titre of phage selected for further purification through endotoxin-depletion.

Endotoxin was removed from the purified phage preparation using the EndoTrap HD 5/1 kit (Hyglos) per the manufacturer's protocol. Here, phage preparation was diluted 1:5 in 20 mM Tris–HCl containing 450 mM NaCl and 0.125 mM $CaCl_2$, passing the phage solution three times through the column. Concentrations of endotoxin in the phage preparations before and after purification were determined using the Endpoint Chromogenic Limulus Amebocyte Lysate (LAL) assay (Lonza), using endotoxin-free reagents and equipment. A high titre phage preparation (10^{11} PFU/mL), generated as previously described, was tested diluted in endotoxin-free water diluted 10^{-8} (10^3 PFU/mL) to reach the detectable range of the kit. Purified phage preparations were tested in duplicate at 1:5 dilution in endotoxin-free water and the concentration interpolated from a standard curve using a 3PL curve fit in GraphPad Prism software.

Study Participants and Epithelial Cell Collection

This study was carried out in accordance with the recommendations of the National Health and Medical Research Council of Australia's National Statement on Ethical Conduct in Human Research with written informed consent was obtained from the parent or guardian of all participants. All participants gave written informed consent in accordance with the Declaration of Helsinki. The study was approved by St. John of God Health Care Human Research Ethics Committee Ref#901 sub-study 901.1050 and by the Princess Margaret Hospital for Children Ethics Committee Ref#1762EPP. Sixteen individual cell cultures derived from children with CF (n = 8) and from healthy non-CF children (n = 8), aged from 0–6 years were collected. Median ages of participants with or without CF were not significantly different (3.0 vs. 3.2 years old, respectively; $p = 0.88$), nor proportions of females in each of these groups (37.5% vs. 50%, respectively; $p = 0.60$). Parental consent was obtained prior to bronchial brushing and cells collected as described previously (Kicic et al., 2006; Sutanto et al., 2011). Epithelial cells were purified by removal of CD68+ cells and the epithelial phenotype confirmed (Lane et al., 2005; Kicic et al., 2006; McNamara et al., 2008). Demographics of the study cohort are shown in **Table 1**.

Cell Cultures

Children with CF had cell samples collected during bronchoscopy as part of their annual clinical surveillance program (Sutanto et al., 2011). In addition, cells from non-CF controls were collected from children during elective non-respiratory related surgery where intubation was required.

Primary airway epithelial cells derived from bronchial brushings were conditionally reprogrammed, a method which we previously reported resulted in cells that retain their phenotype and functionality in culture (Martinovich et al., 2017). Briefly, airway epithelial cells were co-cultured with irradiated fibroblasts and grown on tissue culture-grade flasks that were pre-coated with fibronectin and type I collagen (Kicic et al., 2006). Cells were grown to 90% confluence in pre-coated flasks in culture media for approximately 5 days, and then seeded into 96-well plates at ~20,000–40,000 cells/well in growth media containing bronchial epithelial basal medium (BEBM®; Lonza, Basel, Switzerland) supplemented with SingleQuot additives. All cell cultures were at passage 3 at time of experiments and were maintained at 37°C in an atmosphere of 5% CO_2 under aseptic conditions. Experiments were conducted on multi-layered primary airway epithelial submerged cultures which exhibit typical cobblestone morphology (**Figure 1**).

Stimulation of Cell Cultures

Prior to exposure to phage, media in 96-well plates was changed to starvation media (growth medium minus bovine pituitary extract, epidermal growth factor, and antibiotics) for 24 h. Cells were then exposed to saline control or phage treatments in infection media (media minus bovine pituitary extract and antibiotics). The following treatments were applied to cells as 10% of the medium in 90% v/v infection media: (1) isotonic saline, (2) E79 phage (ratio 1:1 per epithelial cell), and (3) E79 (ratio of 10:1

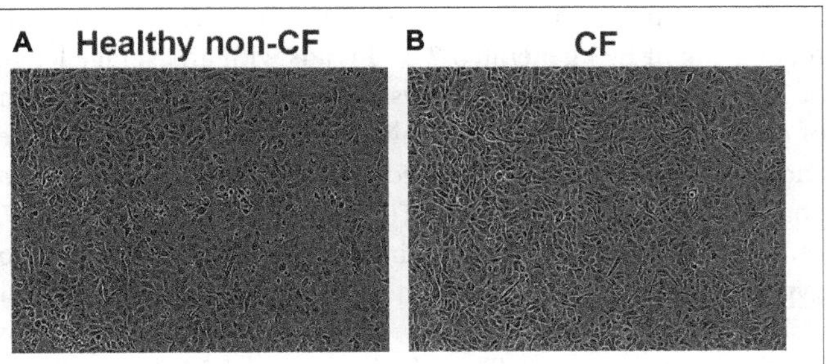

FIGURE 1 | Phase contrast images of confluent primary airways cell cultures obtained using conditionally reprogrammed method. Epithelial cobblestone morphology is typically maintained and observed in both healthy non-CF **(A)** and CF **(B)** primary cell cultures. Representative image of eight subjects per phenotype. Magnification 100×.

per epithelial cell). Cells were then incubated for 48 h at 37°C in 5% CO_2. After exposure, cell supernatant was collected from replicate wells, pooled and frozen at −80°C until batch cytokine analyses were performed. Following removal of supernatant from 96-well plates, cell viability was assessed.

Cytokine Detection in Cell Culture Supernatants

The concentration of IL-8 in culture supernatants was determined using enzyme-linked immunosorbent assays (ELISA; R&D Systems) previously used in our laboratory (Kicic et al., 2016). Values were interpolated from a standard curve with a range of 3.125–200 pg/mL of IL-8. IL-6 was measured in culture supernatants using a time-resolved fluorescence immunoassay as previously described (Taylor et al., 2007; Sutanto et al., 2011) with a minimum detectable value of 3 pg/mL. The concentration of IL-1β in cell culture supernatants was tested using commercially available ELISA kits, according to the manufacturer instructions (eBioscience), with a limit of detection of 2 pg/mL. Fluorescence and absorbance measurements for immunoassays were detected using the ClarioStar plate reader (software version 5.20 R5 from BMG Labtech). Concentrations of cytokines were interpolated from measurements using a standard curve used in the same assay. Data were transformed using the calculation x = log(x) and a 4-parameter logistic curve fit in GraphPad Prism software. Any values falling below the limit of detection were assigned a value of half the lowest detectable concentration multiplied by the dilution factor. Following interpolation of concentrations, they were back-transformed using $x = 10^x$.

Cell Viability and Apoptosis Measurements

Airway epithelial cell viability was determined using the CellTiter 96 Aqueous Non-Radioactive Cell Proliferation Assay Kit (Promega). Following incubation as instructed, absorbance of each well was measured at 492 nm using a plate reader. A control well without cells was used to determine background absorbance. The percentage viability in each treatment well was then compared to the calculated mean control value. Mean values from at least three technical replicate wells were used in final calculations.

Apoptosis was measured in cells exposed to phage for 48 h using a ssDNA apoptosis ELISA Kit (Merck Millipore) as previously described (Sutanto et al., 2011; Kicic et al., 2016). Briefly, following exposure, culture supernatant was removed, and cells were fixed using 200 μL per well of a solution containing 80% methanol and 20% PBS. Plates were then air dried for 30 min at RT and stored at 4°C until batch analyses of apoptosis were performed. The percentage of apoptotic cells compared to untreated controls was then determined where data were normalized to the control apoptosis value for that plate.

Statistical Analyses

Continuous variables were tested for normality using a Shapiro–Wilk test. Since most variables did not follow a normal distribution, non-parametric tests were used. Categorical variables in the CF and healthy non-CF cohorts were compared using a Chi-squared test, and continuous clinical variables were compared using a Mann–Whitney test. Cytokine measurements were presented as both absolute concentrations measured in supernatants adjusted for viable cell numbers, and for the purposes of comparing between the CF and healthy non-CF groups, cytokine levels in phage treated wells were normalized to the saline well as a ratio of 1. Paired data including results from cell culture experiments and bacterial minimum inhibitory concentration assays were compared using a Friedman test or Wilcoxon signed-rank test, comparing phage treatments to the control (saline), with Dunn's post-test applied for multiple comparisons where appropriate. Unpaired data comparing cytokine fold-change in phage-treated wells between CF and HNA were compared using Mann–Whitney tests. All statistical analyses were performed in SPSS v24 (IBM). In all tests, a *p*-value <0.05 was considered statistically significant.

RESULTS

Isolation of Clinically Derived Phage

One *P. aeruginosa* phage (P5) was successfully isolated from patient sputum by direct plating and propagated on patient strain PMH5. Six other phages were observed as plaques on lawns of bacterial isolates derived from CF patients, but could not be successfully propagated to high titre or were unstable at 4°C in storage, and thus were not investigated further. In total, 6/20 (30%) CF-derived *P. aeruginosa* were demonstrated to carry spontaneously inducible lysogenic phages.

Phage Host Ranges

Plaque formation by E79 was observed on lawns of 20/22 (91%) of *P. aeruginosa* strains tested (**Table 2**), making it a strong candidate for further testing as a potential therapeutic phage. F116 and P5 had more limited host ranges (36 and 64% strains susceptible, respectively), and were known (F116) or suspected (P5) temperate phages, and were therefore eliminated from further screening, since these were not considered to be ideal for phage therapy.

TABLE 2 | Host range of phages within the panel of clinical *P. aeruginosa* isolates and PAO1 strain.

P. aeruginosa strain	Colony phenotype	Phage susceptibility		
		E79	F116	P5
PAO1	Smooth	++	++	++
PMH1	Mucoid	++	–	++
PMH2	Smooth	++	–	–
PMH3	Mucoid	++	–	–
PMH4	Mucoid	++	–	+
PMH5	Smooth	++	+	++
PMH6	Rough	++	–	–
PMH7	Mucoid	++	–	+
PMH9	Smooth	–	–	++
PMH10	Mucoid	–	–	++
PMH11	Rough	++	+	++
PMH12	Mucoid	++	–	–
PMH13	Smooth	++	+	++
PMH14	Smooth	++	–	–
PMH15	Mucoid	++	–	–
PMH16	Rough	++	–	–
PMH17	Smooth	++	–	+
PMH18	Rough	++	–	–
PMH19	Mucoid	++	+	+
PMH20	Mucoid	++	++	++
PMH22	Mucoid	++	+	+
PMH23	Rough	++	+	+

++Indicates complete clearing, +indicates partial clearing, –indicates no visible clearing of the bacterial lawn.

E79 Genetic and Morphological Characterization

Both E79 and P5 were confirmed to be double-stranded DNA phages, demonstrated by digestion by *Hind*III and *Bam*HI, respectively (not shown). TEM of E79 identified the phage to have a head diameter of 63.6 ± 3.8 nm, head length of 60.5 ± 5.7 nm, tail width of 8.4 ± 0.8 nm, tail length of 128.1 ± 3.7 nm, and a sheath width of 16.6 ± 2.4 nm. Genome sequencing of E79 generated 2.2 M reads with an average length of 252 bp. The sequencing analysis returned a complete genome of 66,061 bp, with BLASTN analysis revealing 98% query cover and 97% identity to a range of widespread PB1-like *Pseudomonas* phages in the *Myoviridae* family (Ceyssens et al., 2009). The E79 genome contained 96 open reading frames, 75 of which were for hypothetical phage proteins. No virulence factors or antibiotic resistance genes were detected, nor any genes from the host PAO1 bacterial genome. The full sequence of E79 is deposited in GenBank under accession #MH536736.

Phage Purification

Phage fractions were collected from the ion-exchange chromatography column and examined for remaining viable phage. Approximately 80% of the added phage was recovered in the saline fractions collected. Maximal phage recovery occurred from the elution at approximately 450 mM NaCl (**Figure 2B**). The concentration of endotoxin in the filter-sterilized phage (unpurified) and the purified, endotoxin-depleted phage preparations was approximately 10^8 and 1.9 EU/mL, respectively. E79 phage preparations were stored at 4°C and retained the high infective titre for >20 weeks of testing (**Figure 2A**).

Bacterial Growth Inhibition

Growth of clinical *P. aeruginosa* isolates was significantly decreased (median 33% decrease) in the MOI 1:1 (low phage ratio) and MOI of 10:1 (high phage ratio) (median 23% decrease). Of 14 clinical isolates tested, a variety of growth inhibition and clinical antibiotic resistance phenotypes were observed (**Table 3**) with 11 (79%) showing some growth inhibition by E79. Of these, eight (57%) exhibited single or multiple antibiotic-resistance.

Response of Airway Epithelial Cells to Stimulation

Viability of airway epithelial cells from children with CF or healthy non-CF controls was not affected when treated with

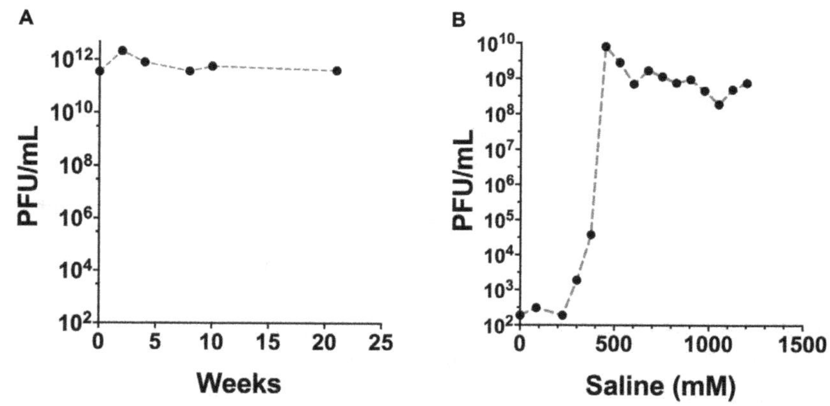

FIGURE 2 | Stability and recovery of E79 phage after purification steps. **(A)** Titre of E79 phage was retained over long term storage at 4°C, determined by the drop-on-plate method using PAO1 as the propagating host strain. **(B)** Recovery of E79 in fractions from ion-exchange chromatography column. Data show average values obtained from three replicate measurements of a single solution.

TABLE 3 | Comparative sensitivity of clinical *P. aeruginosa* isolates to E79 phage at high MOI (10:1 ratio to bacterial cells) or low MOI (1:1 ratio to bacterial cells) and to antibiotics.

Sample ID	Gentamicin	Ceftazidime	Meropenem	Amikacin	Piperacillin	Cefepime	Tobramycin	Ciprofloxacin	Norfloxacin	Timentin	Piperacillin/ Tazobactam	Aztreonam	E79 at low MOI	E79 at high MOI
ARESTCF-1	S	S	S	S	S	S	S	S	S	**I**	S	S	S	S
ARESTCF-2	S	S	S	S	S	S	S	S	S	**I**	S	**I**	**R**	S
ARESTCF-3	S	S	S	S	S	S	S	S	S	S	S	**I**	S	S
ARESTCF-4	S	S	S	S	S	S	S	S	S	S	S	S	S	S
ARESTCF-5	S	S	S	S	S	S	S	S	S	**I**	S	S	S	S
ARESTCF-6	S	S	S	S	S	S	S	S	S	**I**	S	S	S	S
ARESTCF-7	S	S	S	S	S	S	S	S	S	**R**	S	**R**	**R**	**R**
ARESTCF-8	S	S	S	S	S	S	S	S	S	S	S	S	S	S
ARESTCF-9	S	S	S	S	S	S	S	S	S	S	S	S	**R**	**R**
ARESTCF-10	S	S	S	S	S	S	S	S	S	S	S	S	S	S
ARESTCF-11	S	S	S	S	S	S	S	S	S	S	S	**R**	S	S
ARESTCF-12	S	S	S	S	S	S	S	S	S	S	S	S	**R**	**R**
ARESTCF-13	**I**	S	S	S	S	S	S	S	S	S	S	S	**R**	S
ARESTCF-14	S	S	S	S	S	S	S	S	S	S	S	S	S	S

MOI, multiplicity of infection; S, sensitive; I, intermediate; R, resistant. Results with intermediate resistance or resistance are indicated with bolded font and gray shading.

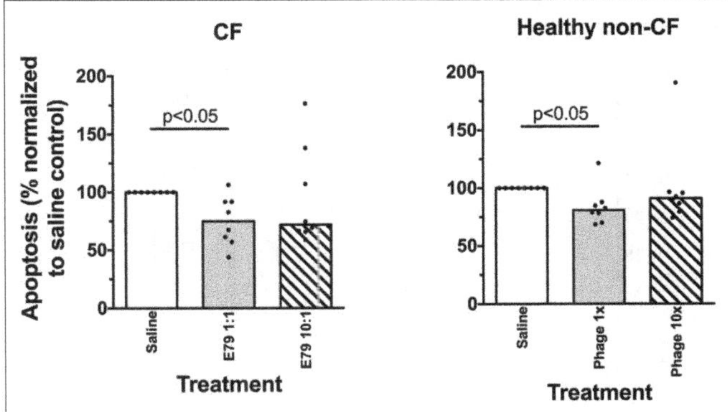

FIGURE 3 | Survival of primary airways cells exposed to phage. Apoptosis in cell cultures exposed to phage at high or low concentration relative to saline controls. Average individual values are shown from three replicate wells, and bars indicate the group median value. Statistically significant differences in Friedman post-tests ($p < 0.05$) are indicated by p-values.

phage at either ratio (data not shown). Similarly, E79 phage did not induce apoptosis in either phenotype at either the low or high phage ratio (**Figure 3**); rather exposure to phage was associated with lower apoptosis levels than observed in control wells.

Comparing 8 non-CF and 8 CF cultures treated with phage suspensions at low or high ratio, there was no induced inflammatory cytokine production (**Figure 4**). Specifically, no significant increase in IL-1β, IL-6, and Il-8 was observed when CF or healthy non-CF cells were treated with low or high phage titres ($p > 0.05$; **Figure 4**).

DISCUSSION

New antibacterial therapies are urgently required to counteract the rise of multidrug-resistant microbes. In this work, we successfully propagated and screened three bacteriophages and identified that the *P. aeruginosa*-infecting phage E79 had the broadest host range of these. Moreover, the protocol utilized to purify phage was successful in removing bacterial contaminants to the extent that no significant apoptosis, or inflammatory cytokine production was detected in either airway epithelial cells from children with CF or healthy non-CF controls after 48 h of co-culture with purified E79 phage. Collectively, this work demonstrates a proof of concept that a screening approach utilizing bacteriophage and primary epithelial cells derived from the CF population could be applied for the development of new therapies for people with CF-associated antibiotic-resistant bacterial lung infections.

Given the association of *P. aeruginosa* airway infections and pulmonary decline in people with CF, early intervention when children are first infected could be critical in preventing lung damage and increase life expectancy (Ranganathan et al., 2017). Inhaled phage therapy is one option that could be utilized in combination with current therapies to improve outcomes. The optimal dosing formulations and regimes would

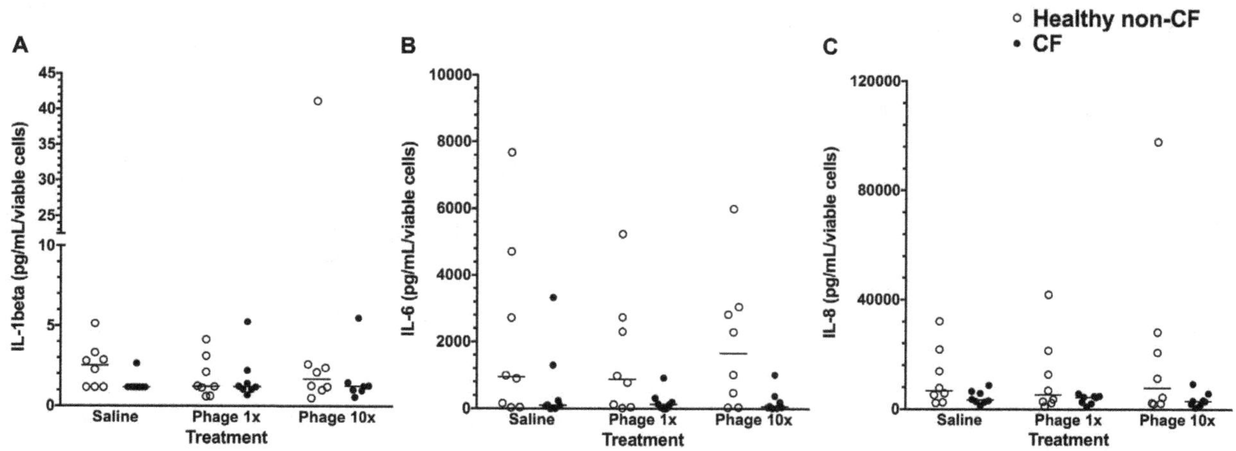

FIGURE 4 | Cytokine production in primary airways cells exposed to phage. Levels of **(A)** IL-1β, **(B)** IL-6, and **(C)** IL-8 cytokines in culture supernatants of cells exposed to treatments for 48 h compared with untreated controls cell. Cytokine concentrations were adjusted for the ratio of viable cells in the phage treatment wells compared with the control well. Data show values for healthy non-CF children (open circles; $n = 8$) or children with CF (closed circles; $n = 8$) representing the mean calculated from three replicate treatment wells per individual. Horizontal lines represent the group (healthy non-CF or CF) median.

need to be determined in clinical trials following identification of ideal phage candidates, using pre-clinical models such as the one described here. A limited number of case studies are described in the literature on treatment of airways infections in children with CF with phage therapy, as well as a number of reports on use in uncontrolled studies in CF and non-CF adults (Sulakvelidze et al., 2001; Kutateladze and Adamia, 2008; Kvachadze et al., 2011; Abedon, 2015; Hoyle et al., 2018). Encouragingly, these early reports suggest that phage therapy may be feasible in the pediatric CF population.

Our pre-clinical screening method demonstrated that almost half of *P. aeruginosa* isolates carried one or more spontaneously released phages. It is likely that these phages were temperate, and therefore may not be ideal for therapeutic use (Hraiech et al., 2015), although we did not confirm this with genome sequencing. Isolation and propagation to high titre proved difficult for most of these phages. The prevalence of non-propagatable isolates in this study is not unique (Serwer et al., 2004), and isolation techniques could be optimized in future, such as inclusion of antibiotics in culture media (Santos et al., 2009). Despite the potential for lysogenic phages to confer resistance to related phages (Labrie et al., 2010; James et al., 2012; van Houte et al., 2016), each bacterial isolate utilized for screening of host ranges here was susceptible to at least one phage tested for activity, indicating that the children from whom the bacteria were isolated could potentially be treated with phage therapy.

We found that the virulent phage, E79, had many ideal characteristics for further development as a therapeutic phage, including stability in high titre preparation, broad infective capacity of clinical *P. aeruginosa* isolates, and lack of known bacterial pathogenicity genes. Indeed, PB1-like phages such as E79 are considered by some to be among the most promising for application in phage therapy (Krylov et al., 2015) due in part to the low frequency of mutation to phage-resistance (Ceyssens et al., 2009). On the other hand, an earlier study suggested that E79 had restricted access to the deeper layers of a biofilm of PAO1 generated on glass (Doolittle et al., 1996), although the authors stated that fluorescently labeling the phage significantly affected infective capacity and that they could not determine whether the decrease in signal deeper in the biofilm was an experimental artifact. In another study, biofilm challenge with E79 resulted in a transient increase at 24 h in biofilm formation, although following further incubation, biofilm decreased (Hosseinidoust et al., 2013). Despite the limitations of extrapolating artificial biofilm methods to human CF lungs, which have very different environmental conditions that might affect bacterial growth, these are important issues to address for phage therapy. Certainly, further characterization would be required for clinical development in a more disease-appropriate model system. Here, to determine bacterial infective capacity, we used a qualitative drop-on-plate assay and an indirect optical density assay of bacterial viability. Whilst these assays may give some indication of a phage's broad infective capacity of various bacterial strains, more accurate prediction of clinical outcomes in patients would ideally involve quantitative measurement of phage activity in a biofilm model, ideally including live/dead cell imaging.

Phage-host dynamics are complex with pharmacokinetic interactions that may not be correctly predicted without including as many components as possible of the phage-bacterial-host cell interaction in a model. *In vivo*, it is predicted that the human immune system would work in a complementary manner to phage to control bacterial growth. Roach et al. (2017) reported that neutrophils are important for immunophage synergy and immunodeficient mice did not respond to phage treatment of *P. aeruginosa* pneumonia in the same manner as immunocompetent mice. Therefore, simple antimicrobial assays may not accurately predict clinical consequences of novel treatments. Given the differences between healthy and CF neutrophil phenotypes (Gray et al., 2018), it is critical to examine immunophage synergy for people with CF in a relevant model for these individuals, and as such it may be possible to include neutrophils or other immune cells in an airways co-culture model. Although we did not include any non-epithelial cells in this model, one major focus was adequate purification of phage preparation. Given that human airways epithelial cells express a range of Toll-like receptors (Ritter et al., 2005), and our work assessed upregulation of downstream cytokines from NF-κB activation, our model was sufficient for this aim. The response of primary cells derived from different children was personalized; though overall, phage preparations did not induce cytokine production, in some individuals, production of inflammatory cytokines in response to phage exposure was elevated when compared to untreated cells. Despite this, as a group (CF or non-CF children) the differences between phage-exposed and control cell cultures were not statistically significant. Therefore, our data suggest that personalized screening approaches may be best to determine the appropriate treatment for people with CF, where grouped results may not be representative of outcomes for all individuals within that group. However, the method used here in this pilot study could be significantly improved in future by one or all of the following: (a) use of air-liquid interface (ALI) in primary respiratory cell cultures, (b) examination of biofilm, (c) addition of professional immune cells in co-culture with respiratory cells, and (d) delivery of aerosolised phage preparations.

The phage purification methods used here were comparable to those used successfully by others, and resulted in depletion of endotoxin and other bacterial signatures that might have activated epithelial cell inflammatory responses. However, it is likely that without extra preparatory steps, host DNA contamination may be an issue for phage preparations (Kleiner et al., 2015). In addition, it is possible that the decreased levels of apoptosis in phage suspension-treated cells compared with saline-exposed cells is a host cell pro-survival response to damage caused by other PAO1 contaminants remaining in the phage preparation (Wu et al., 2011). Given that we did not find any PAO1-associated genes in the E79 genome, our methods to remove free host DNA were successful, and therefore, it may be appropriate to utilize a similar DNase treatment step to avoid potential transfer of host bacterial genes to bacteria in the human airways, as previously suggested (Pirnay et al., 2015). Previous work with other phages has shown different methods of pharmacological preparation affect viability and particle sizing, which are relevant for inhalation of phages (Leung et al., 2016). In the CF lung environment, it will be important to determine the pharmacological formulations that best allow phages to survive the preparation steps and to enter the lungs with optimal aerodynamic properties in an inhaled formulation (Chang et al., 2017). The activity of optimized phage formulations in the lung environment can be investigated using models of the CF airway, although more purification steps should be taken with phage preparations in future.

In this study, of eight clinical isolates of *P. aeruginosa* that displayed some level of resistance to single or multiple antibiotics, seven exhibited E79 phage-susceptibility at the highest MOI tested, while two out of six antibiotic-susceptible isolates were E79 phage-resistant. This preliminary result suggests that the combined use of traditional antibiotics and phages might be a good approach in at least some cases of antibiotic-resistant infections. Rossitto et al. (2018) have noted the limited number of investigations of combined antibiotic-phage treatment, but consider this a promising approach for the future of anti-*P. aeruginosa* therapy in CF. The rate of progress from bench to bedside that might be predicted by the ease with which novel phages are isolated is in fact limited by the uncertainty surrounding their safety. This situation arises, in part, from inadequate characterization of these phages in clinically relevant CF models. Therefore, in future, the process of selecting phages for therapeutic development could be performed as a high-throughput methodology for people with CF, identifying phages that are suitable for their particular infecting bacterial strain and immunological idiosyncrasies, and determining appropriate dosage using appropriate personalized *in vitro* models.

AUTHOR CONTRIBUTIONS

BC, ST, and AK developed the research concept and designed the experiments. ST and AK carried out the experimental work. ST and MO conducted the data analysis. ST wrote the first draft of the manuscript. All authors contributed to the drafting and editing of the manuscript.

FUNDING

This work was funded by the Telethon Kids Institute Blue Sky Research Grant.

ACKNOWLEDGMENTS

We would like to thank Ms. Jessica Hillas for assistance with cell culture and Dr. Richard Allcock for assistance with genome sequencing. We also thank Dr. Rosemary Carzino for technical assistance in providing AREST CF bacterial isolates. We sincerely thank the participants and their families on the Western Australian Epithelial Research Program (WAERP) for their contribution to this study, and the Telethon Kids Institute for supporting part of this work through the Blue Sky Research Grant.

Members of the WAERP

Anthony Kicic, Stephen M. Stick, Darryl A. Knight, Elizabeth Kicic-Starcevich, Luke W. Garratt, Marc Padros-Goosen, Ee-Lyn Tan, Erika N. Sutanto, Kevin Looi, Jessica Hillas, Thomas Iosifidis, Nicole C. Shaw, Samuel T. Montgomery, Kak-Ming Ling, Kelly M. Martincvich, Francis J. Lannigan, Ricardo

Bergesio, Bernard Lee, Shyan Vijaya-Sekeran, Paul Swan, Mairead Heaney, Ian Forsyth, Tobias Schoep, Alexander Larcombe, Monica Hunter, Kate McGee, Nyssa Millington.

Members of the Australian Respiratory Early Surveillance Team for Cystic Fibrosis (AREST CF)

The full membership of the Australian Respiratory Early Surveillance Team for Cystic Fibrosis (AREST CF) is available at www.arestcf.org.

Members of the Australian Respiratory Epithelium Consortium (AusREC)

Anthony Kicic, Stephen M. Stick, Elizabeth Kicic-Starcevich, Luke W. Garratt, Erika N. Sutanto, Kevin Looi, Jessica Hillas, Thomas Iosifidis, Nicole C. Shaw, Samuel T. Montgomery, Kak-Ming Ling, Kelly M. Martinovich, Matthew W-P Poh, Daniel R. Laucirica, Craig Schofield, Samantha McLean, Katherine Landwehr, Emma de Jong, Nigel Farrow, Eugene Roscioli, David Parsons, Darryl A. Knight, Christopher Grainge, Andrew T. Reid, Su-Kim Loo, and Punnam C. Veerati.

REFERENCES

Abedon, S. T. (2015). Phage therapy of pulmonary infections. *Bacteriophage* 5:e1020260. doi: 10.1080/21597081.2015.1020260

Adams, M. (1959). *Bacteriophages.* New York, NY: Interscience Publishers, Inc.

Alemayehu, D., Casey, P. G., McAuliffe, O., Guinane, C. M., Martin, J. G., Shanahan, F., et al. (2012). Bacteriophages ?MR299-2 and ?NH-4 can eliminate *Pseudomonas aeruginosa* in the murine lung and on cystic fibrosis lung airway cells. *mBio* 3:e00029-12. doi: 10.1128/mBio.00029-12

Brettin, T., Davis, J. J., Disz, T., Edwards, R. A., Gerdes, S., Olsen, G. J., et al. (2015). RASTtk: a modular and extensible implementation of the RAST algorithm for building custom annotation pipelines and annotating batches of genomes. *Sci. Rep.* 5:8365. doi: 10.1038/srep08365

Bruttin, A., and Brussow, H. (2005). Human volunteers receiving *Escherichia coli* phage T4 orally: a safety test of phage therapy. *Antimicrob. Agents Chemother.* 49, 2874–2878. doi: 10.1128/AAC.49.7.2874-2878.2005

Ceyssens, P., Miroshnikov, K., Mattheus, W., Krylov, V., Robben, J., Noben, J., et al. (2009). Comparative analysis of the widespread and conserved PB1-like viruses infecting *Pseudomonas aeruginosa. Environ. Microbiol.* 11, 2874–2883. doi: 10.1111/j.1462-2920.2009.02030.x

Chang, R. Y., Wong, J., Mathai, A., Morales, S., Kutter, E., Britton, W., et al. (2017). Production of highly stable spray dried phage formulations for treatment of *Pseudomonas aeruginosa* lung infection. *Eur. J. Pharm. Biopharm.* 121, 1–13. doi: 10.1016/j.ejpb.2017.09.002

CLSI. (2016). *Performance Standards for Antimicrobial Susceptibility Testing. CLSI Supplement M100.* Wayne, PA: Clinical and Laboratory Standards Institute.

Doolittle, M. M., Cooney, J. J., and Caldwell, D. E. (1996). Tracing the interaction of bacteriophage with bacterial biofilms using fluorescent and chromogenic probes. *J. Ind. Microbiol.* 16, 331–341. doi: 10.1007/BF01570111

Dunn, N. W., and Holloway, B. W. (1971). Pleiotropy of p-fluorophenylalanine-resistant and antibiotic hypersensitive mutants of *Pseudomonas aeruginosa. Genet. Res.* 18, 185–197. doi: 10.1017/S0016672300012593

Farrell, P. M., Collins, J., Broderick, L. S., Rock, M. J., Li, Z., Kosorok, M. R., et al. (2009). Association between mucoid *Pseudomonas* infection and bronchiectasis in children with cystic fibrosis. *Radiology* 252, 534–543. doi: 10.1148/radiol.2522081882

Friman, V. P., Ghoul, M., Molin, S., Johansen, H. K., and Buckling, A. (2013). *Pseudomonas aeruginosa* adaptation to lungs of cystic fibrosis patients leads to lowered resistance to phage and protist enemies. *PLoS One* 8:e75380. doi: 10.1371/journal.pone.0075380

Gray, R. D., Hardisty, G., Regan, K. H., Smith, M., Robb, C. T., Duffin, R., et al. (2018). Delayed neutrophil apoptosis enhances NET formation in cystic fibrosis. *Thorax* 73, 134–144. doi: 10.1136/thoraxjnl-2017-210134

Henry, M., Lavigne, R., and Debarbieux, L. (2013). Predicting in vivo efficacy of therapeutic bacteriophages used to treat pulmonary infections. *Antimicrob. Agents Chemother.* 57, 5961–5968. doi: 10.1128/aac.01596-13

Hosseinidoust, Z., Tufenkji, N., and van de Ven, T. G. M. (2013). Formation of biofilms under phage predation: considerations concerning a biofilm increase. *Biofouling* 29, 457–468. doi: 10.1080/08927014.2013.779370

Hoyle, N., Zhvaniya, P., Balarjishvili, N., Bolkvadze, D., Nadareishvili, L., Nizharadze, D., et al. (2018). Phage therapy against *Achromobacter xylosoxidans* lung infection in a patient with cystic fibrosis: a case report. *Res. Microbiol.* doi: 10.1016/j.resmic.2018.05.001 [Epub ahead of print].

Hraiech, S., Brégeon, F., and Rolain, J.-M. (2015). Bacteriophage-based therapy in cystic fibrosis-associated *Pseudomonas aeruginosa* infections: rationale and current status. *Drug Des. Dev. Ther.* 9, 3653–3663. doi: 10.2147/DDDT.S53123

James, C. E., Fothergill, J. L., Kalwij, H., Hall, A. J., Cottell, J., Brockhurst, M. A., et al. (2012). Differential infection properties of three inducible prophages from an epidemic strain of *Pseudomonas aeruginosa. BMC Microbiol.* 12:216. doi: 10.1186/1471-2180-12-216

Kicic, A., Stevens, P. T., Sutanto, E. N., Kicic-Starcevich, E., Ling, K. M., Looi, K., et al. (2016). Impaired airway epithelial cell responses from children with asthma to rhinoviral infection. *Clin. Exp. Allergy* 46, 1441–1455. doi: 10.1111/cea.12767

Kicic, A., Sutanto, E. N., Stevens, P. T., Knight, D. A., and Stick, S. M. (2006). Intrinsic biochemical and functional differences in bronchial epithelial cells of children with asthma. *Am. J. Respir. Crit. Care Med.* 174, 1110–1118. doi: 10.1164/rccm.200603-392OC

Kleiner, M., Hooper, L. V., and Duerkop, B. A. (2015). Evaluation of methods to purify virus-like particles for metagenomic sequencing of intestinal viromes. *BMC Genomics* 16:7. doi: 10.1186/s12864-014-1207-4

Koehler, D. R., Downey, G. P., Sweezey, N. B., Tanswell, A. K., and Hu, J. (2004). Lung inflammation as a therapeutic target in cystic fibrosis. *Am. J. Respir. Cell Mol. Biol.* 31, 377–381. doi: 10.1165/rcmb.2004-0124TR

Krylov, V., Shaburova, O., Pleteneva, E., Krylov, S., Kaplan, A., Burkaltseva, M., et al. (2015). Selection of phages and conditions for the safe phage therapy against *Pseudomonas aeruginosa* infections. *Virol. Sin.* 30, 33–44. doi: 10.1007/s12250-014-3546-3

Kutateladze, M., and Adamia, R. (2008). Phage therapy experience at the Eliava institute. *Med. Mal. Infect.* 38, 426–430. doi: 10.1016/j.medmal.2008.06.023

Kvachadze, L., Balarjishvili, N., Meskhi, T., Tevdoradze, E., Skhirtladze, N., Pataridze, T., et al. (2011). Evaluation of lytic activity of staphylococcal bacteriophage Sb-1 against freshly isolated clinical pathogens. *Microbial. Biotechnol.* 4, 643–650. doi: 10.1111/j.1751-7915.2011.00259.x

Labrie, S. J., Samson, J. E., and Moineau, S. (2010). Bacteriophage resistance mechanisms. *Nat. Rev. Microbiol.* 8, 317–327. doi: 10.1038/nrmicro2315

Lane, C., Burgess, S., Kicic, A., Knight, D., and Stick, S. (2005). The use of non-bronchoscopic brushings to study the paediatric airway. *Respir. Res.* 6:53. doi: 10.1186/1465-9921-6-53

Leung, S. S., Parumasivam, T., Gao, F. G., Carrigy, N. B., Vehring, R., Finlay, W. H., et al. (2016). Production of inhalation phage powders using spray freeze drying and spray drying techniques for treatment of respiratory infections. *Pharm. Res.* 33, 1486–1496. doi: 10.1007/s11095-016-1892-6

Majewska, J., Beta, W., Lecion, D., Hodyra-Stefaniak, K., Klopot, A., Kazmierczak, Z., et al. (2015). Oral application of T4 phage induces weak antibody production in the gut and in the blood. *Viruses* 7, 4783–4799. doi: 10.3390/v7082845

Martinovich, K. M., Iosifidis, T., Buckley, A. G., Looi, K., Ling, K. M., Sutanto, E. N., et al. (2017). Conditionally reprogrammed primary airway epithelial cells maintain morphology, lineage and disease specific functional characteristics. *Sci. Rep.* 7:17971. doi: 10.1038/s41598-017-17952-4

Matsumoto, H., Itoh, Y., Ohta, S., and Terawaki, Y. (1986). A generalized transducing phage of *Pseudomonas cepacia. J. Gen. Microbiol.* 132, 2583–2586. doi: 10.1099/00221287-132-9-2583

McNamara, P. S., Kicic, A., Sutanto, E. N., Stevens, P. T., and Stick, S. M. (2008). Comparison of techniques for obtaining lower airway epithelial cells from children. *Eur. Respir. J.* 32, 763–768. doi: 10.1183/09031936.0016 2507

Merabishvili, M., Pirnay, J. P., Verbeken, G., Chanishvili, N., Tediashvili, M., Lashkhi, N., et al. (2009). Quality-controlled small-scale production of a well-defined bacteriophage cocktail for use in human clinical trials. *PLoS One* 4:e4944. doi: 10.1371/journal.pone.0004944

National Guideline Alliance. (2017). *National Institute for Health and Care Excellence: Clinical Guidelines. Cystic Fibrosis: Diagnosis and Management.* London: National Institute for Health and Care Excellence (UK).

Pillarisetti, N., Williamson, E., Linnane, B., Skoric, B., Robertson, C. F., Robinson, P., et al. (2011). Infection, inflammation, and lung function decline in infants with cystic fibrosis. *Am. J. Respir. Crit. Care Med.* 184, 75–81. doi: 10.1164/rccm.201011-1892OC

Pirnay, J.-P., Blasdel, B. G., Bretaudeau, L., Buckling, A., Chanishvili, N., Clark, J. R., et al. (2015). Quality and safety requirements for sustainable phage therapy products. *Pharm. Res.* 32, 2173–2179. doi: 10.1007/s11095-014-1617-7

Ranganathan, S. C., Hall, G. L., Sly, P. D., Stick, S. M., and Douglas, T. A. (2017). Early lung disease in infants and preschool children with cystic fibrosis. what have we learned and what should we do about it?. *Am. J. Respir. Crit. Care Med.* 195, 1567–1575. doi: 10.1164/rccm.201606-1107CI

Ritter, M., Mennerich, D., Weith, A., and Seither, P. (2005). Characterization of toll-like receptors in primary lung epithelial cells: strong impact of the TLR3 ligand poly(I:C) on the regulation of Toll-like receptors, adaptor proteins and inflammatory response. *J. Inflamm.* 2:16. doi: 10.1186/1476-9255-2-16

Roach, D. R., Leung, C. Y., Henry, M., Morello, E., Singh, D., Di Santo, J. P., et al. (2017). Synergy between the host immune system and bacteriophage is essential for successful phage therapy against an acute respiratory pathogen. *Cell Host Microbe* 22, 38.e4–47.e4. doi: 10.1016/j.chom.2017.06.018

Rossitto, M., Fiscarelli, E. V., and Rosati, P. (2018). Challenges and promises for planning future clinical research into bacteriophage therapy against *Pseudomonas aeruginosa* in cystic fibrosis. An argumentative review. *Front. Microbiol.* 9:775. doi: 10.3389/fmicb.2018.00775

Sahota, J. S., Smith, C. M., Radhakrishnan, P., Winstanley, C., Goderdzishvili, M., Chanishvili, N., et al. (2015). Bacteriophage delivery by nebulization and efficacy against phenotypically diverse *Pseudomonas aeruginosa* from cystic fibrosis patients. *J. Aerosol. Med. Pulm. Drug Deliv.* 28, 353–360. doi: 10.1089/jamp. 2014.1172

Santos, S. B., Carvalho, C. M., Sillankorva, S., Nicolau, A., Ferreira, E. C., and Azeredo, J. (2009). The use of antibiotics to improve phage detection and enumeration by the double-layer agar technique. *BMC Microbiol.* 9:148. doi: 10.1186/1471-2180-9-148

Serwer, P., Hayes, S. J., Zaman, S., Lieman, K., Rolando, M., and Hardies, S. C. (2004). Improved isolation of undersampled bacteriophages: finding of distant terminase genes. *Virology* 329, 412–424. doi: 10.1016/j.virol.2004.08.021

Slayter, H. S., Holloway, B. W., and Hall, C. E. (1964). The structure of *Pseudomonas Aeruginosa* phages B3, E79, and F116. *J. Ultrastruct. Res.* 11, 274–281. doi: 10.1016/S0022-5320(64)90032-2

Sulakvelidze, A., Alavidze, Z., and Morris, J. G. (2001). Bacteriophage therapy. *Antimicrob. Agents Chemother* 45, 649–659. doi: 10.1128/aac.45.3.649-659. 2001

Sutanto, E. N., Kicic, A., Foo, C. J., Stevens, P. T., Mullane, D., Knight, D. A., et al. (2011). Innate inflammatory responses of pediatric cystic fibrosis airway epithelial cells: effects of nonviral and viral stimulation. *Am. J. Respir. Cell Mol. Biol.* 44, 761–767. doi: 10.1165/rcmb.2010-0368OC

Tai, A. S., Kidd, T. J., Whiley, D M., Ramsay, K. A., Buckley, C., Bell, S. C., et al. (2015). Molecular surveillance for carbapenemase genes in carbapenem-resistant *Pseudomonas aeruginosa* in Australian patients with cystic fibrosis. *Pathology* 47, 156–160. doi: 10.1097/pat.0000000000000216

Taylor, A. L., Hale, J., Hales, B. J., Dunstan, J. A., Thomas, W. R., and Prescott, S. L. (2007). FOXP3 mRNA expression at 6 months of age is higher in infants who develop atopic dermatitis, but is not affected by giving probiotics from birth. *Pediatric Allergy Immunol.* 18, 10–19. doi: 10.1111/j.1399-3038.2006.00483.x

Tian, X., Liu, Y., Yang, J., Wang, E., Liu, T., Xu, W., et al. (2016). p.G970D is the most frequent CFTR mutation in Chinese patients with cystic fibrosis. *Hum. Genome Var.* 3:15063. doi: 10.1038/hgv.2015.63

Trend, S., Fonceca, A. M., Ditcham, W. G., Kicic, A., and Cf, A. (2017). The potential of phage therapy in cystic fibrosis: essential human-bacterial-phage interactions and delivery considerations for use in *Pseudomonas aeruginosa*-infected airways. *J. Cyst. Fibros.* 16, 663–670. doi: 10.1016/j.jcf.2017. 06.012

van Houte, S., Buckling, A., and Westra, E. R. (2016). Evolutionary ecology of prokaryotic immune mechanisms. *Microbiol. Mol. Biol. Rev.* 80, 745–763. doi: 10.1128/mmbr.00011-16

World Health Organization (2014). *Antimicrobial Resistance: Global Report on Surveillance.* Geneva: World Health Organization.

Wu, M., Huang, H., Zhang, W., Kannan, S., Weaver, A., McKibben, M., et al. (2011). Host DNA repair proteins in response to *Pseudomonas aeruginosa* in lung epithelial cells and in mice. *Infect. Immun.* 79, 75–87. doi: 10.1128/IAI. 00815-10

16

Trial Refresh: A Case for an Adaptive Platform Trial for Pulmonary Exacerbations of Cystic Fibrosis

Andre Schultz[1,2,3], Julie A. Marsh[3,4], Benjamin R. Saville[5,6], Richard Norman[7], Peter G. Middleton[8], Hugh W. Greville[9], Matthew I. Bellgard[10], Scott M. Berry[5] and Tom Snelling[3,7,11,12]* on behalf of the BEAT CF Investigators*

[1] Faculty of Health and Medical Sciences, The University of Western Australia, Crawley, WA, Australia, [2] Department of Respiratory Medicine, Perth Children's Hospital, Nedlands, WA, Australia, [3] Wesfarmers Centre of Vaccines & Infectious Diseases, Telethon Kids Institute, The University of Western Australia, Nedlands, WA, Australia, [4] School of Population and Global Health, The University of Western Australia, Nedlands, WA, Australia, [5] Berry Consultants, Austin, TX, United States, [6] Department of Biostatistics, Vanderbilt University, Nashville, TN, United States, [7] School of Public Health, Curtin University, Bentley, WA, Australia, [8] Ludwig Engel Centre for Respiratory Research, Westmead Institute for Medical Research, Sydney, NSW, Australia, [9] Department of Thoracic Medicine, Royal Adelaide Hospital, Adelaide, SA, Australia, [10] eResearch Office, Queensland University of Technology, Brisbane, QLD, Australia, [11] Department of Infectious Diseases, Perth Children's Hospital, Nedlands, WA, Australia, [12] Menzies School of Health Research, Charles Darwin University, Darwin, NT, Australia

***Correspondence:**
Andre Schultz
andre.schultz@health.wa.gov.au
Tom Snelling
Tom.Snelling@telethonkids.org.au

Cystic fibrosis is a genetic disease typically characterized by progressive lung damage and premature mortality. Pulmonary exacerbations, or flare-ups of the lung disease, often require hospitalization for intensive treatment. Approximately 25% of patients with cystic fibrosis do not recover their baseline lung function after pulmonary exacerbations. There is a relative paucity of evidence to inform treatment strategies for exacerbations. Compounding this lack of evidence, there are a large number of treatment options already as well as becoming available. This results in significant variability between medication regimens prescribed by different physicians, treatment centers and regions with potentially adverse impact to patients. The conventional strategy is to undertake essential randomized clinical trials to inform treatment decisions and improve outcomes for patients with exacerbations. However, over the past several decades, clinical trials have generally failed to provide information critical to improved treatment and management of exacerbations. Bayesian adaptive platform trials hold the promise of addressing clinical uncertainties and informing treatment. Using modeling and response adaptive randomization, they allow for the evaluation of multiple treatments across different management domains, and progressive improvement in patient outcomes throughout the course of the trial. Bayesian adaptive platform trials require substantial amounts of preparation. Basic preparation includes extensive stakeholder involvement including elicitation of consumer preferences and clinician understanding of the research topic, defining the research questions, determining the best outcome measures, delineating study sub-groups, in depth statistical modeling, designing end-to-end digital solutions seamlessly supporting clinicians, researchers and patients, constructing randomisation algorithms and importantly, defining pre-determined intra-study end-points. This review will discuss the motivation and necessary steps required to embark on a Bayesian adaptive platform trial to optimize medication regimens for the treatment of pulmonary exacerbations of cystic fibrosis.

Keywords: adaptive trial, platform trial, Bayesian, cystic fibrosis, exacerbations, master protocol, response adaptive randomisation

BACKGROUND

Cystic fibrosis (CF) is a genetic disease typically characterized by progressive lung damage and premature mortality. Pulmonary exacerbations, or flare-ups of the lung disease, often require hospitalization for intensive treatment. Pulmonary exacerbations remain an important driver of progressive loss of lung function and premature death in CF. Up to 25% of patients do not recover their baseline lung function, typically measured as the forced expiratory volume in 1 s (FEV1), after an exacerbation (Sanders et al., 2010). Key to improving survival is the prevention of loss of lung function with each exacerbation. Reflecting this, when the James Lind Alliance recently canvassed research priorities from over 1,000 CF consumers from 23 countries, management of CF exacerbations, and specifically identification of the most effective/least toxic antibiotics, figured among their priorities (Rowbotham et al., 2018).

There are grounds for believing that better treatment of exacerbations may reduce the loss of lung function and thus improve survival. There is substantial variation in the rate of decline between individuals, even among those with the same primary genetic mutations. The demonstrated heterogeneity in outcomes among those with access to the same range of treatments (Stephenson et al., 2017), indicates that response may depend on individual patient characteristics or factors present during an exacerbation. Given these considerations, we identify three general questions that need to be addressed in order to improve the management of CF exacerbations: (a) What are the optimal interventions where multiple options exist; (b) How does optimal treatment vary by different patient characteristics; and (c) Do treatments have cumulative or antagonistic effects when used in combination.

Despite considerable research effort, answers to these questions have remained elusive. Antibiotics are a mainstay of the treatment of pulmonary exacerbations. A recent Cochrane review identified 40 studies of antibiotic treatment of CF exacerbations (Hurley et al., 2015). Most studies evaluated only two antibiotics and were small, inconclusive, never replicated, and completed a decade or more ago. The reviewers concluded that "No specific antibiotic combination can be considered to be superior to any other, and neither is there evidence showing that the intravenous route is superior to the inhaled or oral routes" (Hurley et al., 2015). The failure of this review of several decades of research to reach any meaningful conclusion is symptomatic of the challenges of conducting trials in CF. Continuing to undertake conventional trials may never usefully address this clinical uncertainty, and certainly not within a timeframe that will benefit many of the current generation of people with CF.

Recent advances in clinical trial methods can help to evaluate complex interventions for rare conditions like CF. These innovations allow for improved trial efficiency and may be more conducive to participation by patients and clinicians alike. These methods have recognized validity, having been used particularly in commercial cancer trials, accepted for regulatory purposes by both the Food and Drug Administration (Woodcock and LaVange, 2017) and the European Medicines Agency, and published in high impact journals. These methods are being applied in trials of the treatment of breast cancer (I-SPY2) (Park et al., 2016), severe community-acquired pneumonia (REMAP-CAP (NCT02735707)), and brain cancer (GBM-AGILE) (Alexander et al., 2018). Here, we describe the planning for BEAT CF, a Bayesian adaptive platform trial that aims to optimize the management of CF exacerbations.

BEAT CF aims to be an exemplar of the REMAP (randomized, embedded, multi-arm, adaptive, platform) trial approach (Angus, 2015). The key features of BEAT CF are the use of Bayesian statistical inference, flexible sample size, the comparison of several different treatment options simultaneously and in combination, response adaptive randomization, and the evaluation of treatment responses in different types of patient. Key to the successful implementation of BEAT CF will be its nesting within a treatment register, embedding of trial procedures in routine clinical care and a digital health approach that is dynamic to adapt to the informatics and data integration challenges (Bellgard et al., 2017). A core (master) protocol will allow the sequential introduction of new interventions over time, as initial questions are answered. Each of these features will be introduced below, contrasting REMAP trials with more traditional trial approaches, and highlighting the benefits, challenges and limitations inherent in establishing a REMAP trial for a complex clinical domain.

CORE PROTOCOL

A limitation of undertaking sequential disconnected trials is that the lack of standardized eligibility criteria, trial endpoints, subgroup definitions, and comparator treatments makes the aggregation of such data complex and uncertain. The core protocol of a REMAP trial aims to standardize these design elements so that treatment responses can be meaningfully aggregated across trials, across settings and over time. For BEAT CF, we propose to broadly involve clinicians and other domain experts, consumers and other stakeholders in this decision-making. Investment in the development of an overarching core protocol is also intended to prevent *reinventing the wheel* for each trial, improving efficiency through the sharing of infrastructure, and reducing the time to commencement and completion. In addition to standardizing specific design elements, the core protocol can also set out an overarching governance framework, including how the safety of participants is monitored. A core protocol implemented across multiple centers might institute a platform for the ready identification of potentially eligible study participants, facilitating enrolments.

BAYESIAN STATISTICAL INFERENCE

Up until now, most clinical trials, and all trials in managing CF exacerbations, have been traditionally designed trials which have employed frequentist statistical inference. Frequentist statistical inference underlies the vast majority of clinical studies, although thanks to increasing computer processing capacity, there has been a steady resurgence in Bayesian statistical inference in recent years (Green et al., 2015). In brief, frequentist inference assesses the *likelihood* of an observation, such as the observed difference in treatment effect between an investigational and a control treatment if no true difference exists (Berry, 2006). If an observation is very unlikely under this "null hypothesis" (i.e., it would rarely occur just by chance), this is taken as evidence that, to the contrary, a true difference exists. Frequentist inference flips the question of the probability that a difference exists, into a question about the probability of a result if no difference exists. To apply frequentist inference, one needs to be able to enumerate all the possible ways that a trial could have unfolded (that is the possible number of treatment successes and failures across both arms), and this requires many aspects of the design to be fixed in advance (e.g., randomization probabilities, sample sizes, number of treatment arms). If these components are not fixed it may be impossible to enumerate the number of possible ways that a trial may have unfolded and therefore to calculate how "unlikely" an observation is. Fixing the design so as to confine the number of possible outcomes makes the frequentist analysis tractable, but it comes at the cost of lost flexibility. New methods allow the design to be adapted as data accrues according to established rules (Saville et al., 2014), and these rules can be designed to maximize efficiency (including the chance of a conclusive result), or to maximize the chance that participants receive optimal treatment, or both.

Whereas frequentist inference is based solely on the *likelihood of an outcome*, Bayesian inference is directly concerned with the actual question, i.e., the *probability of a difference in treatment effect*, or the most probable values of the true difference in treatment effects. Bayesian inference does this by combining the *likelihood* of the observation for the range of possible treatment differences with the baseline *probability* (or "prior") of those possible treatment differences (Dmitrienko and Wang, 2006). Bayesian inference provides a straight-forward mechanism for updating one's estimate of the most probable range of treatment differences as new observations are made, that is, as data accrues (Connor et al., 2013). Trial designs that are adaptive can unfold in any one of a nearly limitless number of ways, so estimating how "unlikely" a particular result is (that is a particular instance of treatment responses among those who receive an intervention or control) is very hard to determine. The ability to update the probabilities for a range of possible treatment differences as new data accrues therefore makes Bayesian inference very useful for adaptive studies, although it should be noted that adaptive designs based on frequentist inference have also been advocated.

RESPONSE ADAPTIVE RANDOMISATION

When we have surveyed Australian CF clinicians, we have found that, like colleagues in the United States (West et al., 2017), they use a wide range of antibiotics to treat pulmonary exacerbations. Sequentially comparing the relative efficacy of all currently used antibiotics two-at-a-time would take an unfeasibly long time, notwithstanding the complexity of antibiotic combinations. Furthermore, assessing all antibiotics contemporaneously in a multi-arm trial would require an unfeasibly large number of participants. REMAP trials aim to greatly improve the efficiency of multi-arm trials using response adaptive randomisation (RAR). RAR is the progressive, rule-based assignment of an increasing proportion of new participants to interventions which appear most promising, and the potential elimination of those which are demonstrated to be inferior to alternatives options (Berry et al., 2015; Cellamare et al., 2017) (**Box 1**). Rather than having a fixed ratio of treatment assignment across arms, the ratio is updated (or adapted) at predefined intervals based on evidence from accruing data (Connor et al., 2013). At each analysis we will estimate the probability that each treatment, or treatment combination, is superior to all other options for a given patient type. Future treatment assignments will be based on these probabilities such that probability of assignment to a treatment is proportional to the probability that treatment is better than all other options for a given patient type (Connor et al., 2013). Randomization to ineffective treatments may be suspended or entirely eliminated if pre-specified futility boundaries are met (Berry et al., 2015). By assigning progressively more randomized participants to the best strategies and dropping ineffective therapies, it is expected that RAR will produce better patient outcomes for patients who participate in the trial (Connor et al., 2013).

SUBGROUP EFFECTS

One challenge for clinicians when trying to apply clinical trial results to their clinical practice is in determining whether the results are applicable to their own patient population, or indeed to a specific patient at hand. In pulmonary exacerbations, for example, it seems highly plausible that exacerbations represent

BOX 1 | Response adaptive randomisation.

- The progressive, rule-based assignment of an increasing proportion of new participants to interventions which appear most promising.
- The potential elimination of interventions demonstrated to be inferior to available alternatives when pre-specified futility boundaries are met.

a range of pathophysiologic processes, with responses to certain treatments influenced by the predominant process and, in the case of exacerbations caused by infecting bacteria, the species, and susceptibility profile of those bacteria (Doring et al., 2012). However, most trials are only interested in measuring *average* treatment effects of an intervention over a study population, and implicitly assume individuals respond homogenously to different interventions or treatment combinations. If a difference in treatment effects between subgroups is expected, the trialist will need to confine the trial to only the patient group which is expected to respond, or will run parallel trials in each group. If a difference in treatment response is hypothesized but not expected, the trialist can choose to aggregate data across the subgroups unless a statistical test for heterogeneity confirms a difference in treatment effects across subgroups, in which case the results for the two groups are reported separately. The problem with the latter approach is that such tests are relatively insensitive for true differences which can lead to inappropriate pooling of results; the problem with splitting by patient subgroups is that the precision is diluted by ever shrinking sample sizes. This is a problem in CF where the range of potential subgroups and plausible treatment effect modifiers is very large, based on variation in sputum microbiology, disease stage, and prior and concurrent treatment history.

REMAP trials aim to estimate specific treatment responses across a range of predefined patient subgroups much more efficiently than traditional trials. Such subgroups could be defined by factors that plausibly impact on response to treatment, or more specifically, influence the probability of a better response to one treatment than another, for example baseline lung function and airway microbiology status in the case of pulmonary exacerbations. Bayesian modeling can be used to allow the observed treatment response in one group to inform the probable treatment effect in another. Bayesian prior distributions are carefully calibrated to control the amount of *borrowing* of information between respective sub groups, and are verified in the design stage via simulation (Berry and Berry, 2004). This differs from the extreme approaches of complete pooling (i.e., ignoring subgroups effects and estimating a single common treatment effect) or no pooling (i.e., independent estimation of treatment effects in each subgroup). The Bayesian modeling approach can be described as being in between these two extremes, with *partial pooling* of information from patient subgroups. For subgroups with small sample sizes, the estimated subgroup treatment effects tend to be closer to each other. As sample sizes increase within subgroups, estimation of treatment effects may grow apart depending on the observed data within the subgroups.

COMPARISON OF MULTIPLE DIFFERENT TREATMENT OPTIONS SIMULTANEOUSLY

Like most chronic diseases, the management of CF pulmonary exacerbations is complex and multimodal (Elborn, 2016; Waters et al., 2016; West et al., 2017). Traditional trial designs typically do not account for multimodality but instead focus on one or more treatments within a single therapeutic "domain," where domain refers to a set of mutually exclusive treatment options. In the management of pulmonary exacerbations for example, therapeutic domains include the choice and route of antibiotic (both primary/backbone and adjunctive) (West et al., 2017), the use of mucoactive therapies (including dornase alpha, hypertonic saline, and mannitol) (Bakker et al., 2014; Dentice et al., 2016), the use of immune modulators (steroids, non-steroidal anti-inflammatory drugs, and macrolides) (Ghdifan et al., 2010; Lands and Stanojevic, 2016), and type and intensity of airway clearance therapies. Trials that attempt to evaluate a complex multi-modal intervention typically evaluate them as a fixed "bundle"; the limitation of this approach is that it makes it impossible to know which components of the bundle, if any, are effective, which ineffective or deleterious, and whether any combinations are synergistic or antagonistic.

In the REMAP design, participants can be randomly assigned to one of two or more options across each of two or more therapeutic domains. Participants are therefore assigned to one of many possible treatment combinations. This gives rise to a multi-dimensional estimation problem. For example, in a REMAP with three therapeutic domains each with three treatment options, there are 3^3 (twenty seven) combinations and therefore 27 separate treatment effects to be estimated, ignoring any subgroup-specific effects. As for subgroup effects, this multi-dimensional estimation problem is made tractable by the use of Bayesian modeling which allows, for example, the observed treatment outcomes among patients receiving a backbone antibiotic together with one adjunctive antibiotic, to inform the estimated treatment effect of the same backbone antibiotic when given in conjunction with a different adjunctive antibiotic, and *vice versa* (Berry and Berry, 2004).

A PLATFORM TRIAL WITH A DECISION-BASED MASTER PROTOCOL

Most clinical trials are stand-alone, time-limited, and designed to answer a single efficacy or comparative efficacy question. Regardless of whether the trial is conclusive or not, any follow-up or completely new questions usually require the establishment of a new trial. Typically there is little or no transfer of study infrastructure between trials which is wasteful of resources. Also, trials of interventions for CF exacerbations have variously measured different but related outcome measures, such as the absolute or relative improvements in the predicted FEV1, or the proportion of patients returning to some fraction of their "baseline" FEV1, or the reduction in some composite measure of symptoms. Furthermore, trials have measured these endpoints at variable lengths of time after initiation of CF exacerbation therapy. Failure of concurrent and consecutive trials to adopt the same endpoints has made it impossible to compare, let alone aggregate, results across studies. More recently there have been efforts to establish consistent endpoints, or core outcome sets, for trials in cystic fibrosis and other trials (Stanojevic and Ratjen, 2016; West et al., 2017).

A REMAP trial aims to achieve greater efficiency through a core (or master) trial protocol. The core protocol sets out exactly what data are to be collected including the primary and any secondary endpoints, and the procedures around how data is captured and managed, including the trial governance arrangements. Any treatment options which are subject to random assignment are dealt with in a series of appendices to the master protocol, with a therapeutic domain and all treatment options within that domain covered by its own appendix.

This use of a core protocol facilitates consistency in trial endpoints and processes over time. The modular structure of the protocol allows for the domain-specific trial appendices to be modified over time without changing the core protocol; treatment options within a domain can be added or removed according to pre-specified rules and entire domains can be added or removed over time. Once the superiority of a treatment has been established over all other treatments within an existing domain, a new domain with unanswered questions could replace the existing domain (Berry et al., 2015). This circumvents the need for setting up an entirely new clinical trial. For example if the optimal combinations of backbone and adjuvant antibiotics for CF exacerbation have been determined for individual patient sub-groups, a new phase of the study might focus on optimization of immune modifiers, mucoactive agents, airway clearance strategies or other therapeutic domains.

Non-inferiority and equivalence findings can also be evaluated in a REMAP trial. In particular, the study would still result in improvement in care if it was able to eliminate one or more inferior treatment arms, while showing the remaining treatment arms are equivalent. In addition, some treatments may require an efficacy superiority margin to be favored relative to other treatments in the presence of differing toxicity/safety profiles. We are currently investigating various options for incorporating toxicity into the primary analysis and RAR algorithm.

EMBEDDING IN ROUTINE CLINICAL CARE

Despite the potential efficiencies gained through the use of adaptive processes, a REMAP trial must nonetheless enroll a large number and broad range of participants if it is to efficiently address the full range of management questions. For this to occur, a REMAP trial needs to be successfully embedded in routine clinical care. Embedding, in which trial participation occurs seamlessly with delivery of care and with minimal additional impost on either clinician or participant, requires extensive stakeholder involvement in the design and strong buy-in by clinicians and patients. To secure this, REMAP investigators must spend considerable effort eliciting clinician's expert understanding of the subject domain, as well as consumer input into identification of patient-centered study outcomes. Clinicians and patients may be more likely to engage with a trial for which there is prospect of a personal benefit from participation. Unlike traditional trials which are ethically predicated on no expectation of a personal benefit, response adaptive processes of REMAP trials are designed to improve the chances that a participant receives optimal therapy, and minimize the chance of inferior therapy.

Many traditional trials blind the participant, or the outcome assessor, or both, to the treatment assignment, usually through the use of matched placebos or sham treatments. Blinding helps to safeguard against bias that might arise, especially if the clinician, patient or assessor have preconceptions about the relative effectiveness of the treatment options. Complete blinding of participants is typically not feasible in a REMAP owing to the large number and range of therapeutic options evaluated, together with the desire to achieve successful embedding in routine care. In any unblinded study (regardless of equal or response adaptive randomization), there is the risk that patient's or physician's knowledge can affect outcomes. This can be minimized through the choice of objective outcomes such as change in FEV1, especially if the person performing the measurement is, herself, blinded to the treatment assignment. For unblinded studies incorporating RAR, there is additional risk of operational bias resulting from a site's perceived impression of adaptive randomization. Although it would be difficult to measure any such bias that might exist in this setting, we believe that knowledge of the best performing treatments at the site level would only be obvious in settings where there is a dominant treatment receiving greater randomizations across all or most subgroups. In such a setting, the risk of bias may be outweighed by the risk of continued randomization to under-performing arms.

DIGITAL HEALTH SOLUTION CONSIDERATIONS

The implementation of REMAP trials demands a rethink on approaches to data management, flow, sharing and the interfaces necessary to engage with participants, clinicians, and study coordinators. Whereas in conventional trials, paper-based records might be sufficient to manage the workflow and capture trial data, in a REMAP the need for continuous and iterative interaction between clinicians, patients, and statisticians demand digital solutions.

Any solution needs to ensure that data are captured electronically in order to support frequent pre-planned, scheduled analyses. Logic checks need to be built-in and designed to minimize data entry errors and the need for corrections which would otherwise delay analyses. All data needs to be held securely and privacy ensured – potentially identifiable information needs to be held at the site and not accessible to those who are not directly involved in patient care, including researchers. There should be facility for patients (or their parents) to directly enter symptom information, or patient reported outcomes (Napier et al., 2017). It is necessary for the randomisation procedure to accommodate the RAR process – that is, it is essential that any embedded randomisation process must be capable of being updated over time following each analysis. Static randomisation processes, for example those employing fixed randomisation lists, will not be fit-for-purpose.

Lessons learnt from the successful deployment of clinical registries offer insights into the types digital infrastructure required to implement REMAP trials (Bellgard et al., 2013; Lacaze et al., 2017). For instance, patient-centric registries allow patients to securely register through online registration with configurable online informed consent (Bellgard et al., 2012; Napier et al., 2017). Others have demonstrated the potential value of rich and well-collected patient registry data for improving patient decision-making in CF beyond simple rule-based algorithms (Alaa and van der Schaar, 2018). Online clinical reporting forms and participant questionnaires that can be configured by coordinators without software development skills enables the digital health solution to dynamically adapt to requirements (Bellgard et al., 2014). Longitudinal data capture and time-stamped ongoing patient assessments can be captured either by the patient themselves or by the clinician through automated notifications (Bellgard et al., 2015). In addition, patient registry platforms can have multi-lingual support and data elements can be derived allowing logic steps to be incorporated (Napier et al., 2017).

CONSENT

In traditional two-arm trials, once informed consent for participation has been obtained, recording that consent is relatively straight-forward. For a REMAP trial, where a participant may be offered randomisation across a number of therapeutic domains, capturing participant consent is more complex. For example participants might happily accept random assignment of treatment in one domain, but not in another. In some situations, specific treatment options, and possibly entire domains, may not be available in all centers. In the case of a REMAP in managing CF exacerbations, a participant might decline randomisation during one exacerbation, but accept randomisation during a subsequent exacerbation. Furthermore, a participant might never accept random assignment of treatment, but might nonetheless agree to have their treatment and outcome data collected in a treatment register. Consenting to a REMAP is not simply a binary choice to participate or not, and this complex and nuanced consent needs to be captured and efficiently and faithfully reflected in subsequent study processes.

Because of the complex nature of REMAP trial designs, it may not be possible to achieve adequately informed consent at the time of acute illness. It may be necessary to provide detailed education to prospective participants in the non-acute setting. In the case of a REMAP for managing CF exacerbations, for example, an option would be to obtain consent in a dynamic and stepwise fashion. In the first step, prospective participants may be invited to consent to enrolment in a prospective treatment register, in which patients simply agree to allow their treatment and outcome data to be captured to inform future best practice. This could occur in the outpatient setting, and could be supported by extensive education about the REMAP design and processes. Separately, those who are enrolled in the treatment register can then be invited to opt-in to randomized care at the time of pulmonary exacerbations. Because participants will have already received education in the outpatient setting, this additional consent to randomisation can be expedited so as not to unnecessarily disrupt the delivery of care. In this two-level consent process, participants may agree to have their treatment and outcome data captured in the treatment register, but not always (or perhaps never) further consent to receive randomized care of their exacerbations. Similarly, the treating clinician may decide against random treatment assignment for a patient during a given exacerbation. Having patients opting out of randomisation, or their clinicians deciding against random treatment assignment, is an issue found in nearly every randomized clinical trial. Patients who opt out of randomization are not included in the primary analysis. Hence, the generalizability of the primary analysis results is limited to a population of patients who are willing to be randomized. Whereas traditional clinical trials disregard data arising from unrandomized patients as inherently uninformative due to potential bias, it may be possible within the context of a REMAP to utilize this data for hypothesis generation, or possibly even for formal integration into treatment effect estimates.

ETHICS STATEMENT

Similar to all clinical trials BEAT CF will require approval by participating institutions' ethics and governance committees. Such committees will be confronted with a range of innovative features including the novel study design, complex Bayesian statistics, the absence of blinding to allocated treatment, and dynamic consent. Involvement of ethics and governance committees from the early planning stages may help to avoid roadblocks in the approval process. Evidence of extensive consumer involvement in study design and planning may also be looked upon favorably by these committees.

TRIAL EFFICIENCY AND COST

REMAP trials have the potential to be highly cost-efficient as multiple research questions can be addressed simultaneously in a single clinical trial (Berry et al., 2015). Thus, while there are significant initial costs associated with establishing the trial, these costs can be defrayed across many questions of interest. Additionally, the trial platform allows for efficiency with a single data capture and governance platform across multiple centers. If REMAPs are effectively embedded in clinical care the incremental costs of inclusion of additional study sites may be relatively small, and offset by improved effectiveness and cost-efficiency of care. The use of a core protocol allows new domains to be studied without the need to develop an entirely new protocol. While REMAP designs are motivated by the desire to greatly improve the efficiency of clinical comparative effectiveness research, to date these efficiencies remain largely unproven and may only be achieved if a REMAP design aligns with the specific objectives of the study.

LIMITATIONS AND CHALLENGES

Whilst a Bayesian adaptive platform trial many potentially provide many benefits for the study of CF exacerbations, specific challenges still remain. Some of these challenges transcend statistical design. For example, the precise definition of an exacerbation remains controversial (Goss and Burns, 2007; Stenbit and Flume, 2011). The clinical decision to hospitalize for treatment of an exacerbation may vary from one treatment center to another (Johnson et al., 2003) but has been successfully used as a pragmatic definition in clinical trials. Furthermore, the decision to admit to hospital can potentially be standardized between participating study sites (Ferkol et al., 2006). Secondly, exacerbations may have multiple etiologies requiring different optimal treatments (Stenbit and Flume, 2011). However, similar to asthma, different etiologies that result in the same clinical phenomenon (i.e., exacerbation) can usefully be studied as a single entity. Thirdly, the optimal duration of treatment for exacerbations remain contentious (Szentpetery and Flume, 2018) and there is uncertainty about best outcome measure, and timing of the outcome measure, for studying treatment effect. Such challenges face all clinical trials of exacerbations but can be overcome in the CF community where collaborative effort is the norm.

Another challenge for platform trial is population drift that can influence results. This can be addressed with Bayesian modeling that accounts for changes in population over time. Logistical challenges include the need for rapid data accrual to inform adaptations. Digital solutions, discussed above, can be applied to facilitate timely data capture. Many of the abovementioned limitations are discussed elsewhere (Saville and Berry, 2016), alongside the statistical efficiencies obtained through adaptive platform strategies.

IN SUMMARY

There is a need to optimize the management of pulmonary exacerbations of CF, but the traditional clinical trial approach may not be a feasible approach for addressing the multitude of clinical questions. REMAP trial designs may offer a much more effective and efficient approach to finding answers to the many questions confronting CF patients and clinicians. Features include response adaptive randomisation, and the ability to compare multiple different treatment options simultaneously over a range of patient sub-groups. Once the original research questions have been answered, the platform design with a core protocol would facilitate the seamless transition to follow-up questions. For such a trial to be successful for the study of exacerbations of CF the trial will need to be embedded in routine clinical care and innovative digital solutions will be required for implementation. Overall, the challenges are large but the gains for CF could be considerable.

AUTHOR CONTRIBUTIONS

AS co-wrote the first draft of the manuscript and contributed to the writing throughout. JM contributed to writing the first draft. BS and MB wrote sub-sections of the manuscript and contributed the manuscript as a whole. RN, HG, and PM provided expert input into an advanced version of the manuscript. SB provided expert input and oversight. TS acted as senior author by writing large sections of the manuscript and providing oversight and leadership throughout.

FUNDING

BEAT CF is supported by a BHP Blue Sky Award, and funding from the MTPConnect Project Fund Program (PRJ2017-57) and the Australian Medical Research Future Fund (MRFF APP 1152376). The contents of the published material are solely the responsibility of the authors and do not reflect the views of the Australian Government. AS is supported by a National Health and Medical Research Council fellowship (APP1168022). JM is supported by a Telethon-Perth Children's Hospital Research Fund research capacity grant (CRIPTIC). BS and SB are supported by a Channel 7 Telethon Trust Major Beneficiary grant. TS is supported by a National Health and Medical Research Council fellowship (GNT1111657).

REFERENCES

Alaa, A. M., and van der Schaar, M. (2018). Prognostication and risk factors for cystic fibrosis via automated machine learning. *Sci. Rep.* 8:11242. doi: 10.1038/s41598-018-29523-2

Alexander, B. M., Ba, S., Berger, M. S., Berry, D. A., Cavenee, W. K., Chang, S. M., et al. (2018). Adaptive global innovative learning environment for glioblastoma: GBM AGILE. *Clin. Cancer Res.* 24, 737–743. doi: 10.1158/1078-0432.CCR-17-0764

Angus, D. C. (2015). Fusing randomized trials with big data: the key to self-learning health care systems? *JAMA* 314, 767–768. doi: 10.1001/jama.2015.7762

Bakker, E. M., Volpi, S., Salonini, E., Mullinger, B., Kroneberg, P., Bakker, M., et al. (2014). Small airway deposition of dornase alfa during exacerbations in cystic fibrosis; a randomized controlled clinical trial. *Pediatr. Pulmonol.* 49, 154–161. doi: 10.1002/ppul.22800

Bellgard, M., Beroud, C., Parkinson, K., Harris, T., Ayme, S., Baynam, G., et al. (2013). Dispelling myths about rare disease registry system development. *Source Code Biol. Med.* 8:21. doi: 10.1186/1751-0473-8-21

Bellgard, M. I., Chartres, N., Watts, G. F., Wilton, S., Fletcher, S., Hunter, A., et al. (2017). Comprehending the health informatics spectrum: grappling with system entropy and advancing quality clinical research. *Front. Public Health* 5:224. doi: 10.3389/fpubh.2017.00224

Bellgard, M. I., Macgregor, A., Janon, F., Harvey, A., O'Leary, P., Hunter, A., et al. (2012). A modular approach to disease registry design: successful adoption of an internet-based rare disease registry. *Hum. Mutat.* 33, E2356–E2366. doi: 10.1002/humu.22154

Bellgard, M. I., Napier, K., Render, L., Radochonski, M., Lamont, L., Graham, C., et al. (2015). A registry framework enabling patient-centred care. *Stud. Health Technol. Inform.* 214, 8–14.

Bellgard, M. I., Render, L., Radochonski, M., and Hunter, A. (2014). Second generation registry framework. *Source Code Biol. Med.* 9:14. doi: 10.1186/1751-0473-9-14

Berry, D. A. (2006). Bayesian clinical trials. *Nat. Rev. Drug Discov.* 5, 27–36. doi: 10.1038/nrd1927

Berry, S. M., and Berry, D. A. (2004). Accounting for multiplicities in assessing drug safety: a three-level hierarchical mixture model. *Biometrics* 60, 418–426. doi: 10.1111/j.0006-341X.2004.00186.x

Berry, S. M., Connor, J. T., and Lewis, R. J. (2015). The platform trial: an efficient strategy for evaluating multiple treatments. *JAMA* 313, 1619–1620. doi: 10.1001/jama.2015.2316

Cellamare, M., Ventz, S., Baudin, E., Mitnick, C. D., and Trippa, L. (2017). A Bayesian response-adaptive trial in tuberculosis: the endTB trial. *Clin. Trials* 14, 17–28. doi: 10.1177/1740774516665090

Connor, J. T., Elm, J. J., Broglio, K. R., and Esett and Adapt-It Investigators. (2013). Bayesian adaptive trials offer advantages in comparative effectiveness trials: an example in status epilepticus. *J. Clin. Epidemiol.* 66(8 Suppl.), S130–S137. doi: 10.1016/j.jclinepi.02.015

Dentice, R. L., Elkins, M. R., Middleton, P. G., Bishop, J. R., Wark, P. A., Dorahy, D. J., et al. (2016). A randomised trial of hypertonic saline during hospitalisation for exacerbation of cystic fibrosis. *Thorax* 71, 141–147. doi: 10.1136/thoraxjnl-2014-206716

Dmitrienko, A., and Wang, M. D. (2006). Bayesian predictive approach to interim monitoring in clinical trials. *Stat. Med.* 25, 2178–2195. doi: 10.1002/sim.2204

Doring, G., Flume, P., Heijerman, H., and Elborn, J. S. (2012). Treatment of lung infection in patients with cystic fibrosis: current and future strategies. *J. Cyst. Fibros* 11, 461–479. doi: 10.1016/j.jcf.2012.10.004

Elborn, J. S. (2016). Cystic fibrosis. *Lancet* 388, 2519–2531. doi: 10.1016/S0140-6736(16)00576-6

Ferkol, T., Rosenfeld, M., and Milla, C. E. (2006). Cystic fibrosis pulmonary exacerbations. *J. Pediatr.* 148, 259–264. doi: 10.1016/j.jpeds.2005.10.019

Ghdifan, S., Couderc, L., Michelet, I., Leguillon, C., Masseline, B., and Marguet, C. (2010). Bolus methylprednisolone efficacy for uncontrolled exacerbation of cystic fibrosis in children. *Pediatrics* 125, e1259–e1264. doi: 10.1542/peds.2009-2042

Goss, C. H., and Burns, J. L. (2007). Exacerbations in cystic fibrosis. 1: Epidemiology and pathogenesis. *Thorax* 62, 360–367. doi: 10.1136/thx.2006.060889

Green, P. J., Łatuszyński, K., Pereyra, M., and Robert, C. P. (2015). Bayesian computation: a summary of the current state, and samples backwards and forwards. *Stat. Comput.* 25, 835–862. doi: 10.1007/s1122

Hurley, M. N., Prayle, A. P., and Flume, P. (2015). Intravenous antibiotics for pulmonary exacerbations in people with cystic fibrosis. *Coch. Database Syst. Rev.* 30:CD009730. doi: 10.1002/14651858.CD009730.pub2

Johnson, C., Butler, S. M., Konstan, M. W., Morgan, W., and Wohl, M. E. (2003). Factors influencing outcomes in cystic fibrosis: a center-based analysis. *Chest* 123, 20–27. doi: 10.1378/chest.123.1.20

Lacaze, P., Millis, N., Fookes, M., Zurynski, Y., Jaffe, A., Bellgard, M., et al. (2017). Rare disease registries: a call to action. *Intern. Med. J.* 47, 1075–1079. doi: 10.1111/imj.13528

Lands, L. C., and Stanojevic, S. (2016). Oral non-steroidal anti-inflammatory drug therapy for lung disease in cystic fibrosis. *Coch. Database Syst. Rev.* 4:CD001505. doi: 10.1002/14651858.CD001505.pub4

Napier, K. R., Tones, M., Simons, C., Heussler, H., Hunter, A. A., Cross, M., et al. (2017). A web-based, patient driven registry for angelman syndrome: the global angelman syndrome registry. *Orphanet. J. Rare Dis.* 12:134. doi: 10.1186/s13023-017-0686-1

Park, J. W., Liu, M. C., Yee, D., Yau, C., van, L. J., Paoloni, M., et al. (2016). Adaptive randomization of neratinib in early breast cancer. *N. Engl. J. Med.* 375, 11–22. doi: 10.1056/NEJMoa1513750

Rowbotham, N. J., Smith, S., Leighton, P. A., Rayner, O. C., Gathercole, K., Elliott, Z. C., et al. (2018). The top 10 research priorities in cystic fibrosis developed by a partnership between people with CF and healthcare providers. *Thorax* 73, 388–390. doi: 10.1136/thoraxjnl-2017-210473

Sanders, D. B., Bittner, R. C., Rosenfeld, M., Hoffman, L. R., Redding, G. J., and Goss, C. H. (2010). Failure to recover to baseline pulmonary function after cystic fibrosis pulmonary exacerbation. *Am. J. Respir. Crit. Care Med.* 182, 627–632. doi: 10.1164/rccm.200909-1421OC

Saville, B. R., and Berry, S. M. (2016). Efficiencies of platform clinical trials: a vision of the future. *Clin. Trials* 13, 358–366. doi: 10.1177/1740774515626362

Saville, B. R., Connor, J. T., Ayers, G. D., and Alvarez, J. (2014). The utility of Bayesian predictive probabilities for interim monitoring of clinical trials. *Clin. Trials* 11, 485–493. doi: 10.1177/1740774514531352

Stanojevic, S., and Ratjen, F. (2016). Physiologic endpoints for clinical studies for cystic fibrosis. *J. Cyst. Fibros* 15, 416–423. doi: 10.1016/j.jcf.2016.05.014

Stenbit, A. E., and Flume, P. A. (2011). Pulmonary exacerbations in cystic fibrosis. *Curr. Opin. Pulm. Med.* 17, 442–447. doi: 10.1097/MCP.0b013e32834b8c04

Stephenson, A. L., Sykes, J., Stanojevic, S., Quon, B. S., Marshall, B. C., Petren, K., et al. (2017). Survival comparison of patients with cystic fibrosis in canada and the united states: a population-based cohort study. *Ann. Intern. Med.* 166, 537–546. doi: 10.7326/M16-0858

Szentpetery, S., and Flume, P. A. (2018). Optimizing outcomes of pulmonary exacerbations in cystic fibrosis. *Curr. Opin. Pulm. Med.* 24, 606–611. doi: 10.1097/MCP.0000000000000519

Tunney, M. M., Klem, E. R., Fodor, A. A., Gilpin, D. F., Moriarty, T. F., McGrath, S. J., et al. (2011). Use of culture and molecular analysis to determine the effect of antibiotic treatment on microbial community diversity and abundance during exacerbation in patients with cystic fibrosis. *Thorax* 66, 579–584. doi: 10.1136/thx.2010.137281

Waters, V., Stanojevic, S., Klingel, M., Chiang, J., Sonneveld, N., Kukkar, R., et al. (2015). Prolongation of antibiotic treatment for cystic fibrosis pulmonary exacerbations. *J. Cyst. Fibros* 14, 770–776. doi: 10.1016/j.jcf.2015.07.010

Waters, V., Stanojevic, S., and Ratjen, F. (2016). Special considerations for the treatment of pulmonary exacerbations in children with cystic fibrosis. *Expert. Rev. Respir. Med.* doi: 10.1080/17476348.2017.1246963 [Epub ahead of print].

West, N. E., Beckett, V. V., Jain, R., Sanders, D. B., Nick, J. A., Heltshe, S. L., et al. (2017). Standardized treatment of pulmonary exacerbations (STOP) study: physician treatment practices and outcomes for individuals with cystic fibrosis with pulmonary exacerbations. *J. Cyst. Fibros* 16, 600–606. doi: 10.1016/j.jcf.2017.04.003

Woodcock, J., and LaVange, L. M. (2017). Master protocols to study multiple therapies, multiple diseases, or both. *N. Engl. J. Med.* 377, 62–70. doi: 10.1056/NEJMra1510062

17

Gene Therapy for Cystic Fibrosis Lung Disease: Overcoming the Barriers to Translation to the Clinic

Martin Donnelley[1,2,3] and David W. Parsons[1,2,3]*

[1] Robinson Research Institute, University of Adelaide, Adelaide, SA, Australia, [2] Adelaide Medical School, University of Adelaide, Adelaide, SA, Australia, [3] Respiratory and Sleep Medicine, Women's and Children's Hospital, North Adelaide, SA, Australia

***Correspondence:**
Martin Donnelley
martin.donnelley@adelaide.edu.au

Cystic fibrosis (CF) is a progressive, chronic and debilitating genetic disease caused by mutations in the CF Transmembrane-Conductance Regulator (*CFTR*) gene. Unrelenting airway disease begins in infancy and produces a steady deterioration in quality of life, ultimately leading to premature death. While life expectancy has improved, current treatments for CF are neither preventive nor curative. Since the discovery of *CFTR* the vision of correcting the underlying genetic defect – not just treating the symptoms – has been developed to where it is poised to become a transformative technology. Addition of a properly functioning *CFTR* gene into defective airway cells is the only biologically rational way to prevent or treat CF airway disease for *all CFTR* mutation classes. While new gene editing approaches hold exciting promise, airway gene-addition therapy remains the most encouraging therapeutic approach for CF. However, early work has not yet progressed to large-scale clinical trials. For clinical trials to begin in earnest the field must demonstrate that gene therapies are safe in CF lungs; can provide clear health benefits and alter the course of lung disease; can be repeatedly dosed to boost effect; and can be scaled effectively from small animal models into human-sized lungs. Demonstrating the durability of these effects demands relevant CF animal models and accurate and reliable techniques to measure benefit. In this review, illustrated with data from our own studies, we outline recent technological developments and discuss these key questions that we believe must be answered to progress CF airway gene-addition therapies to clinical trials.

Keywords: Cystic fibrosis, rat, mouse, airway, lung, genetic therapies, gene-addition, lobe-targeted delivery

INTRODUCTION

Cystic fibrosis (CF) is an insidious disease that slowly smothers the health and potential of too many young lives. It is the most common fatal genetic disease in the developed world; 1 in 25–30 people with Caucasian ancestry carry a single defective copy of the *CFTR* gene (Cystic Fibrosis Foundation, 2018) and have no symptoms; 1 in ~3000 babies are born with mutations on both alleles, resulting in the disease. CF is a multisystem disease that affects many organs, producing a life expectancy of approximately 40 years (Australian Cystic Fibrosis Data Registry, 2016). Premature death usually results from lung disease, after a lifetime struggling to deal with progressive respiratory failure.

New mutation-specific modulator and corrector pharmaceuticals such as Kalydeco (ivacaftor), Orkambi (lumacaftor/ ivacaftor), and Symdeko (tezacaftor/ ivacaftor) have given substantial benefit to some people with CF. Assuming a patient has the right *CFTR* mutation class, these personalized medicines can increase the presence and/or function of the CFTR protein in the cell, improve lung function, and slow lung disease progression. However, they have been neither preventive nor curative since they do not address the *CFTR* gene defect itself, and some have limited effectiveness. Importantly, the cost of these once-daily medications is prohibitive and likely to be unsustainable, with the health systems in several countries declining to recommend Orkambi for governmental financial support due to poor cost-benefit.

Since CF is a recessive genetic disorder, addition of a single copy of the properly functioning *CFTR* gene into affected CF airway cells is recognized as the only rational and feasible way to prevent or treat CF airway disease (Griesenbach et al., 2016). Gene therapy would provide proper cellular function, regardless of the person's *CFTR* mutation class. The vision for a child born with CF is that treatment with a proven *CFTR* gene-addition therapy at birth would prevent that child ever developing CF lung disease. For those already living with CF, the same therapy would halt progression of their lung disease.

Gene therapies for a range of inherited diseases have now reached the clinic in China (Kim et al., 2008), Europe (Touchot and Flume, 2017), and most recently in the United States where Luxturna, a gene-addition treatment for retinal dystrophy (Russell et al., 2017) was approved by the FDA in Dec 2017 as a prescription medicine (Morrison, 2018). To 2017, there have been almost 2600 gene therapy trials, including 36 for CF (Ginn et al., 2018). Gene therapy is now a therapeutic reality for some genetic diseases, but the challenge for the CF field is to convert the extensive preclinical developments into an effective and safe treatment option for people with CF.

DEVELOPMENTS IN AIRWAY GENE TRANSFER TECHNIQUES

Although gene therapy has the potential to be efficacious for CF, a range of challenges have been identified. Here we describe those challenges and their solutions.

Vector Designs Affect Efficacy

A 12-month, monthly repeat-dose Phase II *CFTR* non-viral (liposome) gene-transfer clinical trial showed significant, albeit modest and transient, lung function benefits in CF patients (Alton et al., 2015). That study confirmed that a *CFTR* gene therapy can correct human CF lung disease, is likely to be safe, have low immunogenicity, and be amenable to repeated dosing. However, due to the poor efficiency and transient response, that group has since concentrated their development efforts on a more efficient lentiviral (LV) gene vector (Alton et al., 2017). Recently, the delivery of *CFTR* mRNA using nanoparticles has been shown to improve chloride channel function in CF mice for 2 weeks, with a superior response compared to liposomal delivery (Robinson et al., 2018). However, the short duration of action may be a barrier to adoption.

Initial CF gene-addition research used adeno- (Ad) and adeno-associated viruses (AAV) as the gene vectors, but these failed the clinical transition process for CF lung disease due to significant side-effects, and/or lack of efficacy and duration (Moss et al., 2007). AAV also has a DNA packaging capacity limit that requires truncation of the CFTR gene, and AAV vector genomes remain largely episomal (not integrated), meaning that gene transfer to terminally differentiated airway cells is transient and rapidly lost with airway cell turnover (Karda et al., 2016). Despite these challenges [well described by Guggino and Cebotaru (2017)] AAV vector development is continuing, including the assessment of alternative serotypes (Steines et al., 2016; Guggino et al., 2017; Duncan et al., 2018). Interestingly, an integrating *piggyBac*/Ad *CFTR* vector was recently shown to phenotypically correct CF pig airways, with the possibility that it could produce extended gene expression (Cooney et al., 2018).

Lentiviral vectors are now one of the lead CF airway gene-addition vectors for therapeutic development because they transduce dividing and non-dividing cells, can be pseudotyped to target specific cell types by altering surface receptor recognition elements, integrate into the host cell chromosome providing lasting benefit, and generate little immune response. LV vectors have been effective in a range of preclinical studies (Copreni et al., 2004; Cmielewski et al., 2014a; Cooney et al., 2016; Alton et al., 2017). Supported by the clinical successes in effectiveness and safety within *ex vivo* CAR-T cell therapies in cancer treatment (Milone and O'Doherty, 2018), we believe that LV vectors are currently the *CFTR* delivery vehicle of choice. The remainder of this article focuses specifically on the barriers of translating LV gene vectors for CF to the clinic.

Physical and Biological Barriers of the Airway Surface Restrict Gene Delivery

The airway epithelium has evolved to protect cells against foreign invaders such as viruses and bacteria. The normal physical host defenses at the airway surface play a leading role in limiting the efficiency of any type of gene transfer into the airway epithelium (Kim et al., 2016). Mucus that covers the epithelial surface traps vector particles, which are then removed from the airway by mucociliary clearance (MCC) efficiently preventing vector particles from reaching vector-relevant receptors on the cell membrane surface (Castellani and Conese, 2010). This situation is exacerbated in CF due to the increased volume and viscosity of the mucus (Duncan et al., 2016). Finally, for vectors designed to target the airway stem cells, known to be a subpopulation of airway basal cells at the deep-lying epithelial basement membrane (Rock et al., 2009), access past the epithelial tight junctions is also needed. These tight junctions separate the luminal surface from the deeper layers, acting as a normal defense against pathogenic particles.

Gene vectors must be able to penetrate the CF mucus barrier and reach the underlying target epithelium and target cells. One recognized approach that enables gene vector particles to reach the relevant airway-surface cell vesicular stomatitis virus (VSV-G) receptors and the basal stem cells, is conditioning the airway epithelium with the compound lysophosphatidylcholine (LPC) prior to gene vector delivery. LPC is a normal component of lung surfactant, and its primary role is to transiently permeabilize airway tight-junctions, and it may also help to solubilize surface mucus and enable greater vector access to airway cells. *In vivo* acute and long-term reporter gene studies have shown the effectiveness of LPC conditioning for enhancing gene expression in mice (Limberis et al., 2002; Stocker et al., 2009; Cmielewski et al., 2014a, 2017). In addition, successful gene expression using the LacZ reporter gene has been achieved in short-term (7 day) studies, transducing the conducting airways in sheep (Liu et al., 2010) (a large lung model), marmosets (Farrow et al., 2013) (a primate model), ferrets (Cmielewski et al., 2014b), and rats (McIntyre et al., 2018).

Reporter gene expression is predominantly in ciliated cells, but the LV vector also reaches the alveolar space where type I and II cells and macrophages are transduced. LPC airway conditioning has enabled transduction of endogenous adult airway stem cells (Farrow et al., 2018), confirming the mechanistic basis for stem-cell-based durable *in vivo* gene expression. These studies showed the potential for life-long replenishment of therapeutic benefit via the emergence of cell lineages that were corrected *in situ* by the purposely transduced airway stem cells. LV vectors can also robustly transduce human airway basal cells *in vitro* (Farrow et al., 2018), and human air liquid interface (ALI) cultures, supporting applicability to human airways.

While much understanding can be gleaned from reporter gene studies, the gene transfer methods must also be demonstrated to effectively alter a CF airway, by delivering the *CFTR* gene. Previous studies have shown that LV vectors can partially correct CFTR function in CF mouse nasal airways (the only site of measurable CF airway functional pathophysiology in mice) (Limberis et al., 2002; Stocker et al., 2009; Cmielewski et al., 2014a). Improvement was significant and extended for at least 12 months after the single *CFTR* vector dose, validating the strength and persistence of benefit possible with a LV vector.

The efficacy of LPC enhancement is also not limited to LV vectors. Helper adenoviral vector studies in pigs have showed strong and extensively distributed reporter gene transfer, with no systemic toxicity or infection reported from use of the combined LPC-hAdv vector aerosol (Cao et al., 2013). However, the key question from these studies remains: can a *CFTR* gene-addition process improve the course of disease in a CF lung?

Suitability of CF Animal Models for CFTR Gene Therapy Research

A range of CF animal models have been developed, with the mouse, pig, ferret and rat the most well characterized (Lavelle et al., 2016; McCarron et al., 2018). Small animal models are ideal for developing gene-addition techniques for CF for cost and handling reasons, and the gene vector volume required to treat the lungs is modest facilitating large well-powered studies. Although many CF mouse models have been developed, the *CFTR* Null mouse does not exhibit lung disease, and the β-ENaC mouse is not suitable for gene-addition therapy development because its lungs contain functional CFTR. The pig (Meyerholz, 2016) and ferret (Sun et al., 2014) models recapitulate human lung disease but exhibit severe gut disease (Meyerholz et al., 2010; Sun et al., 2010) that necessitates intensive husbandry requirements with associated high costs. Lung gene vector dosing requirements prohibit extensive testing in the pig.

Our group recently used CRISPR/Cas9 gene-editing to create colonies of Phe508del (Class II) and 512X CF (Class I) rats (McIntyre et al., 2017). Hallmark CF pathophysiology is consistent with the United States CF rat (Tuggle et al., 2014; Birket et al., 2018), with frequent severe gut obstruction and increased gut motility, as well as poorly developed vas deferens, seminal vesicles & epididymis. As in humans, the phenotype of these two mutations is different. Both have higher mortality than wild-type, with the 512X rats having higher pre- and post-weaning mortality than the Phe508del. Both have a lower average body weight compared to wild-type, although this effect appears to be more pronounced in male animals.

Nasal-airway potential difference (PD) measurements have confirmed altered CFTR airway function in both models. The 512X rats have no response, or a weak response to a chloride-free environment that is consistent with classically defective CFTR function. The Phe508del animals are also significantly different to heterozygote/normal rats, but with an intermediate response consistent with the presence of residual CFTR function seen in the human Phe508del mutation. Since our treatment focus is CF *lung* disease, we are investigating methods of performing PD measurements in the trachea and/or deeper airways, as is possible in humans (Davies et al., 2005), as a method for tracking functional CFTR changes in the CF rat lung.

Improvements in Airway and Lung Function Must Be Measured

Measuring the effects of airway gene therapies on lung and airway health has been a major challenge for all CF research groups, with CFTR channel function typically assessed using transepithelial potential difference measurements, along with Ussing chamber and halide assays. However, these techniques all have limitations, particularly for *in vivo* use in animal models. Fortunately, Phase Contrast X-ray Imaging (PCXI) based approaches have recently been demonstrated to be able to directly measure airway and lung health *in vivo*.

Phase Contrast X-ray Imaging utilizes X-ray refraction to achieve high spatial and temporal resolution as well as excellent airway and lung soft tissue contrast, and has the potential to dramatically reduce radiation doses (Kitchen et al., 2017). Using PCXI it is now possible to measure changes in airway surface liquid (ASL) depth following treatment (Siu et al., 2008; Morgan et al., 2013, 2016), as well as the clearance of micron-sized marker particles on the airway surface by mucociliary clearance (MCC) (Donnelley et al., 2012a,b, 2014, 2017; Gradl et al., 2018). ASL depth and MCC are the two key airway physiological parameters that must show rapid beneficial changes if a CF airway gene therapy is to be considered effective.

Phase Contrast X-ray Imaging -based analyses have now also been developed to provide quantitative measurement of lung function, taking the focus away from the requirement to use qualitative assessment of structure (i.e., via CT imaging) to *infer* function. Structural changes that occur with CF lung disease alter the flow of air in the lung and the regional patterns of lung motion, whether by obstruction that increases airway resistance, or by changes to the lung parenchyma that alter the mechanical properties of the tissue. It follows that abnormal motion of lung regions during respiration is an accurate indicator of disease (Fouras et al., 2012). Lung motion can be tracked by combining velocimetry techniques with the enhanced airway contrast offered by PCXI. This technique can perform pinpoint spirometry – a method referred to as 4DxV – and was developed and validated in β-ENaC mice at the SPring-8 synchrotron (Stahr et al., 2016). It allows local ventilation to be quantitatively measured at every point in the lung, enabling *local* treatment effects to be assessed. The 4DxV imaging methods can now be used in rat lungs at the Imaging and Medical Beamline at the Australian Synchrotron (Murrie et al., 2015), with commercially available turnkey systems now available (4Dx, Melbourne, VIC, Australia).

With long-lived and easily maintained CF rats now available, and the ability to measure changes in airway surface and lung health in only those lung regions that are treated, it is now possible to quantify the short- and long-term effects of contained, local-region dosing of a gene therapy to the lungs of a living CF animal model, without the need for post-mortem lung analyses.

Scalable Vector Production and Precision Delivery Capabilities Are Essential

Translating this gene-addition technology to humans requires larger gene vector volumes, but there are a range of challenges associated with upscaling LV vector production (McCarron et al., 2016). Common methods currently employ adherent cell cultures using cell-factories (Rout-Pitt et al., 2018), however, packed-bed bioreactor approaches can now also yield unconcentrated titres of 10^5–10^6 TU/ml. Once concentrated and purified for *in vivo* use titres in our laboratory are 10^8–10^9 TU/ml. Commercially available, suspension-based production methods such as the LV-MAX™ LV Production System (Gibco) have the potential for scalable production in stirred-tank bioreactors and are animal component-free, important characteristics for establishing LV manufacturing methods for future clinical use (McCarron et al., 2016). In our laboratory unconcentrated LV-MAX™ titres are already greater than 10^6 TU/ml and are easily scalable to human-sized lung doses by using larger bioreactor vessels. However, until stable packaging cell lines can be used, a major barrier to transient transfection systems remains the production of large quantities of plasmid DNA.

To translate successful preclinical developments into humans it is important to determine whether viral gene therapy techniques developed in small animal models are readily translatable to a human-sized lung. Although intended to be beneficial, these LV gene-addition therapies are deliberately designed to induce permanent genetic alterations. It is the authors' opinion that the first LV CF gene vector trials in humans will be accompanied by a heightened level of caution compared to new transient-effect daily pharmaceuticals. We propose that the first lung gene-addition trials with viral vectors in humans must be performed bronchoscopically, to enable precise gene delivery and to examine the gene vector effects in a specific limited region of the lung. This method offers an "exit strategy" – by wedge or lobe excision – should a treatment unexpectedly produce unresolvable or unacceptable serious adverse events. However, until recently this strategy could not be tested in small animal models because bronchoscopic delivery was not possible.

The ability to accurately and precisely deliver fluid doses to a small region of the lung has been almost impossible in small animals such as rats and mice due to the small size of their airways. However, the first reliable bronchoscopic dosing technique that can target pre-selected regions of the rat lung was recently reported (McIntyre et al., 2018), and is based on a 1.1 mm diameter rigid sialendoscope normally used for human salivary duct procedures. This miniature bronchoscope system has light, video vision, two access channels, and can be used to dose fluid into at least the fourth-generation branches of the rat airway in ~200 gram rats. That study showed that rats lungs are amenable to reporter gene delivery and expression at a similar level and with similar cell type distributions across nasal and lung regions as found in mouse studies. *LacZ* expression was present in ciliated and goblet / secretory cells, the two most relevant cell populations on the conducting-airway surface epithelium. However, unlike nasal or tracheal delivery, bronchoscopic delivery limited transduction to only the treated lung lobe/region.

Together, bronchoscopic dosing and bioreactor production methods allow the developments in small animal models to be easily scaled to the levels required for translational to human clinical trials.

THE MAIN CHALLENGES FOR THE FIELD

An effective gene-addition therapy for CF lung disease requires accurate compound delivery to the target location, high levels of transduction, and effective CFTR protein expression in the cells relevant to CF disease. Reliable and relevant measurements of the benefit to the treated region, as well as the whole lung, are essential. However, several challenges remain before genetic therapies for CF lung disease can be translated to the clinic.

Gene Therapy Efficacy Should Be Validated in a CF Lung

The ability of a viral gene-addition vector to adequately modify CF lung disease health and progression has never been demonstrated, but it is the authors' opinion that this is essential prior to human clinical trials. Certainly, the effectiveness of *CFTR* gene-addition *per se* has been validated clinically by the UK CF Gene Therapy Consortium (Alton et al., 2015), and that group has undertaken extensive preparation for clinical trials of lung *CFTR* gene-addition using a SIV LV vector. Although the consortium has not yet reported *in vivo* CFTR functional improvements in a CF animal model, they have approval for human trials (Alton et al., 2017). Similarly, the Iowa United States CF gene therapy research group have used uninfected neonatal CF pigs to examine LV-*CFTR* gene transfer efficacy, but the absence of suitable outcome measures (as described in the previous section) meant that the CF pigs were necessarily humanely killed 2 weeks later for lung-tissue analysis (Cooney et al., 2016). The ability to perform localized delivery of LV-*CFTR* into a diseased CF rat lung, combined with non-invasive PCXI based assessments is expected to enable the first-ever *in vivo* long-duration testing of LV gene addition therapy for CF lung disease. Future long-term studies should also assess survival differences produced by *CFTR* gene-addition, to estimate the likely human therapeutic benefit.

The Safety Profile of LPC and LV Must Be Demonstrated in a CF Lung

The power of gene therapy was illustrated following clinical trials using first generation γ-retroviral vectors, which successfully treated genetic disorders such as SCID-X1. However, they resulted in serious adverse events such as acute lymphoblastic leukemia due to viral promoters that upregulated proto-oncogenes lying close to the integration site (Hacein-Bey-Abina et al., 2008; Howe et al., 2008). LV vectors were subsequently redesigned to improve their safety profile. Those modifications included reducing the amount of native HIV genome in the vector and modifying the viral long terminal repeat (LTR) to remove endogenous viral promoter sequences to render the vectors replication deficient (Yu et al., 1986; Dull et al., 1998). Finally, the viral components required for replication were separated onto separate plasmids and delivered *in trans*. Nonetheless, comprehensive integration site analyses remain essential for vectors destined for clinical trials.

The safety of airway conditioning compounds must also be established. LPC action is transient, dose-controllable, and well-tolerated in *in vivo* animal studies. Despite demonstrating that LPC enables effective gene-addition and is well-tolerated in multiple animal species, it is not known whether the desired transient tight-junction permeabilization in a CF airway, where infective bacteria are normally present, may bring unacceptable risks. Potentially allowing those pathogens access to normally protected sub-surface regions, raises the possibility of additional local or even systemic infections to occur. The theoretical dangers of altering airway barrier function, even transiently, in the infective milieu of a CF lung are obvious. However, LPC has a convincing preclinical history of safe use, so the potential of airway conditioning and gene-addition therapy in humans with CF must not simply be dismissed as too risky in the absence of any evidence. The rule *primum nil nocere,* first do no harm (Smith, 2005), which drives much of the bioethics of medicine, it is not an absolute. For example, acceptance of the harm, pain, and risk from myeloablative conditioning is accepted as an essential conditioning procedure for bone marrow transplantation. These important questions related to the acceptability of airway / lung conditioning are yet to be answered.

Methods to Increase Gene Expression Levels Must Be Developed

The ability to achieve reporter or *CFTR* gene transfer using LV vectors has previously been established, with *in situ* transduction of resident airway basal cells that replenish the airway with transgene-expressing daughter cells the likely basis for this long-term expression. However, in most mice gene expression eventually wanes, and in some reduces to zero after only 6-months (Cmielewski et al., 2014a). This data, and the inherent uncertainties of translating *in vivo* mouse data to a human disease, suggests that it may be beneficial or necessary to produce higher levels of gene expression through initial multi-dosing, or by repeat-dosing if gene expression wanes. However, a host immune response directed against the gene transfer agent may block initial gene expression and/or prevent expression arising from repeated doses. Few studies have examined strategies for effectively re-administering LV vectors to the airways.

Feline immunodeficiency virus (FIV) and simian immunodeficiency virus (SIV) LV vectors have been successfully re-administered to the airways without loss of effectiveness, suggesting LV vectors may evade adaptive immune responses (Sinn et al., 2008; Griesenbach et al., 2012). These vectors were pseudotyped with the GP64 and F/HN envelopes, respectively, which both target receptors located on the apical surface of the airway, so they are unlikely to be able to reach or transduce the basal stem cells located on the basolateral airway surface. The SIV study showed repeat dosing was feasible but did not increase transgene expression. These studies also highlighted that expression levels are highly dependent on the dose timing and the choice of transgene delivered at each dose. The knowledge that patients will continue to benefit from additional doses will revolutionize CF airway gene therapy and pathways to clinical trials.

Dosing Methods Need to Be Optimized in Human-Sized Lungs

The ability to dose human sized lungs must also be established early. Human lungs are substantially larger than in small animal models. They are also differently developed and branched, and cell type distributions and proportions along the conducting airways where CF pathophysiology begins are different. Confirming the feasibility and effectiveness of LV gene-addition techniques in human-sized lungs, such as in pigs or sheep, along with the necessary vector production requirements, is of vital importance.

CONCLUSION

While expensive daily drug-based options for treating the downstream effects of the *CFTR* gene defect are emerging, gene-addition therapies are the only approach with the immediate potential to prevent or halt CF lung disease. Although treatment for pancreatic insufficiency, CF related diabetes and other CF associated pathologies will still be required, by dealing with the fundamental gene defect at its source within airway cells, airway gene therapy can be expected to transform the treatment options for CF lung disease.

A range of proven LV gene vectors and adequate novel vector production techniques have been developed. LPC and LV gene-addition techniques have already been validated in multiple animal models. The production of new animal models such as the CF rat will enable significant advances in CF translational capability, with bronchoscopic delivery techniques able to dose individual lobes of the rat lung. Innovative new non-invasive PCXI-based measurements of airway and lung function can now be used to complement standard measurement techniques.

It is the authors' opinions that key questions that must be answered before airway gene therapy can be translated to the clinic involve clearly demonstrating long-term efficacy and the safety of LPC and LV delivery in a CF lung, the ability to re-dose to boost *CFTR* gene expression levels, and the ability to translate these techniques into human-sized lungs. Together the new capabilities described here will allow these key questions that will enable the translation of airway gene therapy to humans to be answered.

AUTHOR CONTRIBUTIONS

DP and MD contributed to the conception and design of the work and wrote the manuscript.

FUNDING

MD was supported by a Robinson Research Institute Career Development Fellowship. Studies supported by NHMRC Project Grants GNT1079712, GNT1098127, and GNT1160011, grants from the United States CF Foundation, a Fay Fuller Foundation Discovery Grant, CF South Australia, the Women's and Children's Hospital Foundation, and the Cure 4 CF Foundation.

ACKNOWLEDGMENTS

X-ray imaging research was undertaken on the Imaging and Medical Beamline at the Australian Synchrotron, beamline 20XU at the SPring-8 Synchrotron, and at the Munich Compact Light Source. The authors thank Kaye Morgan, Patricia Cmielewski, Nigel Farrow, Juliette Delhove, Alexandra McCarron, Nathan Rout-Pitt and Chantelle McIntyre for their assistance with the studies and their helpful contributions to this paper.

REFERENCES

Alton, E., Armstrong, D. K., Ashby, D., Bayfield, K. J., Bilton, D., Bloomfield, E. V., et al. (2015). Repeated nebulisation of non-viral CFTR gene therapy in patients with cystic fibrosis: a randomised, double-blind, placebo-controlled, phase 2b trial. *Lancet Respir. Med.* 3, 684–691. doi: 10.1016/S2213-2600(15)00245-3

Alton, E. W., Beekman, J. M., Boyd, A. C., Brand, J., Carlon, M. S., Connolly, M. M., et al. (2017). Preparation for a first-in-man lentivirus trial in patients with cystic fibrosis. *Thorax* 72, 137–147. doi: 10.1136/thoraxjnl-2016-208406

Australian Cystic Fibrosis Data Registry (2016). *Australian Cystic Fibrosis Data Registry Annual Report, 2015.* Available at: http://shop.cysticfibrosis.org.au/data-registry

Birket, S. E., Davis, J. M., Fernandez, C. M., Tuggle, K. L., Oden, A. M., Chu, K. K., et al. (2018). Development of an airway mucus defect in the cystic fibrosis rat. *JCI Insight* 3:97199. doi: 10.1172/jci.insight.97199

Cao, H., Machuca, T. N., Yeung, J. C., Wu, J., Du, K., Duan, C., et al. (2013). Efficient gene delivery to pig airway epithelia and submucosal glands using helper-dependent adenoviral vectors. *Mol. Ther. Nucleic Acids* 2:e127. doi: 10.1038/mtna.2013.55

Castellani, S., and Conese, M. (2010). Lentiviral vectors and cystic fibrosis gene therapy. *Viruses* 2, 395–412. doi: 10.3390/v2020395

Cmielewski, P., Donnelley, M., and Parsons, D. W. (2014a). Long-term therapeutic and reporter gene expression in lentiviral vector treated cystic fibrosis mice. *J. Gene Med.* 16, 291–299. doi: 10.1002/jgm.2778

Cmielewski, P., Farrow, N., Donnelley, M., McIntyre, C., Penny-Dimri, J., Kuchel, T., et al. (2014b). Transduction of ferret airway epithelia using a pre-treatment and lentiviral gene vector. *BMC Pulm Med.* 14:183. doi: 10.1186/1471-2466-14-183

Cmielewski, P., Farrow, N., Devereux, S., Parsons, D., and Donnelley, M. (2017). Gene therapy for Cystic Fibrosis: improved delivery techniques and conditioning with lysophosphatidylcholine enhance lentiviral gene transfer in mouse lung airways. *Exp. Lung Res.* 43, 426–433. doi: 10.1080/01902148.2017.1395931

Cooney, A. L., Abou Alaiwa, M. H., Shah, V. S., Bouzek, D. C., Stroik, M. R., Powers, L. S., et al. (2016). Lentiviral-mediated phenotypic correction of cystic fibrosis pigs. *JCI Insight* 1:e88730. doi: 10.1172/jci.insight.88730

Cooney, A. L., Singh, B. K., Loza, L. M., Thornell, I. M., Hippee, C. E., Powers, L. S., et al. (2018). Widespread airway distribution and short-term phenotypic correction of cystic fibrosis pigs following aerosol delivery of piggyBac/adenovirus. *Nucleic Acids Res.* 46, 9591–9600. doi: 10.1093/nar/gky773

Copreni, E., Penzo, M., Carrabino, S., and Conese, M. (2004). Lentivirus-mediated gene transfer to the respiratory epithelium: a promising approach to gene therapy of cystic fibrosis. *Gene Ther.* 11(Suppl. 1), S67–S75. doi: 10.1038/sj.gt.3302372

Cystic Fibrosis Foundation (2018). *What is CF?* Availbale at: https://www.cff.org/What-is-CF/About-Cystic-Fibrosis/

Davies, J. C., Davies, M., McShane, D., Smith, S., Chadwick, S., Jaffe, A., et al. (2005). Potential difference measurements in the lower airway of children with and without cystic fibrosis. *Am. J. Respir. Crit. Care Med.* 171, 1015–1019. doi: 10.1164/rccm.200408-1116OC

Donnelley, M., Morgan, K. S., Awadalla, M., Farrow, N. R., Hall, C., and Parsons, D. W. (2017). High-resolution mucociliary transport measurement in live excised large animal trachea using synchrotron X-ray imaging. *Respir. Res.* 18:95. doi: 10.1186/s12931-017-0573-2

Donnelley, M., Morgan, K. S., Siu, K. K., Farrow, N. R., Stahr, C. S., Boucher, R. C., et al. (2014). Non-invasive airway health assessment: synchrotron imaging reveals effects of rehydrating treatments on mucociliary transit in-vivo. *Sci. Rep.* 4:3689. doi: 10.1038/srep03689

Donnelley, M., Morgan, K. S., Siu, K. K., and Parsons, D. W. (2012a). Dry deposition of pollutant and marker particles onto live mouse airway surfaces enhances monitoring of individual particle mucociliary transit behaviour. *J. Synchrotron. Radiat.* 19(Pt 4), 551–558. doi: 10.1107/S0909049512018250

Donnelley, M., Siu, K. K., Jamison, R. A., and Parsons, D. W. (2012b). Synchrotron phase-contrast X-ray imaging reveals fluid dosing dynamics for gene transfer into mouse airways. *Gene Ther.* 19, 8–14. doi: 10.1038/gt.2011.80

Dull, T., Zufferey, R., Kelly, M., Mandel, R. J., Nguyen, M., Trono, D., et al. (1998). A third-generation lentivirus vector with a conditional packaging system. *J. Virol.* 72, 8463–8471.

Duncan, G. A., Jung, J., Hanes, J., and Suk, J. S. (2016). The mucus barrier to inhaled gene therapy. *Mol. Ther.* 24, 2043–2053. doi: 10.1038/mt.2016.182

Duncan, G. A., Kim, N., Colon-Cortes, Y., Rodriguez, J., Mazur, M., Birket, S. E., et al. (2018). An adeno-associated viral vector capable of penetrating the mucus barrier to inhaled gene therapy. *Mol. Ther. Methods Clin. Dev.* 9, 296–304. doi: 10.1016/j.omtm.2018.03.006

Farrow, N., Donnelley, M., Cmielewski, P., Roscioli, E., Rout-Pitt, N., McIntyre, C., et al. (2018). Role of basal cells in producing persistent lentivirus-mediated airway gene expression. *Hum. Gene Ther.* 29, 653–662. doi: 10.1089/hum.2017.059

Farrow, N., Miller, D., Cmielewski, P., Donnelley, M., Bright, R., and Parsons, D. W. (2013). Airway gene transfer in a non-human primate: lentiviral gene expression in marmoset lungs. *Sci. Rep.* 3:1287. doi: 10.1038/srep01287

Fouras, A., Allison, B. J., Kitchen, M. J., Dubsky, S., Nguyen, J., Hourigan, K., et al. (2012). Altered lung motion is a sensitive indicator of regional lung disease. *Ann. Biomed. Eng.* 40, 1160–1169. doi: 10.1007/s10439-011-0493-0

Ginn, S. L., Amaya, A. K., Alexander, I. E., Edelstein, M., and Abedi, M. R. (2018). Gene therapy clinical trials worldwide to 2017: an update. *J. Gene Med.* 20:e3015. doi: 10.1002/jgm.3015

Gradl, R., Dierolf, M., Gunther, B., Hehn, L., Moller, W., Kutschke, D., et al. (2018). In vivo dynamic phase-contrast X-ray imaging using a compact light source. *Sci. Rep.* 8:6788. doi: 10.1038/s41598-018-24763-8

Griesenbach, U., Davies, J. C., and Alton, E. (2016). Cystic fibrosis gene therapy: a mutation-independent treatment. *Curr. Opin. Pulm. Med.* 22, 602–609. doi: 10.1097/MCP.0000000000000327

Griesenbach, U., Inoue, M., Meng, C., Farley, R., Chan, M., Newman, N. K., et al. (2012). Assessment of F/HN-pseudotyped lentivirus as a clinically relevant vector for lung gene therapy. *Am. J. Respir. Crit. Care Med.* 186, 846–856. doi: 10.1164/rccm.201206-1056OC

Guggino, W. B., Benson, J., Seagrave, J., Yan, Z., Engelhardt, J., Gao, G., et al. (2017). A preclinical study in rhesus macaques for cystic fibrosis to assess gene transfer and transduction by AAV1 and AAV5 with a dual-luciferase reporter system. *Hum. Gene Ther. Clin. Dev.* 28, 145–156. doi: 10.1089/humc.2017.067

Guggino, W. B., and Cebotaru, L. (2017). Adeno-associated Virus (AAV) gene therapy for cystic fibrosis: current barriers and recent developments. *Expert Opin. Biol. Ther.* 17, 1265–1273. doi: 10.1080/14712598.2017.1347630

Hacein-Bey-Abina, S., Garrigue, A., Wang, G. P., Soulier, J., Lim, A., Morillon, E., et al. (2008). Insertional oncogenesis in 4 patients after retrovirus-mediated gene therapy of SCID-X1. *J. Clin. Invest.* 118, 3132–3142. doi: 10.1172/JCI35700

Howe, S. J., Mansour, M. R., Schwarzwaelder, K., Bartholomae, C., Hubank, M., Kempski, H., et al. (2008). Insertional mutagenesis combined with acquired somatic mutations causes leukemogenesis following gene therapy of SCID-X1 patients. *J. Clin. Invest.* 118, 3143–3150. doi: 10.1172/JCI35798

Karda, R., Buckley, S. M. K., and Waddington, S. N. (2016). Gene therapy with adeno-associated virus for cystic fibrosis. *Am. J. Respir. Crit. Care Med.* 193, 234–236. doi: 10.1164/rccm.201510-2024ED

Kim, N., Duncan, G. A., Hanes, J., and Suk, J. S. (2016). Barriers to inhaled gene therapy of obstructive lung diseases: a review. *J. Control. Release* 240, 465–488. doi: 10.1016/j.jconrel.2016.05.031

Kim, S., Peng, Z., and Kaneda, Y. (2008). Current status of gene therapy in Asia. *Mol. Ther.* 16, 237–243. doi: 10.1038/sj.mt.6300336

Kitchen, M. J., Buckley, G. A., Gureyev, T. E., Wallace, M. J., Andres-Thio, N., Uesugi, K., et al. (2017). CT dose reduction factors in the thousands using X-ray phase contrast. *Sci. Rep.* 7:15953. doi: 10.1038/s41598-017-16264-x

Lavelle, G. M., White, M. M., Browne, N., McElvaney, N. G., and Reeves, E. P. (2016). Animal models of cystic fibrosis pathology: phenotypic parallels and divergences. *BioMed. Res. Int.* 2016, 1–14. doi: 10.1155/2016/5258727

Limberis, M., Anson, D. S., Fuller, M., and Parsons, D. W. (2002). Recovery of airway cystic fibrosis transmembrane conductance regulator function in mice with cystic fibrosis after single-dose lentivirus-mediated gene transfer. *Hum. Gene Ther.* 13, 1961–1970. doi: 10.1089/10430340260355365

Liu, C., Wong, E., Miller, D., Smith, G., Anson, D., and Parsons, D. (2010). Lentiviral airway gene transfer in lungs of mice and sheep: successes and challenges. *J. Gene Med.* 12, 647–658. doi: 10.1002/jgm.1481

McCarron, A., Donnelley, M., McIntyre, C., and Parsons, D. (2016). Challenges of up-scaling lentivirus production and processing. *J. Biotechnol.* 240, 23–30. doi: 10.1016/j.jbiotec.2016.10.016

McCarron, A., Donnelley, M., and Parsons, D. (2018). Airway disease phenotypes in animal models of cystic fibrosis. *Respir Res.* 19:54. doi: 10.1186/s12931-018-0750-y

McIntyre, C., Donnelley, M., and Parsons, D. (2017). Generation of new cystic fibrosis rat models in Australia developed using CRISPR/Cas9 genome editing. *Pediatr. Pulmonol.* 52:279.

McIntyre, C., Donnelley, M., Rout-Pitt, N., and Parsons, D. (2018). Lobe-specific gene vector delivery to rat lungs using a miniature bronchoscope. *Hum. Gene Ther. Methods* 29, 228–235. doi: 10.1089/hgtb.2018.050

Meyerholz, D. K. (2016). Lessons learned from the cystic fibrosis pig. *Theriogenology* 86, 427–432. doi: 10.1016/j.theriogenology.2016.04.057

Meyerholz, D. K., Stoltz, D. A., Pezzulo, A. A., and Welsh, M. J. (2010). Pathology of gastrointestinal organs in a porcine model of cystic fibrosis. *Am. J. Pathol.* 176, 1377–1389. doi: 10.2353/ajpath.2010.090849

Milone, M. C., and O'Doherty, U. (2018). Clinical use of lentiviral vectors. *Leukemia* 32, 1529–1541. doi: 10.1038/s41375-018-0106-0

Morgan, K. S., Donnelley, M., Paganin, D. M., Fouras, A., Yagi, N., Suzuki, Y., et al. (2013). Measuring airway surface liquid depth in ex vivo mouse airways by x-ray imaging for the assessment of cystic fibrosis airway therapies. *PLoS One* 8:e55822. doi: 10.1371/journal.pone.0055822

Morgan, K. S., Petersen, T. C., Donnelley, M., Farrow, N., Parsons, D. W., and Paganin, D. M. (2016). Capturing and visualizing transient X-ray wavefront topological features by single-grid phase imaging. *Opt. Express* 24, 24435–24450. doi: 10.1364/OE.24.024435

Morrison, C. (2018). Fresh from the biotech pipeline-2017. *Nat. Biotechnol.* doi: 10.1038/nbt.4068 [Epub ahead of print].

Moss, R. B., Milla, C., Colombo, J., Accurso, F., Zeitlin, P. L., Clancy, J. P., et al. (2007). Repeated aerosolized AAV-CFTR for treatment of cystic fibrosis: a randomized placebo-controlled phase 2B trial. *Hum. Gene Ther.* 18, 726–732. doi: 10.1089/hum.2007.022

Murrie, R. P., Morgan, K. S., Maksimenko, A., Fouras, A., Paganin, D. M., Hall, C., et al. (2015). Live small-animal X-ray lung velocimetry and lung microtomography at the australian synchrotron imaging and medical beamline. *J. Synchrotron. Radiat.* 22, 1049–1055. doi: 10.1107/S1600577515006001

Robinson, E., MacDonald, K. D., Slaughter, K., McKinney, M., Patel, S., Sun, C., et al. (2018). Lipid nanoparticle-delivered chemically modified mRNA restores chloride secretion in cystic fibrosis. *Mol. Ther.* 26, 2034–2046. doi: 10.1016/j.ymthe.2018.05.014

Rock, J. R., Onaitis, M. W., Rawlins, E. L., Lu, Y., Clark, C. P., Xue, Y., et al. (2009). Basal cells as stem cells of the mouse trachea and human airway epithelium. *Proc. Natl. Acad. Sci. U.S.A.* 106, 12771–12775. doi: 10.1073/pnas.0906850106

Rout-Pitt, N., McCarron, A., McIntyre, C., Parsons, D., and Donnelley, M. (2018). Large-scale production of lentiviral vectors using multilayer cell factories. *J. Biol. Methods* 5:15020. doi: 10.14440/jbm.2018.236

Russell, S., Bennett, J., Wellman, J. A., Chung, D. C., Yu, Z. F., Tillman, A., et al. (2017). Efficacy and safety of voretigene neparvovec (AAV2-hRPE65v2) in patients with RPE65-mediated inherited retinal dystrophy: a randomised, controlled, open-label, phase 3 trial. *Lancet* 390, 849–860. doi: 10.1016/S0140-6736(17)31868-8

Sinn, P. L., Arias, A. C., Brogden, K. A., and McCray, P. B. Jr. (2008). Lentivirus vector can be readministered to nasal epithelia without blocking immune responses. *J. Virol.* 82, 10684–10692. doi: 10.1128/JVI.00227-08

Siu, K. K., Morgan, K. S., Paganin, D. M., Boucher, R., Uesugi, K., Yagi, N., et al. (2008). Phase contrast X-ray imaging for the non-invasive detection of airway surfaces and lumen characteristics in mouse models of airway disease. *Eur. J. Radiol.* 68 (Suppl. 3), S22–S26. doi: 10.1016/j.ejrad.2008.04.029

Smith, C. M. (2005). Origin and uses of primum non nocere–above all, do no harm! *J. Clin. Pharmacol.* 45, 371–377. doi: 10.1177/0091270004273680

Stahr, C. S., Samarage, C. R., Donnelley, M., Farrow, N., Morgan, K. S., Zosky, G., et al. (2016). Quantification of heterogeneity in lung disease with image-based pulmonary function testing. *Sci. Rep.* 6:29438. doi: 10.1038/srep29438

Steines, B., Dickey, D. D., Bergen, J., Excoffon, K. J., Weinstein, J. R., Li, X., et al. (2016). CFTR gene transfer with AAV improves early cystic fibrosis pig phenotypes. *JCI Insight* 1:e88728. doi: 10.1172/jci.insight.88728

Stocker, A. G., Kremer, K. L., Koldej, R., Miller, D. S., Anson, D. S., and Parsons, D. W. (2009). Single-dose lentiviral gene transfer for lifetime airway gene expression. *J. Gene Med.* 11, 861–867. doi: 10.1002/jgm.1368

Sun, X., Olivier, A. K., Liang, B., Yi, Y., Sui, H., Evans, T. I. A., et al. (2014). Lung phenotype of juvenile and adult cystic fibrosis transmembrane conductance regulator–knockout ferrets. *Am. J. Respir. Cell Mol. Biol.* 50, 502–512. doi: 10.1165/rcmb.2013-0261OC

Sun, X., Sui, H., Fisher, J. T., Yan, Z., Liu, X., Cho, H.-J., et al. (2010). Disease phenotype of a ferret CFTR-knockout model of cystic fibrosis. *J. Clin. Investig.* 120, 3149–3160. doi: 10.1172/jci43052

Touchot, N., and Flume, M. (2017). Early insights from commercialization of gene therapies in Europe. *Genes (Basel)* 8:78. doi: 10.3390/genes802 0078

Tuggle, K. L., Birket, S. E., Cui, X., Hong, J., Warren, J., Reid, L., et al. (2014). Characterization of defects in ion transport and tissue development in cystic fibrosis transmembrane conductance regulator (CFTR)-knockout rats. *PLoS One* 9:e91253. doi: 10.1371/journal.pone.009 1253

Yu, S. F., von Ruden, T., Kantoff, P. W., Garber, C., Seiberg, M., Ruther, U., et al. (1986). Self-inactivating retroviral vectors designed for transfer of whole genes into mammalian cells. *Proc. Natl. Acad. Sci. U.S.A.* 83, 3194–3198. doi: 10.1073/pnas.83.10.3194

18

Elucidating the Interaction of CF Airway Epithelial Cells and Rhinovirus: Using the Host-Pathogen Relationship to Identify Future Therapeutic Strategies

Kak-Ming Ling[1,2], Luke W. Garratt[2], Timo Lassmann[2], Stephen M. Stick[1,2,3,4†], Anthony Kicic[1,2,3,4,5†], WAERP[1], AusREC[1,6,7] and Australian Respiratory Early Surveillance Team for Cystic Fibrosis[1,3,8,9]*

[1] Paediatrics, Medical School, Faculty of Healthy and Medical Science, University of Western Australia, Nedlands, WA, Australia, [2] Telethon Kids Institute, University of Western Australia, Nedlands, WA, Australia, [3] Department of Respiratory Medicine, Princess Margaret Hospital for Children, Perth, WA, Australia, [4] Centre for Cell Therapy and Regenerative Medicine, School of Medicine and Pharmacology, University of Western Australia, Nedlands, WA, Australia, [5] Occupation and Environment, School of Public Health, Curtin University, Bentley, WA, Australia, [6] Robinson Research Institute, University of Adelaide, Adelaide, SA, Australia, [7] Hunter Medical Research Institute: Priority Research Centre for Asthma and Respiratory Disease, New Lambton Heights, NSW, Australia, [8] Murdoch Children's Research Institute, Melbourne, VIC, Australia, [9] Department of Paediatrics, University of Melbourne, Melbourne, VIC, Australia

***Correspondence:**
Anthony Kicic
anthony.kicic@telethonkids.org.au

† These authors share co-senior authorship*

Chronic lung disease remains the primary cause of mortality in cystic fibrosis (CF). Growing evidence suggests respiratory viral infections are often more severe in CF compared to healthy peers and contributes to pulmonary exacerbations (PEx) and deterioration of lung function. Rhinovirus is the most prevalent respiratory virus detected, particularly during exacerbations in children with CF <5 years old. However, even though rhinoviral infections are likely to be one of the factors initiating the onset of CF lung disease, there is no effective targeted treatment. A better understanding of the innate immune responses by CF airway epithelial cells, the primary site of infection for viruses, is needed to identify why viral infections are more severe in CF. The aim of this review is to present the clinical impact of virus infection in both young children and adults with CF, focusing on rhinovirus infection. Previous *in vitro* and *in vivo* investigations looking at the mechanisms behind virus infection will also be summarized. The review will finish on the potential of transcriptomics to elucidate the host-pathogen responses by CF airway cells to viral infection and identify novel therapeutic targets.

Keywords: cystic fibrosis, airway epithelium, rhinovirus, innate immune response, therapy, transcriptomic

RESPIRATORY INFECTIONS IN THE CYSTIC FIBROSIS LUNG

Chronic obstructive lung disease remains the primary cause of mortality and morbidity in CF (Cutting, 2015). The defective function of the Cystic Fibrosis Transmembrane Conductance Regulator (*CFTR*) gene initiates a lifelong cycle of neutrophilic inflammation, progressive bronchiectasis, mucus obstruction and recurrent microbial infection of the CF airway. These processes typically begin in the first years of life and lead to eventual lung failure during early adulthood. The CF airway environment is vulnerable to colonization by particular bacterial and fungi species including *Haemophilus influenzae*, *Staphylococcus aureus*, *Aspergillus fumigatus*, and *Pseudomonas aeruginosa* (Gangell et al., 2011). Infection by these common pathogens typically trigger neutrophilic responses, however, these fail to eradicate the infection and lead to a sustained release of oxidants and proteases, particularly neutrophil elastase (NE) (Hartl et al., 2007; Painter et al., 2008). This neutrophil-based inflammation has been associated with the progression of structural abnormalities specifically bronchiectasis and air trapping, from as early as 3 months of age (Mott et al., 2012; Sly et al., 2013).

In addition to colonization by bacteria and fungi, the CF airway will be infected with respiratory viruses and viral infections are a major cause of PEx in the pediatric CF population (Goffard et al., 2014; Dijkema et al., 2016). The significance of viral infections in CF has been identified by the advancements in molecular diagnostic technologies to detect virus (Wat, 2015). The prevalence of respiratory viruses during CF PEx can vary from 5% up to 60% (Billard et al., 2017) and include; rhinovirus (RV), influenza A and B, respiratory syncytial virus (RSV), parainfluenza (PIV; Type 1–4), metapneumovirus, coronavirus and adenovirus (Waters and Ratjen, 2015; Flight and Jones, 2017). Earlier work suggested influenza viruses (A & B) (Pribble et al., 1990; Hiatt et al., 1999) and RSV (Abman et al., 1991; Armstrong et al., 1998) were the major cause of PEx in CF. However, studies utilizing more sensitive virological methods in the last 5 years have comprehensively established RV as the most common respiratory virus detected in CF airway (Burns et al., 2012; Wark et al., 2012; Kieninger et al., 2013; Etherington et al., 2014; Dijkema et al., 2016; Stelzer-Braid et al., 2017). Despite numerous studies into the virology of CF airways, the mechanistic link between virus infection, airway inflammation and structural lung disease remains largely unknown. Further investigation into the interaction of these disease components is warranted.

IMPACT OF RV INFECTION IN CF LUNG

A member of the *Picornaviridae* family within the Enterovirus genus, RV features a positive sense single stranded RNA genome ~7.2 kb in length. The airway epithelium is the primary site of RV infection and replication (Vareille et al., 2011). As reviewed by Palmenberg and Gern (2015), 11 viral proteins form the non-enveloped icosahedral structure. The external capsid proteins comprise of VP1, VP2, VP3, while VP4 is located between the interface of capsid protein and RNA genome. These capsid proteins feature a high degree of heterogeneity and consequently the significant antigenic diversity among RV has precluded vaccine development (Glanville and Johnston, 2015; Lewis-Rogers et al., 2017). Currently, there are more than 150 serotypes of RV, which have been classified into 3 species; RV-A, RV-B, and RV-C. Within RV-A and RV-B, strains are clustered into major and minor RV groups based upon their specificity for the intracellular adhesion molecule (ICAM-1) receptor or low-density lipoprotein receptor (LDLR), respectively (Palmenberg, 2017). Recently, the cell receptor for RV-C species has been putatively identified as cadherin related family member 3 (CDHR3), whose expression is largely confined to ciliated cells (Bochkov et al., 2015; Griggs et al., 2017; Palmenberg, 2017).

Rhinovirus infections occur all year round and children experience on average six to eight episodes per year (Worrall, 2011). Although the "common cold" is largely self-limiting, it still poses a burden on the activity and productivity of the general population (Stein, 2017). Additionally, RV infection has a more pronounced effect on vulnerable individuals such as children with CF, as summarized in **Table 1**. These include increased PEx (Asner et al., 2012), more severe respiratory symptoms (Burns et al., 2012; Wark et al., 2012), greater inflammation (Kieninger et al., 2013), reduced quality of life and hospitalization and prolonged antibiotic treatment (Smyth et al., 1995). Prevalence and symptoms of RV infection in patients with CF can vary between cohorts (reviewed by Billard et al., 2017), with some reporting similar rates of RV detection in both children with and without CF (de Almeida et al., 2010; Esposito et al., 2014), while others have reported significant correlations with disease progression in those with CF (Hiatt et al., 1999; van Ewijk et al., 2005). Other features such as age preference, RV serotype, viral load, impact on lung function were assessed in several studies. Susceptibility to particular RV serotype in children with CF requires further investigation due to inconsistent observations (de Almeida et al., 2010; Shah et al., 2015). RV load has been observed to be significantly higher in children with CF (>100 times) when compared to healthy controls and children with asthma (>10 times; Kieninger et al., 2013). This study also illustrated that viral load was negatively correlated to pulmonary function (Kieninger et al., 2013). Cousin et al. (2016) observed that RV-induced PEx in children with CF resulted in failure of pulmonary function recovery for up to 6 weeks. An age preference for RV-associated CF exacerbations has also been reported for young children <5 years old (Stelzer-Braid et al., 2017). However, several other studies have detected a higher frequency of RV in upper and lower airway of adults with CF via screening of sputum and throat swabs (Etherington et al., 2014; Goffard et al., 2014). Adults with CF who have viral associated PEx have been shown to have worse lung function and require more days of intravenous antibiotic treatment (Flight et al., 2014; Goffard et al., 2014). Others have also reported that adult patients who are less responsive to treatment are re-admitted for a subsequent exacerbation within a shorter time frame (Etherington et al., 2014). Finally, Flight et al. (2014) found that RV infection in adults is accompanied by an increased risk of PEx, prolonged antibiotic prescription, higher respiratory symptom scores and heightened level of C-reactive protein. As RV has a large clinical impact on those with CF, it is critical to elucidate how this virus alters host antiviral and inflammatory responses.

AIRWAY EPITHELIUM AND RV INFECTION IN CF

A pseudostratified epithelium lines the surface of the lung (trachea, primary bronchi, secondary bronchi, tertiary bronchi, and bronchioles) and is composed of several cell types including ciliated cells, basal cells, secretory cells and goblet cells. These

TABLE 1 | Summary of clinical studies and outcomes related to Human Rhinovirus infection in CF.

References	Cohorts	Sample Type	Virus Detection								Clinical Data		
			Positive Samples	Detection Method	RV (%)	Influenza (%)	RSV (%)	Parainfluenza (%)	Adenovirus (%)	Others	FEV1	Antibiotic	Hospitalization
Smyth et al., 1995	CF patients (mean age 7.9 years)	Nasopharyngeal Aspirate, Serum Specimen	44/157	Virus Immunofluorescene, Culture, Serology and PCR	58	12	9	12	9	NR	Higher than other virus induced exacerbation	Prolonged treatment	No Difference
Collinson et al., 1996	CF patients (median age 7.3 years)	Nasopharyngeal Specimens	51/119	Virus Culture, PCR	41	NR	NR	NR	NR	NR	Significantly lower	More oral and intravenous antibiotic treatments for those with more infection annually	No Difference
Armstrong et al., 1998	80 infants diagnosed with CF before 12 months of age (31 infatns were hospitalized for persistent respiratory symptoms	BALs/ Nasopharyngeal Samples	14/26	Virus Immunofluorescene, Culture	14.3	14.3	43	28.5	NR	NR	NR	Not for virus infection	Higher
Hiatt et al., 1999	22 infants <2 years of age with CF (30 patient-seasons) and 27 age-matched controls (28 patient-seasons) participated	Nasopharyngeal samples	26/150	Serology, Culture Inoculation	NR	30	23	17	17	27% Picornavirus	NR	NR	RSV infection CF infants has higher rate of hospitalization
Olesen et al., 2006	75 children (media age 8)	Sputum, Laryngeal aspirations	96/606	PCR	87	3	2	6	2	NR	Significantly lower (when excluding HRV infection)	8 patients received antibiotic treatments	NR
Wat et al., 2008	71 CF patients (median age 9)	Nasal swabs and sputum samples	63/138	NASBA	15.9	15.2	2.9	10.9	NR	1% Coronavirus, 36.2% Any	NR	NR	NR
de Almeida et al., 2010	103 CF patients (median age 8.9)	Nasopharyngeal aspirates and nasal mucus specimens, sputum and oropharyngeal samples	203/408	PCR	34.1	1.2	3.7	0.6	0.2	5.9% Enterovirus, 5.6% Human Bocavirus, 4.7 Human Coronavirus, 0.7% Human metapneumovirus	NR	NR	NR

(Continued)

TABLE 1 | Continued

References	Cohorts	Sample Type	Virus Detection								Clinical Data		
			Positive Samples	Detection Method	RV (%)	Influenza (%)	RSV (%)	Parainfluenza (%)	Adenovirus (%)	Others	FEV1	Antibiotic	Hospitalization
Asner et al., 2012	112 CF patients	Mid-turbinate swabs, sputum, throat swab	26/43	Immunofluroescene, multiplex PCR	23	7.6	35	15.4	11.5	34.6% Coxsackie/echovirus, 15.4% Coronavirus, 7.7% Human Metapneumovirus	No Difference	No Difference	No Difference
Stelzer-Braid et al., 2012	37 Participants (median age of 11.4) with CF	Nasal swabs and sputum samples	17/37	Multiplrc PCR	35	2.7	2.7	10.8	NR	2.7% Metapneumovirus; 46% has more than one viral or bacteria pathogen	NR	NR	NR
Kieninger et al., 2013	299 Children (median age 8.2). 195 children with CF (88 stable, 107 exacerbation), 40 children with Non CF Bronchiectasis, 29 children with Asthma and 35 Control Subjects	BALs	73/299	PCR	24.4	NR	NR	NR	NR	NR	Inversely associated with RV load	Increase use of antibiotic when increase respiratory symptoms were recorded	NR
Goffard et al., 2014	46 patients (median age of 29)	Sputum	16/64	PCR	24	3	3	3	NR	8% Coronovirus	No Difference	No Difference	NR
Esposito et al., 2014	47 CF patients with acute pulmonary exacerbation (median age of 16.7) and 31 CF patients in stable clinical condition (median age of 17.3)	Nasopharyngeal Swabs	23/78	PCR	61	17.4	4.3	NR	NR	8.6% Bocavirus, 4.3% Metapeumovirus, 4.3% Enterovirus	No Difference	NR	NR

(Continued)

TABLE 1 | Continued

References	Cohorts	Sample Type	Virus Detection								Clinical Data		
			Positive Samples	Detection Method	RV (%)	Influenza (%)	RSV (%)	Parainfluenza (%)	Adenovirus (%)	Others	FEV1	Antibiotic	Hospitalization
Etherington et al., 2014	180 patients participated ion treatment with intravenous antibiotics for an acute pulmonary exacerbation. 42 patients (media age 26.5) with positive viral detection	Viral Throat Swabs	42/432	PCR	69	19	2.4	4.8	2.4	2.4% Metapneumovirus	Significantly Lower	Intravenous antibiotic for longer period	NR
Flight et al., 2014	100 adults with CF (median age of 28)	Sputum, Nose Swabs and Throat Swabs	191/626	PCR	72.5	6.1	2	2.5	4.1	13.2% Human Metapneumovirus	Lower acute fall in FEV1	Increase number of prescription	NR
Dijkema et al., 2016	20 Children with CF (0–7 years) and age matched healthy control	Nasopharyngeal Swabs	161/352 (only HRV was tested)	Nested PCR, Southern Blotting and Sequencing	45.7	NR	NR	NR	NR	NR	NR	Increase use of antibiotic prophylaxis	NR
Stelzer-Braid et al., 2017	110 children with CF	upper (nasal swab, oropharyngeal suction, and sputum) and lower (bronchoalveolar washings) respiratory tract	59/263 (< 5 years old); 23/202 (older children) only HRV was tested	PCR, Nested PCR	43% (< 5 years old); 12% older children	NR	NR	NR	NR	NR	NR	NR	NR

airway epithelial cells form the first point of contact with inhaled environmental insults, including respiratory viruses. To provide a physical barrier against particulates/pathogens from entering the lung tissue, numerous cell-cell connections are formed including tight junctions, adherent junctions, gap junctions, and desmosomes (Whitsett and Alenghat, 2015). To clear inhaled particles/pathogens, intraepithelial goblet cells, and submucosal glands mucous cells secret mucins. These large glycoproteins bind matter including microbes and allows effective cough clearance by the mucociliary escalator (Foster, 2015). Mucins are transported from the bronchioles to the trachea via beating cilia, expressed by airway epithelial cells of the luminal airway surface (Ma et al., 2018).

Perhaps more significantly for viral pathogens, the airway epithelium plays a crucial role in innate immunity. It has been suggested that the inflammatory responses induced by airway epithelial cells give rise to associated clinical symptoms (Jacobs et al., 2013). RVs can disrupt epithelial tight junctions including zona occludens 1 (ZO-1) protein by stimulating the production of reactive oxygen species (ROS) during viral replication (Unger et al., 2014). Work utilizing airway epithelial cells *in vitro* have shown reduced expression of other tight junction proteins, loss of epithelial integrity, disruption of extracellular matrix and subepithelial fibrosis and induction of proangiogenic molecules which enhance angiogenesis and airway remodeling (Bossios et al., 2005; Leigh et al., 2008; Bochkov et al., 2010; Tacon et al., 2010; Yeo and Jang, 2010; Looi et al., 2018).

The uptake of RV via clathrin-dependent or -independent endocytosis or through micropinocytosis occurs when RV binds to its specific receptors. Upon binding and in a low-pH environment, uncoating of RVs occurs and the virus undergoes conformational changes. The loss of the protein capsid protein VP4, and the externalization of the hydrophobic N-terminal of VP1, facilitates RVs to cross the host cell membrane (Jacobs et al., 2013; Blaas and Fuchs, 2016). Following viral uncoating and membrane rupture, RV "pathogen-associated molecular patterns" (PAMP) are recognized by the host cell via interaction with pattern recognition receptors (PRRs) including; Toll like receptors (TLRs), C-type lectin receptors (CLRs), retinoic acid-inducible gene 1 (RIG-I)-like receptors (RLRs), and nucleotide-binding oligomerization domain-like receptors (NLRs). The signaling pathways induced by TLRs and RLRs are typically host defense antiviral pathways as well as the production of antiviral substances, namely IFNs, B-defensins (Proud et al., 2004), and nitric oxide (Sanders et al., 1998). The airway epithelium also responds to RV infection by activating pro-inflammatory signaling pathways which trigger the release of chemokines and cytokines including IL-8, RANTES/CCL5, and granulocyte-macropahge colony-stimulating factor (GM-CSF), that in turn recruit neutrophils, esoinophils, natural killer cells (NK cells), and macrophages to the infected tissue. IL-6 has an important role in innate immune responses induced by RV infection and IL-6 production has been shown to be inversely correlated to cold symptoms scores and disease severity (Doyle et al., 2010). IL-15 exerts important antiviral and cytotoxic effects and is involved in the activation, differentiation, survival and recruitment of NK cells and CD8+ T cells (Jayaraman et al., 2014). IL-8 has been associated with RV infection as well as cold symptom scores (Gern et al., 2002). Furthermore, it has also been associated with neutrophilic infiltration in sputum (Gern et al., 2000). Taken together, it is evident that innate immune signaling induced by the airway epithelium is essential for effective antiviral responses.

However, in many chronic airway diseases including CF, antiviral responses are defective. Due to the pre-existing genetic defect, normal functions of the CF airway epithelium are often disrupted. As the primary site for virus entry and replication during viral infection, understanding the consequence that lack of CFTR function has on pathophysiology during virus infection is critical for effective disease management. Relevant *in vitro* experimental studies investigating RV infection in CF epithelium have been summarized in **Table 2**. Most studies performed to date assessed cells obtained from adult CF cohorts who had significant disease and structural lung damage. These studies report similar levels of interferon production post infection despite higher viral load being detected (Chattoraj et al., 2011; Dauletbaev et al., 2015). Studying cells from pediatric CF cohorts may generate more relevant data and potentially reveal new insights into early life RV infections that could be exploited therapeutically. Also important is the level of pro-inflammatory cytokines produced by CF epithelium following RV infection. Many studies have reported similar level of IL-8, IL-6, type I, and III IFN production, while others reported higher level of production dependent on virus strain and infectious titer (**Table 2**). These contradictory observations may be due in part to the age of patients involved, disease severity, RV strain, dose, and length of infection. Most studies to date including ours have focused on specific host response targets at the gene or protein level which might not reflect the global innate immune changes during RV infection. The translation of such a targeted approach would be the identification of a single molecule to address a single pathway and ultimately target one downstream effect such as the production of a single cytokine. However, knowing that the interaction of RV and the airway is multifaceted, an alternative approach that addresses this complexity is needed.

PAST AND CURRENT THERAPIES

To date, there have been no studies performed that have focused on potential treatments for RV infection in CF individuals. As RV continues to be the most prevalently detected virus in the all individuals including CF airway, additional evidence is needed to specify its connection with the existing factors such as lack of CFTR and airway inflammation through molecular intermediates and cellular signaling pathways. Common anti-inflammatories including oral corticosteroids and high-dose ibuprofen are unsuitable for treatment in infants and preschool children due to their long-term side effects (Lai et al., 2000; Fennell et al., 2007). Azithromycin may have some interesting antiviral properties, specifically in reducing RV replication via amplification of the IFN pathway-mediated antiviral responses (Schögler et al., 2014). Nevertheless, clinical studies are necessary

TABLE 2 | Summary of *in vitro* studies of Human Rhinovirus infection in CF Airway Epithelium.

Subject	Sampling Sources	RV Serotype	Inoculation Dose	Viral Load	Other Pathogens	Antiviral Cytokines	Inflammatory Cytokines	Apoptosis	References
Adult CF (16–33 years)	BEC (ALI)	RV39	3×10^6 $TCID_{50}$	10^4 TCID50/mL Similar to normal cells	*Pseudomonas aeruginosa* (PA)	RV: IFNβ, λ1, 2 mRNA and protein ↑ Similar to normal cells RV + PA: IFNβ, λ1, 2 mRNA and protein ↓ Only in CF cells	RV: IL8 mRNA ↑ RV + PA: IL-8 mRNA ↑↑ Similar to normal cells	Not measured	Chattoraj et al., 2011
Adult CF (19–41 years)	BEC from explant lung	RV16	MOI 0.1	$>10^4$ copy number Higher in CF	*Pseudomonas aeruginosa* (PA)	RV: IFNβ mRNA↑ Similar to normal cells; OAS1 mRNA↑ Similar to normal cells	RV: IL8 mRNA ↑ Similar to normal cells	Not measured	Dauletbaev et al., 2015
Young children with CF (1–7 years)	AEC	RV1b	MOI 3, 25	~1500 copy/ng RNA	No	Not measured	IL-6 and IL-8 protein ↑ in CF cells only for infection with RV1b of MOI 25 at 48 hours	Reduced compared to normal cells	Sutanto et al., 2011
Children and adults with CF (4.5–48.9 years)	NEC, BEC and cell lines	RV16, RV1b	MOI 2	Not measured	No	Not measured	IL-6, IL-8, IP-10, MCP-1, RANTES↑ Similar to normal cells	Similar apoptosis, ↑necrosis compared to normal cells	Kieninger et al., 2013
Children with CF (3–11 years)	BEC	RV16, RV1b	MOI 4	Not measured	No	RV16: ↓ IFNs (IFN-λ1, IFN-λ2/3 and IFN-β), PRRs (RIG-1 and MDA-5) and ISGs (PKR, OAS1, viperin and MxA). RV1b: ↑ PRRs (TLR3 and RIG-1) and IFN pathway (IFN-λ1 and IFN-λ2/3 compared to normal cells	↑ CXCL8/IL-8, IL-6 and CXCL10/IP-10	Not measured	Schögler et al., 2014

AEC, Airway Epithelial Cells; BEC, Bronchial Epithelial Cells; NEC, Nasal Epithelial Cells.

to elucidate the clinical impact of azithromycin against RV-induced PEx in patients with CF. Vaccination is an important part of CF clinical care, however vaccine development for RV has been rather challenging due to the wide range of antigenic diversity of more than 150 serotypes of RV across three different strains. Technical difficulties in producing sufficient amounts of antigen against multiple RV serotypes using animal models (as reviewed in Del Vecchio et al., 2015) also remains a challenge and as result, the development of a long-lasting RV vaccine has not been successful. This has been further compounded by the lack of a suitable model (other than human) that is fully permissive to RV infection as well as insufficient clinical data to identify and prioritize dominant RV serotypes. In addition, no suitable animal models for CF exhibit complete spectrum of CF phenotype besides CF pig and ferret which are strictly limited for research use (as reviewed in Rosen et al., 2018).

Since vaccination is unavailable, other approaches have been explored in healthy and disease cohorts other than CF. An early approach by Turner et al. (1999) aimed to prevent HRV binding to its receptors via administration of inhaled recombinant soluble ICAM-1 (Tremacamra). Although the reduction in symptom severity and viral shedding were promising, the high costs and dosing regimen recommended (6 times daily) made translation of this therapy into the clinical setting prohibitive (Turner et al., 1999). Targeting viral replication has perhaps been the highest priority in past therapeutic development, where capsid-binding drugs bind to the hydrophobic "pocket" of the viral capsid (reviewed in McKinlay et al., 1992). Pleconaril and Pirodavir were discontinued due to unforeseen side effects and drug efficacy. Reformulated Pleconaril and Vapendavir have completed clinical trials although results have yet to be published [ClinicalTrials.gov (NCT00394914 & NCT01175226)]. A recently discovered compound IMP-1088 offers more promise (Mousnier et al., 2018). This molecule was shown to inhibit human N-myristoyltransferases NMT1 and NMT2, prevent virus assembly and suppress RV replication and infection across various RV strains without inducing cytotoxicity. However, most of this work was demonstrated using cell lines or adult primary cells and further assessment of IMP-1088 on primary cells from young children with CF is necessary. The outcome of such studies would be informative as to whether this compound exerts similar efficacy across all cohorts, as more than 30 polymorphic DNA loci associated with host variation in gene expression called responsereQTLs to rhinovirus infection has been previously reported (Çalişkan et al., 2015).

Alternatively, the roles of type I IFN administration in enhancing the primary antiviral signaling pathway of innate immunity have also been assessed. Early studies involving the prophylactic administration of IFN-α2 or IFN-β were found to demonstrate a reduction in number of RV-induced episodes but no difference in symptom severity or duration (Farr et al., 1984; Hayden et al., 1986; Monto et al., 1986; Sperber et al., 1988). Multiple side effects from high dose administration of IFNs, including nasal bleeding, transient leukopenia and sore throat have also been reported (Sperber et al., 1988). A more recent study assessed low dose IFN-β administration and although antiviral activity was enhanced, it did not aid in reducing cold symptoms of viral induced exacerbations asthma cohorts (Djukanović et al., 2014). Ruuskanen et al. (2014) also suggested that short-term subcutaneous pegylated IFN-α in combination with oral ribavirin treatment rapidly decreased RV RNA in recurrent or chronic rhinovirus infection in immunocompromised patients.

Alternative therapies have not been thoroughly assessed in CF cohorts. While ongoing clinical trials are comprehensive in evaluating the efficacy of CFTR potentiators and correctors for application on mutation specific patients, improvements in infection and inflammation therapies would be highly desirable for all individuals with CF. Indeed, Ivacaftor has been found to reduce sputum *P. aeruginosa* density (>60-fold) and airway inflammation significantly (Hisert et al., 2017). Whether improvements in CFTR folding or function will enhance antiviral responses in children with CF warrant further investigation. Multi-target drug design also holds potential and could be employed to exert both antiviral and anti-inflammation effects. Understanding how host anti-viral and inflammatory responses differ in CF airways, particularly young children, is critical in facilitating the development of new therapeutic treatments that can limit CF disease progression.

NEW THERAPEUTIC FOR RV INFECTIONS

Current therapies directed at RV are mainly focusing on specific viral proteins or inhibition of viral cycle. However, some of these drugs are not effective on drug-resistant viral strains. The current review proposes an alternative approach that focuses on host cellular pathways and factors. To expedite novel therapeutic strategies, investigation on how cellular signaling pathways can be altered by RV infection and how these alterations can be manipulated by new compounds or drugs are crucial for new therapeutic development. The current field of system biology and adoption of high-throughput technologies through transcriptomics not only facilitates characterization of the host-pathogen interaction in a more comprehensive manner, but also aids in understanding how developed and repurposed compounds exert their antiviral properties on RV infection in CF patients.

Knowing viruses can manipulate the host signaling processes and thus altering the host-pathogens interactions (Christiaansen et al., 2015), evaluating the global changes in gene expression during infection via employing gene/transcriptomics could elucidate crucial messages for therapeutic target identification. Transcriptomics is used to study the total RNA output of a cell. Early transcriptomic analyses were performed using microarrays which have customized probes, while current transcriptomic analyses rely on high-throughput RNA sequencing which capture global transcriptome (Mortazavi et al., 2008). These techniques allow analysis for "all molecules" regulated at the gene level. By illustrating their interaction within the cells and the complexities of host-pathogen interactions, enhancing or diminishing specific molecules as well as precise characterization of specific targets can be a more promising therapeutic approach (as reviewed in Cesur and Durmuş, 2018). Generally, computational approaches are used to organize or manage these data sets and interpret the biological inference, including network analysis (such as InnateDB, NetworkAnlayst, and Cytoscape) and pathway analysis (such as Reactome, Kegg Pathway, and Pantherdb).

In the context of host-viral interaction, transcriptomic analysis has been successfully applied to identify the uncharacterized isoforms from wild-type dengue infected host RNA from human hepatoma cells. The authors demonstrated that infection with wild-type dengue virus elicited a different host response compared to infection with a vaccine sensitive strain, highlighting the potential of strain-specific responses (Sessions et al., 2013). Transcriptional profiling of blood specimens from

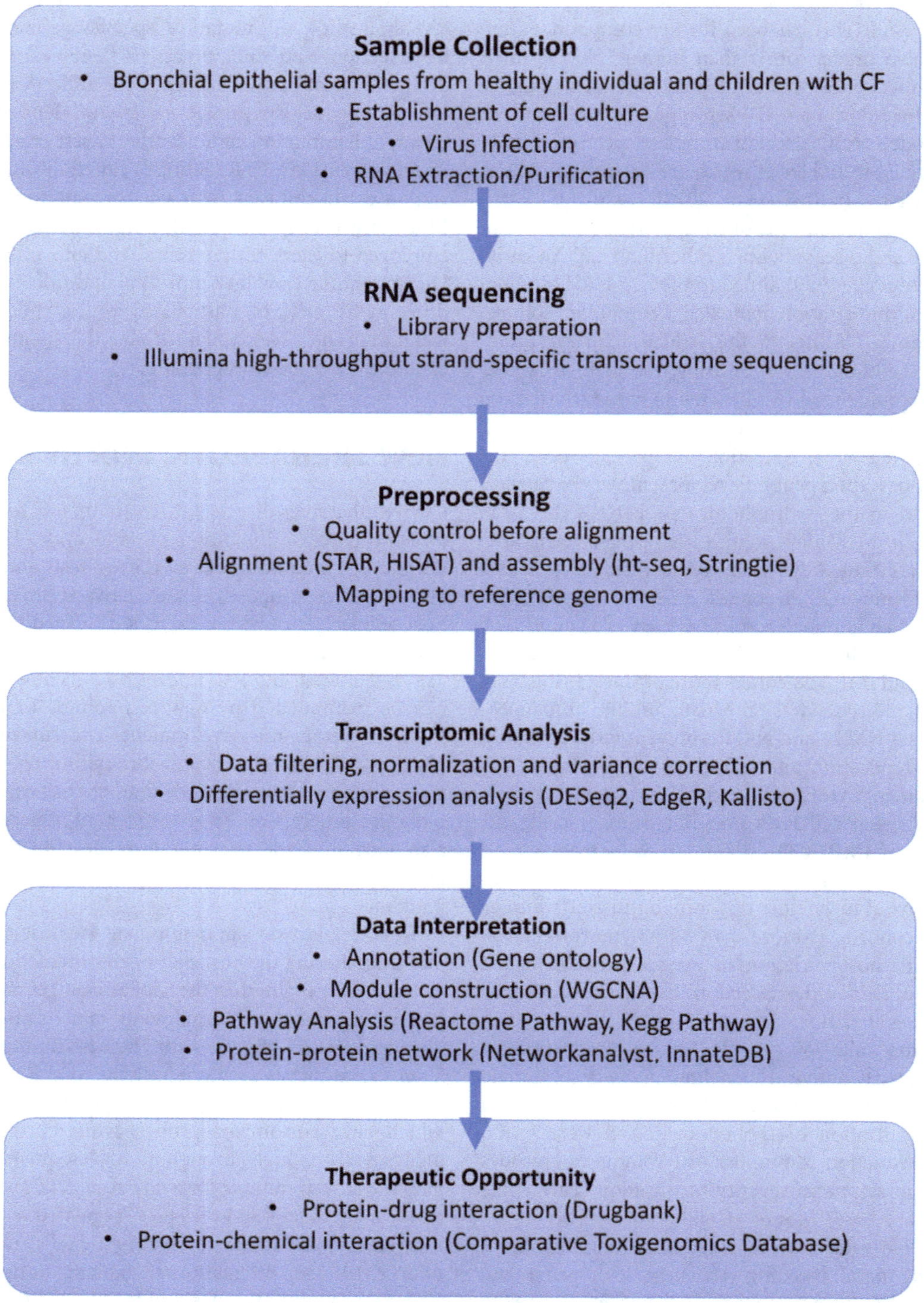

FIGURE 1 | Proposed workflow using transcriptomics to elucidate future treatment for cold virus infection in CF.

symptomatic and asymptomatic patients with RV infection have revealed that individuals with active infection demonstrate a robust transcriptional signature of immune-related genes (Heinonen et al., 2016). In other disease settings including asthma and allergic rhinitis, transcriptomic responses of human respiratory cells to surrogate RV infection [Poly(I:C) stimulation] have potentially identified disease-specific signatures (Wagener et al., 2014). Therefore, it is imperative to assess the global transcript expression and investigate the host-viral interaction, given that CF is a defined genetic disease condition and live RV infection can truly represent an active infection which might involve modification of the host response. This approach is not only applied to protein-coding RNA but also provide insights to critical non-coding RNA such as short non-coding RNAs (miRNAs) and long non-coding RNAs (lncRNAs) which are key regulators for modulation of gene expression (Delpu et al., 2016).

Mapping genes on a complete network allows identification of key hub genes and central genes with high connectivity which exert large effects on signal transduction. Molecular network analysis also allows enrichment of functional modules to identify which area group of genes are cooperatively working together to perform specific biological function and could be associated with disease setting (reviewed by Csermely et al., 2013). Some examples include, the identification of 16 strongly connected hub genes as potential antifungal drug targets against *Candida albicans* (Altwasser et al., 2012), the identification of new key genes for type 1 diabetes (Safari-Alighiarloo et al., 2016) as well as certain cancers (Zaman et al., 2013; Jin et al., 2015). Moreover, omics data has discovered disease modules and revealed substantial inter-patient heterogeneity, highlighting the potential importance of customize treatments to conditions. Numerous algorithms have been introduced to identify disease modules, including ModuleDiscoverer that identified a rodent model of non-alcoholic steatohepatitis (NASH), as well as a severe form of non-alcoholic fatty liver disease (NAFLD) (Vlaic et al., 2018). To maximize the efficacy and treatment outcome, patient individual characteristics, including their genetic profile needs to be considered. Although using biological network analysis can expedite the drug discovery process, the timeline from target identification to clinic application can still be lengthy.

An alternative strategy is to explore drug repurposing. Integrated analysis of disease-gene profiles, pathway analysis, and mining of FDA approved drug databases can be carried out to identify correlations of common pathways with certain compounds or molecules at the network level. Successful examples of drug repurposing based on transcriptomic analyses include the identification of topiramate for the treatment of inflammatory bowel disease (IBD) and cimetidine for the treatment of lung adenocarcinoma (Dudley et al., 2011; Sirota et al., 2011). Using a large-scale expression signature, Lee et al. (2016) have also identified that ivermectin, trifluridine, astemizole, amlodipine, maprotiline, apomorphine, mometasone, and nortriptyline show significant anti-proliferative activity against glioblastoma. With the recent establishment of ImmPort, a data repository that promotes research dataset repurposing (Bhattacharya et al., 2018), the identification of novel targets and repurposed drugs that target these has been accelerated further. Currently, there is paucity of data in CF-related RV-therapy given its impact on CF lung disease and thus new interventions are urgently required. The strategy to repurpose already approved drugs could advance antiviral therapies by reducing cost and improving and quality of life for affected individuals.

CONCLUSION

RV infection remains a significant cause of pulmonary exacerbation in CF. There has been little investigation into antiviral therapies in CF especially in young children who are more susceptible to these types of infection. However, modern virological procedures and omic technologies now facilitate more in-depth studies of the genes and molecular pathways involved in aberrant CF antiviral responses to RV. We propose transcriptomics could be leveraged to elucidate future therapeutic intervention for treatment of rhinovirus infection in CF. For example, a global gene expression profile of bronchial epithelial cells from patients with CF, under baseline conditions and after RV infection will be profiled following next-generation RNA sequencing (**Figure 1**). Sequences can be aligned and mapped to already available reference genomes to identify differentially expressed genes pre- and post-infection. The identified genes could then be annotated using online repositories or libraries to investigate their enriched functional biological pathways. Moreover, networks or subnetworks can then be constructed by mapping identified genes to explore their relationship using curated protein-protein interaction databases. Therapeutic opportunities can also identify by exploring protein-protein interaction and protein-transcription factor, protein-drug interaction as well as chemical interaction databases. Finally, monolayer cell cultures which have previously been found to be more susceptible for RV infection (Bochkov et al., 2010) represent an oversimplified model for the multicellular interactions of epithelial (ciliated cells, goblet cells) and immune cells (dendritic cells, neutrophils). Indeed, functional validation utilizing human *in vitro* 3D airway models (Boda et al., 2018) will be needed to further elucidate to host-pathogen interactions. The emergence of single cell transcriptomics could be used to compliment 3D airway models and accelerate progress in this new era of scientific research. Overall, the advancement of these promising tools should aid in expediting new therapeutic intervention in this sphere.

AUTHOR CONTRIBUTIONS

K-ML, LG, and AK conceptualized the contents of the manuscript. K-ML wrote the first draft of the manuscript. K-ML, LG, TL, SS, and AK contributed to the drafting and editing of the manuscript. WAERP, AusREC, and AREST CF approved the final submission of the manuscript.

ACKNOWLEDGMENTS

The members of Western Australian Epithelial Research Program (WAERP) are: AK, SS, Darryl A. Knight, Elizabeth Kicic-Starcevich, LG, Marc Padros-Goosen, Ee-Lyn Tan, Erika N. Sutanto. Kevin Looi, Jessica Hillas, Thomas Iosifidis, Nicole C. Shaw, Samuel T. Montgomery, K-ML, Kelly M. Martinovich, Francis J. Lannigan, Ricardo Bergesio, Bernard Lee, Shyan Vijaya-Sekeran, Paul Swan, Mairead Heaney, Ian Forsyth, Tobias Schoep, Alexander Larcombe, Monica Hunter, Kate McGee, Nyssa Millington. The full membership of the Australian Respiratory Early Surveillance Team for Cystic Fibrosis (AREST CF) is available at www.arestcf.org. The Australian Respiratory Epithelium Consortium (AusREC) acknowledges the following members; AK, SS, Elizabeth Kicic-Starcevich, LG, Erika N. Sutanto, Kevin Looi, Jessica Hillas, Thomas Iosifidis, Nicole C. Shaw, Samuel T. Montgomery, K-ML, Kelly M. Martinovich, Matthew W.-P. Poh, Daniel R. Laucirica, Craig Schofield, Samantha McLean, Katherine Landwehr, Emma de Jong, Nigel Farrow, Eugene Roscioli, David Parsons, Darryl A. Knight, Christopher Grainge, Andrew T. Reid, Su-Kim Loo, and Punnam C. Veerati. This work was supported by grants from the National Health and Medical Research Council of Australia (NHMRC; APP1069101 and APP1142505) and United States Cystic Fibrosis Foundation (#STICK15A0). SS is a NHMRC Practitioner Fellow. LG is a NHMRC Peter Doherty Fellow.

REFERENCES

Abman, S. H., Ogle, J. W., Harbeck, R. J., Butler-Simon, N., Hammond, K. B., and Accurso, F. J. (1991). Early bacteriologic, immunologic, and clinical courses of young infants with cystic fibrosis identified by neonatal screening. *J. Pediatr.* 119, 211–217. doi: 10.1016/S0022-3476(05)80729-2

Altwasser, R., Linde, J., Buyko, E., Hahn, U., and Guthke, R. (2012). Genome-wide scale-free network inference for *Candida albicans*. *Front. Microbiol.* 3:51. doi: 10.3389/fmicb.2012.00051

Armstrong, D., Grimwood, K., Carlin, J. B., Carzino, R., Hull, J., Olinsky, A., et al. (1998). Severe viral respiratory infections in infants with cystic fibrosis. *Pediatr. Pulmonol.* 26, 371–379. doi: 10.1002/(SICI)1099-0496(199812)26:6<371::AID-PPUL1>3.0.CO;2-N

Asner, S., Waters, V., Solomon, M., Yau, Y., Richardson, S. E., Grasemann, H., et al. (2012). Role of respiratory viruses in pulmonary exacerbations in children with cystic fibrosis. *J. Cyst. Fibros.* 11, 433–439. doi: 10.1016/j.jcf.2012.04.006

Bhattacharya, S., Dunn, P., Thomas, C. G., Smith, B., Schaefer, H., Chen, J., et al. (2018). ImmPort, toward repurposing of open access immunological assay data for translational and clinical research. *Sci. Data* 5:180015. doi: 10.1038/sdata.2018.15

Billard, L., Le Berre, R., Pilorgé, L., Payan, C., Héry-Arnaud, G., and Vallet, S. (2017). Viruses in cystic fibrosis patients' airways. *Crit. Rev. Microbiol.* 43, 690–708. doi: 10.1080/1040841X.2017.1297763

Blaas, D., and Fuchs, R. (2016). Mechanism of human rhinovirus infections. *Mol. Cell. Pediatr.* 3:21. doi: 10.1186/s40348-016-0049-3

Bochkov, Y. A., Hanson, K. M., Keles, S., Brockman-Schneider, R. A., Jarjour, N. N., and Gern, J. E. (2010). Rhinovirus-induced modulation of gene expression in bronchial epithelial cells from subjects with asthma. *Mucosal Immunol.* 3, 69–80. doi: 10.1038/mi.2009.109

Bochkov, Y. A., Watters, K., Ashraf, S., Griggs, T. F., Devries, M. K., Jackson, D. J., et al. (2015). Cadherin-related family member 3, a childhood asthma susceptibility gene product, mediates rhinovirus C binding and replication. *Proc. Natl. Acad. Sci. U.S.A.* 112, 5485–5490. doi: 10.1073/pnas.1421178112

Boda, B., Benaoudia, S., Huang, S., Bonfante, R., Wiszniewski, L., Tseligka, E. D., et al. (2018). Antiviral drug screening by assessing epithelial functions and innate immune responses in human 3D airway epithelium model. *Antiviral Res.* 156, 72–79. doi: 10.1016/J.ANTIVIRAL.2018.06.007

Bossios, A., Psarras, S., Gourgiotis, D., Skevaki, C. L., Constantopoulos, A. G., Saxoni-Papageorgiou, P., et al. (2005). Rhinovirus infection induces cytotoxicity and delays wound healing in bronchial epithelial cells. *Respir. Res.* 6:114. doi: 10.1186/1465-9921-6-114

Burns, J. L., Emerson, J., Kuypers, J., Campbell, A. P., Gibson, R. L., McNamara, S., et al. (2012). Respiratory viruses in children with cystic fibrosis: viral detection and clinical findings. *Influenza Other Respir. Viruses* 6, 218–223. doi: 10.1111/j.1750-2659.2011.00292.x

Çalişkan, M., Baker, S. W., Gilad, Y., and Ober, C. (2015). Host genetic variation influences gene expression response to rhinovirus infection. *PLoS Genet.* 11:e1005111. doi: 10.1371/journal.pgen.1005111

Cesur, M. F., and Durmuş, S. (2018). "Systems biology modeling to study pathogen-host interactions," in *Host-Pathogen Interactions. Methods in Molecular Biology*, eds C. Medina and F. López-Baena (New York, NY: Human Press), 97–112. doi: 10.1007/978-1-4939-7604-1_10

Chattoraj, S. S., Ganesan, S., Jones, A. M., Helm, J. M., Comstock, A. T., Bright-Thomas, R., et al. (2011). Rhinovirus infection liberates planktonic bacteria from biofilm and increases chemokine responses in cystic fibrosis airway epithelial cells. *Thorax* 66, 333–339. doi: 10.1136/thx.2010.151431

Christiaansen, A., Varga, S. M., and Spencer, J. V. (2015). Viral manipulation of the host immune response. *Curr. Opin. Immunol.* 36, 54–60. doi: 10.1016/j.coi.2015.06.012

Collinson, J., Nicholson, K. G., Cancio, E., Ashman, J., Ireland, D. C., Hammersley, V., et al. (1996). Effects of upper respiratory tract infections in patients with cystic fibrosis. *Thorax* 51, 1115–1122. doi: 10.1136/thx.51.11.1115

Cousin, M., Molinari, N., Foulongne, V., Caimmi, D., Vachier, I., Abely, M., et al. (2016). Rhinovirus-associated pulmonary exacerbations show a lack of FEV 1 improvement in children with cystic fibrosis. *Influenza Other Respir. Viruses* 10, 109–112. doi: 10.1111/irv.12353

Csermely, P., Korcsmáros, T., Kiss, H. J. M., London, G., and Nussinov, R. (2013). Structure and dynamics of molecular networks: a novel paradigm of drug discovery: a comprehensive review. *Pharmacol. Ther.* 138, 333–408. doi: 10.1016/j.pharmthera.2013.01.016

Cutting, G. R. (2015). Cystic fibrosis genetics: from molecular understanding to clinical application. *Nat. Rev. Genet.* 16, 45–56. doi: 10.1038/nrg3849

Dauletbaev, N., Das, M., Cammisano, M., Chen, H., Singh, S., Kooi, C., et al. (2015). Rhinovirus load is high despite preserved interferon-β response in cystic fibrosis bronchial epithelial cells. *PLoS ONE* 10:e0143129. doi: 10.1371/journal.pone.0143129

de Almeida, M. B., Zerbinati, R. M., Tateno, A. F., Oliveira, C. M., Romão, R. M., Rodrigues, J. C., et al. (2010). Rhinovirus C and respiratory exacerbations in children with cystic fibrosis. *Emerg. Infect. Dis.* 16, 996–999. doi: 10.3201/eid1606.100063

Del Vecchio, A. M., Branigan, P. J., Barnathan, E. S., Flavin, S. K., Silkoff, P. E., and Turner, R. B. (2015). Utility of animal and *in vivo* experimental infection of humans with rhinoviruses in the development of therapeutic agents for viral exacerbations of asthma and chronic obstructive pulmonary disease. *Pulm. Pharmacol. Ther.* 30, 32–43. doi: 10.1016/J.PUPT.2014.10.005

Delpu, Y., Larrieu, D., Gayral, M., Arvanitis, D., Dufresne, M., Cordelier, P., et al. (2016). "Noncoding RNAs: clinical and therapeutic applications," in *Drug Discovery in Cancer Epigenetics*, eds G. Egger and P. Arimondo (Academic Press), 305–326. doi: 10.1016/B978-0-12-802208-5.00012-6

Dijkema, J. S., Ewijk, B. E., van, Wilbrink, B., Wolfs, T. F. W., Kimpen, J. L. L., and Ent, C. K., van der (2016). Frequency and duration of rhinovirus infections in children with cystic fibrosis and healthy controls: a longitudinal cohort study. *Pediatr. Infect. Dis. J.* 35, 379–383. doi: 10.1097/INF.0000000000001014

Djukanović, R., Harrison, T., Johnston, S. L., Gabbay, F., Wark, P., Thomson, N. C., et al. (2014). The effect of inhaled IFN-β on worsening of asthma symptoms caused by viral infections. A randomized trial. *Am. J. Respir. Crit. Care Med.* 190, 145–154. doi: 10.1164/rccm.201312-2235OC

Doyle, W. J., Casselbrant, M. L., Li-Korotky, H.-S., Doyle, A. P. C., Lo, C.-Y., Turner, R., et al. (2010). The interleukin 6–174 C/C genotype predicts greater rhinovirus illness. *J. Infect. Dis.* 201, 199–206. doi: 10.1086/649559

Dudley, J. T., Sirota, M., Shenoy, M., Pai, R. K., Roedder, S., Chiang, A. P., et al. (2011). Computational repositioning of the anticonvulsant topiramate for inflammatory bowel disease. *Sci. Transl. Med.* 3:96ra76. doi: 10.1126/scitranslmed.3002648

Esposito, S., Daleno, C., Scala, A., Castellazzi, L., Terranova, L., Sferrazza Papa, S., et al. (2014). Impact of rhinovirus nasopharyngeal viral load and viremia on severity of respiratory infections in children. *Eur. J. Clin. Microbiol. Infect. Dis.* 33, 41–48. doi: 10.1007/s10096-013-1926-5

Etherington, C., Naseer, R., Conway, S. P., Whitaker, P., Denton, M., and Peckham, D. G. (2014). The role of respiratory viruses in adult patients with cystic fibrosis receiving intravenous antibiotics for a pulmonary exacerbation. *J. Cyst. Fibros.* 13, 49–55. doi: 10.1016/j.jcf.2013.06.004

Farr, B. M., Gwaltney, J. M., Adams, K. F., and Hayden, F. G. (1984). Intranasal interferon-α2 for prevention of natural rhinovirus colds. *Antimicrob. Agents Chemother.* 26, 31–34. doi: 10.1128/AAC.26.1.31

Fennell, P. B., Quante, J., Wilson, K., Boyle, M., Strunk, R., and Ferkol, T. (2007). Use of high-dose ibuprofen in a pediatric cystic fibrosis center. *J. Cyst. Fibros.* 6, 153–158. doi: 10.1016/j.jcf.2006.06.003

Flight, W., and Jones, A. (2017). The diagnosis and management of respiratory viral infections in cystic fibrosis. *Expert Rev. Respir. Med.* 11, 221–227. doi: 10.1080/17476348.2017.1288102

Flight, W. G., Bright-Thomas, R. J., Tilston, P., Mutton, K. J., Guiver, M., Morris, J., et al. (2014). Incidence and clinical impact of respiratory viruses in adults with cystic fibrosis. *Thorax* 69, 247–253. doi: 10.1136/thoraxjnl-2013-204000

Foster, W. M. (2015). "Mucociliary function," in *Comparative Biology of the Normal Lung, 2nd Edn.*, ed R. A. Parent (Academic Press), 561–579. doi: 10.1016/B978-0-12-404577-4.00029-1

Gangell, C. L., Gard, S. E., Douglas, T. A., Park, J., de Klerk, N. H., Keil, T., et al. (2011). Inflammatory responses to individual microorganisms in the lungs of children with cystic fibrosis. *Clin. Infect. Dis.* 53, 425–432. doi: 10.1093/cid/cir399

Gern, J. E., Martin, M. S., Anklam, K. A., Shen, K., Roberg, K. A., Carlson-Dakes, K. T., et al. (2002). Relationships among specific viral pathogens, virus-induced interleukin-8, and respiratory symptoms in infancy. *Pediatr. Allergy Immunol.* 13, 386–393. doi: 10.1034/j.1399-3038.2002.01093.x

Gern, J. E., Vrtis, R., Grindle, K. A., Swenson, C., and Busse, W. W. (2000). Relationship of upper and lower airway cytokines to outcome experimental rhinovirus infection. *Am. J. Respir. Crit. Care Med.* 162, 2226–2231. doi: 10.1164/ajrccm.162.6.2003019

Glanville, N., and Johnston, S. L. (2015). Challenges in developing a cross-serotype rhinovirus vaccine. *Curr. Opin. Virol.* 11, 83–88. doi: 10.1016/j.coviro.2015.03.004

Goffard, A., Lambert, V., Salleron, J., Herwegh, S., Engelmann, I., Pinel, C., et al. (2014). Virus and cystic fibrosis: rhinoviruses are associated with exacerbations in adult patients. *J. Clin. Virol.* 60, 147–153. doi: 10.1016/j.jcv.2014.02.005

Griggs, T. F., Bochkov, Y. A., Basnet, S., Pasic, T. R., Brockman-Schneider, R. A., Palmenberg, A. C., et al. (2017). Rhinovirus C targets ciliated airway epithelial cells. *Respir. Res.* 18:84. doi: 10.1186/s12931-017-0567-0

Hartl, D., Latzin, P., Hordijk, P., Marcos, V., Rudolph, C., Woischnik, M., et al. (2007). Cleavage of CXCR1 on neutrophils disables bacterial killing in cystic fibrosis lung disease. *Nat. Med.* 13, 1423–1430. doi: 10.1038/nm1690

Hayden, F. G., Albrecht, J. K., Kaiser, D. L., and Gwaltney, J. M. (1986). Prevention of natural colds by contact prophylaxis with intranasal alpha$_2$-interferon. *N. Engl. J. Med.* 314, 71–75. doi: 10.1056/NEJM198601093140202

Heinonen, S., Jartti, T., Garcia, C., Oliva, S., Smitherman, C., Anguiano, E., et al. (2016). Value of host transcriptome analysis. Rhinovirus detect. Symptomatic asymptomatic child. *Am. J. Respir. Crit. Care Med.* 193, 772–782. doi: 10.1164/rccm.201504-0749OC

Hiatt, P. W., Grace, S. C., Kozinetz, C. A., Raboudi, S. H., Treece, D. G., Taber, L. H., et al. (1999). Effects of viral lower respiratory tract infection on lung function in infants with cystic fibrosis. *Pediatrics* 103, 619–626. doi: 10.1542/peds.103.3.619

Hisert, K. B., Heltshe, S. L., Pope, C., Jorth, P., Wu, X., Edwards, R. M., et al. (2017). Restoring cystic fibrosis transmembrane conductance regulator function reduces airway bacteria and inflammation in people with cystic fibrosis and chronic lung infections. *Am. J. Respir. Crit. Care Med.* 195, 1617–1628. doi: 10.1164/rccm.201609-1954OC

Jacobs, S. E., Lamson, D. M., St George, K., and Walsh, T. J. (2013). Human rhinoviruses. *Clin. Microbiol. Rev.* 26, 135–162. doi: 10.1128/CMR.00077-12

Jayaraman, A., Jackson, D. J., Message, S. D., Pearson, R. M., Aniscenko, J., Caramori, G., et al. (2014). IL-15 complexes induce NK- and T-cell responses independent of type i IFN signaling during rhinovirus infection. *Mucosal Immunol.* 7, 1151–1164. doi: 10.1038/mi.2014.2

Jin, B., Wang, W., Du, G., Huang, G. Z., Han, L. T., Tang, Z. Y., et al. (2015). Identifying hub genes and dysregulated pathways in hepatocellular carcinoma. *Eur. Rev. Med. Pharmacol. Sci.* 19, 592–601.

Kieninger, E., Singer, F., Tapparel, C., Alves, M. P., Latzin, P., Tan, H. L., et al. (2013). High rhinovirus burden in lower airways of children with cystic fibrosis. *Chest* 143, 782–790. doi: 10.1378/chest.12-0954

Lai, H.-C., FitzSimmons, S. C., Allen, D. B., Kosorok, M. R., Rosenstein, B. J., Campbell, P. W., et al. (2000). Risk of persistent growth impairment after alternate-day prednisone treatment in children with cystic fibrosis. *N. Engl. J. Med.* 342, 851–859. doi: 10.1056/NEJM200003233421204

Lee, H., Kang, S., and Kim, W. (2016). Drug repositioning for cancer therapy based on large-scale drug-induced transcriptional signatures. *PLoS ONE* 11:e0150460. doi: 10.1371/journal.pone.0150460

Leigh, R., Oyelusi, W., Wiehler, S., Koetzler, R., Zaheer, R. S., Newton, R., et al. (2008). Human rhinovirus infection enhances airway epithelial cell production of growth factors involved in airway remodeling. *J. Allergy Clin. Immunol.* 121, 1238.e4–1245.e4. doi: 10.1016/j.jaci.2008.01.067

Lewis-Rogers, N., Seger, J., and Adler, F. R. (2017). Human rhinovirus diversity and evolution: how strange the change from major to minor. *J. Virol.* 91, e01659–e01616. doi: 10.1128/JVI.01659-16

Looi, K., Buckley, A. G., Rigby, P. J., Garratt, L. W., Iosifidis, T., Zosky, G. R., et al. (2018). Effects of human rhinovirus on epithelial barrier integrity and function in children with asthma. *Clin. Exp. Allergy* 48, 513–524. doi: 10.1111/cea.13097

Ma, J., Rubin, B. K., and Voynow, J. A. (2018). Mucins, mucus, and goblet cells. *Chest* 154, 169–176. doi: 10.1016/j.chest.2017.11.008

McKinlay, M. A., Pevear, D. C., York, N., and Rossmann, M. G. (1992). Treatment of the picornavirus common cold by inhibitors or viral uncoating and attachment. *Annu. Rev. Microbiol.* 46, 635–654. doi: 10.1146/annurev.mi.46.100192.003223

Monto, A. S., Shope, T. C., Schwartz, S. A., and Albrecht, J. K. (1986). Intranasal interferon-alpha 2b for seasonal prophylaxis of respiratory infection. *J. Infect. Dis.* 154, 128–133. doi: 10.1093/infdis/154.1.128

Mortazavi, A., Williams, B. A., McCue, K., Schaeffer, L., and Wold, B. (2008). Mapping and quantifying mammalian transcriptomes by RNA-Seq. *Nat. Methods* 5, 621–628. doi: 10.1038/nmeth.1226

Mott, L. S., Park, J., Murray C. P., Gangell, C. L., De Klerk, N. H., Robinson, P. J., et al. (2012). Progression of early structural lung disease in young children with cystic fibrosis assessed using CT. *Thorax* 67, 509–516. doi: 10.1136/thoraxjnl-2011-200912

Mousnier, A., Bell, A. S., Swieboda, D. P., Morales-Sanfrutos, J., Pérez-Dorado, I., Brannigan, J. A., et al. (2018). Fragment-derived inhibitors of human N-myristoyltransferase block capsid assembly and replication of the common cold virus. *Nat. Chem.* 10, 599–606. doi: 10.1038/s41557-018-0039-2

Olesen, H. V., Nielsen, L. P., and Schiotz, P. O. (2006). Viral and atypical bacterial infections in the outpatient pediatric cystic fibrosis clinic. *Pediatr. Pulmonol.* 41, 1197–1204. doi: 10.1002/ppul.20517

Painter, R. G., Bonvillain, R. W., Valentine, V. G., Lombard, G. A., LaPlace, S. G., Nauseef, W. M., et al. (2008). The role of chloride anion and CFTR in killing of *Pseudomonas aeruginosa* by normal and CF neutrophils. *J. Leukoc. Biol.* 83, 1345–1353. doi: 10.1189/jlb.0907658

Palmenberg, A. C. (2017). Rhinovirus C, asthma, and cell surface expression of virus receptor CDHR3. *J. Virol.* 91:e00072-17. doi: 10.1128/JVI.00072-17

Palmenberg, A. C., and Gern, J. E. (2015). Classification and evolution of human rhinoviruses. *Methods Mol. Biol.* 1221, 1–10. doi: 10.1007/978-1-4939-1571-2_1

Pribble, C. G., Black, P. G., Bosso, J. A., and Turner, R. B. (1990). Clinical manifestations of exacerbations of cystic fibrosis associated with nonbacterial infections. *J. Pediatr.* 117, 200–204. doi: 10.1016/S0022-3476(05)80530-X

Proud, D., Sanders, S. P., and Wiehler, S. (2004). Human rhinovirus infection induces airway epithelial cell production of human beta-defensin 2 both *in vitro* and *in vivo*. *J. Immunol.* 172, 4637–4645. doi: 10.4049/jimmunol.172.7.4637

Rosen, B. H., Chanson, M., Gawenis, L. R., Liu, J., Sofoluwe, A., Zoso, A., et al. (2018). Animal and model systems for studying cystic fibrosis. *J. Cyst. Fibros.* 17, S28–S34. doi: 10.1016/j.jcf.2017.09.001

Ruuskanen, O., Waris, M., and Kainulainen, L. (2014). Treatment of persistent rhinovirus infection with pegylated interferon α2a and ribavirin in patients with hypogammaglobulinemia. *Clin. Infect. Dis.* 58, 1784–1786. doi: 10.1093/cid/ciu169

Safari-Alighiarloo, N., Taghizadeh, M., Tabatabaei, S. M., Shahsavari, S., Namaki, S., Khodakarim, S., et al. (2016). Identification of new key genes for type 1 diabetes through construction and analysis of the protein-protein interaction networks based on blood and pancreatic islet transcriptomes. *J. Diabetes* 9, 764–777. doi: 10.1111/1753-0407.12483

Sanders, S. P., Siekierski, E. S., Porter, J. D., Richards, S. M., and Proud, D. (1998). Nitric oxide inhibits rhinovirus-induced cytokine production and viral replication in a human respiratory epithelial cell line. *J. Virol.* 72, 934–942.

Schögler, A., Kopf, B. S., Edwards, M. R., Johnston, S. L., Casaulta, C., Kieninger, E., et al. (2014). Novel antiviral properties of azithromycin in cystic fibrosis airway epithelial cells. *Eur. Respir. J.* 45, 428–439. doi: 10.1183/09031936.00102014

Sessions, O. M., Tan, Y., Goh, K. C., Liu, Y., Tan, P., Rozen, S., et al. (2013). Host cell transcriptome profile during wild-type and attenuated dengue virus infection. *PLoS Negl. Trop. Dis.* 7:e2107. doi: 10.1371/journal.pntd.0002107

Shah, A., Connelly, M., Whitaker, P., McIntyre, C., Etherington, C., Denton, M., et al. (2015). Pathogenicity of individual rhinovirus species during exacerbations of cystic fibrosis. *Eur. Respir. J.* 45, 1748–1751. doi: 10.1183/09031936.00229114

Sirota, M., Dudley, J. T., Kim, J., Chiang, A. P., Morgan, A. A., Sweet-Cordero, A., et al. (2011). Discovery and preclinical validation of drug indications using compendia of public gene expression data. *Sci. Transl. Med.* 3:96ra77. doi: 10.1126/scitranslmed.3003215

Sly, P. D., Gangell, C. L., Chen, L., Ware, R. S., Ranganathan, S., Mott, L. S., et al. (2013). Risk factors for bronchiectasis in children with cystic fibrosis. *N. Engl. J. Med.* 368, 1963–1970. doi: 10.1056/NEJMoa1301725

Smyth, A. R., Smyth, R. L., Tong, C. Y., Hart, C. A., and Heaf, D. P. (1995). Effect of respiratory virus infections including rhinovirus on clinical status in cystic fibrosis. *Arch. Dis. Child.* 73, 117–120.

Sperber, S. J., Levine, P. A., Innes, D. J., Mills, S. E., and Hayden, F. G. (1988). Tolerance and efficacy of intranasal administration of recombinant β(serine) interferon in healthy adults. *J. Infect. Dis.* 158, 166–175. doi: 10.1093/infdis/158.1.166

Stein, R. A. (2017). Hopes and challenges for the common cold. *Int. J. Clin. Pract.* 71:e12921. doi: 10.1111/ijcp.12921

Stelzer-Braid, S., Johal, H., Skilbeck, K., Steller, A., Alsubie, H., Tovey, E., et al. (2012). Detection of viral and bacterial respiratory pathogens in patients with cystic fibrosis. *J. Virol. Methods* 186, 109–112. doi: 10.1016/j.jviromet.2012.08.008

Stelzer-Braid, S., Liu, N., Doumit, M., D'Cunha, R., Belessis, Y., Jaffe, A., et al. (2017). Association of rhinovirus with exacerbations in young children affected by cystic fibrosis: preliminary data. *J. Med. Virol.* 89, 1494–1497. doi: 10.1002/jmv.24794

Sutanto, E. N., Kicic, A., Foo, C. J., Stevens, P. T., Mullane, D., Knight, D. A., et al. (2011). Innate inflammatory responses of pediatric cystic fibrosis airway epithelial cells: effects of nonviral and viral stimulation. *Am. J. Respir. Cell Mol. Biol.* 44, 761–767. doi: 10.1165/rcmb.2010-0368OC

Tacon, C. E., Wiehler, S., Holden, N. S., Newton, R., Proud, D., and Leigh, R. (2010). Human rhinovirus infection up-regulates MMP-9 production in airway epithelial cells via NF-{kappa}B. *Am. J. Respir. Cell Mol. Biol.* 43, 201–209. doi: 10.1165/rcmb.2009-0216OC

Turner, R. B., Wecker, M. T., Pohl, G., Witek, T. J., McNally, E., St George, R., et al. (1999). Efficacy of tremacamra, a soluble intercellular adhesion molecule 1, for experimental rhinovirus infection: a randomized clinical trial. *JAMA* 281, 1797–1804.

Unger, B. L., Ganesan, S., Comstock, A. T., Faris, A. N., Hershenson, M. B., and Sajjan, U. S. (2014). Nod-Like Receptor X-1 Is Required for Rhinovirus-Induced Barrier Dysfunction in Airway Epithelial Cells. *J. Virol.* 88, 3705–3718. doi: 10.1128/JVI.03039-13

van Ewijk, B. E., van der Zalm, M. M., Wolfs, T. F. W., and van der Ent, C. K. (2005). Viral respiratory infections in cystic fibrosis. *J. Cyst. Fibros.* 4(Suppl. 2), 31–36. doi: 10.1016/j.jcf.2005.05.011

Vareille, M., Kieninger, E., Edwards, M. R., and Regamey, N. (2011). The airway epithelium: soldier in the fight against respiratory viruses. *Clin. Microbiol. Rev.* 24, 210–229. doi: 10.1128/CMR.00014-10

Vlaic, S., Conrad, T., Tokarski-Schnelle, C., Gustafsson, M., Dahmen, U., Guthke, R., et al. (2018). ModuleDiscoverer: identification of regulatory modules in protein-protein interaction networks. *Sci. Rep.* 8:433. doi: 10.1038/s41598-017-18370-2

Wagener, A. H., Zwinderman, A. H., Luiten, S., Fokkens, W. J., Bel, E. H., Sterk, P. J., et al. (2014). dsRNA-induced changes in gene expression profiles of primary nasal and bronchial epithelial cells from patients with asthma, rhinitis and controls. 15:9. doi: 10.1186/1465-9921-15-9

Wark, P. A. B., Tooze, M., Cheese, L., Whitehead, B., Gibson, P. G., Wark, K. F., et al. (2012). Viral infections trigger exacerbations of cystic fibrosis in adults and children. *Eur. Respir. J.* 40, 510–512. doi: 10.1183/09031936.00202311

Wat, D. (ed.). (2015). "Respiratory virus in cystic fibrosis – a review of the literature," in *Cystic Fibrosis in the Light of New Research* (InTechOpen), 143–169. doi: 10.5772/60905

Wat, D., Gelder, C., Hibbitts, S., Cafferty, F., Bowler, I., Pierrepoint, M., et al. (2008). The role of respiratory viruses in cystic fibrosis. *J. Cyst. Fibros.* 7, 320–328. doi: 10.1016/j.jcf.2007.12.002

Waters, V., and Ratjen, F. (2015). Pulmonary exacerbations in children with cystic fibrosis. *Ann. Am. Thorac Soc.* 12 (Suppl 2), S200–S206. doi: 10.1513/AnnalsATS.201502-098AW

Whitsett, J. A., and Alenghat, T. (2015). Respiratory epithelial cells orchestrate pulmonary innate immunity. *Nat. Immunol.* 16, 27–35. doi: 10.1038/ni.3045

Worrall, G. (2011). Common cold. *Can. Fam. Physician* 57, 1289–1290.

Yeo, N.-K., and Jang, Y. J. (2010). Rhinovirus infection-induced alteration of tight junction and adherens junction components in human nasal epithelial cells. *Laryngoscope* 120, 346–352. doi: 10.1002/lary.20764

Zaman, N., Li, L., Jaramillo, M. L., Sun, Z., Tibiche, C., Banville, M., et al. (2013). Signaling network assessment of mutations and copy number variations predict breast cancer subtype-specific drug targets. *Cell Rep.* 5, 216–223. doi: 10.1016/j.celrep.2013.08.028

19

Animal Models in the Pathophysiology of Cystic Fibrosis

*Anna Semaniakou, Roger P. Croll and Valerie Chappe**

Department of Physiology and Biophysics, Faculty of Medicine, Dalhousie University, Halifax, NS, Canada

Correspondence:
Valerie Chappe
valerie.chappe@dal.ca

Our understanding of the multiorgan pathology of cystic fibrosis (CF) has improved impressively during the last decades, but we still lack a full comprehension of the disease progression. Animal models have greatly contributed to the elucidation of specific mechanisms involved in CF pathophysiology and the development of new therapies. Soon after the cloning of the CF transmembrane conductance regulator (*CFTR*) gene in 1989, the first mouse model was generated and this model has dominated *in vivo* CF research ever since. Nonetheless, the failure of murine models to mirror human disease severity in the pancreas and lung has led to the generation of larger animal models such as pigs and ferrets. The following review presents and discusses data from the current animal models used in CF research.

Keywords: cystic fibrosis, CF mice, animals in CF, CF ferrets, CF pigs, CF rats

INTRODUCTION

Cystic fibrosis, is the most common lethal autosomal recessive disorder in the Caucasian population, affecting one in 2,500 to 3,000 newborns and 70,000 people worldwide (C. G. App, Epidemiology). In 1938, CF was differentiated from celiac disease and named "cystic fibrosis of the pancreas" by Andersen (1938; Davis, 2006). Paul di Sant' Agnese, discovered the sweat electrolyte defect, and the standardization of the sweat test in 1959 made the diagnosis of CF accurate (Gibson and Cooke, 1959; Wine, 2010). Thirty years later, Riordan et al. (1989) discovered the gene responsible for CF, (*CFTR*), located on human chromosome 7. In 1989, they established the basic defect to be in a cAMP-regulated chloride channel (Welsh and Smith, 1993). Since then, an explosion of basic and clinical research has led to therapeutic progress, and the median age of survival today ranges from 40 to 53 years old, with the highest in Canada, which is a remarkable improvement from only 6 months in 1938 (Riordan et al., 1989; Rommens et al., 1989).

In addition, CF is caused by the dysfunction or absence of the CFTR channel from the exocrine tissues due to mutations in the gene (Riordan et al., 1989). While more than 2,000 mutations have been reported to date, the most common disease-causing mutation, occurring in 70% of patients, is F508del, a deletion of three nucleotides that results in the loss of phenylalanine (F) at the 508th position on the protein.

Abbreviations: rAAV, adeno-associated virus; AA, amino acid; ATP, adenosine triphosphate; ASL, airway surface liquid; BAL, bacterial alveolar lavage; *Bcc, Burkholderia cepacia* complex; CACC, Ca^{2+}-activated Cl^- channel; CFTR, cystic fibrosis transmembrane conductance regulator protein; *CFTR*, cystic fibrosis transmembrane conductance regulator gene; CF, cystic fibrosis; ENaC, epithelial sodium channel; iFABP, intestinal fatty-acid binding protein promoter; $[Ca^{2+}]_I$, intracellular Ca^{2+}; KO, knockout; LPS, lipopolysaccharides; MI, meconium ileus; MUC5AC, mucin 5AC; MUC5B, mucin 5B; MCC, mucociliary clearance; PI, pancreatic insufficiency, PS, pancreatic sufficient; PD, potential difference; RE, respiratory epithelia; I_{sc}, short-circuit current; SMGs, submucosal glands, Vt, transepithelial voltage; VIP, vasoactive intestinal peptide; WT, wild type.

Respiratory failure is the major cause of death but as a multiorgan disease, CF also causes PI, intestinal obstruction and malabsorption, biliary cirrhosis and congenital bilateral absence of the vas deferens (Durie and Forstner, 1989; Wong, 1998; van der Doef et al., 2011; Wilschanski and Novak, 2013; Lavelle et al., 2016).

Animal models are essential tools for understanding and comprehensively investigating CF pathophysiology. Each model is unique and variably resembles human CF manifestations with variable ortholog CFTR protein identity (**Table 1**). This review describes the availability of various animal models for CF and how useful they are for studying disease manifestation and progression in the lungs, intestines and other affected organs.

MURINE MODELS IN CYSTIC FIBROSIS RESEARCH

The first genetically modified mouse models of CF disease were created 3 years after the identification of the *CFTR* gene by homologous recombination in embryonic stem cells through targeting a mutation to a specific site in the murine genome (Clarke et al., 1994; Gosselin et al., 1998). Cloning of the mouse homolog of the human *CFTR* gene, which is located on mouse chromosome 6, revealed a 78% AA sequence homology to the human CFTR protein (Tata et al., 1991; Ellsworth et al., 2000). To our knowledge, 14 more mouse models have been described in the literature to date with different characteristics, grouping them in two categoriess (**Table 2**) (O'Neal et al., 1993; Ratcliff et al., 1993; Dorin et al., 1994; Colledge et al., 1995; Hasty et al., 1995; van Doorninck et al., 1995; Zeiher et al., 1995; Delaney et al., 1996; Rozmahe et al., 1996; Fisher et al., 2012). The first category consists of those models in which the *CFTR* gene was disrupted using a "replacement strategy" or an "insertional strategy." A replacement strategy causes an interruption of the *CFTR* gene and generates complete nulls ("knockout": KO) with no normal CFTR protein production, while with the "insertional strategy" a low amount (~10%) of normal mouse CFTR mRNA is produced (Davidson and Dorin, 2001; Scholte et al., 2004). The models generated by an "insertional strategy" method are also referred as "residual function" models (Davidson and Dorin, 2001). Phenotypic differences are observed between the absolute nulls and the residual function models due to the low amount of normal *CFTR* expression in the latter.

TABLE 1 | Amino acid identity in CFTR orthologs.

Species	CFTR aa Identity vs. humans	Reference
Mouse	78%	Tata et al., 1991
Pig	93%	Ostedgaard et al., 2007
Ferret	92%	Fisher et al., 2012
Rat	75.5%	Trezise et al., 1992
Zebrafish	55%	Liu et al., 2017
Sheep	91%	Harris, 1997

Percentage of amino acid identity of CFTR orthologs from animal models described in this review, and compared to human CFTR.

The second category contains mouse models that replicate known clinical mutations in CF, such as the Class II F508del ($Cftr^{tm1Eur}$, $Cftr^{tm1Kth}$, and $Cftr^{tm2Cam}$) and Class III, G551D ($Cftr^{tm1G551D}$) (Delaney et al., 1996; Lavelle et al., 2016) utilizing a replacement-gene targeting strategy or a double homologous recombination method, also known as a "hit and run" procedure (Hasty et al., 1991; Davidson and Dorin, 2001). In this category, survival rates, disease severity and pathology vary from model to model. The variations are attributed to different types of mutations, levels of mRNA expression, environmental factors and genetic backgrounds that can be responsible for various levels of activity of modifier genes in the mouse strains used (Tarran et al., 2001; Scholte et al., 2004). Moreover, because CF mutant mice are less fertile than normal mice, breeding CF mutant mice from heterozygous animals is strongly recommended to avoid phenotypic abnormalities and experimental variability (Zeiher et al., 1995). Lastly, gender and age are factors that should be considered especially for studying the progression of lung disease.

In a recent study, McHugh et al. (2018a) generated a G542X CF mouse model with CRISPR/Cas9 gene editing method. 40.9% of founder mice expressed the G542X mutation and this new clone was generated in approximately 3 months, whereas traditional methods using embryonic stem cells, would necessitate 1–2 years to obtain the desired mouse colony. These mice have decreased CFTR expression and a lack of CFTR function in the airways and intestine; they have low survival rates due to intestinal obstruction. Pharmacological read-through of the G542X mutation in this mouse model enables functional CFTR protein production, making this model very interesting for further investigation of non-sense mutations (Than et al., 2016; McHugh et al., 2018b).

Do Cystic Fibrosis Mice Develop Spontaneous Lung Disease?

Progressive lung disease with respiratory failure is a major clinical concern that causes 95% of the morbidity and mortality in patients with CF. Lung disease develops over recurrent exacerbations of pulmonary infections caused by a large spectrum of bacterial species including *Staphylococcus aureus*, *Haemophilus influenza*, *Pseudomonas aeruginosa* and the *Bcc* (Tarran et al., 2001; Festini et al., 2006). *P. aeruginosa* is persistent in human lungs with CF and chronic pulmonary infection is inevitable, despite antibiotic therapies, with biofilm-forming cells of a mucoid phenotype in more severe advanced infections. Spontaneous colonization with the above pathogens has not been detected in mice models unless a pathogen challenge was applied.

Kent et al. (1997) designed a model from a single genetic background (congenic), C57BL/6J $Cftr^{tm1Unc}/Cftr^{tm1Unc}$, that under specific pathogen-free conditions, developed spontaneous and progressive lung disease (Guilbault et al., 2005, 2006). Loss of mucociliary transport, post-bronchiolar hyperinflation of alveoli, and parenchymal interstitial thickening with indication of fibrosis and inflammatory cell recruitment characterize the lung disease in this congenic model (Kent et al., 1997). It also showed reduced control of the *P. aeruginosa* infection. Acinar and alveolar over inflation, reflect small airway obstructions that

TABLE 2 | Murine models used in cystic fibrosis research.

CF mice models	Cftr mRNA	Survival to maturity	Reference
Knockout models (replacement method)			
Cftr$^{tm/Unc}$	No WT mRNA detectable	<5%	Snouwaert et al., 1992
Cftr$^{tm/Cam}$		<5%	Ratcliff et al., 1993
Cftr$^{tm/Hsc}$		25%	Rozmahe et al., 1996
Cftr^{tm3Bay}		40%	Hasty et al., 1995
Cftr^{tm3Uth}		25%	Wilke et al., 2011
Residual function models (insertional method)			
Cftr$^{tm/Hgu}$	10% of WT	90%	Wilke et al., 2011
Cftr$^{tm/Bay}$	<2% of WT	40%	O'Neal et al., 1993
F508del models (replacement-gene targeting method)			
Cftr^{tm2Cam}	30% of WT	<5%	Colledge et al., 1995
Cftr$^{tm/Kth}$	Decreased levels of mutant mRNA in intestine	40%	Zeiher et al., 1995
F508del models (Hit and Run method)			
Cftr$^{tm/Eur}$	Normal level of mutant mRNA	90%	Rozmahe et al., 1996
Models with other mutations			
Cftr^{tm2Hgu} (G551D- replacement-gene targeting method)	50% of WT	65%	Wilke et al., 2011
Cftr^{tm3Hgu} (G480C- Hit and Run method)	Normal level of mutant mRNA	90%	Wilke et al., 2011
Cftr^{tm2Uth} (R117H- replacement-gene targeting)	5–20% of WT	95%	Wilke et al., 2011
Transgenes			
Tg (FABPCFTR): correction of intestinal obstruction	–	1.5–8.5 months	Zhou et al., 1994
Tg (CCSPSsnn 1b): βENaC over-expression (model of CF-lung disease)	–	40%	Wilke et al., 2011
VIP-KO: CF-like phenotype in lung and intestine	Normal level of WT	Normal	Alcolado et al., 2014

Levels of Cftr mRNA expression, compared to WT Cftr mRNA, are indicated when known. Survival rates at maturity refers to after weaning.

are observed in the early stages of CF in humans (Guilbault et al., 2005). Later on, more studies boosted our knowledge with significant observations in CF pulmonary pathology using mice that were not exposed to pathogens. Thus, excessive inflammation was noticed in *Cftr*^{tmr1Hgu} mice, MCC dysfunction in *Cftr*^{tm1Hgu} and *Cftr*^{tm1Unc} mice, goblet cell hyperplasia with ASL depletion in the nasal epithelium of *Cftr*^{tm1Unc} mice, and a distal extension of SMGs in *Cftr*^{tm1Hgu} and *Cftr*^{tm1G551D} mice (Cowley et al., 1997; Zahm et al., 1997; Tarran et al., 2001; Scholte et al., 2004). The *Cftr*^{tm1G551D} model demonstrated defective pulmonary clearance and a high sensitivity to *P. aeruginosa* (McMorran et al., 2001).

To date, many research groups using congenic mice are still trying to develop methods for *P. aeruginosa* inoculation that would mimic chronic infection with this persistent pathogen. Techniques such as intratracheal inoculation of bacteria-loaded agar beads or seaweed alginate must be used to reproduce the human lung phenotype with *P. aeruginosa*.

The fact that CF mice do not develop airway's infections led Shah et al. (2016) to investigate the reasons why mice have functioning airway's host defenses compared to humans and pigs with CF. This interesting study demonstrated that, in addition to the presence of Ca^{+}-activated anion channels, mice also express small amounts (1–10%) of the non-gastric H^{+}/K^{+} adenosine triphosphatase ATP12A transcripts, which catalyzes the hydrolysis of ATP coupled with the exchange of H^{+} and K^{+} ions across the plasma membrane. Consequently, mouse airways, including those in CF models, secrete low levels of H^{+} maintaining the pH of the ASL unaltered. The authors showed that the over-expression of ATP12A in CF mice airways caused acidification of the ASL, impairment of airway host defenses as well as increased amount of bacteria. These data suggest ATP12A as a potential therapeutic target for CF disease treatment (Shah et al., 2016).

Durie et al. (2004) described a promising long-living congenic *Cftr*$^{-/-}$ model bred in the C57BL/6 background that displays the human lung pathology with signs of inflammation, presence of macrophages, tissue damage, and acinar dilation (Durie et al., 2004). Defective bacterial clearance, increased levels of pro-inflammatory factors, and inflammation was demonstrated using *Cftr*^{tm1Unc} and *Cftr*^{tm1G551D} mice (Heeckeren et al., 1997; McMorran et al., 2001; Van Heeckeren et al., 2006). Macrophages are the most commonly found immune cells in the lung that play a significant role in bacteria eradication from the airways through phagocytosis. The input of macrophages polarization and plasticity in CF disease progression is still undefined. Studies in CF mice have shown that macrophages are unable to degrade internalized pathogens such as *P. aeruginosa* and *Bcc* (Bruscia and Bonfield, 2016; Li et al., 2017). More specifically, *Cftr*$^{-/-}$ mice challenged with *P. aeruginosa* had increased IL-8, IL-6, and TNF-alpha levels and decreased IL-10 level, indicating that the absence of CFTR can cause excessive lung inflammation (Bruscia and Bonfield, 2016). Additionally, the number of both alveolar and peritoneal macrophages was high in F508del mice treated with LPS, illustrating their adaptability in the airway environment (Bruscia and Bonfield, 2016). CF mice may not be able to develop acute lung disease as patients with CF do, but they have been successfully used to demonstrate a defective autophagy mechanism which can lead to lung hyper-inflammation (Luciani et al., 2010). An increasing amount of literature on CF macrophages is becoming available (Andersson et al., 2008; Bruscia et al., 2009, 2011; Meyer et al., 2009; Abdulrahman et al., 2011; Sorio et al., 2016; Li et al., 2017).

Zhou et al. (2011) generated a transgenic "β-ENaC" mouse model to recapitulate the pathophysiology of the CF lung. This model, which over-expresses the β subunit of the ENaC with increased Na^+ absorption, presented with ASL depletion, reduced MCC with airway mucus obstruction, goblet cell hyperplasia, chronic lung inflammation, and high mortality related to lung disease (Zhou et al., 2011). Nonetheless, even this interesting model failed to replicate the spontaneous bacterial infection that develops in patients with CF (Zhou et al., 2011).

Overall, while the above-mentioned methods and murine models further our understanding of CF lung abnormalities, they do not provide any information on how the disease starts and the development of early stages of infection and inflammation. Furthermore, the general notion that mice do not show "spontaneous" lung pathology could be misleading. Many factors play a role in this. The short life span of mice and clean or sterile environment under which the experiments are conducted are not comparable with the conditions for human lungs with CF that are continuously challenged with various pathogens along their lifetime. In addition, diverse genetic background is an important factor, while low levels of residual CFTR protein expression in some models affect the disease severity. Moreover, the size of the airways and the presence of a non-CFTR calcium-activated Cl^- channel (CACC) in parallel with CFTR and other dissimilarities in lung disease between humans and mice models (Clarke et al., 1994; Gosselin et al., 1998; Lavelle et al., 2016) can account for differences in resistance to bacteria.

Submucosal Glands to Study Fluid Secretion Defects

Submucosal glands lining the cartilaginous airways are responsible for maintaining sterility in the airways by secreting antimicrobial defenses, such as lysozyme, lactoferrin, defensins, bicarbonate, and others (Salinas et al., 2005; Ianowski et al., 2007). Moreover, they secrete mucus when stimulated with Ca^+ -elevating agonists, for example acetylcholine (ACh) or carbachol (CCh), and/or cAMP agonists, such as forskolin (FSK) or VIP, and contain serous cells that express high levels of CFTR (Borthwick et al., 1999). In CF airway glands, the synergy between cAMP and calcium signaling is lost, and glands do not respond to VIP or FSK. In humans, SMGs extend into the bronchi, while, in mice they are confined to the trachea. Congenic mice models, especially those with a C57BL/6 genetic background, have been used to study SMG dysfunction since these mice show increased airway abnormalities and are prone to infection with *P. aeruginosa.* Grubb and Boucher (1999) mentioned that mice have very few SMGs (Grubb and Boucher, 1999). However, in a study of tracheal SMG secretion in *Cftr*$^{-/-}$ mice, Ianowski et al.(2007) observed that the upper trachea contains only 15–20 airway glands in wild-type (WT) mice and an abundance of glands in CF-KO mice (De Jonge, 2007; Ianowski et al., 2007). Furthermore, they demonstrated that glands from an inbred congenic *Cftr*$^{-/-}$ mouse strain responded to CCh but not to VIP or FSK similar to human CF glands (Ianowski et al., 2007). This study also documented that glands from CF mice did not secrete when they were exposed to chili oil, a treatment that produces secretion through stimulation of sensory nerves and the release of tachykinins, such as substance P. Additionally, it was demonstrated for the first time, that on tracheal SMGs of *Cftr*$^{-/-}$ mice, the substance P-stimulated fluid secretion requires CFTR (Ianowski et al., 2007).

The neuropeptide VIP is abundantly secreted around all exocrine glands including SMGs and sweat glands. It is well known to work in synergy with ACh to regulate secretions (Lundberg et al., 1980; Heinz-Erian et al., 1985, 1986). Interestingly, VIP KO mice generated in the C57BL/6 background demonstrated, *in vivo,* the central role of VIP in CFTR regulation (Chappe and Said, 2012; Alcolado et al., 2014). Originally developed to study airway diseases, such as bronchial asthma (Hamidi et al., 2006; Szema et al., 2006; Said, 2009), VIP-KO mice were used by Alcolado et al. (2014) to demonstrate the molecular link between VIP and CFTR regulation in the airways and small intestines, and observed a CF-like phenotype. The absence of VIP resulted in CFTR intracellular retention. A subsequent loss of CFTR-dependent chloride current was measured in functional assays with an Ussing chamber analysis of the small intestine *ex vivo*. In the lung, lymphocyte aggregation, increased airway secretion, alveolar thickening, and edema were observed. Inflammation and tissue damage observed in VIP-KO mice were attributed, at least in part, to the lack of CFTR-dependent secretions that rely on VIP stimulation of CFTR function. These observations support early findings of a lack of VIPergic innervation of human CF glands.

Nasal and Tracheal Epithelium

Murine CF nasal epithelium exhibits two important characteristics of human CF airways: Na^+ hyper-absorption and a defect in cAMP-mediated Cl^- secretion (Grubb and Boucher, 1999; Tarran et al., 2001). Hyper-absorption of Na^+ was demonstrated *in vivo* with an increased baseline PD across the epithelium that was largely decreased in the presence of the ENaC blocker, amiloride (Grubb et al., 1994; Grubb and Boucher, 1999). In addition, the decreased level or absence of cAMP-stimulated Cl^- conductance was noticed in all murine models except for F508del *Cftr*^{tm1Eur}. As mentioned above, the ~10% residual normal CFTR expression in this model, may allow for a residual Cl^- permeability. In addition, nasal epithelium from *Cftr*^{tm1Unc} and *Cftr*^{tm1Hsc} demonstrates a Cl^- secretory response, which may be due to calcium dependent chloride channel (CACC) (Grubb and Boucher, 1999). The CACC is the prevalent Cl^- channel in murine tracheal epithelium (Rock et al., 2009). The gene that encodes this "pseudo" Cl^- channel is *TMEM16A*, and it was shown to be necessary for maintaining regular ASL levels. Studies on tracheas from *Tmem16a*$^{-/-}$ mice demonstrated more than 60% lower CACC activity and reduced MCC with mucus accumulation (Ousingsawat et al., 2009; Rock et al., 2009).

Despite bioelectric similarities, the murine nasal mucosa is composed of ~40% olfactory epithelia and 60% RE, while the human nasal cavity is lined by more than 95% RE. However, the dominant cell type is the cilia cell, as in humans (Harkema et al., 1991; Tarran et al., 2001). In the *in vivo* analysis of *Cftr*^{tm1Unc}, the nasal septal mucosa demonstrated goblet cell hyperplasia and enlargement correlated with reduced ASL height rather than changes in salt composition (Tarran et al., 2001). A study using *Cftr*^{Hm1G551D} and *Cftr*^{tm1Unc}-*TgN*$^{(FABRCFTR)}$ mouse models was conducted to examine whether the structural changes in nasal mucosa were related to infection and inflammation. Interestingly, they detected features that are comparable with human CF tissues, such as thickening of the RE with an increased number of mucus cells. The conclusion of the study suggested that the changes observed were not a consequence of initial inflammation (Hilliard et al., 2008). Another study from Grubb et al. (2007) using *Cftr*^{tm1Unc} mice reported that an ion transport defect in CF results in progressive morphological and structural changes in the olfactory epithelium of the nasal cavity (Grubb et al., 2007).

The nasal cavity has been used extensively to investigate Cl^- permeability in response to corrector drug treatment by measuring the PD across the nasal epithelium. The murine nasal mucosa appears to offer an excellent model for investigating the abnormal electrophysiological profile of CF epithelial cells and testing potential corrector drugs. The murine trachea has also been used for studying cartilaginous rings alterations in *Cftr*$^{-/-}$ and F508del-CFTR mice. Structural modifications were observed in both newborn and adult CF mice independently of the CFTR absence or protein dysfunction and those changes could be indigenous (Bonvin et al., 2008).

Although the murine nasal cavity closely resembles that of humans and is easily accessible, most studies have rather used murine tracheal SMGs to examine MCC abnormalities and airway submucosal inflammation (Zahm et al., 1997; Grubb et al., 2004; Ianowski et al., 2007). Additionally, data from other animal models reported significant differences in size, density, secretory capacity and fluid secretion defects between nasal and tracheal glands. Ianowski et al. (2007) suggested that the murine trachea is an appropriate tissue for studying airway glands abnormalities in CF (Ianowski et al., 2007). Airway SMGs are found in the proximal trachea of mice. In the cartilaginous rings, CFTR expression is found at the highest levels in SMG serous tubules as reported by Engelhardt et al. (1992). Furthermore, it is well known that serous cells secrete antimicrobial proteins, such as lysozyme and lactoferrin, indicating the importance of tracheal glands in CF disease (Engelhardt et al., 1992). Nevertheless, in murine trachea, the CACC exhibits "CFTR-like" activity and protects CF mice from having the severe lung phenotype that is observed in humans. Consequently, one must ask whether murine tracheal glands are appropriate for studying secretion abnormalities in CF. Until now, there has been no consensus about it.

Cystic Fibrosis Mice Develop Severe Postnatal Intestinal Disease

One of the earliest disease manifestations in CF is the MI in 15–20% of CF newborns and distal intestinal obstruction syndrome in 25% of adults (Zielenski et al., 1999). Moreover, CF mice are characterized by severe intestinal obstructions, including mucus accumulation, goblet cell hyperplasia, and crypt dilatation and elongation, symptoms similar to the human disease manifestations (Grubb and Boucher, 1999; Norkina et al., 2004), which develop postnatally and appear to be the hallmark for all the CF mouse models (Grubb and Gabriel, 1997; Keiser and Engelhardt, 2011) with the exception of only two mouse models (*Cftr*^{tm1HGU} and *Cftr*^{tm1Eur}). The severity of the disease and the survival rate differ among genotypes (Grubb and Gabriel, 1997; Durie et al., 2004; Canale-Zambrano et al., 2007; De Lisle and Borowitz, 2013). The neonatal death rate is ~60% for CF null mice and only 35% for F508del-CFTR. However, this percentage of MI is still high compare to only 10% in the human disease. The *Cftr*^{tm1Eur} and *Cftr*^{tm2Hgu} models, carrying the F508del and G480C mutations, respectively, exhibit intestinal alterations that are not as severe as those in the *CFTR*-KO mice (De Lisle and Borowitz, 2013). The *Cftr*^{tm1G551D} has an approximate 70% survival rate with less severe pathology than the null models (Scholte et al., 2004). A murine F508del model was generated with a replacement-gene targeting method by Colledge et al. (1995) and was suggested to be an accurate model for testing therapeutic drugs. It demonstrated severe meconium obstruction, reduced cAMP-stimulated Cl^- secretion, and the temperature-dependent trafficking defect that is described associated with this mutation in the human disease (Colledge et al., 1995). Tissue sections of the colon and duodenum revealed huge crypt dilation with increased mucus accumulation. As previously mentioned, the genetic background variation and low residual level of expression of normal CFTR proteins have been proposed to explain dissimilarities between models.

Studies have shown that the expression of modifier genes may also be responsible for this intestinal variability. A genetic modifier of MI was detected in chromosome 19 in humans and on mouse chromosome 7 and was shown to be involved in the disease progression in KO mice (Rozmahe et al., 1996; Zielenski et al., 1999; Gyömörey et al., 2000). Norkina et al. (2004), using a DNA microarray, observed the presence of some gene expression associated with inflammation and presence of innate immune cells, such as mast cells and neutrophils, similar to those observed in the intestine of patients with CF (Norkina et al., 2004). Amelioration of the intestinal obstruction and an increase in the survival rate was achieved by the expression of human CFTR cDNA in the intestinal track of *Cftr*^{tm1Unc} mice, under the control of the rat intestinal fatty-acid-binding protein (iFABP) gene promoter. This *Cftr*^{tm1Unc}-*TgN*$^{(FABPCFTR)}$

model enabled long-term studies in the intestine (De Lisle and Borowitz, 2013).

In a recent study, McHugh et al. (2018b) investigated the efficacy of linaclotide in treating intestinal pathophysiology in CF mice carrying the F508del mutation or *Cftr*-KO mice. Linaclotide is a drug that has been approved by FDA to treat chronic idiopathic constipation. This study demonstrated that this drug elevates the amount of fluid in the intestinal lumen and improves intestinal transit, thus prompting the authors to recommend linaclotide as a therapeutic option to treat CF intestinal manifestations (Than et al., 2016; McHugh et al., 2018a).

Electrophysiological studies have confirmed the ion transport abnormalities in CF mice with a similar phenotype to that of the human CF intestine: low or absence of cAMP-mediated Cl^- transport (Grubb and Gabriel, 1997). Moreover, they display a significant reduction in the basal PD and short-circuit current (I_{sc}) (Grubb, 1999).

In summary, the CF murine intestine exhibits many pathophysiological similarities with that in humans with CF. However, it is important to categorize the different mouse models and background strains, the various techniques by which they were generated, the pathogen exposure, and the husbandry conditions during the research before evaluating the intestinal phenotype.

Cystic Fibrosis Mice Develop Mild Pancreatic Disease

In contrast to patients with CF in whom exocrine PI is a major condition, CF mice exhibit only moderate pancreatic changes (Snouwaert et al., 1992). Durie et al. (2004) demonstrated that a long-living CF-KO mouse bred into a congenic C57BL/6 background develops pancreatic pathology similar to humans with presence of inflammatory cells and macrophages and increased acinar volume at an older age (Durie et al., 2004). Surprisingly, mice with the F508del or G551D mutation, do not show any apparent pancreatic disease (Dorin et al., 1992; Colledge et al., 1995; van Doorninck et al., 1995; Delaney et al., 1996). The milder pancreatic disease in mice is attributed first to the lower level of normal CFTR protein expression in the murine pancreas, while high CFTR expression level has been shown in humans (Gray et al., 1995), and second to differences in the CACC channel expression. The CACC is detected in both WT and CF mice alleviating the pancreatic disease progression and perhaps explaining the mild murine pancreatic pathology (Marino et al., 1991; Clarke et al., 1994; Gray et al., 1995; Keiser and Engelhardt, 2011).

Mice Sweat Glands – An Underestimated Tissue in Cystic Fibrosis Research

Increased NaCl reabsorption abnormalities from sweat have been broadly studied with the sweat concentration being the most reliable pathophysiological marker. In mice, sweat glands are present in the palmoplantar skin (paw) (Lu and Fuchs, 2014). This tissue has largely been underutilized in CF research. In humans, sweat glands are controlled by adrenergic, cholinergic, and peptidergic innervation (Heinz-Erian et al., 1985). Heinz-Erian et al. (1985) demonstrated a reduction of VIP, in the sweat glands of patients with CF (Heinz-Erian et al., 1985). They proposed that, since VIP activates the opening of the CFTR channel, enabling the movement of water and Cl^- across epithelium, the lack of VIP innervation could cause low levels of water, Cl^- impermeability, and abnormalities involving other ions that manifest in CF disease. Sato et al. (1994) investigated changes in cholinergic and β-adrenergic responsiveness during the postnatal life and reported that the mouse sweat glands are mainly under cholinergic control and express CFTR. Sweat secretion can be monitored in response to cAMP elevating agonists with activation of either K^+ channels, Cl^- channels, or both. The secretion rates are higher in older animals (over 6-weeks old) but are independent from glandular enlargement. Additionally, Chappe et al. (personal communication) examined VIP expression in sweat glands of F508del mice and found support for the murine sweat glands as a valuable tissue for studying CF disease progression. Sweat glands remain free of infection, do not exhibit morphological alterations and are easy to collect. Accordingly, their use should be further evaluated for studying CF disease development and progression.

PORCINE MODELS IN CYSTIC FIBROSIS RESEARCH

Cystic Fibrosis Pigs Develop Lung Pathology Gradually

The expression of the CACC channel in parallel with the CFTR channel in some mouse organs and the inability of mice to develop "spontaneous" lung disease led investigators to examine the pathology of the CF lung using other animal models. Rogers et al. (2008b) recommended porcine airways as a possible model for CF because of their similar lung anatomy and morphological similarities with humans and identical bioelectric ion properties. Welsh et al. (2001, 2009) (Rogers et al., 2008b; Fisher et al., 2011) developed the first CF pigs with homologous recombination, utilizing adeno-associated virus (rAAV) vectors to target the *CFTR* gene in fibroblasts from fetal pigs. A somatic cell nuclear transfer of these cells into oocytes was made to generate a heterozygous male pig and through heterozygous × heterozygous breeding, $Cftr^{-/-}$ piglets were born (Rogers et al., 2008b).

At birth, the lungs of the $Cftr^{-/-}$ piglets, like those of human CF infants, are normal with no signs of pathology (Rogers et al., 2008c). However, in contrast to control animals, BAL fluid from neonatal CF piglets revealed a large number of different bacterial species (Rogers et al., 2008c; Welsh et al., 2009; Stoltz et al., 2010) and a rapid lung infection, which shows a more severe lung pathology than in patients with CF (Stoltz et al., 2010; Wine, 2010). When lungs from newborn WT and CF piglets were specifically challenged with *S. aureus*, the most common lung pathogen in infants and children with

CF, only the CF piglets had more *S. aureus* than normal (Stoltz et al., 2010). That could be due to abnormalities in the pH of the ASL caused by reduced CFTR-dependent bicarbonate transport as reported by Pezzulo et al. (2012). Newborn *Cftr*$^{-/-}$ pigs were also used to examine macrophage dysfunction and to determine if their defective polarization and function are due to the absence of CFTR, or a consequence of the chronic inflammation and infection. Data from this study suggested that defective macrophages function is present at the onset of the disease and is the cause of inflammation (Paemka et al., 2017). Since the newborn CF pigs do not present signs of lung inflammation at birth, they are considered a good model for studying macrophages dysfunction prior to the beginning of the chronic inflammation.

Importantly, neonatal CF piglets have not been examined after a challenge with *P. aeruginosa*, and hence we do not know if CF pig airways are able to eradicate these bacteria. These data suggest that lungs from newborn CF pigs lack inflammation at birth but are unable to sterilize their lungs, suggesting that infection initiates inflammation (Wine, 2010).

The CF piglets revealed tracheal abnormalities, including narrowed proximal airways with thicker and more discontinuous cartilage, enlarged SMGs, and hyperplasia. Alterations in tracheal smooth muscle of F508del homozygote piglets were milder because of the residual CFTR function (Ostedgaard et al., 2011). These congenital tracheal alterations are similar to airway structural changes that occur in CF infants (Meyerholz et al., 2010a; Stoltz et al., 2015). It is suggested that the loss of CFTR produces tracheal abnormalities that may contribute to CF disease development during postnatal life (Rogers et al., 2008c; Welsh et al., 2009). However, the specific mechanisms for these abnormalities and how the absence of CFTR during development induces these defects are still unknown (Meyerholz et al., 2010a).

While mucociliary transport plays a significant role in maintaining the airways sterile, it is still unknown if in CF it is defective from birth and contributes to the beginning of the disease or if it becomes defective later, contributing to disease progression. A study from Hoegger et al. (2014a), established a new *in vivo* mucociliary transport assay (X-ray-computed tomographic-based method) with newborn pigs, which provides important insight into the pathophysiology of CF, as well as other respiratory diseases, at their early stages. The authors analyzed the movement of particles in bulk, and individually, in the large airways. They found that cilia orientation directs particles to the ventral area of the trachea and to the larynx, while the rate of individual particle's movement was largely heterogynous. They speculate that different mucus properties may account for this heterogeneity (Hoegger et al., 2014a). Moreover, using 350 μm diameter tantalum microdisks, they found that CF SMGs secrete dense mucus strands that remained tethered and prevent the movement of those dense disks. The authors conclude that impaired mucus detachment from SMGs could be an early defect in CF (Hoegger et al., 2014b).

The development of lung disease in CF pigs is not easy to investigate because most of them die from MI that occurs in 100% of the piglets (Rogers et al., 2008c; Welsh et al., 2009; Meyerholz et al., 2010b; Stoltz et al., 2010, 2013; Olivier et al., 2015). A study from Stoltz et al. (2010), performing an ileostomy on CF pigs that survived approximately 2 months or more, demonstrated the presence of structural, bacteriological and inflammatory markers of CF. Part of the airways were characterized by the presence of macrophages, neutrophils and bacteria, similar to those in human airways. Ostedgaard et al. (2011) demonstrated that, despite residual CFTR expression, older *Cftr*$^{F508del/F508del}$ pigs exhibited lung disease similar to humans, rendering the minimal CFTR activity observed (~6% to WT function) insignificant for lung pathogenesis. A study from Shah et al. (2016) demonstrated that CF pigs, like humans, have ASL acidification in contrast to mice. This is thought to be due to ATP12A in absence of CFTR chloride channels. Acidification of the ASL impairs airway defense while ATP12A inhibition, which increases the pH, improves host defense properties of the ASL in CF pigs (Shah et al., 2016).

Although CF pigs recapitulate most of the human manifestations of CF, only a small number have been used for studying CF pathology, mostly due to the difficulty of keeping them alive long enough. Even after an ileostomy or cecostomy to cure MI, 60% of the piglets still had to be euthanized for gastric ulcers (Stoltz et al., 2010; Wine, 2010; Olivier et al., 2015). Long-term research still needs to be conducted to validate the data.

Porcine Submucosal Glands – Excellent for Studying Secretion

Porcine lungs highly express CFTR proteins in the serous cells of SMGs of the cartilaginous airways, and, as in humans, exhibit the same secretion abnormalities in CF animals, with no detected morphological changes (Rogers et al., 2008c; Welsh et al., 2009). Chen et al. (2010) demonstrated a lack of cAMP-mediated Cl^- transport and subsequently impaired bicarbonate (HNO_3^-) transport with an absence of sodium hyper-absorption or reduction in ASL depth (Chen et al., 2010). This finding in CF pigs, with no signs of inflammation at birth, contradicts the hypothesis that Na^+ hyper-absorption might trigger lung disease. The authors suggested that defects in Cl^- and HNO_3^- initiate lung pathology and not deviations in sodium transport (Chen et al., 2010; Stoltz et al., 2015).

Ion transport abnormalities were detected in nasal airway epithelia from CF piglets with a hyperpolarized baseline transepithelial voltage (Vt), while the addition of amiloride (ENaC inhibitor) decreased the Vt in all CF piglets (Rogers et al., 2008a,c; Welsh et al., 2009). Perfusion of the apical membrane with a solution containing low Cl^- concentration and isoproterenol (to elevate cAMP) hyperpolarized nasal Vt in WT and heterozygous but not in *Cftr*$^{-/-}$ pigs (Rogers et al., 2008a,c; Joo et al., 2010). Lastly, perfusion with ATP to stimulate P2Y2 receptors and CACC channels produced further hyper-polarization while the CFTR inhibitor glybenclamide depolarized Vt in *Cftr*$^{+/+}$ and *Cftr*$^{+/-}$ but not in *Cftr*$^{-/-}$ piglets, demonstrating that a lack of CFTR channel function causes electrolyte transport abnormalities in airway epithelia (Rogers et al., 2008c; Welsh et al., 2009). The CFTR selective inhibitor CFTRinh-172 was found to be less effective with the porcine protein compared to the human CFTR (Rogers et al., 2008a). Liu et al. (2007) have reported species-specific differences in airway epithelial electrolyte transport and CFTR function (Liu et al., 2007).

Nasal vs. Tracheal Submucosal Glands

Human CF SMGs only secrete minimally in response to agonists that increase intracellular cAMP alone (VIP and FSK) or slightly to agonists that elevate $[Ca^{2+}]_i$ (substance P and CCh) (Choi et al., 2007). The combination of these two types of agents produce a synergetic response that is lost in CF. Accordingly, Joo et al. (2010) showed that tracheal SMGs from CF piglets did not respond to FSK but did respond to CCh, while substance P proved to be more efficacious in CF pigs than in humans. In contrast to human SMGs, *Cftr*$^{-/-}$ pigs exhibited synergistic secretion which was attributed to CFTR-independent pathways (Joo et al., 2010). Future studies on the specific mechanisms are necessary and would clarify whether this tissue is appropriate for studying fluid secretion defects in CF disease.

Interestingly, a study from Ostedgaard et al. (2017) demonstrated that tracheal SMGs from CF pigs produce mucin 5B (MUC5B) while goblet cells produce mainly mucin 5A (MUC5AC) and moderate MUC5B. The same study suggested that these two types of mucins have different morphologic structures that account for a more effective MCC transport (Ostedgaard et al., 2017).

Cho et al. (2011) described morphological and fluid secretion differences between nasal and tracheal glands in CF piglets. In contrast to tracheal glands, nasal glands were found to be smaller and more numerous than in humans (Cho et al., 2011) with no response to FSK and a moderate response to CCh, while the synergy was almost lost (Joo et al., 2010). These findings are of high interest because, as Rogers et al. (2008c) showed, CF piglets have abnormal ion transport in nasal epithelium (Rogers et al., 2008c) which could contribute to lung pathology in CF when combined with defective fluid secretion from nasal glands.

Intestinal Obstruction Is Fatal in Cystic Fibrosis Piglets

Meconium ileus is 100% fatal for CF pigs and a surgical ileostomy must be performed right after birth so as they can survive longer (Welsh et al., 2009; Meyerholz et al., 2010b; Stoltz et al., 2013). Accordingly, to suppress intestinal obstruction, Stoltz et al. (2013) used the rat intestinal fatty-acid-binding protein promoter (iFABP) to express WT porcine CFTR proteins (pCFTR) in *Cftr*$^{-/-}$ "gut-corrected" pigs (Stoltz et al., 2013). Their data supported the hypothesis that approximately 20% of CFTR expression was adequate to partially restore CFTR-mediated Cl^- transport. Similar to *Cftr*$^{-/-}$ and *Cftr*$^{F508del/F508del}$ pigs, these transgenic animals developed pancreatic, liver, and lung disease and therefore failure to thrive (Stoltz et al., 2013). The expression of CFTR proteins in parts of the intestine, other than in ileum, might be important for improving the MI defect. Gut correction was tested only in neonatal CF pigs and hence it is not known yet if the required amount of CFTR function during adult life would be the same. Nonetheless, while surgical gut correction is not always successful, this transgenic model would be another method for making these animals live long enough (up to 12 months) to study disease progression.

Interestingly, while one would expect less disease severity in *Cftr*$^{F508del/F508del}$ pigs compared to null animals, due to residual function of CFTR (~6% of WT), they still show 100% penetrance of MI, as was reported by Ostedgaard et al. (2011). In general, MI in CF pigs closely resembles the disease in humans, while distinct anatomy or physiology in combination with the differences in genetic background between pigs and humans may account for the dissimilarity of penetrance rate.

Porcine Pancreatic Pathogenesis Is Closely Similar to Humans

Cystic fibrosis pigs closely recapitulate pancreatic pathogenesis of humans CF with varying levels of disease severity among genotypes (Rogers et al., 2008c; Meyerholz et al., 2010b). After surgical correction of MI, PI develops spontaneously in these animals (Keiser and Engelhardt, 2011). The exocrine pancreas in newborn *Cftr*$^{-/-}$ pigs, as in human CF neonates, is smaller than normal, with degenerative lobules containing loose adipose tissue, mild, scattered inflammation, and dilated ducts with eosinophils, neutrophils, and macrophages. The endocrine tissue is intact, spared from the surrounding exocrine destruction with fewer acinar cells and zymogen granules (Rogers et al., 2008c; Welsh et al., 2009; Meyerholz et al., 2010b). Insulin-immunoreactive islets are mostly localized on the intact lobular tissue without alterations in the amount of insulin produced or glucagon cells. The volume and pH of pancreatic fluid are reduced in CF neonatal pigs, as in humans, with increased protein concentration (Gibson-Corley et al., 2016).

Interesting data from Abu-El-Haija et al. (2012) in fetal and newborn *Cftr*$^{-/-}$ and *Cftr*$^{F508del/F508del}$ pigs demonstrated that tissue damage starts *in utero* and pro-inflammatory, complement cascade, pro-apoptotic, and pro-fibrotic pathways are involved (Abu-El-Haija et al., 2012). They noticed elevated activation of the apoptotic caspase-3 pathway in the CF pig pancreas whereas the α-smooth muscle actin, a myofibroblast marker and activator of early fibrosis pathways, was observed in both fetal and newborn pigs. Tissue remodeling with mucus accumulation and duct cell proliferation was observed in the neonatal and not in fetal CF pigs, indicating that these changes do not initiate disease pathogenesis but follow pancreatic damage over time. Compared to *Cftr*$^{-/-}$, *Cftr*$^{F508del/F508del}$ pigs exhibit slightly less severe exocrine pancreatic pathogenesis that may be attributed to the residual CFTR function (Ostedgaard et al., 2011). Future studies that investigate how much CFTR chloride channel function is necessary for the correction of pancreatic disease would be a fundamental knowledge for the progression of CF pathogenesis. Studies in adult CF pigs would be useful and would enhance our understanding of pancreatic damage in humans.

FERRET MODELS IN CYSTIC FIBROSIS RESEARCH

Comparable Lung Pathogenesis With Cystic Fibrosis Patients

The lungs of ferrets share many similarities with human lungs in terms of function and architecture, and like CF pigs, CF ferrets develop spontaneous lung infections soon after birth (Sun et al., 2010, 2014a; Keiser et al., 2015). Similar to pigs, CF ferrets were produced using homologous recombination. The first genetically designed CF ferret was described by Sun et al. (2008), utilizing rAAV-mediated targeting of the *CFTR* gene in fetal fibroblasts followed by nuclear transfer cloning (Sun et al., 2008). The *Cftr*$^{-/-}$ ferrets develop severe lung pathology within the first weeks of life, and like piglets, they are unable to eliminate bacteria. Data from the BAL fluid of newborn CF ferrets revealed various bacterial species including *Streptococcus*, *Staphylococcus* and *Enterococcus* genera while three species of *Pseudomonas* (*P. fluorescents*, *P. putida* and *P. fulva*) were found in low amounts (Sun et al., 2010, 2014a). In addition, macrophages from CF ferrets produce high levels of cytokines after being challenged with pathogens such as *P. aeruginosa*, *Bcc* or challenged with LPS (Bruscia and Bonfield, 2016). Interestingly, a study from Keiser et al. (2015) demonstrated differences in BAL fluid composition from CF and WT animals (Keiser et al., 2015). Levels of lactoferrin and lysozyme were especially increased in the naturally born CF ferrets in contrast to those delivered by C-section, while α_1-antitrypsin and apolipoprotein A1 were reduced following natural birth but remained unaltered in animals delivered by C-section (Keiser et al., 2015). Moreover, proteins related to neutrophil activity were raised in naturally born CF ferrets but absent in those delivered by C-section. The authors measured levels of inflammatory cytokines (IL-1β, IL-8, and TNF-a). They did not find any alteration between C-sectioned CF and non-CF ferrets while the newborn CF animals exhibited lower levels of IL-1β, but IL-8 and TNF-α were higher, similar to infants with CF.

Thus, they concluded that inflammatory dissimilarities in CF ferrets may start *in utero* and result in excessive inflammation during birth, following bacterial exposure (Keiser et al., 2015). These data suggest that innate immunity and inflammatory pathways change under sterile and non-sterile conditions, making these animals a valuable model for studying the early onset and progression of CF disease.

Adult CF ferrets do not show abnormal inflammatory response. However, they have other similarities in lung pathology with humans, such as airway obstruction, thick mucus accumulation, and inflammation (Sun et al., 2014a).

Postnatal Development of Submucosal Glands

In ferrets, as in humans, the CFTR protein is highly expressed in serous cells of SMGs lining their cartilaginous rings. Newborn ferrets do not have ciliated cells or SMGs, but they develop them abundantly a few months after birth (Sun et al., 2014a; Keiser et al., 2015). A study from Keiser et al. (2015) on newborn *Cftr*$^{-/-}$ ferrets reported that tracheal MCC was similar to non-CF ferrets, while ASL height was decreased. Only 1–3 weeks after birth, when MCC rate slightly increases, CF related MCC abnormalities would have an impact on the lung pathology (Keiser et al., 2015). Additionally, Sun et al. (2014a) demonstrated a seven-fold decrease in MCC in adult compared to juvenile *Cftr*$^{-/-}$ ferrets that was attributed to an age-dependent ENaC hyperactivity (Sun et al., 2014a). The unique characteristic of ferret lungs to develop SMGs postnatally suggests the presence of CFTR-independent mechanisms that cause the early lung inflammatory profile and future investigations will be valuable.

Ferret Trachea Is Appropriate for Studying Gland Secretion

Adult ferrets have an abundance of tracheal glands, and like humans, they depend on Cl^- and HCO_3^- for secretion (CFTR-dependent). In adult WT ferret tracheas, Cho et al. (2010) revealed a reduced secretion rate by blocking Cl^- or HCO_3^- in response to VIP or FSK. Additionally, CCh-induced MCC was highly decreased when blocking the Na^+-K^+-$2Cl^-$ (NKCC) co-transporter with bumetanide. The authors showed synergistic secretion when low concentrations of agonists that elevate $[cAMP]_i$ were combined with low concentrations of agonists that elevate $[Ca^{2+}]_i$. Neonatal ferret tracheas contain few cells that express high levels of CFTR since SMGs are not yet developed. Studies on newborn *Cftr*$^{-/-}$ ferrets have shown abnormal fluid secretion from their tracheas in response to FSK and CCh, with higher reduction to FSK stimulation, similar to data from human proximal CF airways (Sun et al., 2010).

As CF ferrets have a similar airway morphology to humans, they are a good model for studying CF pathogenesis. They develop human-like lung disease and CFTR-dependent secretion in trachea, albeit the amiloride-sensitive transepithelial PD was unaltered between CF and non-CF ferret tracheas. However, research in CF ferret fluid secretion is spare, and while it seems a promising animal model, our knowledge has been limited until now.

Intestinal Disease Is More Severe in Ferrets Compared to Humans

Newborn CF ferrets, like CF piglets, present a higher incidence of MI than seen in human infants with CF. Between 50% and 100% of CF ferrets develop MI and die within 36 h due to intestinal obstruction and sepsis (Fisher et al., 2011). Most of CF ferrets that survive MI still fail to thrive soon after birth because of malabsorption. Compared to other animals, they do not have caecum and therefore have less time to digest (Sun et al., 2010). A study from Sun et al. (2014b) in CF ferrets over a month old reported that the small intestine was characterized by a reduction in the height of the villi and mucus accumulation in the crypt with signs of inflammation within the lamina propria and into the epithelium (Sun et al., 2014b). A metagenomic deep sequencing analysis revealed the exacerbation of *Streptococcus*, *Enterococcus*, and *Escherichia* in CF ferret feces, similar to what occurs in CF infants (Sun et al., 2014b). A gut-corrected transgenic model that expresses the *CFTR* gene under the control of the rat fatty acid-binding protein promoter (iFABP), is shown to correct MI in newborn *Cftr*$^{-/-}$ ferrets (Sun et al., 2010). The generation of a F508del-CFTR ferret would be useful to increase our knowledge of CF with the most common mutation.

Pancreatic Insufficiency Occurs the First Months of Life

Newborn *Cftr*$^{-/-}$ ferrets exhibit mild pancreatic pathology, similar to CF human infants, and are characterized by swollen acini and ducts with eosinophilic zymogen material, moderate alterations and pancreatic lesions observed in approximately 75% of *Cftr*$^{-/-}$ ferrets (Keiser and Engelhardt, 2011; Sun et al., 2014b). Olivier et al. (2012) demonstrated that neonatal CF ferrets exhibited elevated apoptosis in exocrine ducts and acini suggesting that pancreatic inflammation starts very early in life. Within the first month of life and before adulthood, the pancreas undergoes rapid tissue deterioration with destruction of acini, duct dilatation and evidence of inflammatory cells (neutrophils, macrophages and lymphocytes) (Olivier et al., 2012). Similar to patients with CF, 85% of adult CF ferrets present a loss of exocrine pancreas with fibrosis and islet remodeling. Interestingly, a small percentage of CF ferrets, like patients with CF, are born PS with light pancreatic pathology while they have normal growth and fecal elastase-1 (EL1) levels (Sun et al., 2014b). This finding demonstrates that, as in patients with CF, modifier genes could be responsible for this small percentage of PS. Additionally, adult CF ferrets exhibit disorganized islets, characterized by large clusters that contain an abundance of β and α cells as occurs in the pancreas of humans with CF (Olivier et al., 2012). In general, CF ferrets share many features of human pancreatic disease, and their ability to exhibit variability of disease severity at birth and in adulthood makes them an excellent model for testing potential therapies and examining the specific mechanisms for PI in CF.

LUNG AND INTESTINE OBSERVATIONS IN A RECENT CYSTIC FIBROSIS RAT MODEL

The first CF rat model was generated by Tuggle et al. (2014) with the use of the zinc-finger endonuclease technique. Rats are an appealing model for studying airway defects in CF because they share many characteristics consistent with humans. In contrast to mice, where SMGs are only located at the proximal trachea, rats SMGs extend to bronchi as in humans. The *Cftr*$^{-/-}$ rats, shortly after birth, exhibit congenital tracheal defects with a reduction in the cartilage and tracheal gland area (Tuggle et al., 2014). Nasal PD measurements demonstrated loss of Cl^- permeability in response to FSK, suggesting that the absence of CFTR chloride channels changes electrophysiological features in the rat (Tuggle et al., 2014). Additionally, young CF rats revealed reduced amounts of ASL in distal airways, similar to humans, while BAL fluid was free of inflammatory markers. The decreased ASL levels were not accompanied with Na^+ hyper-absorption suggesting that ASL regulation was CFTR and not ENaC dependent (Tuggle et al., 2014). Young CF rats did not show rapid pulmonary pathology progression, while the sterile environmental conditions under which they were kept may have had an effect (Tuggle et al., 2014). Future studies that will examine disease progression in adult CF rats housed in a natural environment will clarify the role of ASL depletion in airway obstruction. The presence of an increased number of dilated mucus cells was noticed in the proximal nasal epithelium, adding another similarity with the human pathology.

A study from Tipirneni et al. (2017) investigated nasal septal epithelial cultures from *Cftr*$^{-/-}$ rats and demonstrated that they would be a useful model for *in vitro* sinosal ion transport studies. The authors demonstrated that those cell cultures have comparable *Cftr* gene expression and nasal electrophysiological properties to nasal septal epithelial cultures from human and mice, while being more responsive to ion transport modulators (Tipirneni et al., 2017). Moreover, a recent study from Birket et al. (2018) demonstrated that the development of the SMGs is delayed in the *Cftr*$^{-/-}$ rats but only when the SMGs are fully developed, elevated mucus viscosity and impaired mucociliary transport were observed. Hyperacidic pH and changes in the periciliary layer, however, happen before SMGs develop. Importantly, blocking bicarbonate transport increased mucus viscosity. Additional studies on secretion abnormalities in tracheal glands using CF rats will add important information.

In addition, 70% of *Cftr*$^{-/-}$ rats mortality is due to intestinal obstruction between weaning and 42 days after birth in contrast to piglets and ferrets that suffered from severe intestinal obstruction at birth. Their small intestine was characterized by crypt dilation and mucus accumulation (Tuggle et al., 2014).

While CF rats do not spontaneously develop lung or pancreatic disease during their first 6-weeks of life, they are a good model for investigating bone growth and its direct link to CFTR, without the presence of other disease manifestations such as airway disease. Accordingly, Stalvey et al. (2017) examined the role of CFTR loss on bone growth using young *Cftr*$^{-/-}$ rats by measuring their femur length, bone histomorphometry and cartilaginous growth plates as well as the concentration of serum IGF-I. Deficiency in IGF-I can cause changes in cartilage growth. They found that in absence of the *CFTR* gene, rats show reduced growth and bone content. Also, IGF-I concentration in the serum of *Cftr*$^{-/-}$ rats (a marker also used in non-CF children with bone disease) is decreased, which may explain changes in the growth plate (Stalvey et al., 2017).

In general, the *Cftr*$^{-/-}$ rat is a promising model for long-term studies of CF disease manifestations. Although it is in the early stages, this model could be the base for generating CF rats with disease-causing mutations that would allow investigations of CFTR protein trafficking or gating defects and CFTR correctors and potentiators.

CYSTIC FIBROSIS ZEBRAFISH – A UNIQUE MODEL OF PANCREATIC DISEASE PROGRESSION IN ALL DEVELOPMENTAL STAGES

Zebrafish have been valued as an outstanding tiny research model for studying human diseases. They are inexpensive, and can be generated in large numbers, while requiring minimal housing and handling conditions (Phillips and Westerfield, 2014). Moreover, zebrafish CFTR chloride channels responds similarly to most agonists and antagonists of the human CFTR due to its high homology. Data have demonstrated that the absence of CFTR in zebrafish hinders the development of Kupffer's vesicle (KV), a basic ciliated organ, which determines lateralization in an early developmental zebrafish stage, emphasizing the importance of CFTR function in fluid secretion (Navis and Bagnat, 2015).

The first zebrafish CF model was produced by Navis and Bagnat (2015) using transgenic zebrafish mutant lines. They reported that CFTR was localized on the apical membrane of pancreatic ducts and investigated the absence of CFTR in zebrafish pancreas during various developmental stages suggesting comparable disease pathology as in humans. They reported that most of CF larval zebrafish started to die approximately 10 days post fertilization (dpf), suggesting that pancreatic dysfunction starts early in life. By 16 dpf, pancreatic tissue was partially damaged and neutrophil presence was slightly evident while by 20 dpf, the pancreas was remarkably disrupted. Pancreatic ducts contained mucus, and they were encircled by fibrotic tissue instead of acinar and were highly infiltrated with neutrophils. Additionally, the islets appeared widespread, abundant and diminished in size. The CF zebrafish model closely resembles pancreatic pathogenesis in human adults with CF suggesting that a mild PI may start early in life. Additional studies examining the specific mechanisms that cause pancreatic disease early in life, the role of the inflammatory factors in disease progression, and the ion transport abnormalities using the zebrafish model would be very valuable tools for pancreatic pathogenesis in CF.

SHEEP CF MODEL – A BRIEF DESCRIPTION OF AN ATTRACTIVE UNDERVALUED MODEL

The sheep model is not a commonly used model for studying CF disease compared to mice, pigs and ferrets, respectively. However, at the molecular level, the sheep *CFTR* gene is 91% homologous with the human *CFTR* while at protein level, they have 95% resemblance (Harris, 1997). Many researchers have used an ovine model for studying respiratory diseases such as asthma and chronic obstructive pulmonary disease (COPD) since anatomically, functionally and electrophysiologically sheep airways parallels those of humans (Abraham, 2008; Allen et al., 2009). It has been utilized for examining secretion abnormalities, testing the effect of small molecules as a potential therapy for lung disease and for gene therapy (Cai et al., 2015). Apart from the lung pathology, CFTR protein expression in sheep pancreas mirrors human levels. As a large animal, in combination with its long lifespan, it could be appropriate for therapeutic trials. Generation of a CF ovine model utilizing somatic cell cloning was not successful in the past due to failure of homologous recombination in sheep fibroblasts. In 2018, Fan et al. generated the first *Cftr*$^{-/-}$ sheep model using the CRISPR/Cas9 genome editing and somatic cell nuclear transfer methods. The newborn *Cftr*$^{-/-}$ sheep demonstrated severe intestinal obstruction similar to the MI noticed in approximately 15% of human babies with CF. The pancreas was characterized by hypoplasia and fibrosis similar to humans with CF. This pancreatic hypoplasia was common in both KO and heterozygous sheep. Interestingly, lungs of newborn *Cftr*$^{-/-}$ sheep had minimal signs of disease which is an important feature that enables investigations of early disease progression (Fan et al., 2018). Production of a CF sheep model gave rise to a new chapter of large animals as useful models for novel therapeutic approaches.

DISCUSSION

Despite recent research progress, our understanding of CF pathogenesis is still incomplete. Many questions remain unanswered and CF continues to be a fatal disease. Cell-culture models have been shown to be useful for pre-clinical trials but they lack the structural complexity of intact organs (Scholte et al., 2006; Rogers et al., 2008c; Cutting, 2015). Much of the knowledge on CF pathophysiology that we have today derives from animal models and especially from the wide variability of gene-targeted mouse models. Most of the studies repeatedly note that mice models, in contrast to pigs and ferrets, do not spontaneously develop lung disease as do humans. However, depending on the strain, such as congenic models with the C57BL/6 background, they have the advantage of surviving longer from intestinal disease and are susceptible to lung infection with pathogens, mainly the most persistent *P. aeruginosa*. Pigs and ferrets exhibit similar lung function and architecture with humans and at birth they lack inflammation, and they are unable to eradicate bacteria (Rogers et al., 2008c; Stoltz et al., 2010; Sun et al., 2010; Wine, 2010; Ostedgaard et al., 2011). The disadvantage of these models is the difficulty of keeping them alive long enough since, approximately 48 h after birth they die from intestinal obstruction and a surgical ileostomy is mandatory but not always successful. Consequently, while most of the studies report a lung pathology similar to that in patients with CF, they are only based on experiments that have been conducted in very few animals, mostly newborn (Rogers et al., 2008c; Joo et al., 2010; Stoltz et al., 2010; Sun et al., 2010, 2014a; Wine, 2010; Ostedgaard et al., 2011; Keiser et al., 2015).

Mice SMGs, contrary to those in rats that extend into the bronchi, are confined to the trachea, but they are abundant and identical in structure to those in humans. Despite the bioelectric similarities of murine nasal SMGs with those in humans, tracheal glands are widely utilized due to the highest expression levels of CFTR proteins, whereas studies on *Cftr*$^{-/-}$ mice have demonstrated secretion defects. Tracheal glands from

CF pigs also exhibit secretion defects but they do not completely lose synergy as mice or newborn CF ferrets do (Joo et al., 2010). Secretion defects are restricted only in newborn CF ferrets and CF pigs, in contrast to mice, while studies in CF ferret nasal glands have not been done yet (Sun et al., 2010, 2014a; Keiser et al., 2015). The dominance of the CACC channel in mice airways, intestine and pancreas, in parallel with CFTR proteins, alleviate the severity of the disease pathogenesis compared to other models. Intestinal pathology can be fatal for some CF mice, causing death a few days after birth or around the time of weaning (Davidson and Dorin, 2001). The disease severity varies among strains and although it is more severe than in humans, CF mice intestine still exhibit the same pathophysiological abnormalities, and they are considered a good model for studying human intestinal disease.

In addition, MI is fatal for both CF piglets and ferrets with a penetrance of 100% and 50–100%, respectively, while the occurrence in human infants with CF is only moderate at 15–20%. The generation of transgenic mice, pigs, and ferrets with tissue-corrected *CFTR* gene expression under the control of the iFABP gene promoter alleviates intestinal obstruction with no effects on the other organs. Interestingly, milder pancreatic disease is observed in CF mice, while CF pigs and ferrets that survived from MI demonstrated human-like disease. However, studies in adult pigs and ferrets are limited. The first CF zebrafish model enabled the examination of pancreatic pathogenesis in all developmental stages, demonstrating that a mild pancreatic disease starts early in life (Navis and Bagnat, 2015).

Although human CF is characterized by salty sweat, eccrine sweat glands are underestimated in the above CF animal models. Pigs use mud baths to cool their body (Rogers et al., 2008a) as they have very few sweat glands, which are in the nose, while ferrets do not sweat at all. Importantly, mice have sweat glands in their paws, this is a promising tissue for studying CF disease which should be further evaluated.

CONCLUSION

In conclusion, while various animal models present different advantages for studying different aspects of the disease, there is no single animal model available yet that completely replicates the complexity of CF in humans. Each model presents pros and cons and combining findings from various organs studied in different models provides important clues for our understanding of the CF disease pathogenesis and progression.

AUTHOR CONTRIBUTIONS

AS wrote the paper. All authors contributed to the review of appropriate literature and preparation of the manuscript.

ACKNOWLEDGMENTS

The authors would like to thank Drs. Emmanuelle Brochiero, Younes Anini, and Yassine El Hiani for their input and interesting discussions on this topic. AS was supported by CFF grant.

REFERENCES

Abdulrahman, B. A., Khweek, A. A., Akhter, A., Caution, K., Kotrange, S., Abdelaziz, D. H., et al. (2011). Autophagy stimulation by rapamycin suppresses lung inflammation and infection by Burkholderia cenocepacia in a model of cystic fibrosis. *Autophagy* 7, 1359–1370. doi: 10.4161/auto.7.11.17660

Abraham, W. M. (2008). Modeling of asthma, COPD and cystic fibrosis in sheep. *Pulm. Pharmacol. Ther.* 21, 743–754. doi: 10.1016/j.pupt.2008.01.010

Abu-El-Haija, M., Ramachandran, S., Meyerholz, D. K., Abu-El-Haija, M., Griffin, M., Giriyappa, R. L., et al. (2012). Pancreatic damage in fetal and newborn cystic fibrosis pigs involves the activation of inflammatory and remodeling pathways. *Am. J. Pathol.* 181, 499–507. doi: 10.1016/j.ajpath.2012.04.024

Alcolado, N. G., Conrad, D. J., Poroca, D., Li, M., Alshafie, W., Chappe, F. G., et al. (2014). Cystic fibrosis transmembrane conductance regulator dysfunction in VIP knockout mice. *Am. J. Physiol. Cell Physiol.* 307, C195–C207. doi: 10.1152/ajpcell.00293.2013

Allen, J. E., Bischof, R. J., Chang, H. Y. S., Hirota, J. A., Hirst, S. J., Inman, M. D., et al. (2009). Animal models of airway inflammation and airway smooth muscle remodelling in asthma. *Pulm. Pharmacol. Ther.* 22, 455–465. doi: 10.1016/j.pupt.2009.04.001

Andersen, D. H. (1938). Cystic fibrosis of the pancreas and its relation to celiac disease: a clinical and pathologic study. *Am. J. Dis. Child.* 56, 344–399. doi: 10.1001/archpedi.1938.01980140114013

Andersson, C., Zaman, M. M., Jones, A. B., and Freedman, S. D. (2008). Alterations in immune response and PPAR/LXR regulation in cystic fibrosis macrophages. *J. Cyst. Fibros.* 7, 68–78. doi: 10.1016/j.jcf.2007.05.004

Birket, S. E., Davis, J. M., Fernandez, C. M., Tuggle, K. L., Oden, A. M., Chu, K. K., et al. (2018). Development of an airway mucus defect in the cystic fibrosis rat. *JCI Insight* doi: 10.1172/jci.insight.97199 [Epub ahead of print].

Bonvin, E., Le Rouzic, P., Bernaudin, J., Cottart, C., Vandebrouck, C., Crié, A., et al. (2008). Congenital tracheal malformation in cystic fibrosis transmembrane conductance regulator deficient mice. *J. Physiol.* 586, 3231–3243. doi: 10.1113/jphysiol.2008.150763

Borthwick, D. W., West, J. D., Keighren, M. A., Flockhart, J. H., Innes, B. A., and Dorin, J. R. (1999). Murine submucosal glands are clonally derived and show a cystic fibrosis gene-dependent distribution pattern. *Am. J. Respir. Cell Mol. Biol.* 20, 1181–1189. doi: 10.1165/ajrcmb.20.6.3475

Bruscia, E. M., and Bonfield, T. L. (2016). Cystic fibrosis lung immunity: the role of the macrophage. *J. Innate Immun.* 8, 550–563. doi: 10.1159/000446825

Bruscia, E. M., Zhang, P. X., Ferreira, E., Caputo, C., Emerson, J. W., Tuck, D., et al. (2009). Macrophages directly contribute to the exaggerated inflammatory response in cystic fibrosis transmembrane conductance regulator-/- mice. *Am. J. Respir. Cell Mol. Biol.* 40, 295–304. doi: 10.1165/rcmb.2008-0170OC

Bruscia, E. M., Zhang, P. X., Satoh, A., Caputo, C., Medzhitov, R., Shenoy, A., et al. (2011). Abnormal trafficking and degradation of TLR4 underlie the elevated inflammatory response in cystic fibrosis. *J. Immunol.* 186, 6990–6998. doi: 10.4049/jimmunol.1100396

Cai, Z., Palmai-Pallag, T., Khuituan, P., Mutolo, M. J., Boinot, C., Liu, B., et al. (2015). Impact of the F508del mutation on ovine CFTR, a Cl- channel with enhanced conductance and ATP-dependent gating. *J. Physiol.* 593, 2427–2446. doi: 10.1113/JP270227

Canale-Zambrano, J. C., Poffenberger, M. C., Cory, S. M., Humes, D. G., and Haston, C. K. (2007). Intestinal phenotype of variable-weight cystic fibrosis knockout mice. *Am. J. Physiol. Gastrointest. Liver Physiol.* 293, G222–G229. doi: 10.1152/ajpgi.00405.2006

Chappe, V., and Said, S. I. (2012). "VIP as a corrector of CFTR trafficking and membrane stability," in *Cystic Fibrosis-Renewed Hopes through Research*, ed. D. Sriramulu (London: InTech).

Chen, J., Stoltz, D. A., Karp, P. H., Ernst, S. E., Pezzulo, A. A., Moninger, T. O., et al. (2010). Loss of anion transport without increased sodium absorption characterizes newborn porcine cystic fibrosis airway epithelia. *Cell* 143, 911–923. doi: 10.1016/j.cell.2010.11.029

Cho, H., Joo, N. S., and Wine, J. J. (2011). Defective fluid secretion from submucosal glands of nasal turbinates from CFTR-/-and CFTRΔF508/ΔF508 Pigs. *PLoS One* 6:e24424. doi: 10.1371/journal.pone.0024424

Cho, H. J., Joo, N. S., and Wine, J. J. (2010). Mucus secretion from individual submucosal glands of the ferret trachea. *Am. J. Physiol. Lung Cell. Mol. Physiol.* 299, L124–L136. doi: 10.1152/ajplung.00049.2010

Choi, J. Y., Joo, N. S., Krouse, M. E., Wu, J. V., Robbins, R. C., Ianowski, J. P., et al. (2007). Synergistic airway gland mucus secretion in response to vasoactive intestinal peptide and carbachol is lost in cystic fibrosis. *J. Clin. Invest.* 117, 3118–3127. doi: 10.1172/JCI31992

Clarke, L. L., Grubb, B. R., Yankaskas, J. R., Cotton, C. U., McKenzie, A., and Boucher, R. C. (1994). Relationship of a non-cystic fibrosis transmembrane conductance regulator-mediated chloride conductance to organ-level disease in Cftr(-/-) mice. *Proc. Natl. Acad. Sci. U.S.A.* 91, 479–483. doi: 10.1073/pnas.91.2.479

Colledge, W. H., Abella, B. S., Southern, K. W., Ratcliff, R., Jiang, C., Cheng, S. H., et al. (1995). Generation and characterization of a ΔF508 cystic fibrosis mouse model. *Nat. Genet.* 10, 445–452. doi: 10.1038/ng0895-445

Cowley, E. A., Wang, C. G., Gosselin, D., Radzioch, D., and Eidelman, D. H. (1997). Mucociliary clearance in cystic fibrosis knockout mice infected with *Pseudomonas aeruginosa*. *Eur. Respir. J.* 10, 2312–2318. doi: 10.1183/09031936.97.10102312

Cutting, G. R. (2015). Cystic fibrosis genetics: from molecular understanding to clinical application. *Nat. Rev. Genet.* 16, 45–56. doi: 10.1038/nrg3849

Davidson, D. J., and Dorin, J. R. (2001). The CF mouse: an important tool for studying cystic fibrosis. *Expert Rev. Mol. Med.* 3, 1–27.

Davis, P. B. (2006). Cystic fibrosis since 1938. *Am. J. Respir. Crit. Care Med.* 173, 475–482. doi: 10.1164/rccm.200505-840OE

De Jonge, H. R. (2007). Cystic fibrosis mice rehabilitated for studies of airway gland dysfunction. *J. Physiol.* 580, 7–8. doi: 10.1113/jphysiol.2007.129361

De Lisle, R. C., and Borowitz, D. (2013). The cystic fibrosis intestine. *Cold Spring Harb. Perspect. Med.* 3:a009753. doi: 10.1101/cshperspect.a009753

Delaney, S. J., Alton, E., Smith, S. N., Lunn, D. P., Farley, R., Lovelock, P., et al. (1996). Cystic fibrosis mice carrying the missense mutation G551D replicate human genotype / phenotype correlations. *EMBO J.* 15, 955–963. doi: 10.1002/j.1460-2075.1996.tb00432.x

Dorin, J., Stevenson, B., Fleming, S., Alton, E., Dickinson, P., and Porteous, D. (1994). Long-term survival of the exon 10 insertional cystic fibrosis mutant mouse is a consequence of low level residual wild-type Cftr gene expression. *Mamm. Genome* 5, 465–472. doi: 10.1007/BF00369314

Dorin, J. R., Dickinson, P., Alton, E. W., Smith, S. N., Geddes, D. M., Stevenson, B. J., et al. (1992). Cystic fibrosis in the mouse by targeted insertional mutagenesis. *Nature* 359, 211–215. doi: 10.1038/359211a0

Durie, P. R., and Forstner, G. G. (1989). Pathophysiology of the exocrine pancreas in cystic fibrosis. *J. R. Soc. Med.* 82(Suppl. 16), 2–10.

Durie, P. R., Kent, G., Phillips, M. J., and Ackerley, C. A. (2004). Characteristic multiorgan pathology of cystic fibrosis in a long-living cystic fibrosis transmembrane regulator knockout murine model. *Am. J. Pathol.* 164, 1481–1493. doi: 10.1016/S0002-9440(10)63234-8

Ellsworth, R. E., Jamison, D. C., Touchman, J. W., Chissoe, S. L., Braden Maduro, V. V., Bouffard, G. G., et al. (2000). Comparative genomic sequence analysis of the human and mouse cystic fibrosis transmembrane conductance regulator genes. *Proc. Natl. Acad. Sci. U.S.A.* 97, 1172–1177. doi: 10.1073/pnas.97.3.1172

Engelhardt, J. F., Yankaskas, J. R., Ernst, S. A., Yang, Y., Marino, C. R., Boucher, R. C., et al. (1992). Submucosal glands are the predominant site of CFTR expression in the human bronchus. *Nat. Genet.* 2, 240–248. doi: 10.1038/ng1192-240

Fan, Z., Perisse, I. V., Cotton, C. U., Regouski, M., Meng, Q., Domb, C., et al. (2018). A sheep model of cystic fibrosis generated by CRISPR/Cas9 disruption of the CFTR gene. *JCI Insight* doi: 10.1172/jci.insight.123529 [Epub ahead of print].

Festini, F., Buzzetti, R., Bassi, C., Braggion, C., Salvatore, D., Taccetti, G., et al. (2006). Isolation measures for prevention of infection with respiratory pathogens in cystic fibrosis: a systematic review. *J. Hosp. Infect.* 64, 1–6. doi: 10.1016/j.jhin.2006.02.021

Fisher, J. T., Liu, X., Yan, Z., Luo, M., Zhang, Y., Zhou, W., et al. (2012). Comparative processing and function of human and ferret cystic fibrosis transmembrane conductance regulator. *J. Biol. Chem.* 287, 21673–21685. doi: 10.1074/jbc.M111.336537

Fisher, J. T., Zhang, Y., and Engelhardt, J. F. (2011). Comparative biology of cystic fibrosis animal models. *Methods Mol. Biol.* 742, 311–334. doi: 10.1007/978-1-61779-120-8_19

Gibson, L. E., and Cooke, R. E. (1959). A test for concentration of electrolytes in sweat in cystic fibrosis of the pancreas utilizing pilocarpine by iontophoresis. *Pediatrics* 23, 545–549.

Gibson-Corley, K. N., Meyerholz, D. K., and Engelhardt, J. F. (2016). Pancreatic pathophysiology in cystic fibrosis. *J. Pathol.* 238, 311–320. doi: 10.1002/path.4634

Gosselin, D., Stevenson, M. M., Cowley, E. A., Griesenbach, U., Eidelman, D. H., BoulÉ, M., et al. (1998). Impaired ability of CFTR knockout mice to control lung infection with *Pseudomonas aeruginosa*. *Am. J. Respir. Crit. Care Med.* 157, 1253–1262. doi: 10.1164/ajrccm.157.4.9702081

Gray, M. A., Winpenny, J. P., Verdon, B., McAlroy, H., and Argent, B. E. (1995). Chloride channels and cystic fibrosis of the pancreas. *Biosci. Rep.* 15, 531–541. doi: 10.1007/BF01204355

Grubb, B. R. (1999). Ion transport across the normal and CF neonatal murine intestine. *Am. J. Physiol.* 277(1 Pt 1), G167–G174. doi: 10.1152/ajpgi.1999.277.1.G167

Grubb, B. R., and Boucher, R. C. (1999). Pathophysiology of gene-targeted mouse models for cystic fibrosis. *Physiol. Rev.* 79, S193–S214. doi: 10.1152/physrev.1999.79.1.S193

Grubb, B. R., and Gabriel, S. E. (1997). Intestinal physiology and pathology in gene-targeted mouse models of cystic fibrosis. *Am. J. Physiol.* 273(2 Pt 1), G258–G266. doi: 10.1152/ajpgi.1997.273.2.G258

Grubb, B. R., Jones, J. H., and Boucher, R. C. (2004). Mucociliary transport determined by in vivo microdialysis in the airways of normal and CF mice. *Am. J. Physiol. Lung Cell. Mol. Physiol.* 286, L588–L595. doi: 10.1152/ajplung.00302.2003

Grubb, B. R., Rogers, T. D., Kulaga, H. M., Burns, K. A., Wonsetler, R. L., Reed, R. R., et al. (2007). Olfactory epithelia exhibit progressive functional and morphological defects in CF mice. *Am. J. Physiol. Cell Physiol.* 293, C574–C583. doi: 10.1152/ajpcell.00106.2007

Grubb, B. R., Vick, R. N., and Boucher, R. C. (1994). Hyperabsorption of Na^+ and raised Ca(2+)-mediated Cl- secretion in nasal epithelia of CF mice. *Am. J. Physiol.* 266(5 Pt 1), C1478–C1483. doi: 10.1152/ajpcell.1994.266.5.C1478

Guilbault, C., Martin, P., Houle, D., Boghdady, M., Guiot, M., Marion, D., et al. (2005). Cystic fibrosis lung disease following infection with *Pseudomonas aeruginosa* in Cftr knockout mice using novel non-invasive direct pulmonary infection technique. *Lab. Anim.* 39, 336–352. doi: 10.1258/0023677054306944

Guilbault, C., Novak, J. P., Martin, P., Boghdady, M. L., Saeed, Z., Guiot, M. C., et al. (2006). Distinct pattern of lung gene expression in the Cftr-KO mice developing spontaneous lung disease compared with their littermate controls. *Physiol. Genomics* 25, 179–193. doi: 10.1152/physiolgenomics.00206.2005

Gyömörey, K., Rozmahel, R., and Bear, C. E. (2000). Amelioration of intestinal disease severity in cystic fibrosis mice is associated with improved chloride secretory capacity. *Pediatr. Res.* 48, 731–734. doi: 10.1203/00006450-200012000-00005

Hamidi, S., Szema, A., Lyubsky, S., Dickman, K., Degene, A., Mathew, S., et al. (2006). Clues to VIP function from knockout mice. *Ann. N. Y. Acad. Sci.* 1070, 5–9. doi: 10.1196/annals.1317.035

Harkema, J., Mariassy, A., George, J. S., Hyde, D., and Plopper, C. (1991). Epithelial cells of the conducting airways: a species comparison. *Lung Biol. Health Dis.* 55, 3–39.

Harris, A. (1997). Towards an ovine model of cystic fibrosis. *Hum. Mol. Genet.* 6, 2191–2193. doi: 10.1093/hmg/6.13.2191

Hasty, P., O'Neal, W. K., Liu, K., Morris, A. P., Bebok, Z., Shumyatsky, G. B., et al. (1995). Severe phenotype in mice with termination mutation in exon 2 of cystic fibrosis gene. *Somat. Cell Mol. Genet.* 21, 177–187. doi: 10.1007/BF02254769

Hasty, P., Ramírez-Solis, R., Krumlauf, R., and Bradley, A. (1991). Introduction of a subtle mutation into the Hox-2.6 locus in embryonic stem cells. *Nature* 350, 243–246. doi: 10.1038/350243a0

Heeckeren, A., Walenga, R., Konstan, M. W., Bonfield, T., Davis, P. B., and Ferkol, T. (1997). Excessive inflammatory response of cystic fibrosis mice to bronchopulmonary infection with *Pseudomonas aeruginosa*. *J. Clin. Invest.* 100, 2810–2815. doi: 10.1172/JCI119828

Heinz-Erian, P., Dey, R. D., Flux, M., and Said, S. I. (1985). Deficient vasoactive intestinal peptide innervation in the sweat glands of cystic fibrosis patients. *Science* 229, 1407–1408. doi: 10.1126/science.4035357

Heinz-Erian, P., Paul, S., and Said, S. I. (1986). Receptors for vasoactive intestinal peptide on isolated human sweat glands. *Peptides* 7, 151–154. doi: 10.1016/0196-9781(86)90178-6

Hilliard, T. N., Zhu, J., Farley, R., Escudero-Garcia, S., Wainwright, B. J., Jeffery, P. K., et al. (2008). Nasal abnormalities in cystic fibrosis mice independent of infection and inflammation. *Am. J. Respir. Cell Mol. Biol.* 39, 19–25. doi: 10.1165/rcmb.2007-0284OC

Hoegger, M. J., Awadalla, M., Namati, E., Itani, O. A., Fischer, A. J., Tucker, A. J., et al. (2014a). Assessing mucociliary transport of single particles in vivo shows variable speed and preference for the ventral trachea in newborn pigs. *Proc. Natl. Acad. Sci. U.S.A.* 111, 2355–2360. doi: 10.1073/pnas.1323633111

Hoegger, M. J., Fischer, A. J., McMenimen, J. D., Ostedgaard, L. S., Tucker, A. J., Awadalla, M. A., et al. (2014b). Impaired mucus detachment disrupts mucociliary transport in a piglet model of cystic fibrosis. *Science* 345, 818–822. doi: 10.1126/science.1255825

Ianowski, J. P., Choi, J. Y., Wine, J. J., and Hanrahan, J. W. (2007). Mucus secretion by single tracheal submucosal glands from normal and cystic fibrosis transmembrane conductance regulator knockout mice. *J. Physiol.* 580, 301–314. doi: 10.1113/jphysiol.2006.123653

Joo, N. S., Cho, H. J., Khansaheb, M., and Wine, J. J. (2010). Hyposecretion of fluid from tracheal submucosal glands of CFTR-deficient pigs. *J. Clin. Invest.* 120, 3161–3166. doi: 10.1172/JCI43466

Keiser, N. W., Birket, S. E., Evans, I. A., Tyler, S. R., Crooke, A. K., Sun, X., et al. (2015). Defective innate immunity and hyperinflammation in newborn cystic fibrosis transmembrane conductance regulator–knockout ferret lungs. *Am. J. Respir. Cell Mol. Biol.* 52, 683–694. doi: 10.1165/rcmb.2014-0250OC

Keiser, N. W., and Engelhardt, J. F. (2011). New animal models of cystic fibrosis: what are they teaching us? *Curr. Opin. Pulm. Med.* 17, 478–483. doi: 10.1097/MCP.0b013e32834b14c9

Kent, G., Iles, R., Bear, C. E., Huan, L. J., Griesenbach, U., McKerlie, C., et al. (1997). Lung disease in mice with cystic fibrosis. *J. Clin. Invest.* 100, 3060–3069. doi: 10.1172/JCI119861

Lavelle, G. M., White, M. M., Browne, N., McElvaney, N. G., and Reeves, E. P. (2016). Animal models of cystic fibrosis pathology: phenotypic parallels and divergences. *Biomed Res. Int.* 2016:5258727. doi: 10.1155/2016/5258727

Li, C., Wu, Y., Riehle, A., Ma, J., Kamler, M., Gulbins, E., et al. (2017). *Staphylococcus aureus* survives in cystic fibrosis macrophages, forming a reservoir for chronic pneumonia. *Infect. Immun.* 85:e00883-816. doi: 10.1128/IAI.00883-16

Liu, X., Luo, M., Zhang, L., Ding, W., Yan, Z., and Engelhardt, J. F. (2007). Bioelectric properties of chloride channels in human, pig, ferret, and mouse airway epithelia. *Am. J. Respir. Cell Mol. Biol.* 36, 313–323. doi: 10.1165/rcmb.2006-0286OC

Liu, F., Zhang, Z., Csanády, L., Gadsby, D. C., and Chen, J. (2017). Molecular structure of the human CFTR ion channel. *Cell* 169, 85–95. doi: 10.1016/j.cell.2017.02.024

Lu, C., and Fuchs, E. (2014). Sweat gland progenitors in development, homeostasis, and wound repair. *Cold Spring Harb. Perspect. Med.* 4:a015222. doi: 10.1101/cshperspect.a015222

Luciani, A., Villella, V. R., Esposito, S., Brunetti-Pierri, N., Medina, D., Settembre, C., et al. (2010). Defective CFTR induces aggresome formation and lung inflammation in cystic fibrosis through ROS-mediated autophagy inhibition. *Nat. Cell Biol.* 12, 863–875. doi: 10.1038/ncb2090

Lundberg, J. M., Anggard, A., Fahrenkrug, J., Hokfelt, T., and Mutt, V. (1980). Vasoactive intestinal polypeptide in cholinergic neurons of exocrine glands: functional significance of coexisting transmitters for vasodilation and secretion. *Proc. Natl. Acad. Sci. U.S.A.* 77, 1651–1655. doi: 10.1073/pnas.77.3.1651

Marino, C. R., Matovcik, L. M., Gorelick, F. S., and Cohn, J. A. (1991). Localization of the cystic fibrosis transmembrane conductance regulator in pancreas. *J. Clin. Invest.* 88, 712–716. doi: 10.1172/JCI115358

McHugh, D. R., Cotton, C. U., Moss, F. J., Vitko, M., Valerio, D. M., Kelley, T. J., et al. (2018a). Linaclotide improves gastrointestinal transit in cystic fibrosis mice by inhibiting sodium/hydrogen exchanger 3. *Am. J. Physiol. Gastrointest. Liver Physiol.* doi: 10.1152/ajpgi.00261.2017 [Epub ahead of print].

McHugh, D. R., Steele, M. S., Valerio, D. M., Miron, A., Mann, R. J., LePage, D. F., et al. (2018b). A G542X cystic fibrosis mouse model for examining nonsense mutation directed therapies. *PLoS One* 13:e0199573. doi: 10.1371/journal.pone.0199573

McMorran, B. J., Palmer, J. S., Lunn, D. P., Oceandy, D., Costelloe, E. O., Thomas, G. R., et al. (2001). G551D CF mice display an abnormal host response and have impaired clearance of *Pseudomonas* lung disease. *Am. J. Physiol. Lung Cell. Mol. Physiol.* 281, L740–L747. doi: 10.1152/ajplung.2001.281.3.L740

Meyer, M., Huaux, F., Gavilanes, X., Van Den Brûle, S., Lebecque, P., Lo Re, S., et al. (2009). Azithromycin reduces exaggerated cytokine production by M1 alveolar macrophages in cystic fibrosis. *Am. J. Respir. Cell Mol. Biol.* 41, 590–602. doi: 10.1165/rcmb.2008-0155OC

Meyerholz, D. K., Stoltz, D. A., Namati, E., Ramachandran, S., Pezzulo, A. A., Smith, A. R., et al. (2010a). Loss of cystic fibrosis transmembrane conductance regulator function produces abnormalities in tracheal development in neonatal pigs and young children. *Am. J. Respir. Crit. Care Med.* 182, 1251–1261. doi: 10.1164/rccm.201004-0643OC

Meyerholz, D. K., Stoltz, D. A., Pezzulo, A. A., and Welsh, M. J. (2010b). Pathology of gastrointestinal organs in a porcine model of cystic fibrosis. *Am. J. Pathol.* 176, 1377–1389. doi: 10.2353/ajpath.2010.090849

Navis, A., and Bagnat, M. (2015). Loss of Cftr function leads to pancreatic destruction in larval zebrafish. *Dev. Biol.* 399, 237–248. doi: 10.1016/j.ydbio.2014.12.034

Norkina, O., Kaur, S., Ziemer, D., and De Lisle, R. C. (2004). Inflammation of the cystic fibrosis mouse small intestine. *Am. J. Physiol. Gastrointest. Liver Physiol.* 286, G1032–G1041. doi: 10.1152/ajpgi.00473.2003

Olivier, A. K., Gibson-Corley, K. N., and Meyerholz, D. K. (2015). Animal models of gastrointestinal and liver diseases. animal models of cystic fibrosis: gastrointestinal, pancreatic, and hepatobiliary disease and pathophysiology. *Am. J. Physiol. Gastrointest. Liver Physiol.* 308, G459–G471. doi: 10.1152/ajpgi.00146.2014

Olivier, A. K., Yi, Y., Sun, X., Sui, H., Liang, B., Hu, S., et al. (2012). Abnormal endocrine pancreas function at birth in cystic fibrosis ferrets. *J. Clin. Invest.* 122, 3755–3768. doi: 10.1172/JCI60610

O'Neal, W. K., Hasty, P., McCray, P. B. Jr., Casey, B., RiveraPérez, J., Welsh, M. J., et al. (1993). A severe phenotype in mice with a duplication of exon 3 in the cystic fibrosis locus. *Hum. Mol. Genet.* 2, 1561–1569. doi: 10.1093/hmg/2.10.1561

Ostedgaard, L. S., Meyerholz, D. K., Chen, J. H., Pezzulo, A. A., Karp, P. H., Rokhlina, T., et al. (2011). The DeltaF508 mutation causes CFTR misprocessing and cystic fibrosis-like disease in pigs. *Sci. Transl. Med.* 3:74ra24. doi: 10.1126/scitranslmed.3001868

Ostedgaard, L. S., Moninger, T. O., McMenimen, J. D., Sawin, N. M., Parker, C. P., Thornell, I. M., et al. (2017). Gel-forming mucins form distinct morphologic structures in airways. *Proc. Natl. Acad. Sci. U.S.A.* 114, 6842–6847. doi: 10.1073/pnas.1703228114

Ostedgaard, L. S., Rogers, C. S., Dong, Q., Randak, C. O., Vermeer, D. W., Rokhlina, T., et al. (2007). Processing and function of CFTR-deltaF508 are species-dependent. *Proc. Natl. Acad. Sci. U.S.A.* 104, 15370–15375. doi: 10.1073/pnas.0706974104

Ousingsawat, J., Martins, J. R., Schreiber, R., Rock, J. R., Harfe, B. D., and Kunzelmann, K. (2009). Loss of TMEM16A causes a defect in epithelial Ca^{2+}-dependent chloride transport. *J. Biol. Chem.* 284, 28698–28703. doi: 10.1074/jbc.M109.012120

Paemka, L., McCullagh, B. N., Alaiwa, M. H. A., Stoltz, D. A., Dong, Q., Randak, C. O., et al. (2017). Monocyte derived macrophages from CF pigs exhibit increased inflammatory responses at birth. *J. Cyst. Fibros.* 16, 471–474. doi: 10.1016/j.jcf.2017.03.007

Pezzulo, A. A., Tang, X. X., Hoegger, M. J., Alaiwa, M. H. A., Ramachandran, S., Moninger, T. O., et al. (2012). Reduced airway surface pH impairs bacterial killing in the porcine cystic fibrosis lung. *Nature* 487, 109–113. doi: 10.1038/nature11130

Phillips, J. B., and Westerfield, M. (2014). Zebrafish models in translational research: tipping the scales toward advancements in human health. *Dis. Models Mech.* 7, 739–743. doi: 10.1242/dmm.015545

Ratcliff, R., Evans, M. J., Cuthbert, A. W., MacVinish, L. J., Foster, D., Anderson, J. R., et al. (1993). Production of a severe cystic fibrosis mutation in mice by gene targeting. *Nat. Genet.* 4, 35–41. doi: 10.1038/ng0593-35

Riordan, J. R., Rommens, J. M., Kerem, B., Alon, N., Rozmahel, R., Grzelczak, Z., et al. (1989). Identification of the cystic fibrosis gene: cloning and characterization of complementary DNA. *Science* 245, 1066–1073. doi: 10.1126/science.2475911

Rock, J. R., O'Neal, W. K., Gabriel, S. E., Randell, S. H., Harfe, B. D., Boucher, R. C., et al. (2009). Transmembrane protein 16A (TMEM16A) is a Ca^{2+}-regulated Cl- secretory channel in mouse airways. *J. Biol. Chem.* 284, 14875–14880. doi: 10.1074/jbc.C109.000869

Rogers, C. S., Abraham, W. M., Brogden, K. A., Engelhardt, J. F., Fisher, J. T., McCray, P. B. Jr., et al. (2008a). The porcine lung as a potential model for cystic fibrosis. *Am. J. Physiol. Lung Cell. Mol. Physiol.* 295, L240–L263. doi: 10.1152/ajplung.90203.2008

Rogers, C. S., Hao, Y., Rokhlina, T., Samuel, M., Stoltz, D. A., Li, Y., et al. (2008b). Production of CFTR-Null and CFTR-DeltaF508 heterozygous pigs by adeno-associated virus-mediated gene targeting and somatic cell nuclear transfer. *J. Clin. Invest.* 118, 1571–1577. doi: 10.1172/JCI34773

Rogers, C. S., Stoltz, D. A., Meyerholz, D. K., Ostedgaard, L. S., Rokhlina, T., Taft, P. J., et al. (2008c). Disruption of the CFTR gene produces a model of cystic fibrosis in newborn pigs. *Science* 321, 1837–1841. doi: 10.1126/science.1163600

Rommens, J. M., Iannuzzi, M. C., Kerem, B., Drumm, M. L., Melmer, G., Dean, M., et al. (1989). Identification of the cystic fibrosis gene: chromosome walking and jumping. *Science* 245, 1059–1065. doi: 10.1126/science.2772657

Rozmahe, R., Wilschanski, M., Matin, A., Plyte, S., Oliver, M., Auerbach, W., et al. (1996). Modulation of disease severity in cystic fibrosis transmembrane conductance regulator deficient mice by a secondary genetic factor. *Nat. Genet.* 12, 280–287. doi: 10.1038/ng0396-280

Said, S. I. (2009). Animal models of airway hyperresponsiveness. *Eur. Respir. J.* 33, 217–218. doi: 10.1183/09031936.00131008

Salinas, D., Haggie, P. M., Thiagarajah, J. R., Song, Y., Rosbe, K., Finkbeiner, W. E., et al. (2005). Submucosal gland dysfunction as a primary defect in cystic fibrosis. *FASEB J.* 19, 431–433. doi: 10.1096/fj.04-2879fje

Sato, K., Cavallin, S., Sato, K. T., and Sato, F. (1994). Secretion of ions and pharmacological responsiveness in the mouse paw sweat gland. *Clin. Sci.* 86, 133–139.

Scholte, B. J., Colledge, W. H., Wilke, M., and de Jonge, H. (2006). Cellular and animal models of cystic fibrosis, tools for drug discovery. *Drug Discov. Today Dis. Models* 3, 251–259. doi: 10.1016/j.ddmod.2006.09.003

Scholte, B. J., Davidson, D. J., Wilke, M., and De Jonge, H. R. (2004). Animal models of cystic fibrosis. *J. Cyst. Fibros.* 3, 183–190. doi: 10.1016/j.jcf.2004.05.039

Shah, V. S., Meyerholz, D. K., Tang, X. X., Reznikov, L., Alaiwa, M. A., Ernst, S. E., et al. (2016). Airway acidification initiates host defense abnormalities in cystic fibrosis mice. *Science* 351, 503–507. doi: 10.1126/science.aad5589

Snouwaert, J. N., Brigman, K. K., Latour, A. M., Malouf, N. N., Boucher, R. C., Smithies, O., et al. (1992). An animal model for cystic fibrosis made by gene targeting. *Science* 257, 1083–1088. doi: 10.1126/science.257.5073.1083

Sorio, C., Montresor, A., Bolomini-Vittori, M., Caldrer, S., Rossi, B., Dusi, S., et al. (2016). Mutations of cystic fibrosis transmembrane conductance regulator gene cause a monocyte-selective adhesion deficiency. *Am. J. Respir. Crit. Care Med.* 193, 1123–1133. doi: 10.1164/rccm.201510-1922OC

Stalvey, M. S., Havasi, V., Tuggle, K. L., Wang, D., Birket, S., Rowe, S. M., et al. (2017). Reduced bone length, growth plate thickness, bone content, and IGF-I as a model for poor growth in the CFTR-deficient rat. *PLoS One* 12:e0188497. doi: 10.1371/journal.pone.0188497

Stoltz, D. A., Meyerholz, D. K., Pezzulo, A. A., Ramachandran, S., Rogan, M. P., Davis, G. J., et al. (2010). Cystic fibrosis pigs develop lung disease and exhibit defective bacterial eradication at birth. *Sci. Transl. Med.* 2:29ra31. doi: 10.1126/scitranslmed.3000928

Stoltz, D. A., Meyerholz, D. K., and Welsh, M. J. (2015). Origins of cystic fibrosis lung disease. *N. Engl. J. Med.* 372, 351–362. doi: 10.1056/NEJMra1300109

Stoltz, D. A., Rokhlina, T., Ernst, S. E., Pezzulo, A. A., Ostedgaard, L. S., Karp, P. H., et al. (2013). Intestinal CFTR expression alleviates meconium ileus in cystic fibrosis pigs. *J. Clin. Invest.* 123, 2685–2693. doi: 10.1172/JCI68867

Sun, X., Olivier, A. K., Liang, B., Yi, Y., Sui, H., Evans, T. I., et al. (2014a). Lung phenotype of juvenile and adult cystic fibrosis transmembrane conductance regulator-knockout ferrets. *Am. J. Respir. Cell Mol. Biol.* 50, 502–512. doi: 10.1165/rcmb.2013-0261OC

Sun, X., Olivier, A. K., Yi, Y., Pope, C. E., Hayden, H. S., Liang, B., et al. (2014b). Gastrointestinal pathology in juvenile and adult CFTR-knockout ferrets. *Am. J. Pathol.* 184, 1309–1322. doi: 10.1016/j.ajpath.2014.01.035

Sun, X., Sui, H., Fisher, J. T., Yan, Z., Liu, X., Cho, H. J., et al. (2010). Disease phenotype of a ferret CFTR-knockout model of cystic fibrosis. *J. Clin. Invest.* 120, 3149–3160. doi: 10.1172/JCI43052

Sun, X., Yan, Z., Yi, Y., Li, Z., Lei, D., Rogers, C. S., et al. (2008). Adeno-associated virus-targeted disruption of the CFTR gene in cloned ferrets. *J. Clin. Invest.* 118, 1578–1583. doi: 10.1172/JCI34599

Szema, A. M., Hamidi, S. A., Lyubsky, S., Dickman, K. G., Mathew, S., Abdel-Razek, T., et al. (2006). Mice lacking the VIP gene show airway hyperresponsiveness and airway inflammation, partially reversible by VIP. *Am. J. Physiol. Lung Cell. Mol. Physiol.* 291, L880–L886. doi: 10.1152/ajplung.00499.2005

Tarran, R., Grubb, B., Parsons, D., Picher, M., Hirsh, A., Davis, C., et al. (2001). The CF salt controversy: in vivo observations and therapeutic approaches. *Mol. Cell* 8, 149–158. doi: 10.1016/S1097-2765(01)00286-6

Tata, F., Stanier, P., Wicking, C., Halford, S., Kruyer, H., Lench, N. J., et al. (1991). Cloning the mouse homolog of the human cystic fibrosis transmembrane conductance regulator gene. *Genomics* 10, 301–307. doi: 10.1016/0888-7543(91)90312-3

Than, B. L. N., Linnekamp, J. F., Starr, T. K., Largaespada, D. A., Rod, A., Zhang, Y., et al. (2016). CFTR is a tumor suppressor gene in murine and human intestinal cancer. *Oncogene* 35, 4179–4187. doi: 10.1038/onc.2015.483

Tipirneni, K. E., Cho, D. Y., Skinner, D. F., Zhang, S., Mackey, C., Lim, D. J., et al. (2017). Characterization of primary rat nasal epithelial cultures in CFTR knockout rats as a model for CF sinus disease. *Laryngoscope* 127, E384–E391. doi: 10.1002/lary.26720

Trezise, A. E., Szpirer, C., and Buchwald, M. (1992). Localization of the gene encoding the cystic fibrosis transmembrane conductance regulator (CFTR) in the rat to chromosome 4 and implications for the evolution of mammalian chromosomes. *Genomics* 14, 869–874. doi: 10.1016/S0888-7543(05)80107-7

Tuggle, K. L., Birket, S. E., Cui, X., Hong, J., Warren, J., Reid, L., et al. (2014). Characterization of defects in ion transport and tissue development in cystic fibrosis transmembrane conductance regulator (CFTR)-knockout rats. *PLoS One* 9:e91253. doi: 10.1371/journal.pone.0091253

van der Doef, H. P., Kokke, F. T., van der Ent, C. K., and Houwen, R. H. (2011). Intestinal obstruction syndromes in cystic fibrosis: meconium ileus, distal intestinal obstruction syndrome, and constipation. *Curr. Gastroenterol. Rep.* 13, 265–270. doi: 10.1007/s11894-011-0185-9

van Doorninck, J. H., French, P. J., Verbeek, E., Peters, R., Morreau, H., Bijman, J., et al. (1995). A mouse model for the cystic fibrosis delta F508 mutation. *EMBO J.* 14, 4403–4411. doi: 10.1002/j.1460-2075.1995.tb00119.x

Van Heeckeren, A. M., Schluchter, M. D., Xue, W., and Davis, P. B. (2006). Response to acute lung infection with mucoid *Pseudomonas aeruginosa* in cystic fibrosis mice. *Am. J. Respir. Crit. Care Med.* 173, 288–296. doi: 10.1164/rccm.200506-917OC

Welsh, M. J., Ramsey, B. W., Accurso, F., Cutting, G. R., Scriver, C. R., Beaudet, A. L., et al. (2001). *The Metabolic and Molecular Basis of Inherited Disease*, 8th Edn. New York, NY: McGraw-Hill, 5121–5189.

Welsh, M. J., Rogers, C. S., Stoltz, D. A., Meyerholz, D. K., and Prather, R. S. (2009). Development of a porcine model of cystic fibrosis. *Trans. Am. Clin. Climatol. Assoc.* 120, 149–162.

Welsh, M. J., and Smith, A. E. (1993). Molecular mechanism of CFTR chloride channel dysfunction in cystic fibrosis. *Cell* 73, 1251–1254. doi: 10.1016/0092-8674(93)90353-R

Wilke, M., Buijs-Offerman, R. M., Aarbiou, J., Colledge, W. H., Sheppard, D. N., Touqui, L., et al. (2011). Mouse models of cystic fibrosis: phenotypic analysis and research applications. *J. Cyst. Fibros.* 10, S152–S171. doi: 10.1016/S1569-1993(11)60020-9

Wilschanski, M., and Novak, I. (2013). The cystic fibrosis of exocrine pancreas. *Cold Spring Harb. Perspect. Med.* 3:a009746. doi: 10.1101/cshperspect.a009746

Wine, J. J. (2010). The development of lung disease in cystic fibrosis pigs. *Sci. Transl. Med.* 2:29s20.

Wong, P. Y. (1998). CFTR gene and male fertility. *Mol. Hum. Reprod.* 4, 107–110. doi: 10.1093/molehr/4.2.107

Zahm, J. M., Gaillard, D., Dupuit, F., Hinnrasky, J., Porteous, D., Dorin, J. R., et al. (1997). Early alterations in airway mucociliary clearance and inflammation of the *Lamina propria* in CF mice. *Am. J. Physiol.* 272(3 Pt 1), C853–C859. doi: 10.1152/ajpcell.1997.272.3.C853

Zeiher, B. G., Eichwald, E., Zabner, J., Smith, J. J., Puga, A. P., McCray, P. B., et al. (1995). A mouse model for the delta F508 allele of cystic fibrosis. *J. Clin. Invest.* 96, 2051–2064. doi: 10.1172/JCI118253

Zhou, L., Dey, C. R., Wert, S. E., DuVall, M. D., Frizzell, R. A., and Whitsett, J. A. (1994). Correction of lethal intestinal defect in a mouse model of cystic fibrosis by human CFTR. *Science* 266, 1705–1708. doi: 10.1126/science.7527588

Zhou, Z., Duerr, J., Johannesson, B., Schubert, S. C., Treis, D., Harm, M., et al. (2011). The ENaC-overexpressing mouse as a model of cystic fibrosis lung disease. *J. Cyst. Fibros.* 10, S172–S182. doi: 10.1016/S1569-1993(11)60021-0

Zielenski, J., Corey, M., Rozmahel, R., Markiewicz, D., Aznarez, I., Casals, T., et al. (1999). Detection of a cystic fibrosis modifier locus for meconium ileus on human chromosome 19q13. *Nat. Genet.* 22, 128–129. doi: 10.1038/9635

Permissions

All chapters in this book were first published by Frontiers; hereby published with permission under the Creative Commons Attribution License or equivalent. Every chapter published in this book has been scrutinized by our experts. Their significance has been extensively debated. The topics covered herein carry significant findings which will fuel the growth of the discipline. They may even be implemented as practical applications or may be referred to as a beginning point for another development.

The contributors of this book come from diverse backgrounds, making this book a truly international effort. This book will bring forth new frontiers with its revolutionizing research information and detailed analysis of the nascent developments around the world.

We would like to thank all the contributing authors for lending their expertise to make the book truly unique. They have played a crucial role in the development of this book. Without their invaluable contributions this book wouldn't have been possible. They have made vital efforts to compile up to date information on the varied aspects of this subject to make this book a valuable addition to the collection of many professionals and students.

This book was conceptualized with the vision of imparting up-to-date information and advanced data in this field. To ensure the same, a matchless editorial board was set up. Every individual on the board went through rigorous rounds of assessment to prove their worth. After which they invested a large part of their time researching and compiling the most relevant data for our readers.

The editorial board has been involved in producing this book since its inception. They have spent rigorous hours researching and exploring the diverse topics which have resulted in the successful publishing of this book. They have passed on their knowledge of decades through this book. To expedite this challenging task, the publisher supported the team at every step. A small team of assistant editors was also appointed to further simplify the editing procedure and attain best results for the readers.

Apart from the editorial board, the designing team has also invested a significant amount of their time in understanding the subject and creating the most relevant covers. They scrutinized every image to scout for the most suitable representation of the subject and create an appropriate cover for the book.

The publishing team has been an ardent support to the editorial, designing and production team. Their endless efforts to recruit the best for this project, has resulted in the accomplishment of this book. They are a veteran in the field of academics and their pool of knowledge is as vast as their experience in printing. Their expertise and guidance has proved useful at every step. Their uncompromising quality standards have made this book an exceptional effort. Their encouragement from time to time has been an inspiration for everyone.

The publisher and the editorial board hope that this book will prove to be a valuable piece of knowledge for researchers, students, practitioners and scholars across the globe.

List of Contributors

Carlos M. Farinha
Biosystems and Integrative Sciences Institute, Faculty of Sciences, University of Lisboa, Campo Grande, Portugal

Agnieszka Swiatecka-Urban
Department of Nephrology, Children's Hospital of Pittsburgh, Pittsburgh, PA, United States

Daniel F. Cruz
Biosystems and Integrative Sciences Institute, Faculty of Sciences, University of Lisboa, Campo Grande, Portugal
Department of Nephrology, Children's Hospital of Pittsburgh, Pittsburgh, PA, United States

Emanuela Pesce, Elvira Sondo, Loretta Ferrera, Valeria Tomati, Emanuela Caci and Nicoletta Pedemonte
U.O.C. Genetica Medica, IRCCS Istituto Giannina Gaslini, Genoa, Italy

Paolo Scudieri, Ilaria Musante, Mario Renda, Diego di Bernardo and Luis J. V. Galietta
Telethon Institute of Genetics and Medicine, Pozzuoli, Italy

Nesrine Baatallah, Nathalie Servel and Alexandre Hinzpeter
INSERM, U1151, Institut Necker Enfants Malades, Paris, France
Université Paris Descartes, Paris, France

Cláudia Almeida Loureiro, Ana Margarida Matos, Peter Jordan and Paulo Matos
BioISI—Biosystems & Integrative Sciences Institute, Faculty of Sciences, University of Lisbon, Lisbon, Portugal
Department of Human Genetics, National Health Institute "Dr. Ricardo Jorge," Lisbon, Portugal

João D. Santos, Carlos M. Farinha and Francisco R. Pinto
BioISI—Biosystems & Integrative Sciences Institute, Faculty of Sciences, University of Lisbon, Lisbon, Portugal
Department of Chemistry and Biochemistry, Faculty of Sciences, University of Lisbon, Lisbon, Portugal

Nikhil T. Awatade, Sharon L. Wong and Shafagh A. Waters
Faculty of Medicine, School of Women's and Children's Health, University of New South Wales, Sydney, NSW, Australia
Molecular and Integrative Cystic Fibrosis Research Centre (miCF_RC), School of Medical Sciences, Faculty of Medicine, University of New South Wales, Sydney, NSW, Australia

Chris K. Hewson
Faculty of Medicine, School of Women's and Children's Health, University of New South Wales, Sydney, NSW, Australia
Molecular and Integrative Cystic Fibrosis Research Centre (miCF_RC), School of Medical Sciences, Faculty of Medicine, University of New South Wales, Sydney, NSW, Australia
School of Biotechnology and Biomolecular Sciences, University of New South Wales, Sydney, NSW, Australia

Laura K. Fawcett and Adam Jaffe
Faculty of Medicine, School of Women's and Children's Health, University of New South Wales, Sydney, NSW, Australia
Molecular and Integrative Cystic Fibrosis Research Centre (miCF_RC), School of Medical Sciences, Faculty of Medicine, University of New South Wales, Sydney, NSW, Australia
Department of Respiratory Medicine, Sydney Children's Hospital, Sydney, NSW, Australia

Anthony Kicic
Centre for Child Health Research, Telethon Kids Institute, The University of Western Australia, Nedlands, WA, Australia
Occupation and Environment, School of Public Health, Curtin University, Bentley, WA, Australia
Faculty of Health and Medical Sciences, The University of Western Australia, Nedlands, WA, Australia
Department of Respiratory and Sleep Medicine, Perth Children's Hospital, Nedlands, WA, Australia
Centre for Cell Therapy and Regenerative Medicine, School of Medicine and Pharmacology, The University of Western Australia, Nedlands, WA, Australia

Elizabeth Matthes, Julie Goepp, Carolina Martini, Jiajie Shan and Jie Liao
Department of Physiology, McGill University, Montréal, QC, Canada
Cystic Fibrosis Translational Research Centre, McGill University, Montréal, QC, Canada

John W. Hanrahan
Department of Physiology, McGill University, Montréal, QC, Canada
Cystic Fibrosis Translational Research Centre, McGill University, Montréal, QC, Canada
Research Institute of the McGill University Health Centre, McGill University, Montréal, QC, Canada

David Y. Thomas
Cystic Fibrosis Translational Research Centre, McGill University, Montréal, QC, Canada
Department of Biochemistry, McGill University, Montréal, QC, Canada

Maarten Gees, Sara Musch, Steven Van der Plas, Anne-Sophie Wesse, Ann Vandevelde, Katleen Verdonck, Oscar Mammoliti, Kathleen Sonck, Pieter Stouten, Mia Jans, Jan Van der Schueren, Luc Nelles, Martin Andrews and Katja Conrath
Galapagos NV, Mechelen, Belgium

Tzyh-Chang Hwang
Department of Medical Pharmacology and Physiology, University of Missouri, Columbia, MO, United States

Andrew M. Swensen
AbbVie, North Chicago, IL, United States

Pauline Bardin, Florence Sonneville and Olivier Tabary
INSERM UMR-S938, Centre de Recherche Saint Antoine, Faculté des Sciences, Sorbonne Université, Paris, France

Harriet Corvol
INSERM UMR-S938, Centre de Recherche Saint Antoine, Faculté des Sciences, Sorbonne Université, Paris, France
Paediatric Respiratory Department, Hôpital Trousseau, Assistance Publique - Hôpitaux de Paris, Paris, France

Anita Balázs and Marcus A. Mall
Department of Pediatric Pulmonology, Immunology and Intensive Care Medicine, Charité - Universitätsmedizin Berlin, Berlin, Germany
Berlin Institute of Health, Berlin, Germany
German Center for Lung Research, Giessen, Germany

Manish Bodas
Department of Medicine, University of Oklahoma, Oklahoma City, OK, United States

Neeraj Vij
Department of Pediatric Pulmonary Medicine, Johns Hopkins University School of Medicine, Baltimore, MD, United States
4Dx Limited, Los Angeles, CA, United States
VIJ Biotech LLC, Baltimore, MD, United States

Karl Kunzelmann, Jiraporn Ousingsawat, Inês Cabrita, Rainer Schreiber and Roberta Benedetto
Institut für Physiologie, Universität Regensburg, Regensburg, Germany

Tereza Doušová
Department of Pediatrics, Second Faculty of Medicine, University Hospital Motol, Charles University in Prague, Prague, Czechia

Melanie Janda
Institute of Molecular Animal Breeding and Biotechnology, Ludwig-Maximilians-Universität München, Munich, Germany

Andrea Bähr
Institute of Molecular Animal Breeding and Biotechnology, Ludwig-Maximilians-Universität München, Munich, Germany
Innere Medizin I, Klinikum Rechts der Isar der TU München, München, Germany

Claudia Cossu, Michele Fiore, Debora Baroni and Oscar Moran
Istituto di Biofisica, Consiglio Nazionale Delle Ricerche, Genova, Italy

Valeria Capurro and Emanuela Caci
U.O.C. Genetica Medica, Istituto Giannina Gaslini, Genova, Italy

Maria Garcia-Valverde and Roberto Quesada
Departamento de Química, Facultad de Ciencias, Universidad de Burgos, Burgos, Spain

Ambra Gianotti, Livia Delpiano and Emanuela Caci
U.O.C. Genetica Medica, IRCSS Istituto Giannina Gaslini, Genoa, Italy

Ryosuke Fukuda and Tsukasa Okiyoneda
Department of Biomedical Chemistry, School of Science and Technology, Kwansei Gakuin University, Nishinomiya, Japan

Andrew Berical and Finn Hawkins
Center for Regenerative Medicine, Boston Medical Center and Boston University, Boston, MA, United States
The Pulmonary Center, Boston University School of Medicine, Boston, MA, United States

Rhianna E. Lee
Cystic Fibrosis Research Center, Marsico Lung Institute, University of North Carolina at Chapel Hill, Chapel Hill, NC, United States

Scott H. Randell
Cystic Fibrosis Research Center, Marsico Lung Institute, University of North Carolina at Chapel Hill, Chapel Hill, NC, United States
Department of Cell Biology and Physiology, University of North Carolina at Chapel Hill, Chapel Hill, NC, United States

Stephanie Trend
Telethon Kids Institute, Perth, WA, Australia
Division of Paediatrics, School of Biomedical Sciences, The University of Western Australia, Perth, WA, Australia

Barbara J. Chang
The Marshall Centre for Infectious Diseases Research and Training, School of Biomedical Sciences, The University of Western Australia, Perth, WA, Australia

Mark O'Dea
School of Veterinary and Life Sciences, Murdoch University, Perth, WA, Australia

Stephen M. Stick
Telethon Kids Institute, Perth, WA, Australia
Division of Paediatrics, School of Biomedical Sciences, The University of Western Australia, Perth, WA, Australia
Department of Respiratory Medicine, Perth Children's Hospital, Perth, WA, Australia
Centre for Cell Therapy and Regenerative Medicine, School of Medicine and Pharmacology, The University of Western Australia and Harry Perkins Institute of Medical Research, Perth, WA, Australia

Anthony Kicic
Telethon Kids Institute, Perth, WA, Australia
Division of Paediatrics, School of Biomedical Sciences, The University of Western Australia, Perth, WA, Australia
Department of Respiratory Medicine, Perth Children's Hospital, Perth, WA, Australia
Centre for Cell Therapy and Regenerative Medicine, School of Medicine and Pharmacology, The University of Western Australia and Harry Perkins Institute of Medical Research, Perth, WA, Australia
Occupation and the Environment, School of Public Health, Curtin University, Perth, WA, Australia

Andre Schultz
Faculty of Health and Medical Sciences, The University of Western Australia, Crawley, WA, Australia
Department of Respiratory Medicine, Perth Children's Hospital, Nedlands, WA, Australia
Wesfarmers Centre of Vaccines & Infectious Diseases, Telethon Kids Institute, The University of Western Australia, Nedlands, WA, Australia

Julie A. Marsh
Wesfarmers Centre of Vaccines & Infectious Diseases, Telethon Kids Institute, The University of Western Australia, Nedlands, WA, Australia
School of Population and Global Health, The University of Western Australia, Nedlands, WA, Australia

Scott M. Berry
Berry Consultants, Austin, TX, United States

Benjamin R. Saville
Berry Consultants, Austin, TX, United States
Department of Biostatistics, Vanderbilt University, Nashville, TN, United States

Richard Norman
School of Public Health, Curtin University, Bentley, WA, Australia

Peter G. Middleton
Ludwig Engel Centre for Respiratory Research, Westmead Institute for Medical Research, Sydney, NSW, Australia

Hugh W. Greville
Department of Thoracic Medicine, Royal Adelaide Hospital, Adelaide, SA, Australia

Matthew I. Bellgard
eResearch Office, Queensland University of Technology, Brisbane, QLD, Australia

Tom Snelling
Wesfarmers Centre of Vaccines & Infectious Diseases, Telethon Kids Institute, The University of Western Australia, Nedlands, WA, Australia
School of Public Health, Curtin University, Bentley, WA, Australia
Department of Infectious Diseases, Perth Children's Hospital, Nedlands, WA, Australia
Menzies School of Health Research, Charles Darwin University, Darwin, NT, Australia

Martin Donnelley and David W. Parsons
Robinson Research Institute, University of Adelaide, Adelaide, SA, Australia
Adelaide Medical School, University of Adelaide, Adelaide, SA, Australia
Respiratory and Sleep Medicine, Women's and Children's Hospital, North Adelaide, SA, Australia

Ming Ling
Paediatrics, Medical School, Faculty of Healthy and Medical Science, University of Western Australia, Nedlands, WA, Australia
Telethon Kids Institute, University of Western Australia, Nedlands, WA, Australia

Luke W. Garratt and Timo Lassmann
Telethon Kids Institute, University of Western Australia, Nedlands, WA, Australia

Stephen M. Stick
Paediatrics, Medical School, Faculty of Healthy and Medical Science, University of Western Australia, Nedlands, WA, Australia
Telethon Kids Institute, University of Western Australia, Nedlands, WA, Australia
Department of Respiratory Medicine, Princess Margaret Hospital for Children, Perth, WA, Australia
Centre for Cell Therapy and Regenerative Medicine, School of Medicine and Pharmacology, University of Western Australia, Nedlands, WA, Australia

Anthony Kicic
Paediatrics, Medical School, Faculty of Healthy and Medical Science, University of Western Australia, Nedlands, WA, Australia
Telethon Kids Institute, University of Western Australia, Nedlands, WA, Australia
Department of Respiratory Medicine, Princess Margaret Hospital for Children, Perth, WA, Australia
Centre for Cell Therapy and Regenerative Medicine, School of Medicine and Pharmacology, University of Western Australia, Nedlands, WA, Australia
Occupation and Environment, School of Public Health, Curtin University, Bentley, WA, Australia

Anna Semaniakou, Roger P. Croll and Valerie Chappe
Department of Physiology and Biophysics, Faculty of Medicine, Dalhousie University, Halifax, NS, Canada

Index

A

Airway Epithelium, 43-44, 46, 49, 81, 105-107, 109, 120, 136-137, 139, 142, 144-145, 157-158, 162-165, 167-168, 189, 194, 196-197, 201-202

Airway Plugging, 105-107, 109

Amino Acid, 2-4, 26, 84, 209-210

Anionophores, 123-127, 129, 131-134

Anoctamins, 109, 117, 119-121

Antibiotics, 7, 22, 41, 52, 73, 101, 135, 139-140, 158, 169-170, 172, 175-177, 179, 181-182, 184, 187, 200, 207

Apoptosis, 1, 5-8, 100, 120-121, 134, 169-170, 173, 175, 177-178, 202, 218

Asthma, 83, 85-87, 96-97, 100, 103, 105, 109, 111-112, 114, 116-119, 121, 158, 165, 178, 186, 196-197, 199, 203, 206-208, 212, 219-220,

Autophagy, 9, 11-12, 17-18, 20-21, 25-26, 37, 82, 92-104, 154, 156, 212, 220, 222

Autosomal Recessive Disease, 136

B

Bacterial Infections, 43, 93, 97, 106, 123, 136, 157, 169

Brevenal, 112, 115

Bronchiectasis, 83, 85-86, 89, 158, 170, 172, 178, 196-197, 199, 208

Bronchoalveolar Lavage, 41, 43, 45-46, 167

Bronchoconstriction, 100, 105-106, 115

C

Calnexin, 12, 24, 38, 148, 155

Cell Culture, 22, 43, 48, 51, 58, 137, 139-141, 160, 165-166, 173, 177,

Cell Membrane, 7, 61-62, 72-73, 124, 133, 135, 157, 189, 201

Chloride Channel, 11, 26, 39, 48, 72-74, 80-86, 88-89, 95, 103, 105-106, 117-118, 120-122, 134-136, 145, 147, 155, 209, 212, 216

Ciliated Cells, 43-44, 46, 105, 107, 109, 111, 159, 162, 164, 166, 190, 197, 217

Combination Therapy, 42, 60, 95, 104, 148

Corrector Drugs, 51, 53, 57, 94, 213

Cysteamine, 94-97, 100-101, 103-104

Cystic Fibrosis, 2, 4, 7-9, 11, 24-27, 38-41, 44, 48-51, 55, 58-60, 69-73, 76-77, 80-83, 87-93, 100-106, 117-124, 133-136, 147-149, 153-157, 165-170, 172, 178-181, 183, 186-188, 193-196, 206-211, 213-214, 216-223

Cytosol, 2, 16, 149

D

Denufosol, 105, 112, 115, 119-120

Disease Phenotype, 47, 87

Duodenum, 84, 87, 213

E

Electrophysiology, 52, 60

Endocytic Trafficking, 1, 4-6, 153-154

Endocytosis, 4-5, 7-9, 18, 26, 37, 39, 79, 90, 149-151, 154-156, 201

Endoplasmic Reticulum, 3, 9, 11, 25-27, 38, 42, 85, 111, 148, 154-155

Epithelial Cells, 2, 7, 9, 11, 15, 19, 23, 25-27, 36, 39, 41, 43, 47-53, 55-58, 60-66, 69, 74, 80-82, 84-85, 87-91, 96, 104-111, 116, 119, 134-137, 139-142, 144, 147, 152-158, 160, 172, 174-175, 177-179, 196, 201-202, 205-206, 208, 213

Etiology, 28, 40, 99

Exocrine Organs, 40, 72

Exocytosis, 105, 107, 111

F

Forskolin, 13-15, 22-23, 30, 37, 41, 44, 46-47, 53-57, 61-62, 64, 66-68, 84, 131, 138, 142-143, 146, 162, 212

G

Gastrointestinal Tract, 48-49, 72

Genetic Disease, 72, 95, 123, 157, 170, 180-181, 188, 205, 226

Genistein, 13-15, 22-23, 53-56, 131, 135, 138, 142-143, 146

Glycosylation, 84, 90-91, 149-150

Goblet Cells, 44, 109-111, 144-145, 159, 197, 201, 205, 207, 216

H

Homeostasis, 18, 81, 85, 92, 136, 154, 222

I

Idebenone, 112-113, 120

Infertility, 1, 6-8

Inflammatory Airway Disease, 105-106

Interactome, 1, 3-4, 7, 27-28, 38-39, 152

Ionocytes, 44, 49, 109, 111, 119, 159, 162, 167

Ivacaftor, 7-9, 25-26, 39, 41-42, 48-50, 57-58, 60, 69-71, 73, 80-82, 84, 86, 90, 95, 101-102, 104, 107, 118-121, 124, 135, 137-138, 142-143, 145-147, 152-153, 155, 158, 166-168, 189, 203

K

Kinases, 1-2, 4-5, 8-9, 28, 39, 77, 85, 90, 108, 118, 151, 155

L

Lung Disease, 26, 40, 43, 50, 58-59, 81, 86, 88-93, 95-101, 103, 105-109, 114-115, 117, 121, 137, 150, 154, 157-158, 160-161, 163-165, 167-168, 179-181, 187-194, 196-197, 205, 207, 210-212, 214-217, 219, 221-224

Lungs, 2, 11, 38, 40, 51, 60-61, 72-74, 77, 80, 83-84, 93-97, 99, 103, 106, 157-158, 160, 163, 165, 176-178, 188, 190-194, 207, 210, 212, 214-215, 217, 219, 222

Lysosome, 13, 20, 39, 149

M

Meconium Ileus, 59, 86-88, 91, 121, 209, 216, 223-224
Morbidity, 40, 73, 86, 93, 196, 210
Mucus Plugging, 72, 87-88, 106-107, 115, 117
Mucus Secretion, 43, 105, 107, 109, 111-112, 115, 117, 221
Multiorgan Disease, 83, 210

N

Nasal Cells, 111, 136, 140
Network Biology, 27-28, 36, 38
Neurodegeneration, 1, 6-9, 102
Neuroendocrine Cells, 158-161, 168
Neutrophilic Inflammation, 93, 196

P

Pancreas, 2, 11, 40, 73, 83-84, 87-88, 90, 157, 161, 209, 214, 216, 218-222, 224
Pancreatic Insufficiency, 86-88, 193, 209, 218
Pathogenesis, 18, 41, 43, 49, 81, 86, 92, 94-106, 117, 119, 158, 160, 187, 215-217, 219-220
Pathology, 9, 49, 72, 74, 82, 84, 98, 106, 137, 170, 179, 194, 209-223
Penicillin, 22, 52, 61, 125, 138
Phage Therapy, 169-170, 173, 175-176, 178-179
Phenylalanine, 7, 11, 73, 92-93, 209
Phosphatases, 1, 8, 10, 28
Phosphorylation, 1-2, 4-5, 7-10, 15, 27-28, 35, 39, 62, 85, 149, 151, 153-154, 156
Plasma Membrane, 2, 5, 7, 11, 13, 16, 19-22, 25-28, 38-39, 42, 47, 59, 63, 68-69, 73, 84-86, 88-89, 91-94, 98, 102, 105, 107-109, 111, 120-121, 148, 154-155, 211
Precision Medicine, 48, 51-52, 56-58, 158
Prodigiosin, 123-125, 130-131, 134-135
Proline, 2, 4, 9
Proteasome, 11, 13, 20, 25, 39, 88, 92-93, 96, 101, 154
Proteostasis, 42, 49, 92-93, 95-97, 99-103, 151-152, 154
Pseudomonas Aeruginosa, 81, 93, 100-101, 150, 153, 155, 169-170, 178-179, 207, 210, 221-223
Purinergic Receptors, 109, 111

R

Reactive Oxygen Species, 94, 112, 201
Resveratrol, 112, 115, 117

S

Streptomycin, 22, 52, 61, 125, 138

T

Talniflumate, 114, 116, 119, 121
Tezacaftor, 7, 9, 42, 49-50, 60, 70, 95, 101, 103, 107, 118-121, 158, 166-167, 189
Therapeutic Efficacy, 42, 99, 152-153
Transmembrane Protein, 1, 5, 73, 121-122, 155, 223
Tyrosine, 1-10, 27-28, 31, 34, 39, 151, 154-155

U

Ubiquitination, 11, 13, 20-21, 24-25, 34, 85, 90, 93, 98, 148-154

Y

Yellow Fluorescent Protein, 12, 61, 125

www.ingramcontent.com/pod-product-compliance
Lightning Source LLC
LaVergne TN
LVHW082208200926
848484LV00008B/2231